TEXTBOOK OF VETERINARY TOXICOLOGY

HARPAL SINGH SANDHU
Professor-cum-Head
Department of Veterinary Pharmacology & Toxicology
College of Veterinary Science
Guru Angad Dev Veterinary and Animal Sciences University
Ludhiana – 141 004
INDIA

RAJINDER SINGH BRAR
Professor-cum-Head
Department of Veterinary Pathology
College of Veterinary Science
Guru Angad Dev Veterinary and Animal Sciences University
Ludhiana – 141 004
INDIA

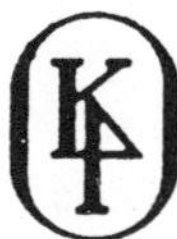

KALYANI PUBLISHERS
LUDHIANA - NEW DELHI - NOIDA (U.P.) - HYDERABAD
CHENNAI - KOLKATA - CUTTACK - GUWAHATI - KOCHI

KALYANI PUBLISHERS

Head Office

B-3251/B, Street No. 5, Backside Sandhu Tower, Gurdev Nagar
Ludhiana-141 001 • Ph. : 0161-2760031, 2745756
E-mail : kalyanibooks@yahoo.co.in • **Website** : www.kalyanipublishers.co.in

Administrative Office

4779/23, Ansari Road, Daryaganj, **New Delhi**-110 002 • Ph. : 011-23271469, 23274393
E-mail : kalyani_delhi@kalyanipublishers.in

Works

B-16, Sector-8, **NOIDA** (U.P.)

Branches

1, Mahalakshmi Street, T. Nagar, **Chennai**-600 017 • Ph. : 044-24344684
Gopabandhu Lane, Behind Govt. Bus Stand, Badambadi
Cuttack-753012 (Odisha) • Ph. : 0671-2311391
4-3-65/2/A, Behind HVS Public School, Raghunath Bagh
Sultan Bazar, **Hyderabad**-500 095 • Ph. : 040-24750368
10/2B, Ramanath Mazumdar Street, **Kolkata**-700 009 • Ph. : 033-22416024
Arunalaya, 1st Floor, Saraswati Road, Pan Bazar, **Guwahati**-781 001 • Ph. : 0361-2731274
Koratti Parambil House, Convent Road, **Kochi**-682035 • Ph. : 0484-2367189
No. 24 + 25, Ist Floor, Hameed Shah Complex, Cubbonpet Main Road, **Bengaluru**-560 002

R 34431 05
T 39613 05

First Edition, 2000
Second Edition, 2009
Reprinted 2019, 2021, 2024

Typesetting & Diagrams by : **Pyramid Enterprises,** Jalandhar-144001

ISBN 978-81-272-4860-4

PRINTED IN INDIA

At **Diamond Agencies Pvt. Ltd.**, B-125, Sec. 63, NOIDA

TEXTBOOK OF VETERINARY TOXICOLOGY

"We think caged birds sing, when indeed they cry."

— **John Webster** (1580-1632)

PREFACE TO THE SECOND EDITION

I expect to pass through this world but once; any good, therefore, that I can do, or any kindness I can show to any fellow creature, let me do it now; let me not defer or neglect it, for I shall not pass this way again.

– Stephen Grellet (1773-1855)

Toxicology is expanding and growing at an unprecedented pace. Every year, hundreds of new synthetic compounds including pesticides, drugs, plastics and other household and laboratory chemicals are introduced in market. Many of these chemicals have improved our living standards by providing benefits which were not known earlier, but some of these have also added to the diseases and miseries little known to man-kind earlier. Although a lot remains to be done in comprehending the adverse effects of many older and newer chemicals on living systems, remarkable contributions have been made recently in understanding the action of some toxicants at the molecular level. Furthermore, better diagnosis of some previously unrecognized intoxications have contributed to the field of veterinary toxicology. Accordingly, we decided to publish the up-dated version of the Textbook of Veterinary Toxicology. The encouraging reception accorded to the first edition of this book has also encouraged us to bring out an up-dated and expanded version of the book on veterinary toxicology.

The new edition of the book has been divided into 2 sections consisting of 20 chapters. All the previous chapters have been extensively revised and some have been reorganised. A chapter on absorption, distribution and excretion of toxicants has been added. Additional figures and photographs have been included for better comprehension of the subject. Selected references for further reading have been provided at the end of each chapter. Though the book has been enlarged, we hope it is still manageable and will enhance the usefulness of the book. The present edition has been prepared mainly to suit the specific needs of undergraduate and graduate veterinary students, teachers and practising veterinarians.

We are thankful to our colleagues, students and readers for providing feedback and useful suggestions. We are grateful to the Authorities of Guru Angad Dev Veterinary and Animal Sciences University, Ludhina for providing excellent academic atmosphere to pen this book. We appreciate M/s Kalyani Publishers, Ludhiana-New Delhi for their patience, cooperation and meticulous work in printing and publishing this work. We are also thankful to M/s Pyramid Enterprises, Jalandhar for the excellent composing and setting of the text. Finally our deepest and heartfelt gratitude to our family members as without their moral support and love, this book would not have been completed.

H.S.Sandhu
R.S.Brar

PREFACE TO THE FIRST EDITION

A wide range of chemicals and drugs are used in the crop protection and animal welfare programmes. Pest control chemicals and fertilizers are used on large scale in the agriculture and public health sectors without much concern about their harmful effects on the people and animal health. Mechanisation and industrial growth have further added to the existing problems. All these have made the animals highly susceptible to their adverse effects. According to a survey, approximately 10 per cent of the veterinary clinical practice is devoted to the diagnosis and treatment of poisoning in animals. Therefore, this book is written with the purpose of providing comprehensive text dealing with the problems associated with the undesirable effects of man-made and natural toxicants. This book is designed primarily according to the guidelines of Veterinary Council of India (V.C.I.) for the professional course of B.V.Sc. & A.H. programme, and may also be useful to the practising veterinarians and our colleagues form allied disciplines.

Although there is a wide range of toxicants from various sources, the emphasis for the present purpose is on a range of toxicants that are present in the animal surroundings. While doing so, efforts have been made to provide adequate, balanced and up-to-date information on the subject without making the book unduly voluminous. For easy comprehension, the book has been written in easy and simple language. Important points have been highlighted and confusions have been avoided by comparing important diagnostic features of the toxicants. Many figures and photographs have been included to aid understanding of important features of toxicants.

We sincerely hope that this book will cater to the needs of the students and also help teachers and practising veterinarians. We welcome suggestions, criticisms and comments from readers. The cooperation and help of M/s Kalyani publishers, Ludhiana-New Delhi to bring out this book is highly appreciated.

H.S.Sandhu
R.S.Brar

NOTICE

This publication is designed to provide accurate and authoritative information in regard to the subject matter covered. However, in view of the possibility of human error or modifications in the ever-changing biological science, the information given may not necessarily be accurate or complete in every respect. Some therapeutic agents described in this book may also not have specific approval by the regulatory authorities for use in conditions and dosage for which they have been recommended. Therefore, readers are encouraged to confirm the information contained herewith other sources, particularly that of drug administration and medical procedure. The manufacturer's guidelines and the package insert for each therapeutic agent should be consulted before the drug in used in animals. Neither the authors nor the publisher assumes any responsibility for any injury and/or damage to animals or property arising from this publication.

LIST OF ABBREVIATIONS AND SYMBOLS

Å — Angstrom (unit)
ACh — Acetylcholine
AChE — Acetylcholinesterase
ADI — Acceptable daily intake
ADP — Adenosine diphosphate
AKP — Alkaline phosphatase
δ-ALA — δ-aminolevulinate
ALT — Alanine aminotransferase
ANTU — Alphanaphthylthiourea
As — Arsenic
AST — Aspartate aminotransferase
ATA — Alimentary toxic aleukia
ATP — Adenosine triphosphate
BAL — British anti-Lewisite
BAPN — β-N-(L-glutamyl) aminopropionitrile
BBB — Blood-brain barrier
BHC — Benzene hexachloride
BP — Blood pressure / Benzo (a) pyrene
BUN — Blood urea nitrogen
C — Centigrade (Celsius)
Ca — Calcium
CCl_4 — Carbon tetrachloride
Cd — Cadmium
CO — Carbon monoxide
CO_2 — Carbon dioxide
COHb — Carboxyhaemoglobin
CNS — Central nervous system
CS_2 — Carbon disulphide
CSF — Cerebrospinal fluid
CTX — Ciguatoxin
Cu — Copper
2,4-D — 2,4-Dichlorophenoxyacetic acid
Da — Dalton
DAM — Diacetyl monoxime
DAS — Diacetoxyscirpenol
DBCP — Dibromochloropropane
DDA — Dichlorodiphenylacetic acid
DDE — Dichlorodiphenyldichloroethylene
DDT — Dichlorodiphenyltrichloroethane
DFP — Diisopropyl fluorophosphate
DMSA — Dimercaptosuccinic acid
DNA — Deoxyribonucleic acid
DNOC — Dinitro-o-cresol
DNP — Dinitrophenol
DON — Dioxynivalenol
DSMA — Disodium methanearsonate
E — Effect
EDB — Ethylene dibromide
EDTA — Ethylenediamine tetra-acetic acid
EEG — Electroencephalogram
e.g. — exempli gratia; for example
ELISA — Enzyme-linked immunosorbent assay
E_{max} — Maximal Effect
EPN — O-ethyl-O-p-nitrophenyl phenylphosphorothioate
etc. — et cetera; and the rest, or and so on
F — Fahrenheit, Fluoride / Fluorine
FAO — Food and Agriculture Organisation
FDA — Food and Drug Administration
g — gramme (s)
GABA — Gamma-aminobutyric acid
GI — Gastrointestinal
GIT — Gastrointestinal tract
GMP — Guanosine-5'-monophosphate
GSH — Glutathione
Gy — Gray
Hb — Haemoglobin
HCl — Hydrochloric acid / Hydrochloride
HCN — Hydrogen cyanide / Hydrocyanate/ Hydrocyanic acid
Hg — Mercury
H_2O_2 — Hydrogen peroxide
HPLC — High performance liquid chromatography
5-HT — 5-Hydroxytryptamine
i.e. — id est; that is
Ig — Immunoglobulin
I.M. — Intramuscular (ly)
I.P. — Intraperitoneal (y)
I.U. — International unit (s)
I.V. — Intravenous (ly)
K — Potassium
K_D — Dissociation constant
kDa — Kilo-Dalton
Kg — Kilogramme (s)
L — Litre (s)
LC_{50} — Lethal concentration-50
LD_{50} — Lethal dose-50
LDH — Lactate dehydrogenase
M — Molar / Microsomal
MAC — Minimum alveolar concentration
MAO — Monoamine oxidase
MDSA — Mesodimercaptosuccinic acid
MCPA — 2-methyl-4-chlorophenoxyacetic acid
MCPB — 2-methyl-4-chlorophenoxybutyric acid
mEq — Milliequivalent (s)
Met-Hb — Methaemoglobin

MFO — Mixed function oxidase
4-MI — 4-Methylimidazole
Min — Minute (s)
ml — millilitre (s)
MLD — Median lethal dose
Mo — Molybdenum
MSG — Monosodium glutamate
MSMA — Monosodium methanearsonate
M.U. — Mouse unit (s)
Na — Sodium
NaOH — Sodium hydroxide
NaCl — Sodium chloride
NAD — Nicotinamide adenine dinucleotide
NADH — Nicotinamide adenine dinucleotide, reduced form
NADP — Nicotinamide adenine dinucleotide phosphate
NADPH — Nicotinamide adenine dinucleotide phosphate, reduced form
NaF — Sodium fluoride
NED — Normal equivalent distribution
NH_3 — Ammonia
NM — Non-microsomal
NO — Nitric oxide
NO_2 — Nitrogen dioxide
NO_2^- — Nitrite
NO_3^- — Nitrate
N_2O_4 — Nitrogen tetroxide
NPN — Non-protein nitrogen
NSAID — Non-steroidal anti-inflammatory drug
O — Atomic / Nascent oxygen
O_2 — Oxygen
O_3 — Ozone
OC — Organochlorine
OCI — Organochlorine insecticide
ODAP — β-N-Oxalyl-L-α, β-diaminopropionic acid
OP — Organophosphorus / Organophosphate
OPI — Organophosphorus insecticide
OPIDN — Organophosphate induced delayed neuropathy
PAH — Polyaromatic hydrocarbon
2-PAM — Pyridine-2-aldoxime
PAN — Peroxyacetyl nitrate
PAPS — 3′-phosphoadenosine-5′-phosphosulphate
Pb — Lead
PBB — Polybrominated biphenyl
PCB — Polychlorinated biphenyl
PCP — Pentachlorophenol
PCV — Packed cell volume
PG — Prostaglandin
pg — picogramme (s)
pH — Negative logarithm of hydrogen ion activity
PH_3 — Phosphine
PO — per os / Oral
ppb — part (s) per billion
ppm — part (s) per million
PSP — Paralytic shell fish
PVC — Polyvinyl chloride
Rad — Radiation absorbed dose
RBC — Red blood cell
Rem — Radiation equivalent man
RNA — Ribonucleic acid
SAM — S-Adenosyl methionine
SAH_C — S-Adenosyl homocysteine
S.C. — Subcutaneous (ly)
SDH — Succinate dehydrogenase
Se — Selenium
SH — Sulphydryl / Thiol group
S.I. — System International (d' Unites)
SO_2 — Sulphur dioxide
S_2O_3 — Sulphur trioxide
Sp/Spp. — Species (singular) / Species (plural)
2,4,5-T — 2, 4, 5-trichlorophenoxyacetic acid
TCA — Tricarboxylic acid
TCDD — Tetrachlorodibenzo-p-dioxine
TDS — Total dissolved solids
TEPP — Tetraethylpyrophosphate
THM — Trihalomethane
T.I. — Therapeutic index
TLC — Thin-layer chromatography
TTX — Tetrodotoxin
TXA_2 — Thromboxane A_2
UDPG — Uridine diphosphate glucose
UDPGA — Uridine diphosphateglucuronic acid
μg — microgramme(s)
μm — micrometre(s)
UV — Ultra violet
Vit. — Vitamin
viz. — videlicet; namely
WHO — World Health Organization
Zn — Zinc
Zn_3P_2 — Zinc phosphide
α — Alpha
β — Beta
δ — Delta
γ — Gamma
° — degree (s)
~ — approximately
> — greater than
< — less than
/ — per
% — per cent

CONTENTS

SECTION-I

GENERAL TOXICOLOGY

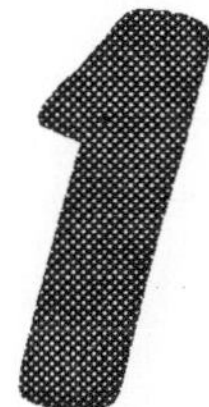

INTRODUCTION

Toxicology as a branch of science deals with understanding the harmful effects of chemical and physical agents on people, animals, wildlife and environment. The science of toxicology is as old as human civilization. Since ancient times, people have learned how to protect themselves from the harmful effects of plants and animals. They also knew how to use poisons to destroy their enemies. In modern era, toxicology helps in understanding in depth the nature and mechanism of the effects of poisons and in invention of their specific antidotes. Along with other sciences, toxicology contributes in development of safer chemicals to be used as drugs, food additives, pesticides and industrial chemicals.

DEFINITIONS AND TERMINOLOGY

I. TOXICOLOGY AND ITS SUB-DISCIPLINES

1. Toxicology: Toxicology (Greek words: toxicon = poison, logos = to study) may be defined in different ways like:

It is a science of poisons.

It is a science of adverse effects of chemicals on living organisms.

It is the study of poisons that include their physical and chemical properties, detection and identification, biological effects, treatment and prevention of disease conditions produced by them.

2. Sub-disciplines of Toxicology: Toxicology has following major sub-disciplines:

a. Aquatic Toxicology: It deals with the study of adverse effects of chemicals discharged into marine and fresh water on aquatic organisms and aquatic ecosystem. It is largely a study of water pollution and its ecological effects.

b. Clinical Toxicology: It deals with the cause, diagnosis, treatment and clinical management of diseases that are caused by or are associated with toxic substances.

c. Developmental Toxicology: It deals with the study of harmful effects of chemicals and drugs on the development of an organism. Manifestations of developmental toxicity include structural malformations, growth retardation, functional impairment, and/ or death of an organism.

d. Ecotoxicology: It is a more specialized area of environmental toxicology that deals with the effects of environmental pollutants on populations and communities of living organisms. Ecotoxicology in general considers effects of pollutants on organisms other than humans.

e. Environmental Toxicology: It deals with the effects of pollutants on the environment (food, water, air or soil) and their prevention. Its subspecialties could include ecotoxicology, aquatic toxicology, etc.

f. Food Toxicology: It deals with natural contaminants, food and feed additives, and toxic and chemoprotective effects of compounds in food.

g. Forensic Toxicology: It deals with the medical and legal (medicolegal/veterolegal) aspects of the harmful effects of chemicals on man and animals. It is basically a hybrid of analytical chemistry and fundamental toxicological principles which help in establishing the cause of death and elucidating its circumstances in a post-mortem investigation.

h. Formal Toxicology: It deals with the formal toxicological studies which are pre-requisite for release of a new drug /chemical e.g. calculation of LD_{50} and minimum toxic dose.

i. Genetic Toxicology: It deals with the study of interaction of toxicants with the process of hereditary.

j. Industrial Toxicology: It deals with the clinical study of workers of industries and environment around them.

k. Occupational Toxicology: It deals with assessing the potential of adverse effects from chemicals in occupational environment and the recommendations of appropriate protective and precautionary measures.

l. Regulatory Toxicology: It deals with administrative functions concerned with the development and interpretation of mandatory toxicology testing programmes and controlling the use, distribution and availability of chemicals used commercially and therapeutically. For example, Food and Drug Administration (FDA) regulates drugs, cosmetics and food additives.

m. Toxicodynamics : It deals with the study of biochemical and physiological effects of toxicants and their mechanisms of action.

n. Toxicokinetics: It deals with the study of absorption, distribution, metabolism and excretion of toxicants in the body.

o. Toxicovigilance: It deals with process of identification, investigation, and evaluation of various toxic effects in the community with a view of taking measures to reduce or control exposures involving the substances that produce these effects.

p. Toxinology: It deals with assessing the toxicity of substances of plant and animal origin and those produced by pathogenic bacteria.

q. Veterinary Toxicology: It deals with the cause, diagnosis and management of established poisonings in domestic and wild animals.

II. TOXICANT AND TYPES OF TOXICANT

a. Poison: Poison may be defined in different ways such as:

A poison is any substance that causes deleterious effects in a living organism.

A poison is any substance or matter which when applied either externally or internally produces ill effects on health or entirely destroys the life.

However, it is difficult to define a poison in true sense because whether a substance is poison or not depends on many factors viz. dose, species, route of exposure, etc. Almost any substance is harmful at some dose and, at the same time is harmless at a very low dose (See for detail Chapter 8, Factors influencing toxicity).

b. Toxicant: Toxicant is synonym of poison and is a more professional term.

c. Toxins: These are special types of poison that are produced by living organisms in small quantities. These are generally classified as biotoxins. Toxins are of following types:

(i) Phytotoxins : These are toxins produced by plants.

(ii) Mycotoxins : These are toxins produced by fungi.

(iii) Zootoxins : These are toxins produced by lower animals. These toxins may have genus name as prefix, e.g. bufotoxin from the toxic toad.

(iv) Bacteriotoxins : These are toxins produced by bacteria. These may be endotoxins (found within bacterial cells) or exotoxins (elaborated from bacterial cells).

d. Venom : Venom is a toxicant synthesised in a specialised gland and ejected by the process of biting or stinging. Venom is also a zootoxin but is transmitted by the process of biting or stinging.

e. Pollutant: It is any undesirable solid, liquid or gaseous matter resulting from the discharge or admixture of noxious materials that contaminate the environment and contributes to pollution.

f. Systemic toxicant: It is a toxicant that affects the entire body or many organs rather than a specific site. For example, potassium cyanide is a systemic toxicant that affects virtually every cell and organ in the body by interfering with the cell's ability to utilize oxygen.

g. Organ toxicant: It is a toxicant that affects only specific organs or tissues (may be called tissue toxicant) while not producing damage to the body as a whole. For example, benzene is a specific organ toxicant in that it is primarily toxic to the blood-forming tissues.

h. Xenobiotic: It is any substance, harmful or not, that is foreign to the body.

III. TOXICITY

1. Toxicity and Toxic Effects

a. Toxicity: It is a state of being poisonous or it is the extent, quality or degree of being poisonous.

It is also used as general term to indicate adverse effects or signs produced by toxicants in the organisms.

b. Toxicosis: It is the condition or disease state that results from exposure to a toxicant. The term toxicosis is often used interchangeably with the term of poisoning or intoxication.

c. Toxic effects: These are undesirable effects produced by a toxicant/drug which are detrimental to either survival or normal functioning of the individual.

d. Side effects: These are undesirable effects which result from the normal pharmacological actions of a drug. These effects may not be detrimental or harmful to the individual.

e. Selective toxicity: It is the toxicity produced by a chemical to one kind of living matter without harming another form of life even though the two may exist in intimate contact.

2. Toxicity in Relation to Frequency and Duration of Exposure

a. Acute toxicity: The toxic effects produced by a single dose or multiple doses during 24 hour period.

b. Subacute toxicity: It is the study of repeated exposure of a toxicant and its effects for 30 days or less.

c. Subchronic toxicity: It is the study of repeated exposure of a toxicant and its effects for 1 to 3 months.

d. Chronic toxicity: It is the study of repeated exposure of a toxicant and its effects for 3 months or more.

3. Toxicity in Relation to Time of Development and Duration of Induced Effects

a. Transient or reversible or temporary toxicity: It is the toxicity or harmful effect that remains for short duration of time, e.g. narcosis produced by organic solvents.

b. Persistent or permanent or irreversible toxicity : It is the toxicity or its harmful effects which persists throughout the life span of an individual and are of permanent nature, e.g. scarring of skin produced by corrosives, and testicular injury produced by dibromo-chloropropane.

c. Immediate toxicity: It is the toxicity that develops shortly after a single exposure to a toxicant e.g., cyanide poisoning.

d. Latent or delayed toxicity: It is the toxicity or harmful effect which has late onset of action, e.g. peripheral neuropathy produced by some organophosphorus insecticides.

e. Cumulative toxicity: It is progressive toxicity or harmful effect produced by summation of incremental injury resulting from successive exposures, e.g. liver fibrosis produced by ethanol.

IV. DOSE AND RELATED TERMS

a. Dose: It is the total or absolute quantity or amount of a substance applied or administered all at one time to an individual to get the desired pharmacological or toxicological response.

b. Lethal dose (LD) : It is the lowest dose that causes death in any animal during the period of observation. Various percentages can be attached to the LD value to indicate doses required to kill 1% (LD_1), 50% (LD_{50}) or 99% (LD_{99}) of the test animals in the population.

c. Median lethal dose (MLD) or Lethal Dose-50 (LD_{50}) : It is the dose of a toxicant that is lethal to 50 per cent of the animals exposed to it under defined conditions like species, route of exposure and duration of exposure. It is a commonly used measure of toxicity.

d. Lethal concentration (LC) : It is the lowest concentration of a compound in feed (or in water in case of fish) that causes death. It is expressed as milligrammes of compound per kilogramme of feed (or water).

e. Lethal concentration-50 (LC_{50}) : It is the concentration of a toxicant in feed or water that is lethal to 50 per cent of exposed animals to it. It mainly expresses acute lethal toxicity.

f. No observed effect level (NOEL): It is the highest dose level/concentration of a substance that under defined conditions of exposure causes no effect (alteration) on morphology, functional capacity, growth, development or life span of the test animals.

g. No observed adverse effect level (NOAEL): It is the highest dose level/ concentration of a substance that under defined conditions of exposure causes no observable/ detectable adverse effect on the morphology, functional capacity, growth, development or life span of the test animals. NOAEL is a variant of NOEL that specifies only that the effect in question is adverse.

h. Maximum allowable (admissible, acceptable) concentration (MAC): It is a regulatory value defining the upper limit of concentration of certain atmospheric contaminants allowed in the ambient air of the workplace.

i. Maximum residue limit / Maximum residue level (MRL): It is the maximum amount of a pesticide or drug (mainly veterinary pharmaceutical) residue that is legally permitted or recognised as acceptable in or on food commodities and animal feeds. Although both the terms have the same meaning, in practice the term maximum residue limit is used for the pesticide residue, while the term maximum residue level is applicable for the drug residue.

j. Maximum tolerated dose (MTD): It is the highest dose or amount of a substance that causes the toxic effects but no mortality in the test organisms. In chronic toxicity study, the MTD can cause limited toxic effects in the test organism, but it should not decrease the body weight more than 10% compared with control group or produce the overt toxicity (death of cells or organ dysfunction). The value is often denoted by LD_0.

k. Maximum tolerated concentration (MTC): It is the highest concentration of a substance in an environment medium that causes the toxic symptoms and no mortality in the test organisms.

l. Absolute lethal dose (LD_{100}): It the lowest dose of a substance that under defined conditions is lethal to 100 per cent exposed animals. The value is dependent on the number of organisms used in its assessment.

m. Absolute lethal concentration (LC_{100}): It is the lowest concentration of a substance in an environment medium that under defined conditions is lethal to 100 per cent exposed organisms or species.

n. Acceptable daily intake (ADI): It is the estimated amount of a substance in food or drinking water that can be ingested daily over a lifetime by humans without appreciable health risk. Acceptable daily intake is normally used for food additives (the term tolerable daily intake is used for contaminants).

V. MISCELLANEOUS TERMS

a. Risk: It is the expected frequency of occurrence of a harmful effect (death, injury or loss) arising from exposure to a chemical or physical agent under specified conditions.

b. Hazard: It is the qualitative description of the adverse effect resulting from a particular chemical or physical agent with no regard to dose or exposure. The term hazard is related to the risk, but it mainly expresses likelihood or probability of danger, irrespective of dose or exposure.

c. Tolerance: It is a state or condition when size of the dose required in producing a toxic effect increases upon repeated exposure. Or

It is a state of decreased responsiveness to the toxic effect of a chemical resulting from prior exposure to that compound or structurally related compound.

d. Acceptable risk: It is the probability of suffering a disease or injury during exposure to a substance, which is considered to be small but acceptable to the individual.

e. Accidental exposure: It is the unintentional contact with a chemical or physical agent that results in the harmful effect.

HISTORY OF TOXICOLOGY

Toxicology in a variety of specialised and primitive forms has been a relevant part of the history of man. Earliest man was well aware of the toxic effects of animal venoms and poisonous plants. Many scientific works carried out during the 19th and 20th centuries have led to increased public awareness that chemicals and drugs used for various purposes may not only be beneficial, but also be injurious to health.

1. Ancient Toxicology: In the early days of civilization, humans in their search for safer foods and habitat have discovered a number of poisonous plants and animals. The earliest records on toxicology are available in the form of ancient books on mythology and legendry, archaeological literature and history books.

a. Ebers Papyrus (1550 B.C.) : The Ebers Papyrus is perhaps the earliest medical record which contains a number of disease conditions and prescriptions employed in Egyptian medicine at that time. Many of these contain recognised poisons, e.g. aconite, an arrow poison of the ancient time; and opium both as a poison and antidote.

b. Hippocrates (460-375 B.C.) : Hippocrates is regarded as the "Father of Rational Medicine". The Hippocratic School formed by a group of physicians providing an ethical basis for the practice of therapeutics also knew of lead, mercury, copper, antimony, etc. as poisons and had some knowledge of their properties. They advocated vomiting to prevent absorption of poisons.

c. Pedanius Dioscorides (50-100 A.D.): He was a Greek army physician who served in the court of the Roman emperor Nero. He was first to classify poisons according to their origin like animal, vegetable and mineral poisons. His classification of natural substances as being toxic or therapeutic is valid still today. Dioscorides is famous for writing a five volume book *De Materia Medica* that is a precursor to all modern pharmacopeias, and is one of the most influential herbal books in history.

d. Geber Ibn Hajar (702-765 A.D.) : He was a Persian writer who classified drugs and poisons of his time and recognised that the difference between a drug and a poison is a matter of dose. Any drug can be toxic if given in large amounts.

e. Moshe ben Maimon (1135-1204): He was a famous Swiss Philosopher, who published the famous book "Treatise on poisons and their antidotes" in 1198 describing the treatment of poisonings from insects, snakes and dogs. His continual efforts to protect against poisonings led to discovery and development of several prevention and antidotal measures.

f. Paracelsus (1493-1541): He was a famous German physician who distinguished a poison from a remedy. He gave the great statement "All substances are poisons; there is none which is not poison. The right dose differentiates a poison and a remedy". This statement laid the foundation of the modern concept of the 'dose-response relationship' and the 'therapeutic index' developed later.

2. Modern Toxicology: Modern toxicology is a relatively young science based on the scientific work carried out by numerous dedicated workers. It is the outcome of rational thinking, experimentation, relationship between dose and therapeutics as compared with toxic, and responses to chemicals. Advances made in all allied disciplines contributed to the better understanding of effects of a number of toxicants in humans and animals.

a. Friedrich Serturner (1783-1841) : He was a German pharmacist who isolated the specific narcotic substance from opium and named it morphine after Morpheus, the Roman God of sleep. Its isolation allowed physicians to prescribe painkillers in regulated dosages.

b. M.J.B. Orfila (1787-1853) : He was a Spanish physician who is considered as 'Father of Toxicology'. He established toxicology as a discipline distinct from others and defined toxicology as the study of poisons. He also attempted to make a systemic correlation between the chemical and biological information of then known poisons and devised methods for detecting poisons. In 1813, he published the results of many toxicological experiments under the title of "Toxicologic Generale" and advocated the necessity of chemical analysis for medicolegal cases. Orfila became very proficient in the chemistry of crime scene investigation and was an early promoter of chemical evidence in the courtroom.

c. Francois Magendie (1783-1855) : He was a pioneer French experimental physiologist and toxicologist who researched the different motor functions of the body in relation to the spine, as well as nerves within it. He also described the effects and uses of morphine, emetine, quinine, strychnine, and other alkaloids, for which he is also called the "Father of Experimental Pharmacology".

d. Louis Lewin (1854-1929) : He was a German scientist who took up the task of classifying drugs and plants in accordance to their psychological effects. He also published many articles and books dealing with toxicology of methyl alcohol, ethyl alcohol, chloroform, opium, and some other chemicals. His important publications are "Toxicologist's view of world history" and "A textbook of toxicology."

e. Paul Hermann Muller : He discovered the insecticidal properties of DDT in 1939 and along with his team introduced other chlorinated hydrocarbon insecticides. He was awarded the Nobel Prize in Physiology or Medicine in 1948 "for his discovery of the high efficiency of DDT as a contact poison against several arthropods."

f. Gerhard Schrader (1903-1990): He was a German chemist who accidentally developed the toxic nerve agents sarin, tabun, soman, and cyclosarin while attempting to develop new insecticides. Schrader and his team, thus, introduced a new class of synthetic insecticides, the organophosphorus insecticides, and defined the structural requirements for insecticidal activity of anticholinesterase compounds. He is also called the "Father of the nerve agents"..

SCOPE OF TOXICOLOGY

The modern toxicology is a multidisciplinary science. It has expanded largely in last few decades to cope with the pressure created by addition of numerous manufactured chemicals through food additives, industrial wastes, drugs, radioactive substances and pesticides. The future of the toxicologist is very bright because this science will further expand as people and animals will continue to be poisoned by more and different chemicals. The contributions and activities of toxicologists are diverse and widespread. Modern toxicology contributes to physiology and pharmacology, environmental sciences, clinical medicine, legal medicine, occupational medicine and hygiene, veterinary medicine, experimental pathology and safety evaluation. Although the importance of toxicology in these professions and disciplines varies greatly, they are incomplete without toxicology. On the other hand, contributions made by various disciplines in the development of toxicology cannot be negated. Therefore, over the years, various specialized sub disciplines of toxicology have been recognised and are being added every year.

Table 1.1: Some important developments in the field of toxicology since 1800 AD.

Year	Scientist(s)	Development
1832	James Marsh	Developed the first chemical test for identifying arsenic, called the Marsh test.
1842	Hugo Reinsch	Developed a series of tests for detecting arsenic and mercury.
1847	Ascanio Sobrero	Discovered nitroglycerine, a powerful explosive and vasodilator.
1850	Claude Bernard	Described the mechanism of action of strychnine and identified site of action of curare.
1851	Stas-Otto	Developed the method of extraction and separation of alkaloids.
1855	Friedrich Gaedcke	First isolated cocaine from leaves of *Erythroxylon coca.*
1869	Theodore G. Wormley	Wrote the first American book 'Microchemistry of Poisons' dedicated to poisons.
1869	Oswald Schmiedeberg	Isolated muscarine from *Amanita muscaria.*
1930	–	Food and Drug Administration (FDA) was founded to regulate the content and safety of consumer drugs and food.
1934	K.K.Chen	Demonstrated antagonistic effect of sodium nitrite and sodium thiosulphate in cyanide poisoning.
1945	R.A. Peters, L.A.Stocken, and R.H.S.Thompson	Developed dimercaprol as an antidote to arsenic containing war gases (lewisite).
1946	Judah Hirsch Quastel	Developed 2, 4-D, the first widely used systemic or hormone herbicide.

Contd...

Year	Scientist(s)	Development
1959-1960's	–	Thalidomide disaster occurred in Europe, which produced thousands of birth defects.
1962	Rachel Carson	Started crusade against the use of DDT and published the great book *"Silent Spring"*.
1970	–	Environmental Protection Agency (EPA) was founded.
1971	Louis J. Casarett and John Doull	Published the first modern Toxicology Textbook titled '*Toxicology: The Basic Science of Poisons*'.
1980	–	International Union of Toxicology (IUTOX) was founded.
1984	–	Bhopal Disaster occurred due to accidental release of methyl isocyanate killing thousands and injuring 100s of people.
1986	–	Chernobyl nuclear power plant accident occurred in Soviet Union spreading radioactive debris over several countries.

BIBLIOGRAPHY

Ballantyne B, Marrs T and Turner P (1995) Fundamentals of toxicology. In: General and Applied Toxicology. Ballantyne B, Marrs T and Turner P (Eds.) p 3. Macmillan Press Ltd., London.

Brown SA and Davis LE (2001) Veterinary Pharmacology: An introduction to the discipline. In: Veterinary Pharmacology and Therapeutics. 8th edn. Adams H R (Ed.) p. 3. Iowa State Univ. Press, Iowa.

Gallo MA (1996) History and scope of toxicology. In: Casarett and Doull's Toxicology: The Basic science of Poisons. 5th edn. Klaassen CD (Ed.) p 3. McGraw Hill Companies Inc., New York.

Garg SK (2000) Veterinary Toxicology. CBS Publishers & Distributors, New Delhi.

Gilbert SG and Hayes T (2006) History of Toxicology: Milestones and Discoveries. (http://www.asmalldoseof.org/historyoftox/index.php).

Hatch RC (1982) Veterinary toxicology: Introduction. In: John's Veterinary Pharmacology and Therapeutics. 5th edn. Booth NH and McDonald LE (Eds.) p 927. Kalyani Publishers, Ludhiana-New Delhi.

Hodgson E, Mailman RB and Chambers JE (1999) Dictionary of Toxicology. 2nd edn. Macmillan Reference Ltd., London.

Hughes WW (1996) Essentials of Environmental Toxicology. Taylor & Francis, Washington.

IUPAC (1993) Commission of Toxicology: Glossary for chemists of terms used in toxicology. *Pure Appl. Chem.* 65 : 2003.

Klaassen CD (2001) Principles of toxicology and treatment of poisoning. In: Goodman & Gilman's The Pharmacological Basis of Therapeutics. 10th edn. Hardman JG, Limbird LE and Gilman AG (Eds.). p 67. The McGraw-Hill Companies Inc., New York.

Lu FC and Kacew S (2002) Lu's Basic Toxicology: Fundamentals, Target Organs and Risk Assessment. Taylor & Francis, New York.

Osweiler GD (1996) Toxicology. Williams and Wilkins, Philadelphia.

Osweiler GD (1999) Introduction to toxicology. In: Veterinary Toxicology. Beasley V (Ed.) p. 2. International Veterinary Information Service, Ithaca NY (www.ivis.org).

Radeleff RD (1970) Veterinary Toxicology. 2nd edn. Lea and Febiger, Philadelphia.

Schiefer HB, Irvine DG and Buzik SC (1997) Understanding Toxicology: Chemicals, Theirs Benefits and Risks. CRC Press, Boca Ratton.

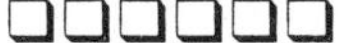

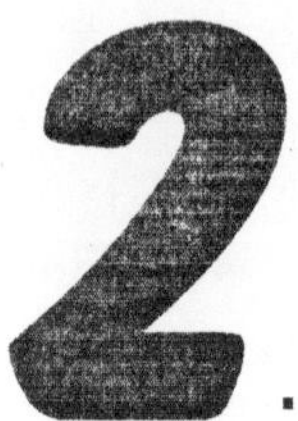

SOURCES OF POISONING

Malicious poisoning
Accidental poisoning
Natural sources
Man-made sources

Poisoning may occur from numerous sources. In humans, poisoning may be malicious, accidental, intentional, or as an occupational hazard, but in animals it is generally either malicious or accidental.

I. MALICIOUS POISONING

Malicious poisoning is unlawful or criminal killing of animals by administering certain toxic substances. It is generally motivated by ill-will or hatred against the animal or its owner and is mostly carried out by mixing certain toxic substances in the food or feed of animal or by the forceful administration of poison to the animal. Incidence of malicious poisoning in animals is on rise and is a matter of great concern. Numerous cases of malicious poisoning in animals are recorded every year. In most cases, the toxicant employed is almost a readily available compound, e.g. insecticide, datura, strychnine, arsenic and warfarin.

II. ACCIDENTAL POISONING

Accidental poisoning may occur when animal takes some toxicant accidentally or is added unintentionally in its feed, fodder or drinking water. Poisoning through ingestion of contaminated feed and water with toxicants, industrial effluents, insecticides, household products, etc. are common in animals. Such toxicants come from either natural sources or man-made sources.

1. Natural Sources

From the earliest times, natural sources provide many important toxicants. Most of these natural toxicants enter the body through food chain.

a. Plants: Despite the existence of literally hundreds of toxic plants, plant intoxication is less important except as a local problem. Toxic plants (e.g. lantana, datura and oleander) are often refused by animals as they may have repulsive smell or contain highly irritant juices and are eaten only when other herbage is scarce. Plants, crops, or grasses grown in areas rich in some minerals (e.g. molybdenum and selenium) also become toxic due to heavy accumulation of these minerals in the plants.

b. Animals: Accidental biting or stinging by poisonous reptiles, amphibians, arachnids or insects (e.g. snakes, spiders, scorpions, toads and bees) often leads to poisoning in animals. Snake bite in animals generally occurs while grazing or hunting, while exposure to toad is seen when dogs or cats attack or mouth the poisonous amphibian.

c. Microorganisms: Toxins produced by certain organisms like fungi and bacteria are highly toxic to animals. Contamination of food and feed with mycotoxins (e.g. aflatoxins and rubratoxins) and bacteriotoxins (e.g. botulinum toxin) is a frequent cause of poisoning in animals. Some of the toxins of marine organisms like dinoflagellates are known to accumulate in food chains. Some bacteria produce poisonous gases (e.g. ammonia and hydrogen sulphide).

d. Minerals: Minerals are dangerous when they contaminate water or when accumulate in plants from mineral rich soil. Poisoning may occur in animals after continuous ingestion of forages, feed, or water high in mineral contents like arsenic, selenium, fluoride, molybdenum and copper. Excessive use of mineral supplements or mineral mixture containing rock phosphates may also cause fluorosis in animals.

2. Man-made Sources

Man-made toxicants are the most common source of poisoning to animals and human beings as they are readily available and some are potentially toxic. Poisoning from man-made toxicants can be avoided by providing the domestic animals with a clean and protected environment.

a. Industrial wastes: Contamination of water reservoir and herbage by industrial effluents and wastes (e.g., chromium, nickel, lead and polychlorinated biphenyls) often leads to outbreak of poisonings among animals. Besides this, industrial gases, vapours, and dusts (e.g., sulphur dioxide, nitrogen dioxide and chlorine) also produce adverse effects on the health of animals.

b. Agrochemicals: Agrochemicals constitute the biggest source of accidental poisoning in all species. Careless and excessive use of pesticides in farms, lawns and houses is responsible for innumerable cases of fatal poisoning in animals. Rat baits (rodenticides) are the worst offenders in small animals and birds. Other important agrochemicals causing intoxication in animals are aluminium phosphide, fertilizers and fungicides.

c. Household products: Numerous commonly used household chemicals and substances like disinfectants (mainly phenol), solvents, cleaners and spot removers, and naphthalene may cause intoxication in domestic animals, especially pets. Most domestic materials can be used with relatively little risk (following the label directions), but when used in a wrong manner, some are extremely toxic.

d. Therapeutic agents: Use of therapeutic agents in improper dosage, by improper route or in improper species often gives rise to toxic effects. Toxic reactions occasionally seen following the use of correct dosage and route are mainly due to idiosyncrasy or impurities in drugs. Indiscriminate use of safe drugs may also lead to toxic and undesirable effects in animals. Use of human drugs without safety data in animals is another source of intoxication in animals (e.g. paracetamol in cats).

e. Food and feed: Almost any food/feed given in excess will cause harmful effects. Excessive and regular use of food and feed additives like saccharin are known to produce adverse effects in laboratories animals and may have similar effects in humans and animals. Introduction of genetically modified (GM) food has generated a new controversy regarding the safety of such foods. It is simply not possible to guarantee that any food, including GM food, is absolutely safe for all individuals.

f. Environmental pollution: Many of the adverse effects seen in humans and animals today are only due to increasing environmental pollution. Excessive use of automobiles, synthetic chemicals, and fossils fuels, etc. has added several hazardous substances (e.g. carbon monoxide, lead, dioxins and pesticides) in environment, thus producing ill-effects on the health of both humans and animals. Animals are exposed to these pollutants through the air they breathe, the food they eat, and the water they drink.

g. Improper management practices: Improper management conditions often accelerate the toxic effects of toxicants. Poor ventilation, overcrowding, and diet deficient in essential nutrients aggravate toxic effects of certain poisons. Burning of coal and other fossil fuels in closed, poorly ventilated sheds and barns during winter may lead to carbon monoxide intoxication in animals.

BIBLIOGRAPHY

Bartik M and Piskac A (1981) Veterinary Toxicology. Elsevier Scientific Publishing Company, Amsterdam.

Clarke ECG and Clarke ML (1967) Garner's Veterinary Toxicology. 3rd edn. Williams and Wilkins, Baltimore.

Garg SK (2000) Veterinary Toxicology. CBS Publishers & Distributors, New Delhi.

Loomis TA (1978) Essentials of Toxicology. 3rd edn. Lea and Febiger, Philadelphia.

Radeleff RD (1970) Veterinary Toxicology. 2nd edn. Lea and Febiger, Philadelphia.

❑❑❑❑❑❑

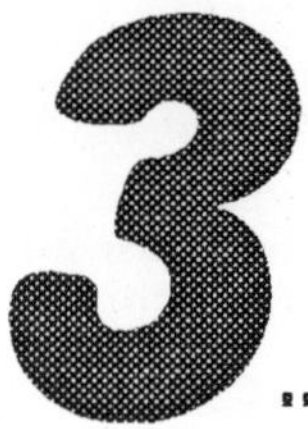

CLASSIFICATION OF TOXICANTS

Classification of toxicants based on
- Source of toxicants
- Physical state of toxicants
- Target organ/system
- Chemical nature/structure
  - Inorganic toxicants
  - Organic toxicants
- Analytical behaviour of toxicants
- Toxic effects
- Uses
- Toxicity/Poisoning potential
- Mechanism of action
- Environmental and public health consideration

Toxic agents are classified in number of ways depending on the interests and needs of the classifier. Dioscorides (50-100 A.D.) classified substances using general characteristics i.e. whether they are toxic or therapeutic. M.J.B. Orfila (1787-1853) classified substances as being of animal, vegetable or mineral origin. However, no single classification is applicable for the entire spectrum of toxic agents and hence combinations of classification systems based on several factors may be needed to provide the best rating system. Classification systems that take into account both the chemical and biological properties of the agent, and the exposure characteristics are most likely to be useful for toxicology in general. Many classification schemes presently available for toxic agents are based on following points:

1. Source of Toxicants

a. Plant toxicants, e.g. morphine, curare and strychnine.

b. Animal toxicants, e.g. toxins (zootoxins) and venoms.

c. Mineral toxicants, e.g., copper, lead, selenium and iron.

d. Synthetic toxicants, e.g. organophosphates, polychlorinated biphenyls and aluminium phosphide.

2. Physical State of Toxicants

a. Gaseous toxicants, e.g. hydrocyanic acid (HCN), sulphur dioxide, carbon monoxide and phosphine.

b. Liquid toxicants, e.g. sulphuric acid, carbon disulphide and nicotine.

c. Solid toxicants, e.g. strychnine, opium and atropine.

d. Dust toxicants, e.g. asbestos dust, silicon dust and metallic dusts.

3. Target Organ/System : It is difficult to classify a toxicant on the basis of its target organ or system as it may affect other systems also. The action on the primary site has been taken as a basis of classification in the present scheme.

a. Neurotoxicants, e.g. organophosphorus insecticides, barbiturates, strychnine and nicotine.

b. Hepatotoxicants, e.g. carbon tetrachloride, aflatoxins, phenol and *Lantana camara*.

c. Nephrotoxicants, e.g. heavy metals (lead, arsenic, cadmium) and oxalates.

d. Pulmonotoxicants, e.g. alpha-naphthylthiourea (ANTU), hydrogen sulphide and ammonia gas.

e. Haematotoxicants, e.g. warfarin, carbon monoxide, phenothiazine and snake venom (pit viper venom).

f. Dermatotoxicants, e.g. coal tar compounds (petroleum oils), heavy metals (arsenic, mercury), p-tertiarybutyl phenol.

4. Chemical Nature / Structure of Toxicants

a. **Inorganic toxicants:** These include metals, metalloids, non-metals and their salts and derivatives, acids and alkalis.

i. Metals, e.g. lead, copper, mercury and antimony.

ii. Non-metals, e.g. phosphorus, sulphur, chlorine and nitrate/nitrite.

iii. Acids and alkalis, e.g. hydrochloric acid, sulphuric acid and potassium hydroxide.

b. **Organic toxicants:** These include all carbon compounds other than the oxides of carbon, the carbonates, and the metallic carbides and cyanides.

i. Hydrocarbons, e.g. cyclopropane, benzene, paraffin and naphthalene.

ii. Halogenated hydrocarbons, e.g. chloroform, BHC, DDT and carbon tetrachloride.

iii. Alcohols and phenols, e.g. methyl alcohol, ethyl alcohol, phenol, cresol and pentachlorophenol.

iv. Ethers, e.g. diethyl ether and divinyl ether.

v. Aldehydes and ketones, e.g. formaldehyde and paraldehyde.

vi. Organic acids, e.g. formic acid, phenoxy acetic acid and salicylic acid.

vii. Esters, e.g. organophosphorus insecticides and suxamethonium.

viii. Amines, e.g. adrenaline, ephedrine and amphetamine.

ix. Amides, e.g. phenacetin and sulphonamides.

x. Glycosides, e.g. digitalis and cyanogenetic glycosides.

xi. Alkaloids, e.g. nicotine, atropine and strychnine.

xii. Proteins, e.g. ricin, crotin and abrin.

5. Analytical Behaviour of Toxicants : Toxicants can be classified into separate characteristic groups according to the analytical procedures involved. In the Stas-Otto scheme, toxicants have been divided into the following groups.

a. Volatile toxicants, e.g. hydrocyanic acid, alcohols, acetone, phenol and chloral hydrate.

b. Extractive toxicants

i. Toxicants extractable by ether from acid solution, e.g. organic acids and nitrocompounds.

ii. Toxicants extractable by ether from alkaline solution e.g. alkaloids.

c. Metals and metalloids, e.g. copper, mercury, zinc, silver and antimony.

6. Toxic Effects : It is difficult to classify toxicants on the basis of toxic effects as a single compound may have number of effects.

a. Carcinogens, e.g. thiouracil, vinyl chloride and nickel.

b. Mutagens, e.g. ethyl methane sulphonate, UV light, nitrogen mustards and nitroso compounds.

c. Teratogens, e.g. phenylmercuric acetate, triazines and thalidomide.

d. Clastogens e.g. UV light and caffeine.

7. Uses

a. Insecticides, e.g. organophosphorus insecticides, carbamates and pyrethroids.

b. Fungicides, e.g. captan, folpet and pentachlorophenol.

c. Herbicides, e.g. triazine, paraquat and 2,4-D.

d. Rodenticides, e.g. warfarin, fluoroacetate and red squill.

e. Food additives

i. Preservatives, e.g. benzoic acid and sodium bisulphite.

ii. Antioxidants, e.g. ascorbic acid.

iii. Emulsifying agents, e.g. cholic acid and desoxycholic acid.

iv. Colouring agents, e.g. amaranth and tartrazine.

v. Anticaking agents, e.g. aluminium-calcium silicate.

8. Toxicity/Poisoning Potential

Group	Lethal dose
a. Extremely toxic	< 1 mg/kg
b. Highly toxic	1-50 mg/kg
c. Moderately toxic	50-500 mg/kg
d. Slightly toxic	0.5-5 g/kg
e. Practically non-toxic	5-15 g/kg
f. Relatively harmless	> 15 g/kg.

9. Mechanism of Action

a. Anticholinesterase agents /cholinesterase inhibitors, e.g. organophosphorus insecticides and carbamates.

b. Sulphydryl (-SH) inhibitors, e.g. mercury and arsenic.

c. Protoplasmic toxicants, e.g. heavy metals.

d. Corrosive toxicants, e.g. caustic alkalis, acids, heavy metals and irritant gases.

e. Methaemoglobin producers, e.g. nitrate/nitrite, chlorates and naphthalene.

f. Inhibitors of cytochrome oxidase, e.g. cyanide.

g. Inhibitors of Krebs cycle, e.g. fluoroacetate.

h. Uncoupler of oxidative phosphorylation, e.g. dinitrophenols and chlorophenol fungicides.

10. Environmental and Public Health Consideration

a. Air pollutants, e.g. carbon monoxide, ozone and sulphur dioxide.

b. Water pollutants e.g. polychlorinated biphenyls, pesticides and heavy metals.

c. Food and feed contaminants, e.g. antibiotics, pesticides, mycotoxins and lectins.

d. Radiation hazards, e.g. X-rays, gamma-rays and radioactive materials.

BIBLIOGRAPHY

Bartik M and Piskac A (1981) Veterinary Toxicology. Elsevier Scientific Publishing Company, Amsterdam.

Clarke ECG and Clarke ML (1967) Garner's Veterinary Toxicology. 3rd edn. Williams and Wilkins, Baltimore.

Garg SK (2000) Veterinary Toxicology. CBS Publishers & Distributors, New Delhi.

Loomis TA (1978) Essentials of Toxicology. 3rd edn. Lea and Febiger, Philadelphia.

Hughes WW (1996) Essentials of Environmental Toxicology. Taylor & Francis, Washington.

Radeleff RD (1970) Veterinary Toxicology. 2nd edn. Lea and Febiger, Philadelphia.

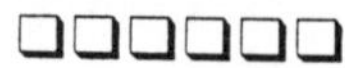

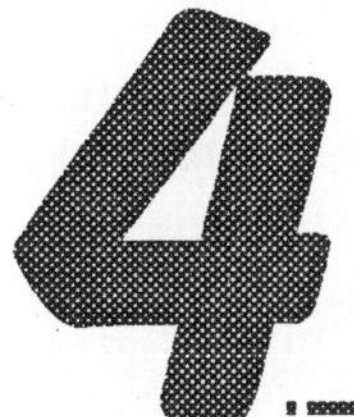

ABSORPTION, DISTRIBUTION AND EXCRETION OF TOXICANTS

Toxicants exert their effect only when they interact with specific receptor or target sites, which may be located at distant organs. To reach the target site, the toxicant must have to be absorbed effectively into blood stream, distributed efficiently to site of action, and subsequently metabolised and excreted from the body. The processes of absorption and distribution are responsible for placement or deployment of the toxicant in the body, and metabolism and excretion for elimination of the toxicant from the body. All these toxicokinetic processes involve movement of toxicant across biological membranes.

PROCESSES OF CELLULAR TRANSPORT OF XENOBIOTICS

Toxicants and other xenobiotics cross biological membranes by several processes, which have been broadly divided into two groups - simple transport and specialised transport. The simple transport consists of diffusion and filtration, while the specialised transport system consists of active transport, facilitated transport and pinocytosis.

I. SIMPLE TRANSPORT

1. Diffusion

Diffusion (Simple diffusion or passive diffusion) is the most important process by which a xenobiotic crosses the biological membranes. In diffusion, the toxicant present in the aqueous medium at one end of the biological membrane partitions and dissolves in the lipid phase of the membrane and finally leaves it by dissolving again in the aqueous medium at the other side of the membrane. The simple diffusion is meant for only lipid soluble substances because they dissolve rapidly in the lipoid matrix of the membranes and hence diffuse quickly. The unionised (undissociated) agents also penetrate biological membranes by diffusion because the unionised form is usually much more lipid soluble than the ionised form.

Simple diffusion process is energy independent and non-saturable. The xenobiotic molecules always diffuse from a region of higher concentration to lower concentration (along the concentration gradient or down hill movement) until equilibrium is attained. A xenobiotic that can exist in both ionised and unionised forms approaches equilibrium only by transfer of its unionised form. Thus the rate of diffusion depends primarily on the magnitude of concentration gradient across the membrane and the degree of lipid solubility (lipid to water partition coefficient). Diffusion is also affected to variable extents by molecular weight of xenobiotic, thickness of membrane and surface area of absorbing surface.

The pH-partition hypothesis: Most toxicants are weak acids or weak bases and exist in physiological solutions in both ionised and unionised forms. The amount of toxicant that exists in unionised or ionised form is a function of its pK_a (negative logarithm of dissociation constant) and the pH of the fluid in which it is dissolved. When the pH of fluid is same as the pK_a value of the drug, the ratio of unionised to ionised forms is 1:1 (therefore, pK_a is numerically equal to the pH at which compound is 50% ionised). As the pK_a value is a characteristic of the compound (pK_a value is a constant for an acid or a base), the degree of its ionisation depends primarily on the pH of the medium. The relative amount of ionised and unionised compound in the body fluid at a particular pH and the per cent of compound ionised at this pH can be determined by Henderson-Hasselbalch equation:

For weak acidic compound

$$pK_a - pH = \log \frac{\text{Conc. of unionised compound}}{\text{Conc. of ionised compound}}$$

$$\%\ \text{ionised compound} = \frac{100}{1 + \text{antilog}\,(pK_a - pH)}$$

For weak basic compound

$$pH - pK_a = \log \frac{\text{Conc. of unionised compound}}{\text{Conc. of ionised compound}}$$

$$\%\ \text{ionised compound} = \frac{100}{1 + \text{antilog}\,(pH - pK_a)}$$

2. Filtration

Filtration (pore filtration) is the simple passage of xenobiotics through pores or channels in the membrane. The process is important in the transfer of many small (Mol. wt. < 100), polar and non-polar substances. The driving force for filtration is constituted by the hydrostatic pressure or the osmotic differences across the membrane due to which water flows through the aqueous pores. This passive (energy independent) bulk fluid movement carries or drags solute molecules through the pores in the moving stream, provided that the soluble molecules are smaller than the diameter of pores or aqueous channels.

Permeation through water-filled channels is of lesser importance for most toxicants because majority of cell membranes (e.g., intestinal mucosa, tissue cells, and erythrocytes) have very small pores (4 Å). However, capillary endothelial cells (except those in brain) have large pores (40 Å) and many large molecules can filter through them. Filtration is of particular importance in renal excretion (glomerular filtration) of toxicants, removal of toxicants from cerebrospinal fluid, and passage of toxicants across hepatic sinusoidal membrane.

II. SPECIALISED TRANSPORT

1. Active Transport

Active transport is an energy dependent transport system in which the solute takes help of a carrier to cross the barrier imposed by lipid bilayer. The carrier is mostly a membrane protein (e.g., enzymes) that binds reversibly with the solute molecule on exterior membrane surface to form the carrier-solute complex. This carrier-solute complex then traverses across the membrane to other side where it dissociates and discharges the solute molecule (Figure 4.1). The carrier then returns to its original site to repeat the cycle by accepting a fresh molecule of solute. The movement of solute occurs against the concentration or electrochemical gradient (from lower to higher concentration; up-hill movement), therefore, the process requires expenditure of energy. After transportation of the solute, energy is also required to energise the carrier for repeating the cycle.

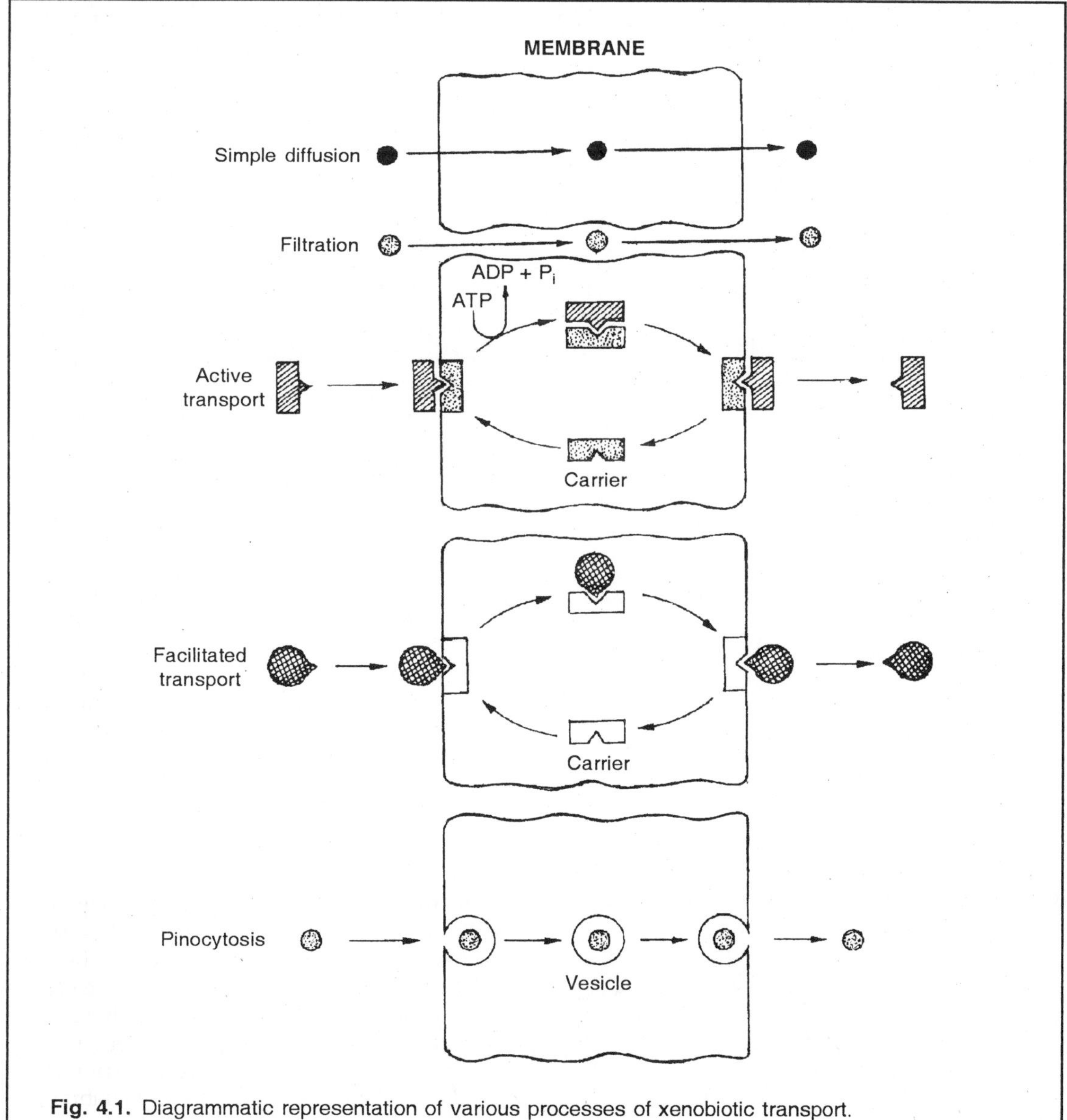

Fig. 4.1. Diagrammatic representation of various processes of xenobiotic transport.
Abbreviations : ATP = adenosine triphosphate; ADP = adenosine diphosphate ; P_i = phosphate

Unlike simple diffusion and filtration, the active transport is a structure specific process i.e. the carriers possess special affinity for and transport xenobiotics of specific chemical structures only. Generally, these carriers have special affinity for essential nutrients like sodium, potassium, glucose, and certain amino acids and vitamins. Because the number of carriers is limited in biological membranes, the process often becomes saturated, particularly at high concentrations of xenobiotics due to non-availability of free carriers. As the carriers are also structure specific, the transport process is subject to competition between agents having similar structures. The active transport is not very common in body because it occurs from selected sites, which are rich in number of carriers.

Table 4.1: Comparative features of simple diffusion and active transport processes.

Features	Simple diffusion	Active transport
1. Energy	Energy independent (passive process)	Energy dependent (active process)
2. Carrier	Not required	Required
3. Movement of substance	Along concentration gradient (down-hill movement)	Against concentration gradient (up-hill movement)
4. Saturation	Non-saturable process	Saturable process
5. Structure specificity	Not required	Required
6. Competitive inhibition	Does no occur	May occur
7. Nature and type of substance	Lipid soluble and unionised	Mainly hydrophilic, polar and electrolyte
8. Occurrence	Wide occurrence in body	Limited to certain sites

2. Facilitated Transport

Facilitated transport is a carrier mediated transport system that operates along the concentration gradient (down-hill movement). Although in this type of transport a carrier facilitates movement of xenobiotic across the membrane, but the driving force is the concentration gradient. Hence it does not require energy and is a passive process. The facilitated transport proceeds more rapidly than the simple diffusion, and can translocate non-diffusible substances. Similar to active transport, it is structure specific and saturable process and is subject to competition between agents having similar structures. Facilitated transport is not a major process for xenobiotic transport.

3. Pinocytosis

Pinocytosis is a minor transport mechanism, which involves engulfing extra cellular materials within a segment of the cell membrane to form saccules or vesicles. These vesicles are then pinched-off intracellularly (interiorised or internalised) and transported across cell membranes where they release the engulfed substance. Pinocytosis, like active transport, requires expenditure of cellular energy and shows structure selectivity (although of low order) and competitive and saturation kinetics. Pinocytosis is responsible for the cellular uptake of macromolecular nutrients like fats, starch, proteins, oil soluble vitamins (e.g., A, D, E and K). Pinocytosis contributes little to transport of most toxicants.

ABSORPTION

Absorption is defined as the process of movement of unchanged compound from its site of administration or exposure to the blood stream. Except for the intravascular routes (intravenous and/or intraarterial), absorption is a prerequisite for all systemic routes because a xenobiotic can exert its action only when it comes into blood circulation from site of exposure. During this process, the xenobiotic has to cross the biological membranes. Both the rate and the extent of absorption are important because they determine the duration and intensity of toxicant action. A toxicant that is completely but slowly absorbed may fail to show toxic effect as the minimum toxic concentration is never reached. On the contrary, a rapidly and completely absorbed toxicant attains the threshold level easily to elicit its toxic effect. Absorption can occur by following routes :

1. Oral Route

The gastrointestinal tract is the most important route of absorption since a majority of acute poisonings involve ingestion. Absorption of toxicants can take place along the entire GI tract, even in the mouth and rectum. The effective barrier to ingested toxicants is the epithelial lining of gastrointestinal tract. The ways in which toxicants cross GI mucous membranes are governed by the fundamental principles of xenobiotic transport as discussed earlier. Lipid soluble and unionised compounds are readily absorbed by diffusion from stomach as well as intestine at rates proportional to their lipid: water coefficient. Some toxicants are small enough to undergo filtration through the pores in the membranes. Uptake of some toxicants may occur via specialized transport systems meant for endogenous ions and nutrients. For example, thallium is absorbed by the iron transport system and lead by the calcium carrier. Particles appear to enter intestinal cells by process of pinocytosis.

Presence of food in the GI tract often dilutes the toxicant and retards its absorption. For example, ethanol and methanol are rapidly absorbed after ingestion, but presence of food in GI tract retards their absorption. Reduced motility and decreased gastric emptying time may also decrease absorption, but not to any significant effect. Gastrointestinal fluids usually promote disintegration (breakdown of solid dosage forms into small particles) and dissolution (solid to liquid phase) of xenobiotics, but may inactivate some toxicants (e.g. some organophosphates). Biotransformation within the ruminal and intestinal lumen by microflora or within the mucosa by host enzyme systems also retards xenobiotic absorption and makes certain compounds ineffective orally (e.g. catecholamines). Absorption of compounds can also be greatly affected by other concurrently ingested compounds e.g. antacids decrease solubility and absorption of tetracyclines by formation of insoluble complexes.

2. Pulmonary Route/Inhalation

Noxious gases, toxic fumes and particulates are absorbed through lungs after inhalation. The lipid soluble volatile and gaseous toxicants (e.g. hydrocyanic acid and chloroform) are absorbed practically instantaneously from lungs because they have relatively high lipid to water coefficients and generally are small molecules. The large surface area of alveoli, high permeability of alveolar epithelium and rich perfusion rate also facilitate their rapid absorption. Water soluble gases like ammonia and chlorine also produce immediate signs but they primarily irritate the upper respiratory tract mucosa. In case of aerosols and particulates, the toxicant delivery to lungs is largely dependent of the particle size of the compound. Larger particles remain confined to the upper respiratory tract and do not reach the pulmonary tree, whereas very small particles (≤ 0.6 microns) reach deep into the respiratory tract and may undergo rapid absorption from alveoli. Large particles are mostly deposited in the nasopharynx and are absorbed either through the regional epithelium or through GI tract epithelium after they are swallowed along the mucus.

3. Topical Route

Toxicants may be absorbed through the skin or mucous membranes after topical exposure. Systemic absorption after dermal exposure depends primarily on lipid solubility of the compound i.e. lipid soluble compounds generally penetrate the skin or mucous membranes more rapidly (e.g. some organophosphates) than the lipid insoluble compounds. In general, absorption of toxicants through intact skin is poor because the keratinised epidermis behaves like a barrier. Inflammation, cuts, rashes, mild burns, etc. promote toxicant absorption through skin because these conditions destroy the epidermis. Organic solvents such as carbon tetrachloride, methanol, and others which are present as vehicles for some formulations may also enhance dermal absorption of toxicants. Application of tourniquets or ice may retard absorption of poisons like snake venoms. Some agents like nerve gases, chloroform and insecticides can be absorbed by intact skin in sufficient quantity to produce systemic toxicity.

Absorption of most toxicants through mucous membranes is usually more rapid than the skin because mucous membranes are thin and highly vascular. Systemic absorption through mucous membranes often results in rapid toxic effects.

4. Parenteral Routes

Parenteral routes are not important means of toxicant exposure under natural conditions, except in malfunctioning infusion devices, incorrect dosage calculation or malicious poisoning. However, parenteral routes like intravenous, intramuscular, subcutaneous, or intrperitoneal are frequently employed by scientists to study toxic effects of drugs and chemicals in laboratory animals. Toxicant absorption from intramuscular and subcutaneous sites is rapid as toxicants are deposited directly in vicinity of the capillaries, which are highly porous and do not obstruct absorption of even large lipid insoluble or ionised compounds. Lipid soluble compounds pass readily across the whole surface of the capillary endothelium. Intravenous route is a major route of drug administration for drug abusers in human medicine.

DISTRIBUTION

Distribution may be defined as a process by which xenobiotics leave the blood stream and enter the extravascular fluid and tissues. Distribution is an important toxicokinetic process because it determines the transport of toxicants to their site of action, to other sites, and to organs of metabolism and excretion. The extent to which a toxicant is distributed to a particular tissue or organ depends largely on its ability to penetrate the capillary endothelium and diffuse across the cell membrane. Factors that affect distribution of a xenobiotic to body organs include physico-chemical properties of compound, binding to plasma and tissue proteins, blood flow through organs, special compartments and barriers, availability of specialised transport systems, disease state, etc.

1. Physicochemical Properties of Toxicant

Distribution of a toxicant to different body tissues is greatly influenced by certain physico-chemical characteristics of the compound. Almost all compounds having molecular weight less than 500 to 600 Da easily cross the capillary membrane to penetrate into the extracellular fluids (except in CNS) because junctions between the capillary endothelial cells are not tight. A compound that is lipid soluble and unionised at blood and extracellular fluid pH permeates the cell more rapidly than a polar and ionised compound. Small, water-soluble molecules and ions of size below 50 Da enter the cell through aqueous filled channels, whereas those of larger size are restricted unless a specialised transport system exists for them.

2. Binding to Plasma and Tissue Proteins:

a. Binding to plasma proteins: Xenobiotics are transported in the circulating blood in two forms - free form and bound to plasma proteins. The free form of toxicants is active, diffusible, and available for metabolism and excretion, whereas the protein bound form is inactive, non-diffusible, and not available for metabolism or excretion as it cannot pass through capillaries and cell membranes because of larger size. Plasma protein binding of toxicants generally involves weak chemical bonds and is a reversible process. Extent of binding is a characteristic of the compound and generally remains fixed for a toxicant within a wide range of concentration. The binding of individual compounds range from nil or very little (e.g., antipyrin) to very high (e.g., warfarin). The plasma protein binding mainly serves as a reservoir, which supplies free compound whenever required.

Free form ◄------► Protein bound form

A large variety of toxicants ranging from weak acids, neutral compounds, and weak bases bind to plasma proteins. Acidic compounds generally bind to plasma albumin and basic compounds to α_1-acid glycoproteins; binding to other plasma proteins (e.g., lipoproteins and globulins) occurs to a much smaller extent. Groups of toxicants that bind to same site may compete with each other for the binding site and show xenobiotic-displacement interaction. A compound with a greater affinity for plasma proteins can displace weakly bound compound from its binding sites and elevate the free compound concentration with resultant toxicity. For example, the antidiabetic drugs bound to plasma proteins can be displaced by sulphonamides, which have greater affinity for the plasma proteins.

b. Binding to tissue proteins: A toxicant may bind to one or more of the several tissue components and may get accumulated there. A toxicant is said to be localised in tissue, if its concentration in that tissue exceeds the concentration in plasma. The tissue-toxicant binding is usually specific (i.e. a particular type a toxicant binds only at a specific tissue/organ) (Table 4.2) and hence it precipitates tissue toxicity. Binding of the toxicant with the tissue may be reversible, where the tissue acts as storage site, or it may be irreversible. The irreversible binding usually occurs as a result of chemical activation of the toxicant, which attaches strongly to the tissue protein by covalent chemical bonding and produces toxicity. For example, paracetamol and chloroform metabolites bind covalently with liver resulting in hepatotoxicity and binding of sulphoxide of chlorpromazine to retina of Hounds breed of dog leads to retinopathy. Bone is a major site for storage of many toxicants including fluoride, lead and strontium.

Table 4.2: List of selected drugs and toxicants having affinity for specific organ/tissue.

Organ / Tissue	Drug(s)
Liver	Chloroquine, paracetamol and epoxides of halogenated hydrocarbons.
Lungs	Imipramine, chlorpromazine and antihistamines.
Kidneys	Heavy metals (mercury, lead, cadmium) and digoxin.
Thyroid	Iodine.
Skin	Chloroquine and phenothiazines.
Eye (retina)	Chloroquine and sulphoxide of chlorpromazine.
Bone and Teeth	Tetracyclines, fluoride and heavy metals (lead).
Adipose tissue	Thiopentone, minocycline and DDT.
Hair	Arsenicals.

3. Blood Flow and Organ Size

The rate of blood flow to tissue capillaries varies widely as a result of unequal distribution of cardiac output to various organs. In addition to the physico-chemical properties of compound and plasma protein binding, the toxicant distribution to a particular organ or tissue depends on the size of tissue (tissue volume) and tissue perfusion rate (volume of blood that flows per unit time per unit volume of tissue). Highly perfused organs such as lungs, kidneys, liver, heart, adrenals, and brain are rapidly equilibrated with lipid soluble toxicants. Muscle and skin are moderately perfused, so they equilibrate slowly with the toxicant present in blood. Adipose tissues, bones and teeth being poorly perfused, take longer to get distributed with the same compound.

4. Specialised Compartments and Barriers

Some organs/areas of the body are not readily accessible to toxicants because their anatomical make-up poses permeability restriction to xenobiotics. These barriers include blood-brain barrier, blood-CSF barrier and placental barrier.

a. Blood-brain barrier: The blood brain barrier is located in the capillaries of brain. The blood-brain barrier (BBB) is constituted by tight and overlapping capillary endothelial cells that lack pores or gaps, a continuous basement membrane, and an envelop formed by 'perivascular foot processes' of astrocyte cells that encircle about 85% of the surface areas of brain capillaries. Since the BBB is a lipoidal barrier, it allows only those toxicants that have high to moderate oil/water partition coefficient. Lipid insoluble, ionised or polar toxicants generally fail to enter the CNS. For example, the lipid soluble methyl mercury readily enters the brain to produce CNS toxicity, but the lipid insoluble inorganic mercury compound does not readily gain entry into brain and produce nephrotoxicity. There are certain specific sites in brain like chemoreceptor trigger zone (CTZ) and posterior lobe of hypothalamus where the BBB does not exist, and at these sites brain may be exposed to some lipid insoluble and polar toxicants.

b. Blood-cerebrospinal fluid barrier: The blood-cerebrospinal fluid (CSF) barrier is formed mainly by the choroid plexus of lateral, third and fourth ventricles. Unlike capillary endothelial cells in brain, the capillary endothelium that lines the choroid plexus have open junctions or gaps, but the choroidal cells are joined to each other by tight junctions. In general, the blood-CSF barrier has permeability characteristics similar to that of BBB and it allows only lipid soluble toxicants to enter the CSF.

c. Placental barrier: The maternal and foetal blood vessels are separated by a layer of trophoblastic cells that together constitute the placental barrier. The characteristics of this lipid barrier are generally the same as of blood-brain barrier. Lipid soluble toxicants pass freely into foetal circulation by diffusion and water-soluble toxicants or essential nutrients cross the placental barrier by carrier mediated transport system. However, the placental barrier is not as effective as the blood-brain barrier.

d. Other barriers: The prostrate, testicles, and globe of eyes contain barriers that prevent toxicant penetration into these tissues. Lipid soluble compounds can penetrate and reach these structures freely, whereas water-soluble compounds entry is restricted. The membrane of erythrocyte acts as a barrier against the penetration of inorganic mercury compounds but not that of alkyl mercury.

5. Availability of Specialised Transport System

Some toxicants are concentrated in some tissues as a result of their uptake by specialised transport systems. For example, iodine is actively concentrated into the thyroid cells.

6. Disease States

Distribution characteristics of several toxicants are altered in disease states. In meningitis and encephalitis, the blood-brain barrier becomes more permeable and several polar antibiotics like penicillin-G, which do not normally cross it, gain access to the brain. In hypoalbuminaemia, plasma protein binding of xenobiotics may be reduced and high concentration of free toxicants is attained. In cong' stive heart failure or shock, the perfusion rate in the entire body decreases that affect distribution of toxicants.

EXCRETION

Excretion may be defined as a process by which toxicants and/or their metabolites are irreversibly transferred from body to external environment. Excretion is thus important in termination of action of toxicants. Excretory organs (except lungs) excrete water soluble and ionised compounds more effectively than the lipid soluble and unionised compounds. Lipid soluble compounds have to be converted into water soluble forms by process of metabolism to facilitate their excretion from the body.

ROUTES OF EXCRETION

Toxicants are excreted in their unchanged form or as metabolites by several routes including the kidneys, lungs, biliary system, intestine, etc. Excretion of drugs or toxicants by kidneys, the principal organ of excretion, is called renal excretion; excretion by organs other than kidneys is known as extra-renal or non-renal excretion.

1. Renal Excretion

Renal excretion is the most important route of xenobiotic excretion. The kidney removes toxicants from body by the same mechanisms as those used in the removal of end-products of normal metabolism. Agents that are water soluble, non-volatile, and small in molecular size are excreted in the urine. The amount of toxicant or its metabolite excreted in urine depends on the sum total of three processes: glomerular filtration, tubular secretion and tubular reabsorption (Figure 4.2). The first two processes remove toxicants from the plasma, whereas the third process reabsorbs toxicants and returns them to the plasma.

a. Glomerular filtration: It is a non-selective and unidirectional process by virtue of which all non-protein bound compounds (whether lipid soluble or water soluble, unionised or ionised) are filtered through glomerular membranes into the renal tubules. Toxicants that are protein bound (Mol.wt. > 65,000) are not passed into glomerular filtrate because of their big size. The driving force for filtration through the glomerulus is the hydrostatic pressure of the blood flowing in the capillaries. Therefore, glomerular filtration of a toxicant depends mainly on its plasma protein binding and renal blood flow. Once a toxicant enters the glomerular filtrate, it is either reabsorbed across the tubular cells if it is lipid soluble and unionised or remains in the tubular fluid and excreted if it is water soluble, ionised and polar compound.

b. Tubular secretion: Tubular secretion (active tubular secretion) is a carrier-mediated process by which some toxicants and/or their metabolites are actively secreted from blood into the tubular lumen. This transport is against concentration or electrochemical gradient, energy dependent, capacity limited and saturable process. Binding of plasma proteins usually does not hinder tubular secretion of a toxicant because as the free toxicant is removed and transported across the tubular epithelium, immediate dissociation of the toxicant-protein complex occurs and the free form is again available for secretion. Active secretion is unaffected by changes in pH, but is dependent on the renal blood flow.

Two active tubular systems have been identified for organic electrolyte compounds, one for acidic compounds (e.g., penicillins and salicylic acid) and other for basic compounds (e.g., morphine and catecholamines). Both systems are relatively non-selective and independent of each other. Both systems are bidirectional i.e. they can transport their substrates from blood to tubular fluid and *vice-versa*. However for most toxicants and their metabolites, secretion into the tubular lumen predominates, whereas for endogenous substances like uric acid the reabsorption predominates. The active secretion decreases with aging, leading to an increase in the duration of toxicants eliminated primarily by the kidneys.

c. Tubular reabsorption: Tubular reabsorption is a process by which toxicants and/or their metabolites are transported from tubular fluid back into the capillary network. It generally occurs after glomerular filtration of toxicants and takes place all along the renal tubule. Contrary to the tubular secretion, the reabsorption results in increase in the half-life of toxicants. Tubular reabsorption is further of two types - passive and active tubular reabsorption.

Passive tubular reabsorption: It is a passive process by which lipid soluble and unionised toxicants are reabsorbed after they are filtered at the glomerulus. The driving force for such a process is the concentration gradient established by reabsorption of water along with sodium and other inorganic ions. Because most toxicants are weak acids or weak bases, the pK_a of the compound and the pH of the urine in tubular fluid determine the degree of ionisation and hence extent of diffusion through the lipoidal tubular membrane. According to the pH-partition hypothesis, weak bases ionise more and are absorbed less in acidic urine, whereas weak acids ionise more and are absorbed less in alkaline urine. Thus, acidification or alkalinisation of urine may alter the rate of excretion of such toxicants because of ion-trapping in the tubular fluid. This principle is utilised for facilitating elimination of some toxicants in poisoning. For

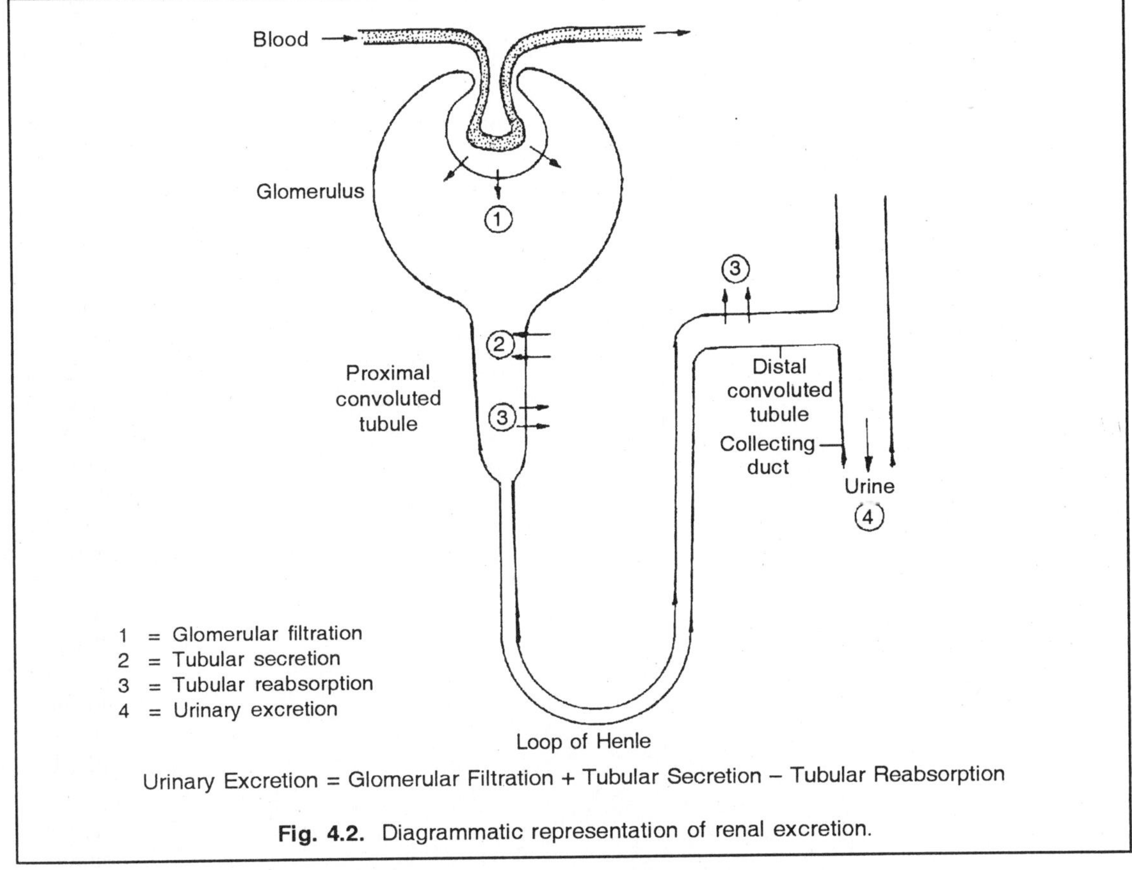

Fig. 4.2. Diagrammatic representation of renal excretion.

example, urine is acidified in poisoning with basic toxicants (e.g. morphine and amphetamine) and alkalinised in poisoning with acidic toxicants (e.g. barbiturates and salicylates). Variation in normal urine pH in domestic animals (carnivores = 5.5 to 7.0, herbivores = 7.0 to 8.0) may also affect the degree of ionisation and hence passive reabsorption of toxicants.

Active tubular reabsorption: Active tubular reabsorption is commonly seen with some endogenous substances or nutrients such as glucose, amino acids, etc., which the body needs to conserve. Very few toxicants are known to undergo active renal tubular reabsorption.

2. Extra-Renal Excretion :

a. Faecal excretion: Faecal excretion is a major pathway for the elimination of toxicants from the body. Faecal excretion is important for unabsorbed poison that remains in GI tract after ingestion and also that is metabolised in liver after absorption and excreted in the intestine.

Non-absorbed ingesta: The non-absorbed portion of xenobiotics contributes to the faecal excretion of most toxicants to some extent because it is rare for 100 per cent of a toxicant to be absorbed after ingestion. In addition to non-absorbed toxicants, varying proportions of nutrients and xenobiotics that are present in food pass through GI tract unabsorbed, contributing to faecal excretion.

Biliary excretion: Biliary route is perhaps the most important contributing source to the faecal excretion of toxicants and their metabolites. In biliary excretion, the toxicant and/or its metabolites are excreted by hepatocytes into the bile canaliculi and ultimately into the duodenum via the bile. Biliary excretion of toxicants may occur both passively and actively (mainly). Biliary excretion is mainly determined by polarity of the substance – greater the polarity, better is the biliary excretion. Metabolites, particularly water-soluble conjugates, are more excreted in bile than the parent compounds. Relatively large molecules are preferentially eliminated in the bile. Accordingly, glucuronide conjugates are mainly and glutathione conjugates are exclusively excreted via the bile. For a toxicant to be excreted unchanged in the bile, it must have highly polar functional groups. Non-ionised toxicant should also be highly polar for biliary excretion (e.g. cardiac glycosides). The relative importance of biliary excretion depends on the type of toxicant and the species involved.

After biliary excretion, some of the conjugated metabolites, especially glucuronide conjugates, are deconjugated by intestinal bacteria and the released lipid soluble parent compound is reabsorbed into the circulation. The reabsorbed compound is again carried to the liver for secretion via bile into the intestine. This phenomenon of toxicant cycling between intestine and liver is called 'enterohepatic cycling or enterohepatic circulation'. Such a recycling process continues until the toxicant is further biotransformed in the liver or is excreted in the urine, or both. The toxicants which are excreted via bile in the intestine but do not undergo enterohepatic cycling are finally excreted in the faeces. The enterohepatic cycling is an important phenomenon that prolongs the duration of action of several drugs and toxicants (e.g., digoxin and some benzodiazepines).

Intestinal excretion: Excretion of compounds or their metabolites into the GI tract is a minor route of xenobiotic elimination. The intestinal excretion is considered a reverse of GI absorption in which xenobiotics may passively diffuse from the blood into the lumen of GI tract. Toxicants excreted in the GI tract may undergo recycling (e.g., morphine) or are eliminated in faeces. Intestinal excretion is a relatively slow process and is considered important for compounds that have low rates of biotransformation and/or low renal or biliary excretion.

b. Pulmonary excretion: The lungs are involved in the elimination of toxicants that exist in a gaseous phase at body temperature. No specialized transport system has been described for pulmonary excretion of toxicants and simple diffusion appears to be the major pathway. Gases and volatile liquids such as inhalation anaesthetics, hydrocyanic acid and carbon monoxide are rapidly absorbed and excreted through the lungs. In general, pulmonary elimination of gases is inversely proportional to the rate of their absorption. For example, gases that are not very soluble in blood such as nitrous oxide are excreted rapidly, whereas highly soluble compounds such as chloroform are excreted slowly because of their storage in the adipose tissue and the limited ventilation volume. Compounds like ethanol that also have high solubility in blood and tissues are diffusion. The rate of elimination of a gas with high solubility in blood is ventilation limited, whereas that of a gas with low solubility in blood is perfusion limited.

c. Mammary excretion: Excretion of xenobiotics in milk is a minor route of toxicant elimination, but it is important because poisoning of mother can affect the suckling young ones. Presence of toxic substances in milk is also important from public health point of view as poisoning of dairy animals may affect the human consumers. Most toxicants enter milk by passive diffusion. As milk is acidic (pH 6.5 to 7.0) relative to plasma (pH 7.4), weakly basic toxicants concentrate more in milk. Since milk contains proteins, some toxicants excreted in milk can bind to milk proteins. Lipophilic toxicants such as DDT, PCBs, dioxins, and furans diffuse along the fats from plasma into the mammary gland and milk can be a major route of their excretion. Metals chemically similar to calcium, like lead, and chelating agents that form complexes with calcium also can be excreted into milk to a considerable extent.

d. Salivary excretion: Excretion of toxicants in saliva is of lesser importance. It occurs primarily by passive diffusion process and, therefore, is predictable on the basis of the pH-partition hypothesis. Toxicants excreted in saliva can undergo cycling in a fashion similar to enterohepatic cycling.

e. Other routes of excretion: Insignificant amounts of some drugs and toxicants (e.g., salicylic acid, alcohol and heavy metals) are excreted through skin via sweat. Toxicants can also be excreted via the lachrymal fluid, intestinal fluid, genital secretions, and tracheobronchial secretions. The heavy metals (e.g., arsenicals) may be detected in hair and nails. Desquamation or loss of epithelial cells in the epidermis permits excretion of toxicants through the skin.

BIBLIOGRAPHY

Adams H R (2001) Veterinary Pharmacology and Therapeutics. 8th edn. Iowa State Univ. Press, Iowa.

Ahrens F A (1996) The National Veterinary Medical Series for Independent Study: Pharmacology. Williams & Wilkins, Baltimore.

Aiello S E (1998) The Merck Veterinary Manual. 8th edn. Merck & Co., New Jersey.

Baggot JD (1977) Principles of Drug Disposition in Domestic Animals. W. B. Saunders, Philadelphia.

Brahmankar DM and Jaiswal SB (1995) Biopharmaceutics and Pharmacokinetics A Treatise. Vallabh Prakashan, Delhi.

Brown SA (2001) Pharmacokinetics: Disposition and fate of drugs in the body. In: Veterinary Pharmacology and Therapeutics. 8th edn. Adams H R (Ed.) p. 15. Iowa State Univ. Press, Iowa.

Cohen Y (1978) Advances in Pharmacology and Therapeutics. Toxicology. Vol 10. Proceedings of the 7th International Congress of Pharmacology. Paris 1978. Pergamon Press, Oxford.

Lu FC and Kacew S (2002) Lu's Basic Toxicology: Fundamentals, Target Organs and Risk Assessment. Taylor & Francis, New York.

Osweiler GD (1996) Toxicology. Williams and Wilkins, Philadelphia.

Radeleff RD (1970) Veterinary Toxicology. 2nd edn. Lea and Febiger, Philadelphia.

Renwick AG (1995) Toxicokinetics. In: General and Applied Toxicology. Ballantyne B, Marrs T and Turner P (Eds.) p 111. Macmillan Press Ltd., London.

Rozman KK and Klaassen CD (1996) Absorption, distribution, and excretion of toxicants. In: Casarett and Doull's Toxicology: The Basic science of Poisons. 5th edn. Klaassen CD (Ed.) p 91. McGraw Hill Companies Inc., New York.

Smith J (2005) Drug discovery for molecular science: An introduction to ADME/Toxicology 2. (http://www. chemie.uni-erlangen.de/clark/smith/teaching html).

Wilkinson GR (2001) Pharmacokinetics: The dynamics of drug absorption, distribution, and elimination. In: Goodman & Gilman's The Pharmacological Basis of Therapeutics. 10th edn. Hardman JG, Limbird LE and Gilman AG (Eds.) p 3. The McGraw-Hill Companies Inc., New York.

❑❑❑❑❑❑

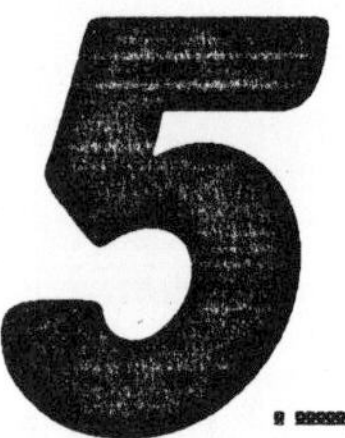

BIOTRANSFORMATION OF TOXICANTS

Biotransformation or Metabolism may be defined as the conversion from one chemical form of a substance to another. It may also be defined as the sum of biochemical changes occurring to a substance within the body. Both metabolism and biotransformation terms are used interchangeably and carry same meaning, particularly when applied to xenobiotics. The primary function of metabolism is to transforms a lipid soluble and non-polar compound to water soluble and polar compound so that it is readily excreted from the body. This is because only water-soluble substances undergo excretion, whereas lipid soluble substances are passively reabsorbed from renal or extra-renal excretory sites into the blood by virtue of their lipophilicity. It has been observed that if a lipid soluble substance is not converted into a water-soluble form, it may remain in body for very long period (weeks, months or years) and may precipitate toxic reaction. Thus metabolism limits the life of a substance in the body and protects the organism from ill-effects of xenobiotics.

Biotransformation: It is a specific term used for chemical transformation of xenobiotics in the body/living organism.

Metabolism: It is a general term used for chemical transformation of xenobiotics and endogenous nutrients (e.g., proteins, carbohydrates and fats) within or outside the body.

Xenobiotics: These are all chemical substances that are not nutrient for body (foreign to body) and which enter the body through ingestion, inhalation or dermal exposure. They include drugs, industrial chemicals, pesticides, pollutants, plant and animal toxins, etc.

Functions of Biotransformation

Biotransformation performs the following functions:

a. It causes conversion of an active compound to inactive or less active metabolite(s) called inactivation or detoxification. For example,

i. Phenobarbitone ⟶ p-hydroxy-phenobarbitone

ii. DDT ⟶ DDE and DDA

b. It causes conversion of an active compound to more active metabolite(s) called bioactivation or toxication. For example,

i. Malathion ⟶ Malaoxon

ii. Acetonitrile ⟶ Cyanide

c. It causes conversion of an inactive compound (i.e. pro-drug or precursor compound) to active metabolite(s) called activation. For example,

i. Phenacetin ⟶ Paracetamol

ii. Thiocyanates ⟶ Cyanide
(Pro-insecticide) (Insecticide)

d. It causes conversion of an active compound to equally active metabolite(s) (no change in activity). For example,

i. Dicrotophos ⟶ Monocrotophos

ii. Digitoxin ⟶ Digoxin.

e. It causes conversion of an active compound to active metabolite(s) having entirely different pharmacological/toxicological activity (change in activity). For example,

i. Iproniazid ⟶ Isoniazid
(Antidepressant) (Antitubercular)

ii. Aflatoxin B_1 ⟶ Aflatoxin M_1
(Hepatotoxin) (Carcinogen)

Xenobiotic Metabolising Organs

Liver is the primary site for metabolism of almost all xenobiotics as it is relatively rich in a large variety of enzymes. It is called hepatic metabolism. Metabolism by organs other than liver (called extrahepatic metabolism) is of lesser importance because low levels of metabolising enzymes are present in such tissues. The order of drug metabolising ability of various organs is: liver > lungs > kidneys > intestine > placenta > adrenals > skin. Some other organs i.e. brain, testes, muscles, and spleen also metabolise compounds to smaller extent. Within a given cell, most xenobiotic-metabolising activity is found in the endoplasmic reticulum (ER) and the cytosol. Metabolism can also occur in mitochondria, nuclear envelope and plasma membrane. The xenobiotic metabolising enzymes in the endoplasmic reticulum (that results in microsomes on differential centrifugation) are often known as microsomal enzymes.

Xenobiotic Metabolising Enzymes

A large number of enzymes in animals are capable of metabolising drugs/toxicants. These enzymes are located mainly in liver. These enzymes can be divided into two main groups: microsomal and non-microsomal enzymes.

a. Microsomal enzymes : The endoplasmic reticulum (especially smooth ER) of liver and other tissues (kidneys and GI tract) contain several enzymes for biotransformation. When a cell is homogenised and differentially centrifuged, the endoplasmic reticulum breaks down to small vesicles known as microsomes. All enzymes present in the microsomes are called microsomal enzymes. Endoplasmic reticulum (microsomes) contains large number of enzymes like monooxygenases (most important) and other enzymes related to phospholipid metabolism, cholesterol synthesis, glucuronide conjugation, hydration of epoxides, ester cleavage, etc. Microsomal enzymes catalyse glucuronide conjugation, most of the oxidative reactions and some reductive and hydrolytic reactions. The monooxygenases and glucuronyl transferase are important microsomal enzymes. Microsomal enzymes are inducible by drugs, toxicants, diets and other factors.

b. Non-microsomal enzymes: Enzymes occurring in organelles/sites other than microsomes are called non-microsomal enzymes. These are usually present in the cytoplasm, plasma and mitochondria. Non-microsomal biotransformation of xenobiotics occurs primarily in the liver, and also in plasma, GI tract and other tissues. Non-microsomal enzymes catalyse all conjugation reactions except glucuronide conjugation and some of the oxidation, reduction and hydrolytic reactions of xenobiotics. Individual variations in the rates of biotransformation of xenobiotics are about the same for non-microsomal enzymes as for microsomal enzymes. None of the non-microsomal enzymes involved in xenobiotic metabolism is known to be inducible.

PATHWAYS OF BIOTRANSFORMATION

There are two major pathways/phases of xenobiotic biotransformation: Phase I and Phase II.

a. Phase I reactions: Phase I (non-synthetic or non-conjugative phase) includes reactions which catalyse oxidation, reduction and hydrolysis of xenobiotics. In phase I reactions, small polar functional groups like – OH, $-NH_2$, –SH, –COOH, etc. are either added or unmasked (if already present) on the otherwise lipid soluble compounds so that the resulting products may undergo phase II reactions. Phase I reactions generally precede phase II reactions.

b. Phase II reactions: Phase II (synthetic or conjugative phase) includes reactions that catalyze conjugation of xenobiotics or their phase I metabolites with endogenous substances like glucuronic acid, sulphate, methyl, glutathione, amino acids, etc. Phase II products, called conjugates, are water-soluble metabolites, which are readily excreted from the body.

Phase I reactions result in inactivation (mostly), no change in activity, or bioactivation, whereas phase II reactions generally result in inactivation (in some cases may cause bioactivation). Phase II reactions are also called synthetic reactions, in contrast to the asynthetic phase I reactions, because the outcome of conjugative processes are generally products with increased molecular size and altered physico-chemical properties (it appears as if a new substance is synthesised). Some compounds pass through phase I reactions and then phase II reactions, others through either of one phase only (Figure 5.1). Most compounds are metabolised by many reactions, simultaneously or sequentially, therefore a range of metabolites can be formed from a single compound simultaneously or one after the other in the body. The rate of biotransformation and the type of biotransformation of toxicant often differ from one species of animal to another and even from one strain to another, a fact that often accounts for difference of toxic response in these animals. The various phase I and phase II reactions are listed in Table 5.1.

I. PHASE I REACTIONS

1. Oxidation

Phase I oxidative reactions are the most important metabolic reactions, as energy in animals is primarily derived by oxidative combustion of organic molecules containing carbon and hydrogen atoms. These reactions increase hydrophilicity of xenobiotics by introducing polar functional groups such as -OH. Oxidative metabolism is mainly carried out by the microsomal monooxygenases or mixed function oxidase (MFO) system and produces metabolites that may be inactive (mostly) or active. Some of the oxidation reactions are also catalysed by non-microsomal enzymes like aldehyde dehydrogenase, xanthine oxidase and monoamine oxidase.

Monooxygenases/Mixed function oxidases : The hepatic endoplasmic reticulum contains an important group of oxidative enzymes called monooxygenases or mixed function oxidases (MFOs). Such enzymes require both molecular

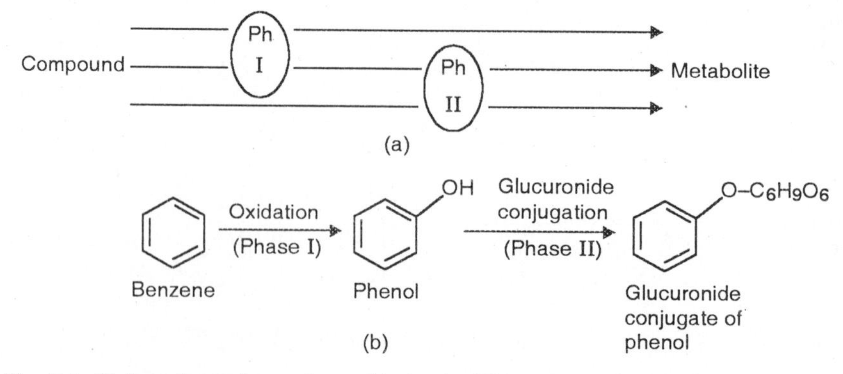

Fig. 5.1. Biotransformations of xenobiotics by Phase I and/or phase II reaction(s).
a. General reaction b. Biotransformation of benzene

oxygen (O_2) and reduced nicotinamide adenine dinucleotide phosphate (NADPH). Mixed function oxidase name was proposed in order to characterise the mixed function of the oxygen molecule. The term monooxygenases for these enzymes was used as they incorporate only one atom of molecular oxygen (O_2) into the organic substrate with concomitant reduction of the second oxygen atom to water.

The multienzyme mixed function oxidase system located in the ER of hepatic cells is composed of an electron transfer chain consisting of three components having two main enzymes.

i. A heme protein known as cytochrome P-450. It is a terminal oxidase enzyme system which plays an important role of transferring an oxygen atom to the substrate RH and converts it to ROH.

ii. A second enzyme, a flavoprotein, is known as cytochrome P-450 reductase (or cytochrome C reductase). It is a NADPH dependent enzyme and functions as an electron carrier, catalysing the reduction of cytochrome P-450 to ferrous form by transferring an electron from NADPH.

iii. A heat stable, lipid component is known as phosphatidylcholine. Its function is to facilitate electron transfer from NADPH to cytochrome P-450.

The overall stoichiometry of the reaction involving the substrate RH which yields the product ROH, is given by the following reaction:

$$RH + O_2 + NADPH + H^+ \longrightarrow ROH + H_2O + NADP^+$$

The most important component of mixed function oxidases is the cytochrome P-450, because it binds to substrate and activates oxygen. The cytochrome P-450 enzymes are widely distributed across all living creatures and carry out a number of oxidative reactions. The name cytochrome P-450 is given to this group of proteins because their reduced form binds with carbon monoxide to form a complex, which has maximum absorbance at 450 nm. Depending upon the extent of amino acid sequence homology, the cytochrome P-450 (CYP) enzymes superfamily contains a number of isoenzymes, the relative amount of which differs among species and among individuals of the same species. Each individual CYP isoform appears to have characteristic substrate specificity based on structural features of the substrate, although considerable overlapping is present. In human beings, of the 1000 currently known cytochrome P-450s, about 50 are functionally active.

Steps in the oxidation of xenobiotics: Various steps as shown in Fig. 5.2 are:

1. Substrate RH binds to the oxidised form of the cytochrome P-450 (Fe^{+++}) to form a complex.

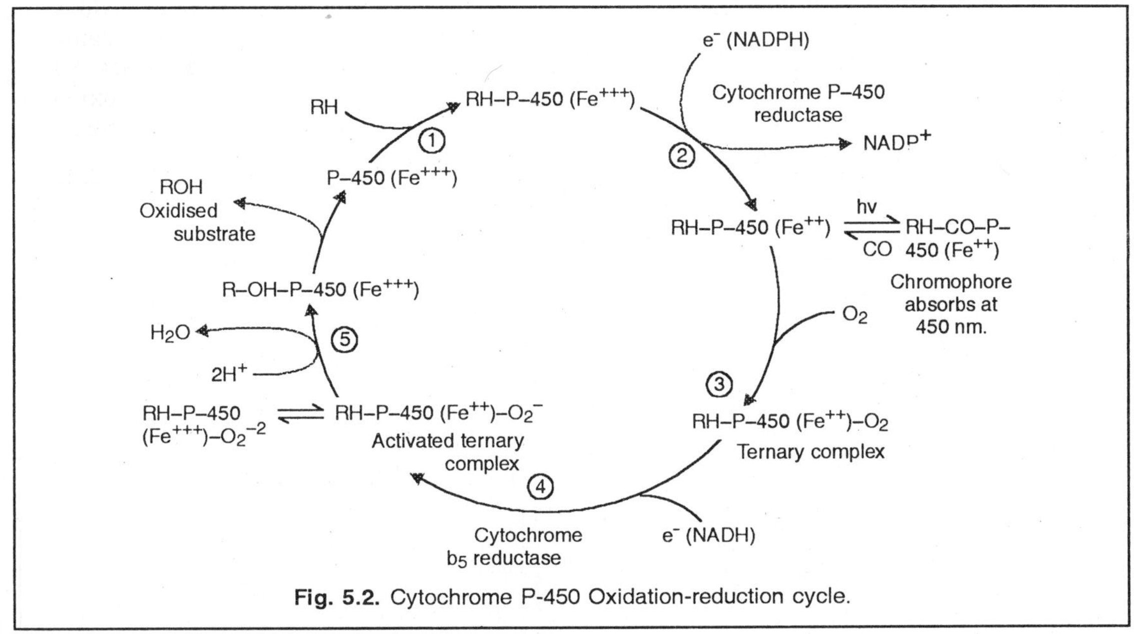

Fig. 5.2. Cytochrome P-450 Oxidation-reduction cycle.

2. Cytochrome P-450 reductase transfers one electron from NADPH to the complex to form reduced (Fe^{++})-P-450-substrate complex. This step is considered to be the rate limiting step in the overall oxidation of xenobiotics.
3. The reduced enzyme-substrate complex combines with a molecule of oxygen (O_2) to form a ternary complex.
4. The ternary complex combines with a second electron supplied by NADH by the same NADPH flavoprotein reductase or NADH-cytochrome b_5 reductase to form a ternary activated oxygen P-450 substrate complex.
5. In a series of steps in the presence of two protons (H^+), one atom of oxygen from the activated oxygen complex is transferred to the substrate to yield the oxidised substrate (R-OH) and the other atom forms water. The free oxidised form of cytochrome P-450 is regenerated and is ready to attach to another molecule of substrate.

In vitro, the MFO system is active only when reaction medium is supplemented with NADPH in the presence of molecular oxygen. The wide distribution of cytochrome P-450 containing MFOs in various organs makes it the most important group of enzymes involved in the biotransformation of xenobiotics.

Type of Oxidative Reactions

Oxidative reactions are mainly carried out by microsomal enzymes and appear to have a similar mechanism when considered in terms of addition of oxygen and supply of electrons to cytochrome P-450. However, these enzymes are mostly non-specific, and both substrates and products fall into many chemical classes. Some of the oxidation reactions are catalysed by non-microsomal enzymes (e.g. aldehyde dehydrogenase, xanthine oxidase and monoamine oxidase). Thus it is convenient to summarise their activities on the basis of the chemical reactions. At the same time, it should be recalled that these reactions are similar and may overlap.

a. Dealkylation : The removal of an alkyl group attached to amide nitrogen or to a heteroatom (such as oxygen) is a frequently encountered reaction.

i. N-dealkylation : Alkyl groups attached directly to nitrogen atom in nitrogen bearing compounds are capable of undergoing N-dealkylation reactions. Due to the presence of N-alkyl groups virtually in all carbamate insecticides, N-dealkylation reaction is important for this group of insecticides. It is also important for some organophosphorus insecticides.

ii. O-dealkylation : This reaction is similar to N-dealkylation. The O-containing functional groups (analogous to amines and amides in N-dealkylation) are ethers and esters; however, only the ethers undergo O-dealkylation. This reaction generally leads to formation of active metabolites (e.g. phenacetin to paracetamol, codeine to morphine).

iii. S-dealkylation: The mechanism of S-dealkylation of thioethers (RSR′) is analogous to

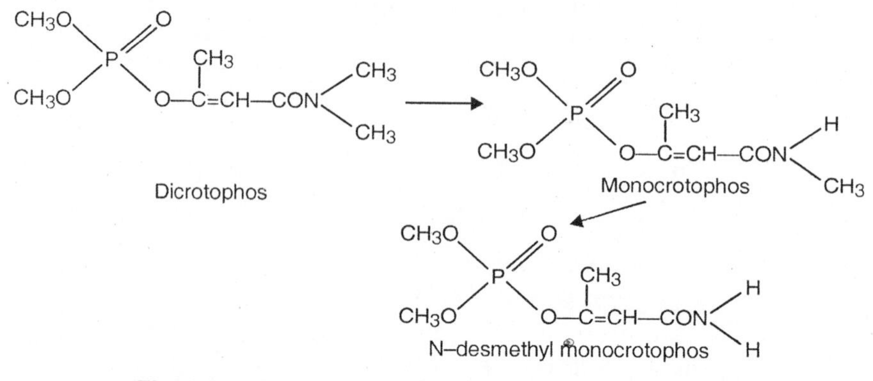

Fig. 5.3. N-dealkylation of dicrotophos and monocrotophos.

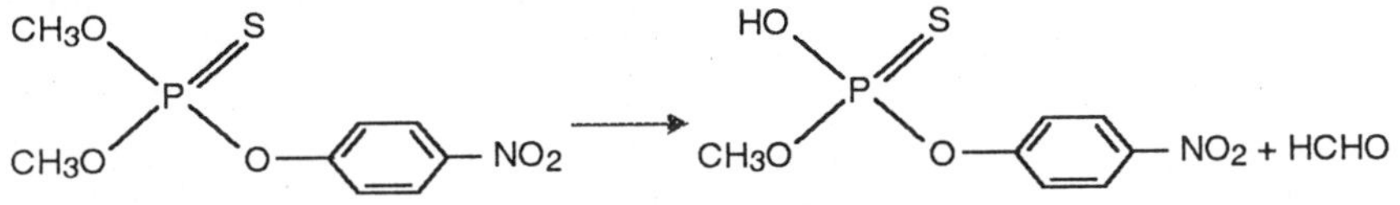

Methyl parathion → Desmethyl parathion + HCHO (Formaldehyde.)

Fig. 5.4. O-dealkylation of methyl-parathion.

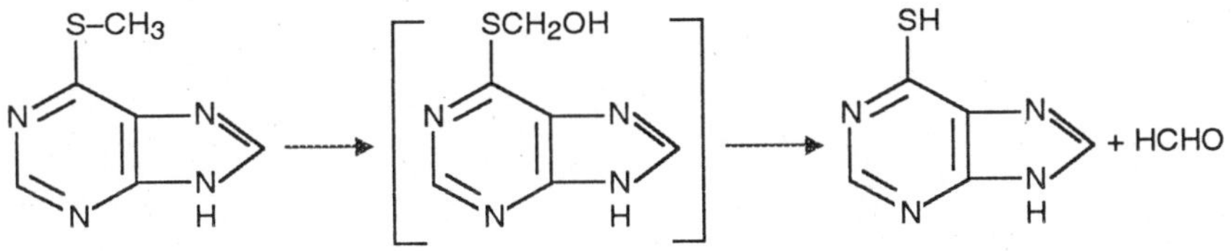

6–Methyl mercaptopurine → [Hydroxylated intermediate] → 6–Mercapto-purine + HCHO (Formal-dehyde)

Fig. 5.5. S-dealkylation of 6-methyl mercaptopurine.

N-dealkylation. The C-S bond cleavage results in the formation of a thiol (RSH) and a carbonyl product (formaldehyde or acetaldehyde).

b. Desulphuration : The replacement of a sulphur atom by an oxygen atom is commonly observed in thioamides (RCSNHR′), thionates and thioates. The process represents activation rather than a detoxification.

The insecticidal activity of malathion is largely due to malaoxon formed by enzymatic oxidation of –P=S to –P=O. The phosphates are the active inhibitors of acetylcholinesterase enzyme.

c. Hydroxylation :

i. Aromatic hydroxylation: It involves addition of an oxygen atom across a double bond in the aromatic compound. This reaction proceeds via formation of a reactive intermediate arene oxide (epoxide).

ii. Aliphatic hydroxylation : Aliphatic hydroxylation results from the insertion of the

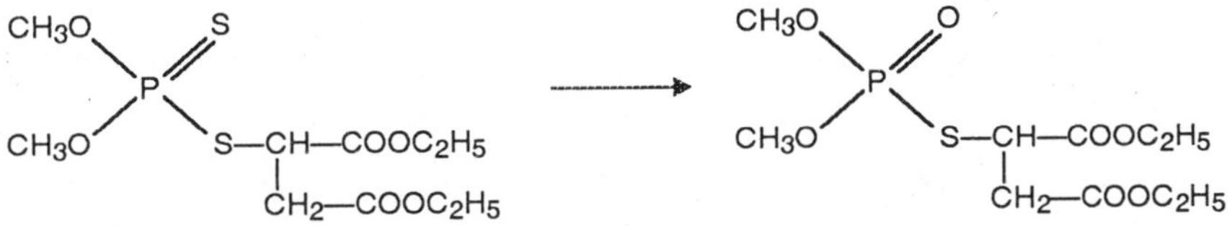

Malathion → Malaoxon

Fig. 5.6. Desulphuration of malathion into malaoxon.

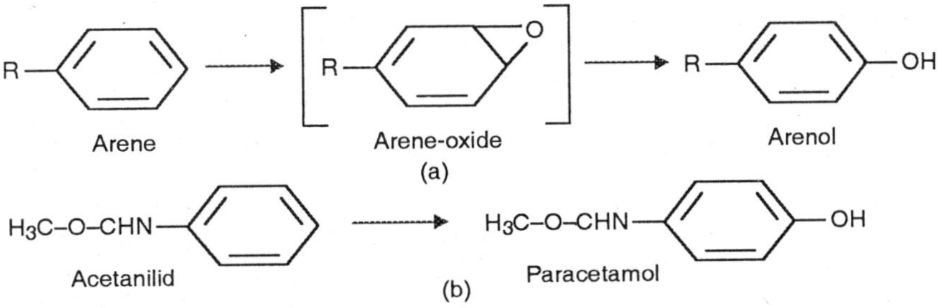

(a) Arene → [Arene-oxide] → Arenol

(b) Acetanilid → Paracetamol

Fig. 5.7. Aromatic hydroxylation of arene into arenol.
a. General reaction b. Biotransformation of acetanilid.

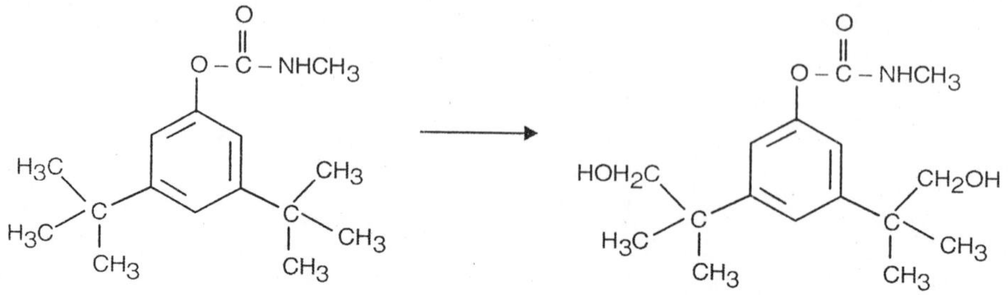

Fig. 5.8. Aliphatic hydroxylation of butacarb.

oxygen atom into a carbon-hydrogen bond.

$$R-CH_2-CH_2-CH_3 \longrightarrow R-CH_2-\underset{\displaystyle OH}{\underset{|}{CH}}-CH_3$$

Aliphatic C–H bonds not adjacent to hetero atoms such as sulphur, oxygen or nitrogen are potential targets for microsomal hydroxylations. This may result in metabolites which are less active, similar active or more active than the parent compound.

iii. Heterocyclic ring-hydroxylation : Oxidation of non-aromatic C=C (double bond) is analogous to aromatic hydroxylation i.e. it proceeds via formation of epoxides to yield 1, 2-dihydrodiols. It is called olefinic oxidation. Epoxides of olefinic hydroxylation are not as reactive as aromatic epoxides.

iv. N-hydroxylation : It occurs by the addition of an oxygen atom to an unshared electron pair on the nitrogen atom.

d. Oxidation (Oxide formation)

i. N-oxidation (N-oxide formation) : N-oxides are formed only by nitrogen atoms having basic properties like amines (not amides). N-oxide products are highly water soluble and are excreted in urine. They are, however, susceptible to reduction to the corresponding amine.

ii. S-oxidation (Sulphoxidation) : It is another important biological activation process in which

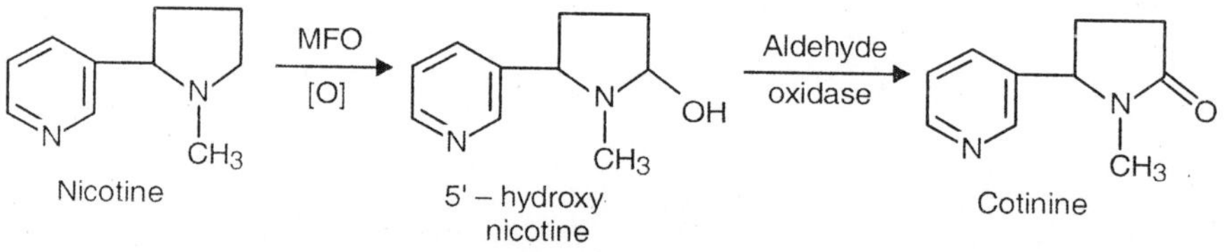

Fig. 5.9. Heterocyclic ring hydroxylation of nicotine.

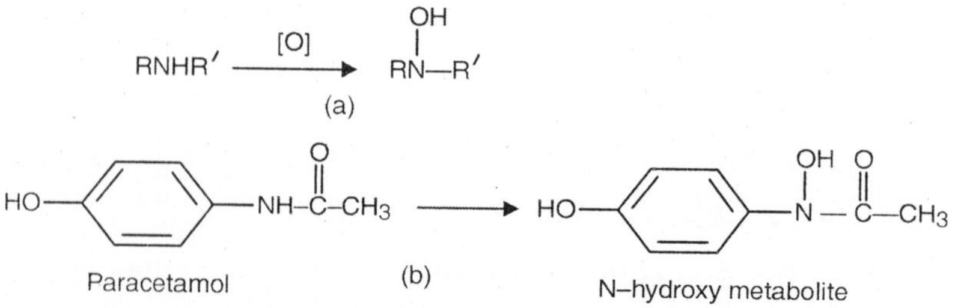

Fig. 5.10. N-hydroxylation of xenobiotics.
(a) General reaction (b) N-hydroxylation of paracetamol.

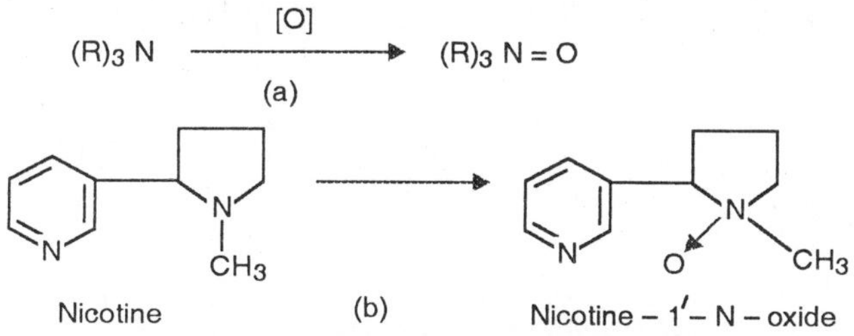

Fig. 5.11. N-oxidation of xenobiotics.
(a) General reaction. (b)Biotransformation of nicotine.

oxygen is added to the unshared electron pair on the sulphur atom e.g. organophosphorus insecticides. However, in some cases this may lead to detoxification. S-oxidation reactions yield sulphoxides which may be further oxidised to sulphones (RSO_2R). Generally the formation of sulphoxide is rapid than that of the sulphone.

e. Epoxidation (Epoxide formation) : Epoxidation occurs by addition of an oxygen atom across the double bond. Formation of unstable epoxides as intermediates is seen in oxidative hydroxylation with many compounds. However, formation of stable epoxide also occurs with some cyclodiene insecticides. Epoxides are usually more toxic than their precursor compounds.

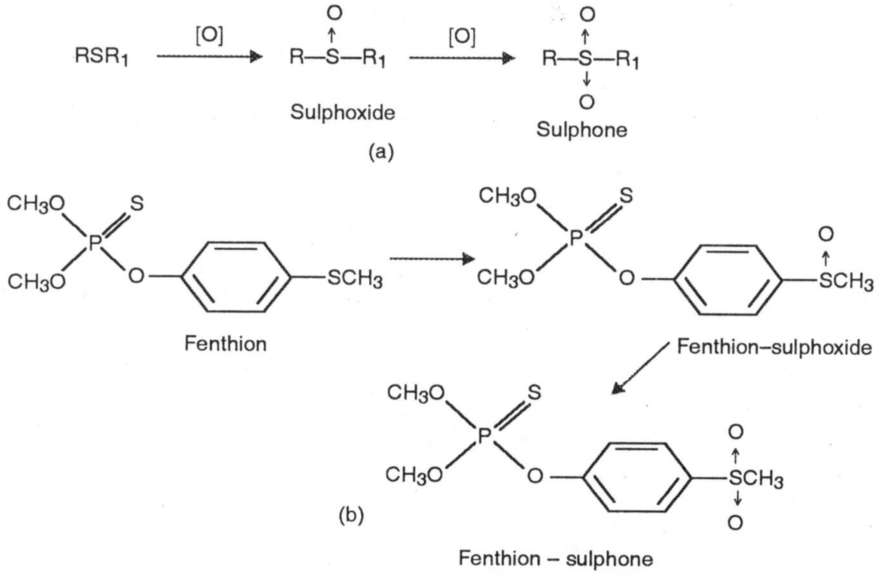

Fig. 5.12. S-oxidation of xenobiotics.
(a) General reaction (b) Biotransformation of fenthion.

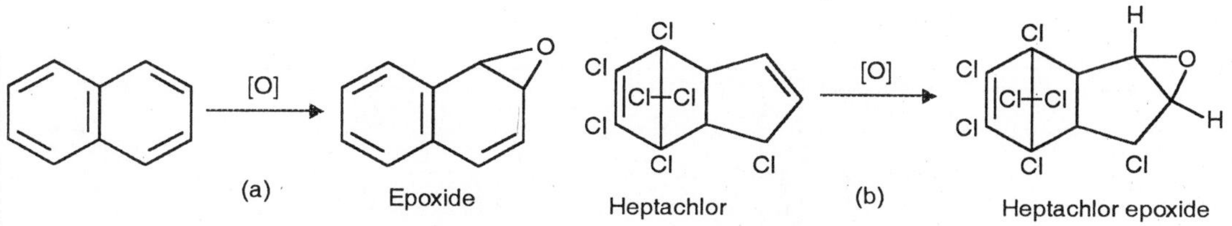

Fig. 5.13. Epoxidation of xenobiotics.
(a) General reaction (b) Biotransformation of heptachlor.

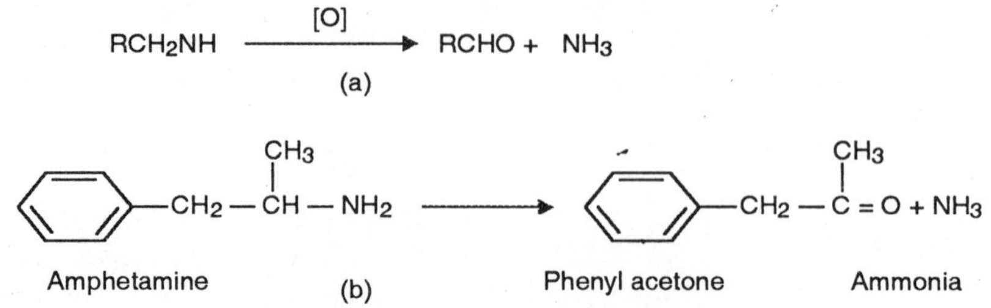

$$RCH_2NH \xrightarrow{[O]} RCHO + NH_3$$

(a)

$$C_6H_5-CH_2-CH(CH_3)-NH_2 \longrightarrow C_6H_5-CH_2-C(CH_3)=O + NH_3$$

Amphetamine (b) Phenyl acetone Ammonia

Fig. 5.14. Deamination of xenobiotics.
(a) General reaction (b) Biotransformation of amphetamine.

f. Deamination : Deamination of primary and secondary amines is also catalysed by microsomal enzymes. Primary aliphatic amines readily undergo deamination, while secondary and tertiary amines are deaminated only when bulky groups are attached to nitrogen. Aromatic and alicyclic amines are resistant to deamination.

g. Alcohol and aldehyde oxidation: These reactions are mainly catalysed by non-microsomal enzymes, dehydrogenases. Primary and secondary alcohols and aldehydes undergo oxidation relatively easily but tertiary alcohols, ketones and carboxylic acids are resistant. In case of ethanol, oxidation to acetaldehyde is reversible and further oxidation of acetaldehyde to acetic acid (carboxylic acid) is very rapid so that acetaldehyde should not accumulate in the body as it is highly toxic.

h. Miscellaneous oxidative reactions

i. Oxidative dehalogenation : This reaction is common with halogen containing drugs such as chloroform. Dehalogenation of chloroform yields phosgene which may result in electrophiles capable of covalent binding to tissues.

2. Reduction

Reduction is acceptance of one or more electron(s) or their equivalent from another substrate. Detoxification of xenobiotics via reductive routes is much less important than the oxidative systems in higher animals and plants but it is gaining importance in the environment. Biotransformation by reduction is also capable of generating polar functional groups such as hydroxy and amino groups which can undergo further biotransformation or conjugation. Many reductive reactions are exact opposite of oxidative reactions. For example,

Alcohol dehydrogenation ⟷ Carbonyl reduction

N-oxidation ⟷ Amine oxide reduction

a. Reduction of N-compounds: The N-containing functional groups that commonly

$$\underset{\text{Ethanol}}{CH_3CH_2OH} + NAD^+ \underset{\text{dehydrogenase}}{\overset{\text{Alcohol}}{\rightleftharpoons}} \underset{\text{Acetaldehyde}}{CH_3CHO} + NADH + H^+$$

$$\underset{\text{Acetaldehyde}}{CH_3CHO} + NAD^+ + H_2O \xrightarrow[\text{dehydrogenase}]{\text{Aldehyde}} \underset{\text{Acetic acid}}{CH_3COOH} + NADH + H^+$$

Fig. 5.15. Oxidation of ethanol (alcohol) and acetaldehyde (aldehyde) by non-microsomal dehydrogenases.

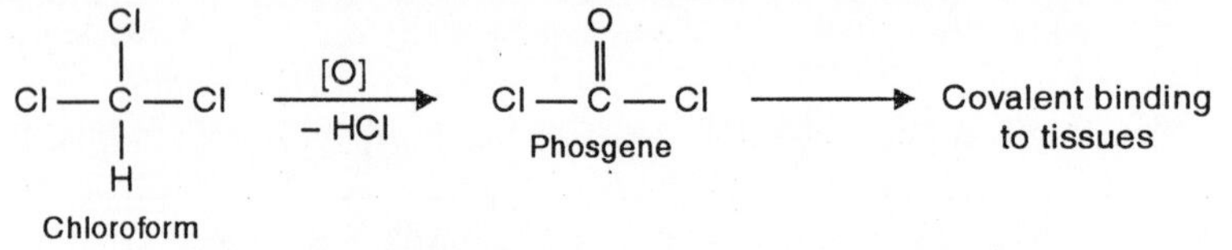

$$\underset{\text{Chloroform}}{CHCl_3} \xrightarrow[-\,HCl]{[O]} \underset{\text{Phosgene}}{Cl-C(=O)-Cl} \longrightarrow \text{Covalent binding to tissues}$$

Fig. 5.16. Oxidative dehalogenation of chloroform.

RNO_2 → $RN = O$ → RNHOH → RNH_2
Nitro Nitroso Hydroxylamine Amine
(a)

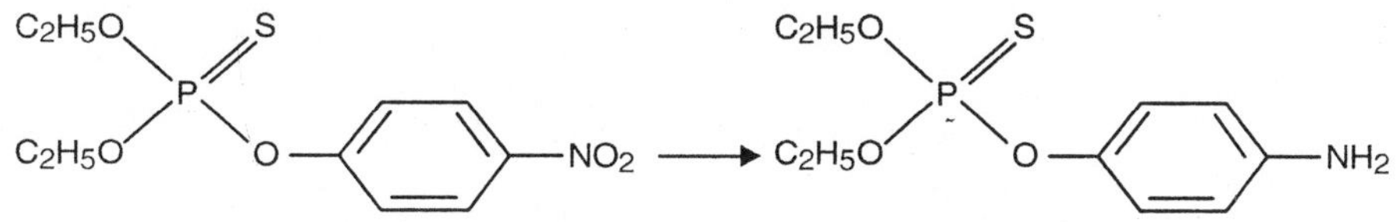

Parathion (b) Aminoparathion

Fig. 5.17. Nitro-reduction of xenobiotics.
(a) General reaction (b) Biotransformation of parathion.

undergo bioreduction are nitro, azo and N-oxide. Such reactions are usually reverse of oxidation.

i. Nitro-reduction: Reduction of nitro groups proceeds via formation of nitroso and hydroxylamine intermediates to yield amines.

ii. Azo-reduction : Reduction of azo compounds can be catalysed either directly by NADPH-cytochrome C reductase or in conjunction with cytochrome P-450 in a complete monoxygenase system. Reduction of azo compounds yield primary amines via formation of hydrazo intermediate (–NH–NH–) which undergoes cleavage at N–N bonds.

b. Reduction of carbonyls (aldehyde and ketones) : Aliphatic aldehydes and ketones undergo extensive bioreduction, whereas, esters, acids and amides are least reactive. Among aldehydes and ketones, several ketones undergo reduction as this result in more polar metabolites. The reaction is usually catalysed by non-microsomal enzymes called aldo-keto reductases :

i. Aliphatic aldehyde ii. Aliphatic ketone

R–N=N–R′ → R–NH–HN–R′ → $RNH_2 + H_2NR'$
Azo Hydrazo Amines
(a)

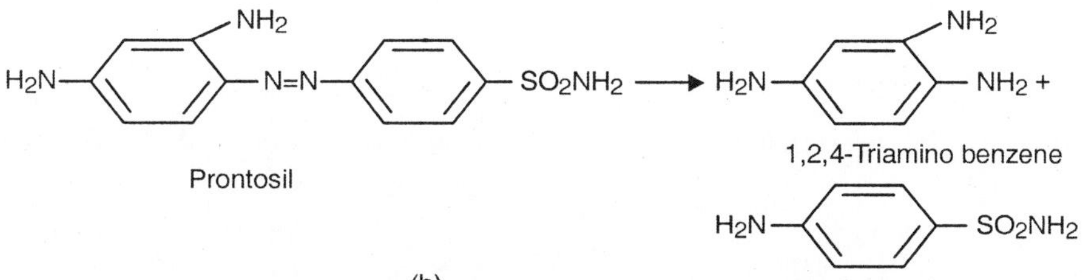

Prontosil → 1,2,4-Triamino benzene + Sulphanilamide
(b)

Fig. 5.18. Azo-reduction of xenobiotics.
(a) General reaction (b) Biotransformation of prontosil.

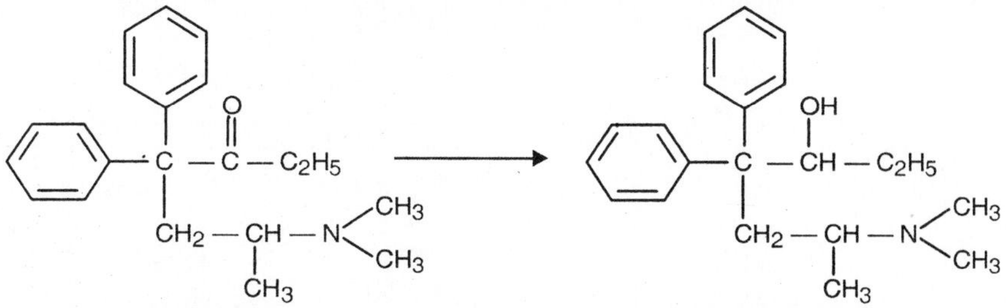

Methadone → Methadol

Fig. 5.19. Reduction of methadone (aliphatic ketone).

Table 5.1: Types of biotransformation reactions.

Phase	Reaction	Type of reaction	Type of enzyme
Phase I	1. Oxidation	*a.* Dealkylation	
		i. N-dealkylation	M
		ii. O-dealkylation	M
		iii. S-dealkylation	M
		b. Desulphuration	
		c. Hydroxylation	
		i. Aliphatic hydroxylation	M
		ii. Aromatic hydroxylation	M
		iii. Heterocyclic ring hydroxylation	M
		iv. N-hydroxylation	M
		d. Oxidation (oxide formation)	
		i. N-oxidation	M
		ii. S-oxidation	M
		e. Epoxidation or epoxide formation	M
		f. Deamination	M
		g. Alcohol oxidation	M, NM
		h. Aldehyde oxidation	NM
		i. Miscellaneous oxidative reactions	M, NM
	2. Reduction	*a.* Azo-reduction	M
		b. Nitro-reduction	M,NM
		c. Carbonyl reduction	NM
	3. Hydrolysis	*a.* Hydrolysis of esters	M, NM
		b. Hydrolysis of amides	M, NM
		c. Hydrolytic dehalogenation	M
Phase II	1. Glucuronide conjugation		M
	2. Sulphate conjugation		NM (cytosol)
	3. Methyl conjugation		NM (cytosol)
	4. Glutathione conjugation and mercapturic acid formation		NM (cytosol)
	5. Acetyl conjugation		NM (mitochndria)
	6. Conjugation with amino acids		NM
	7. Conjugation with thiosulphate		NM
	8. Miscellaneous conjugation reactions		NM

M = Microsomal enzymes; NM = Non-microsomal enzymes

3. Hydrolysis

The hydrolytic reactions differ from oxidative and reductive reactions in three aspects:

i. The reaction does not involve change in the state of oxidation of the substrate.

ii. The reaction results in a large chemical change in the substrate brought about by loss of relatively large fragment(s) of the molecule.

iii. The hydrolytic enzymes that metabolise xenobiotics are the same that act on endogenous substrates and their activity is not confined to only liver as they are found in many other organs including kidneys and intestine.

Hydrolytic enzymes catalyse a number of functional groups like esters, ethers, amides and hydrazides.

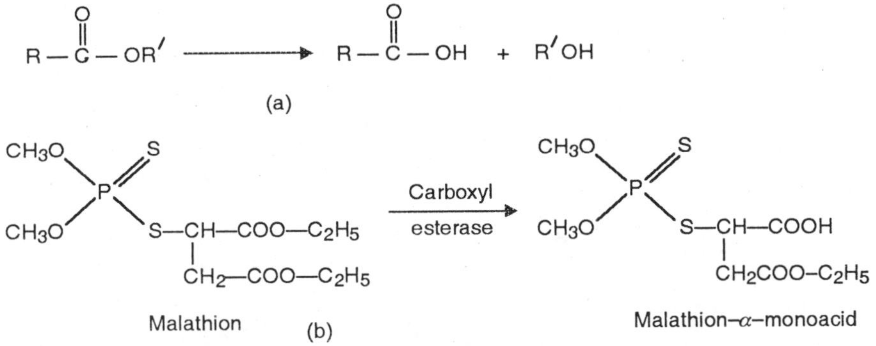

$$R-\overset{O}{\overset{\|}{C}}-OR' \longrightarrow R-\overset{O}{\overset{\|}{C}}-OH + R'OH$$

(a)

$$(CH_3O)_2P(=S)-S-CH(COO-C_2H_5)-CH_2-COO-C_2H_5 \xrightarrow[\text{esterase}]{\text{Carboxyl}} (CH_3O)_2P(=S)-S-CH(COOH)-CH_2COO-C_2H_5$$

Malathion (b) Malathion-α-monoacid

Fig. 5.20. De-esterification (hydrolysis) of xenobiotics.
(a) General reaction. (b) Biotransformation of malathion.

a. Hydrolysis of esters (De-esterification) : Esters are hydrolysed by a variety of non-specific esterases in liver, plasma, GI tract and other tissues. Esters on hydrolysis yield alcohol and carboxylic acid which may undergo a variety of conjugations. Depending on the substrate specificity, the esterases have been named as arylesterase (hydrolyse aromatic esters), carboxylesterase (hydrolyse aliphatic esters), cholinesterase (hydrolyse esters in which alcohol moiety is choline) and acetylesterase (hydrolyse esters in which acid moiety is acetic acid).

b. Hydrolysis of amides (Deamidation) : The hydrolytic cleavage of amide linkages involves C–N cleavage to yield carboxylic acid and amine (or NH_3) with help of enzyme amidases. In general, enzymatic hydrolysis of amides occurs more slowly than esters, probably as a result of the lack of substrate specificity.

B. PHASE-II / CONJUGATION REACTIONS

Phase II or conjugation (Latin, conjugatus = yoked together) reactions involve combination of the xenobioitc or its phase I metabolite with an endogenous substance to form a highly polar product. The product or metabolite formed after a conjugative reaction thus contains two parts: exocon and endocon. The exocon is derived from exogenous compound or xenobiotic and endocon is derived from endogenous substance. Conjugation reactions have high energy requirement and they often utilise suitable enzymes for the reactions. The process of conjugation is generally considered as one of the detoxification mechanisms (not always) as these usually result in more polar products, which can be excreted efficiently from the body.

The endogenous substances (endocons) for conjugation reactions are derived mainly from

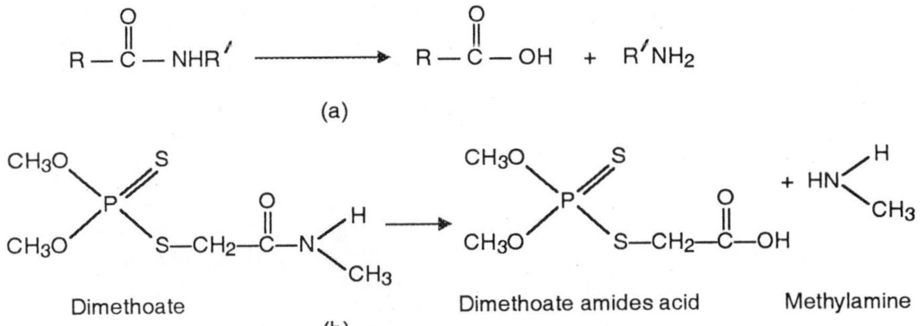

$$R-\overset{O}{\overset{\|}{C}}-NHR' \longrightarrow R-\overset{O}{\overset{\|}{C}}-OH + R'NH_2$$

(a)

$$(CH_3O)_2P(=S)-S-CH_2-\overset{O}{\overset{\|}{C}}-N(H)CH_3 \longrightarrow (CH_3O)_2P(=S)-S-CH_2-\overset{O}{\overset{\|}{C}}-OH + HN(H)CH_3$$

Dimethoate Dimethoate amides acid Methylamine

(b)

Fig. 5.21. Deamidation (hydrolysis of amides) of xenobiotics.
(a) General reaction. (b) Biotransformation of dimethoate.

carbohydrates or amino acids and usually possess large molecular size. They are strongly polar or ionic in nature in order to render the substrate water-soluble. The molecular weight of the conjugate (metabolite) is important for determining its route of excretion. High molecular weight conjugates are excreted predominantly in bile (e.g., glutathione exclusively, glucuronide mainly), while low molecular weight conjugates are excreted mainly in the urine. As the availability of endogenous conjugating substance is limited in the body, saturation of this process is possible and the unconjugated drug/metabolite may precipitate toxicity.

1. Glucuronic Acid Conjugation/ Glucuronidation

The process of conjugation of exogenous substances with carbohydrates is common in animal and plant species. Conjugation with glucuronic acid (glucuronide conjugation or glucuronidation) is the most common and most important phase II reaction in vertebrates, except in cats and fish. The biochemical donor (cofactor) of glucuronic acid is uridine diphosphate α-D-glucuronic acid (UDPGA) and the reaction is carried out by microsomal enzyme uridine diphosphate-glucuronyl transferase (UDP-glucuronyl transferase). In cats, there is reduced transferase activity, while in fish there is deficiency of endogenous glucuronic acid donor. The UDPGA is synthesised in the liver and other tissues from uridine diphosphate-glucose (UDPG) by a specific enzyme UDPG-dehydrogenase located in soluble fraction. Once UDPGA is formed, glucuronidation takes place primarily in hepatocytes, the functional cells of the liver. In this, carbon 1 of glucuronic acid in the form of UDPGA is activated to nucleophilic attack by the oxygen, sulphur or nitrogen groups on substrates. In UDPGA, the bond between C-1 of glucuronic acid and the phosphate group of UDP is of the α-configuration but during reaction with substrates there is inversion of configuration leading to glucuronide derivatives that have a β-configuration. A large number of functional groups are capable of forming oxygen, nitrogen and sulphur glucuronides. Carbon glucuronides have also been detected in some cases.

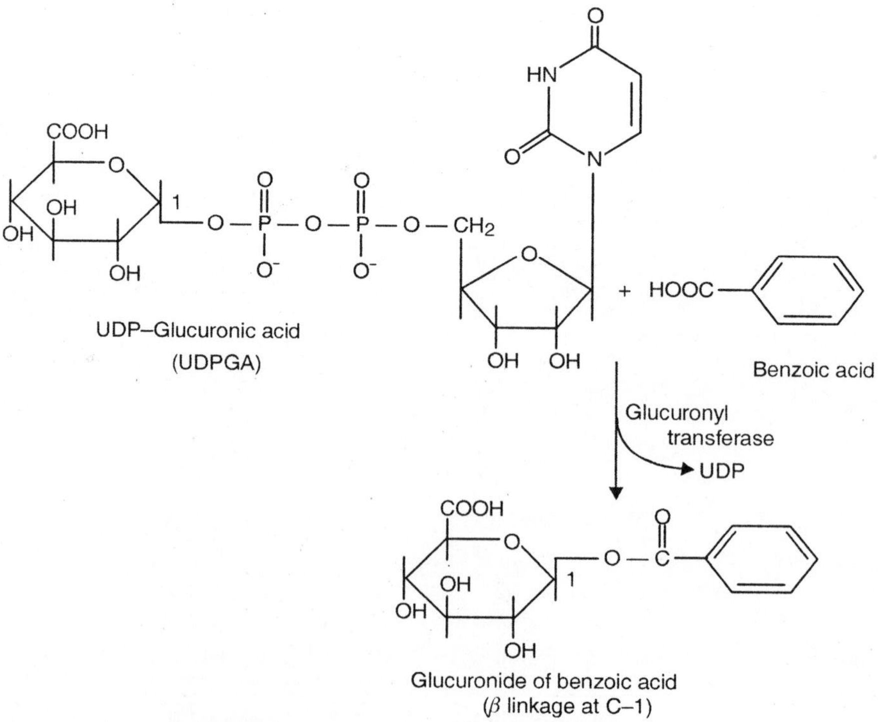

Fig. 5.22. Glucuronide conjugation of benzoic acid.

Several functional groups viz. alcohols, acids, amines can combine easily. Certain endogenous compounds such as steroids, bilirubin, catechols and thyroxin also form glucuronides. The glucuronic derivatives of foreign compounds are then excreted in bile or urine depending on the molecular weight and polarity. The metabolites with a large molecular weight (MW > 350) and less water solubility are more often excreted in bile.

Glucuronyl transferase: The UDP-glucuronyl transferase (E.C. 2.4.1.17) exists as a lipid-protein complex within cells. It is present in endoplasmic reticulum (microsomes) of most tissues, but liver is the most active site of glucuronide synthesis. Glucuronidation capacity of liver and other organs is very low in new born animals. This enzyme can be induced like other microsomal enzymes, but inhibition is not as common as induction.

Deconjugation: Deconjugation is the process by which a glucuronic acid conjugated metabolite is again biotransformed in body to release the free xenobiotic or its active metabolite. The deconjugation is carried out by the enzyme β-glucuronidase mostly in the bile or intestine and the released free xenobiotic or its active metabolite undergoes enterohepatic cycle. The enterohepatic cycle often prolongs the toxic effect of xenobiotics by recycling them in the body. Deconjugation process may also produce toxic effect at sites where some xenobiotics normally do not reach because by this process they gain entry into such tissues and accumulate in quantities sufficient to elicit a toxic response. For example, certain urinary bladder carcinogens are conjugated with glucuronic acid in the liver and then deconjugated in the urinary tract by β-glucuronidase to release carcinogenic metabolite resulting in bladder cancer.

2. Conjugation with Sulphate (Sulphoconjugation or Sulphation)

Conjugation with sulphate is similar to glucuronidation but is catalysed by non-microsomal enzymes. The endogenous donor of the sulphate group is 3′-phosphoadenosine-5′-phosphosulphate (PAPS), an activated form of sulphate. Sulphotransferase enzymes located in the soluble fraction of cell catalyse the transfer of the sulphate from PAPS to the acceptor. The resulting conjugates of hydroxyl and amino groups are

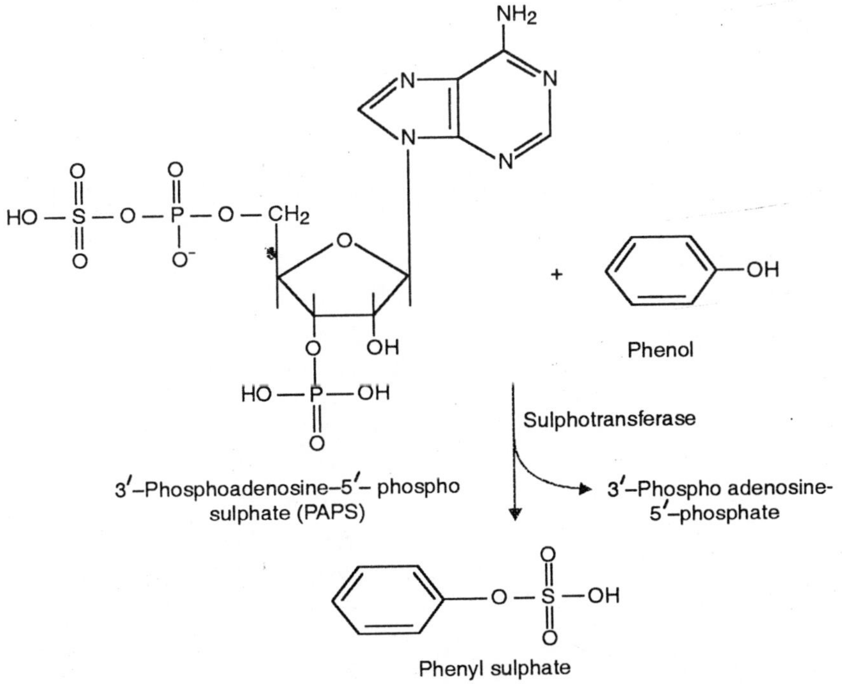

Fig. 5.23. Sulphate conjugation of phenol.

called sulphate ester conjugates or ethereal sulphates. Sulphate conjugates thus formed are more water soluble and rapidly excreted from the body. Sulphate conjugation occurs less commonly than glucuronidation in most domestic animals as the cofactor (PAPS) that transfers sulphate to the substrate is easily depleted (glucuronidation is abundant due to high availability of UDPGA in liver). In the cat, where glucuronidation of phenols is less, ethereal sulphate conjugation is important. Unlike glucuronic acid conjugates that are eliminated in bile, the highly polar sulphate conjugates are readily excreted in the urine.

The biochemistry of sulphate conjugation is complex and not well understood. Some substrates are conjugated readily by most species, while others are conjugated only by selected species. Some of the conjugates may be eliminated directly from the body, while others are further metabolised. Functional groups capable of forming sulphate conjugates include phenols, alcohols, arylamines, N-hydroxylamines and N-hydroxyamides. Some endogenous substances can also undergo sulphation e.g. steroids, biogenic amines. Although the chemical types of exogenous compounds undergoing sulphate conjugation is varied, the most common reactants are phenolic and aliphatic hydroxyl groups and also amino groups. Generally sulphate conjugates are very acidic and are quite susceptible to acid hydrolysis.

Deconjugation : Sulphate conjugates may be hydrolysed by a widely distributed group of enzymes called sulphatases. Sulphate conjugation of xenobiotics, like glucuronidation, may alter the distribution and persistence of the chemicals in body and they often enter the enterohepatic cycle where they may undergo repeated hydrolysis and reconjugation until excreted in the urine.

3. Conjugation with Methyl Group (Methylation)

Conjugation with methyl group (methyl conjugation or methylation) involves transfer of a methyl group (-CH_3) from the cofactor S-adenosyl methionine (SAM) to the acceptor substrate by various methyl transferase enzymes. The methyl group bound to sulphonium ion in SAM has considerable carbonium ion character and is transferred by nucleophilic attack of the alcohol oxygen, amine nitrogen and sulphydryl group on the methyl group giving methylated substrate as product. A number of enzymes (methyl

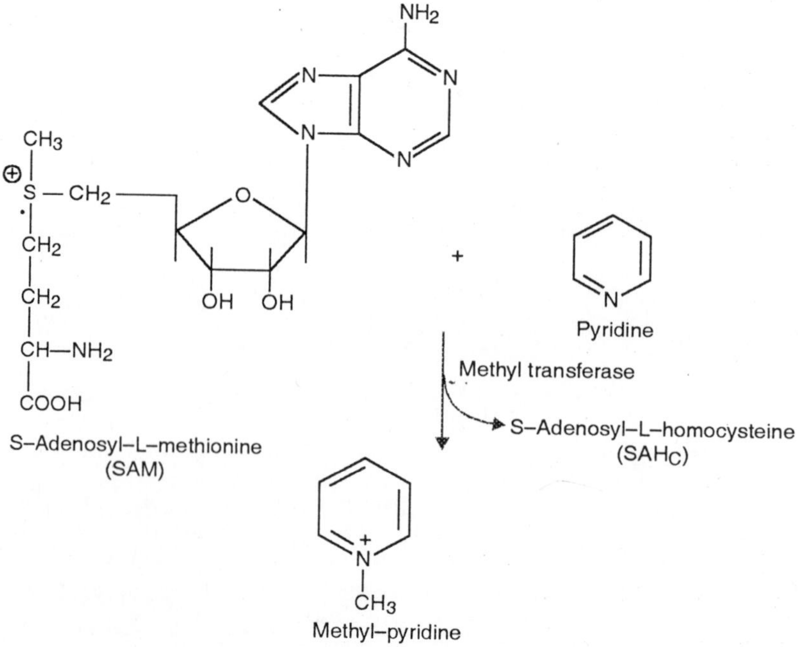

Fig. 5.24. Methyl conjugation of pyridine.

transferases) carry out methylation, some of which are specific.

Methylation reaction differs from general characteristics of phase II reactions in several ways:

(*i*) The metabolites formed are not polar or water soluble.

(*ii*) The metabolites may have equal or greater activity than the parent compound.

(*iii*) The reaction is of lesser importance for xenobiotics but more important for biosynthesis (e.g. adrenaline and melatonin) and inactivation (e.g. noradrenaline and histamine) of endogenous amines.

Nevertheless, methylation is still considered a phase II reaction. The functional groups involved in methylation reactions are amines (aromatic and aliphatic), phenols, N-heterocycles and sulphydryl containing compounds. These reactions are mostly of type N-methylation, O-methylation, etc.

4. Conjugation with Glutathione and Mercapturic Acid Formation

Conjugation with glutathione (glutathione conjugation) and mercapturic acid formation is a minor but important metabolic pathway in animals. Glutathione (GSH, G = glutathione and SH = active –SH group) is a tripeptide having glutamic acid, cysteine and glycine. Glutathione has strong nucleophilic character due to the presence of a –SH (thiol) group in its structure as a result of which it conjugates with electrophilic substrates, a number of which are potentially toxic compounds. The interaction between the substrate and the GSH is catalysed by enzyme glutathione-S-transferase, which is located in the soluble fraction of liver homogenates.

Although only restricted numbers of chemicals undergo glutathione conjugation in comparison to glucuronide and sulphate conjugations, it is considered an important detoxification route in both animals and plants. Many highly electrophilic metabolites that have a tendency to react with tissue nucleophilic groups such as –OH, $-NH_2$ and -SH and precipitate toxicities such as tissue necrosis, carcinogenesis, mutagenesis, teratogenesis, etc., react with glutathione in body. Conjugation with glutathione, thus, protects the tissues from such reactive moieties.

Glutathione conjugation differs from other conjugation reactions in that the process does not require initial activation of the cofactor or the substrate as the GSH which is a nucleophile itself is highly reactive towards an electrophilic substrate. The glutathione conjugate due to high molecular weight is predominantly excreted in the bile and not as such in the urine. For excretion in urine, it undergoes further cleavage (metabolism) to form mercapturic acid. The mercapturic acid formation

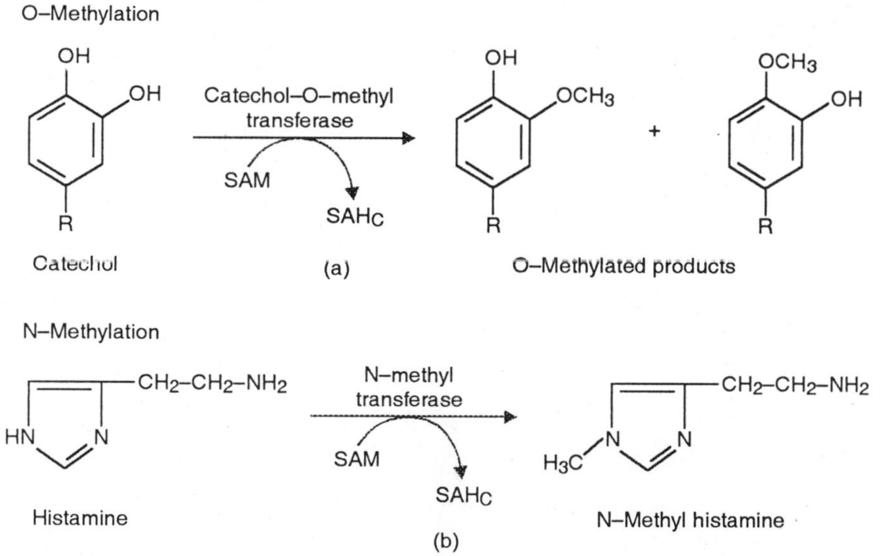

Fig. 5.25. O-methylation and N-methylation biotransformation of xenobiotics and endogenous substances. (a) Biotransformation of catechols (general reaction) (b) Biotransformation of histamine.

is catalysed first by enzyme γ-glutamyl transpeptidase (or glutathionase) to release free glutamyl residue (glutamic acid), then by enzyme cysteinyl glycinase (a peptidase) to release free glycine, and finally N-acetylation of cysteine conjugate by the enzyme N-acetylase to form S-substituted N-acetyl cysteine product called mercapturic acid. The mercapturic acid due to low molecular weight is excreted in the urine. The cofactor for acetylation reaction is acetyl coenzyme–A.

5. Conjugation with Acetyl Group (Acetylation)

Conjugation with acetyl group (acetylation) is common reaction of aromatic primary amines, hydrazines, sulphonamides and certain primary aliphatic amines. The general sequence of reaction is similar to that for α-amino acid conjugation and enzymes are non-microsomal N-acetyl transferases. The cofactor for these reactions is acetyl coenzyme A. The N-acetyl transferase enzymes are located in the soluble fraction of cell of various tissues and catalyse the transfer of acetyl group from acetyl coenzyme–A, resulting in formation of amide in case of amines. There are multiple forms of N-acetyl transferase enzymes in animal tissues. Dogs and foxes do not acetylate the aromatic amino groups due to deficiency of arylamine acetyltransferase enzyme.

Acetylation is not a true detoxification process because occasionally it results in decrease in water solubility of an amine and, thus, increases in its

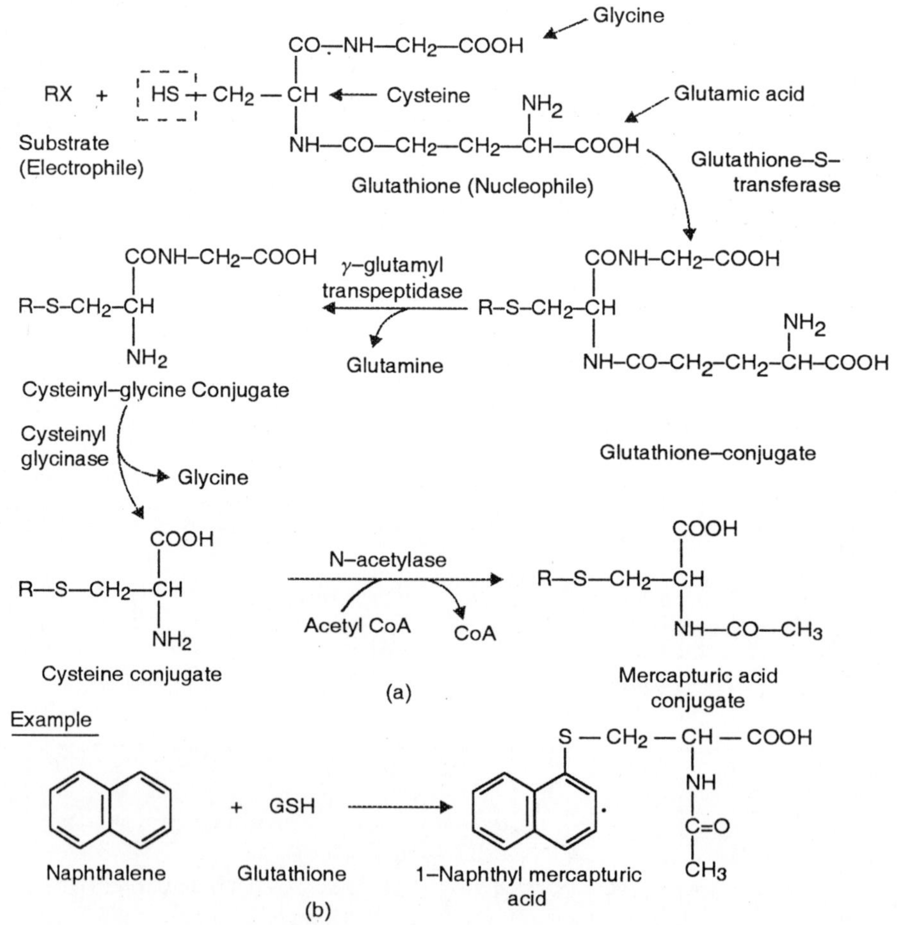

RX + HS–CH₂–CH(–CO–NH–CH₂–COOH)(–NH–CO–CH₂–CH₂–CH(NH₂)–COOH)
Substrate (Electrophile) | Glutathione (Nucleophile) | Glycine | Cysteine | Glutamic acid
Glutathione–S–transferase → Glutathione–conjugate: R–S–CH₂–CH(CONH–CH₂–COOH)(NH–CO–CH₂–CH₂–CH(NH₂)–COOH)
γ–glutamyl transpeptidase → Glutamine
Cysteinyl–glycine Conjugate: R–S–CH₂–CH(CONH–CH₂–COOH)(NH₂)
Cysteinyl glycinase → Glycine
Cysteine conjugate: R–S–CH₂–CH(COOH)(NH₂)
N–acetylase (Acetyl CoA → CoA)
Mercapturic acid conjugate: R–S–CH₂–CH(COOH)(NH–CO–CH₃)
(a)

Example

Naphthalene + GSH (Glutathione) → 1–Naphthyl mercapturic acid (S–CH₂–CH(NH–C(=O)–CH₃)–COOH)
(b)

Fig. 5.26. Glutatione conjugation and mercapturic acid formation of xenobiotics. (a) General reaction (b) Biotransformation of naphthalene.

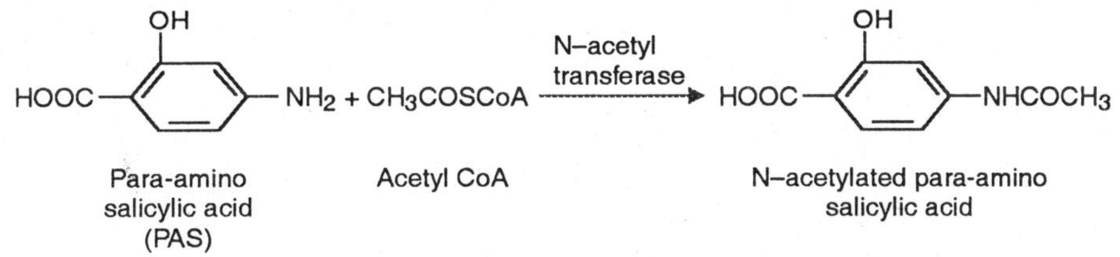

$HOOC-C_6H_3(OH)-NH_2 + CH_3COSCoA \xrightarrow{\text{N-acetyl transferase}} HOOC-C_6H_3(OH)-NHCOCH_3$

Para-amino salicylic acid (PAS) — Acetyl CoA — N-acetylated para-amino salicylic acid

Fig. 5.27. Acetyl-conjugation of para-aminosalicylic acid.

toxicity (e.g. sulphonamides and isoniazid). Acetylation is the primary route of biotransformation of sulphonamide compounds. In human beings, there are ethnic variations in the N-acetylation for certain substrates i.e. slow acetylators and fast acetylators. Among Eskimos, 95% people are fast acetylators and 5% are slow acetylators. Similar to deglucuronidation and desulphuration, there are enzymes in animal tissues that carry out the deacetylation of amines. The degree to which a particular animal species excretes foreign amines as acetyl conjugates depends on the relative rates of acetylation and deacetylation of these compounds.

6. Conjugation with Amino Acids (Amino Acid Conjugation)

Conjugation with amino acids occurs to limited extent in animals because of less availability of amino acids. The substrate in amino acid conjugation is generally an acid (aromatic in particular) and the reaction product is an amide. The most important conjugation reactions involve amino acid glycine; conjugation with glutamine in man and ornithine in birds is also seen. Conjugation with other amino acids like aspartic acid, serine and taurine are uncommon. The type of reaction is different from that seen in glucuronidation or sulphation because in amino acid conjugation the substrate is activated and not the donor (i.e. there is activation of carboxylic acid drug substrate with ATP and coenzyme A to form an acyl CoA intermediate).

Amino acid conjugation occurs extensively in liver mitochondria and thus can be used to estimate hepatic functions. The diagnostic marker used is benzoic acid that on conjugation with glycine yields hippuric acid, which is rapidly excreted in the urine. Thus the rate and extent of urinary excretion of hippuric acid following oral or intravenous administration of benzoic acid indicates functioning of liver. A decrease output indicates hepatic disorder.

In some species there is competition between glucuronidation and amino acid conjugation for metabolism of the aromatic acids. The degree to which glucuronide formation or amino acid conjugation predominates depends on the animal species and structure of the acid.

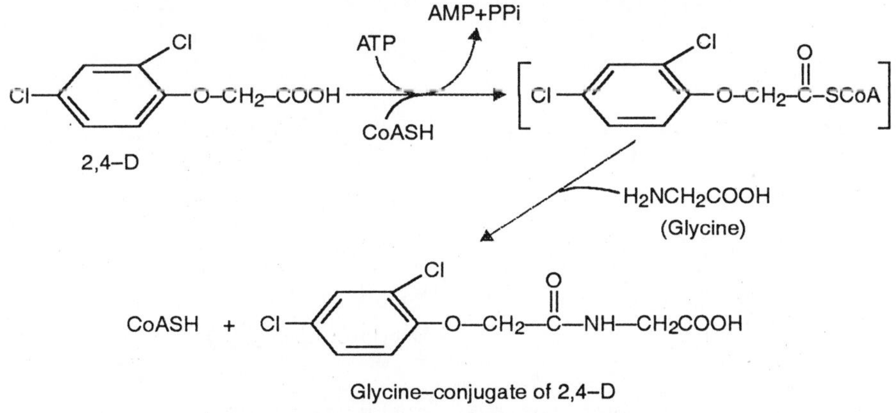

$Cl-C_6H_3(Cl)-O-CH_2-COOH \xrightarrow[\text{CoASH}]{\text{ATP} \rightarrow \text{AMP+PPi}} [Cl-C_6H_3(Cl)-O-CH_2-C(=O)-SCoA]$

2,4-D

$\xrightarrow{H_2NCH_2COOH \text{ (Glycine)}} CoASH + Cl-C_6H_3(Cl)-O-CH_2-C(=O)-NH-CH_2COOH$

Glycine-conjugate of 2,4-D

Fig. 5.28. Glycine conjugation of 2,4-D.

7. Conjugation with Thiosulphate

Conjugation with thiosulphate is an important reaction in the detoxification of cyanide. Conjugation of cyanide ion involves transfer of sulphur atom from the thiosulphate to the cyanide ion in presence of a mitochondrial enzyme rhodanese to form inactive thiocyanate. Thiocyanate formed is much less toxic than the cyanide (true detoxification) and it is excreted in urine.

$$CN^- + S_2O_3^{-2} \xrightarrow{\text{rhodanese}} SCN^- + SO_3^{-2}$$

(cyanide) (thiosulphate) (thiocyanate) (sulphite)

Fig. 5.29. Conjugation of cyanide with thiosulphate.

Complex Nature of Biotransformation

Phase I and phase II pathways and various reactions are often discussed separately but in body toxicants generally undergo several types of biotransformation reactions simultaneously with a number of enzyme systems acting consecutively or concurrently on a substrate or metabolite of that substrate. Thus many metabolites can be formed from a single substrate simultaneously or one after the other in the body. For example, benzene biotransformation (Fig. 5.30) results in number of metabolites from different metabolic pathways.

INDUCTION AND INHIBITION OF METABOLISING ENZYMES

Induction of Metabolising Enzymes

Several drugs and chemicals have ability to increase the metabolising activity of enzymes called enzyme induction. These chemicals known as enzyme inducers mainly interact with DNA and increase the synthesis of microsomal enzyme proteins, especially cytochrome P-450 and glucuronyl transferase. As a result, there is enhanced metabolism of endogenous substances (e.g. sex steroids) and xenobiotics metabolised by microsomal enzymes. Some compounds (e.g. carbamazepine and rifampicin) may stimulate their

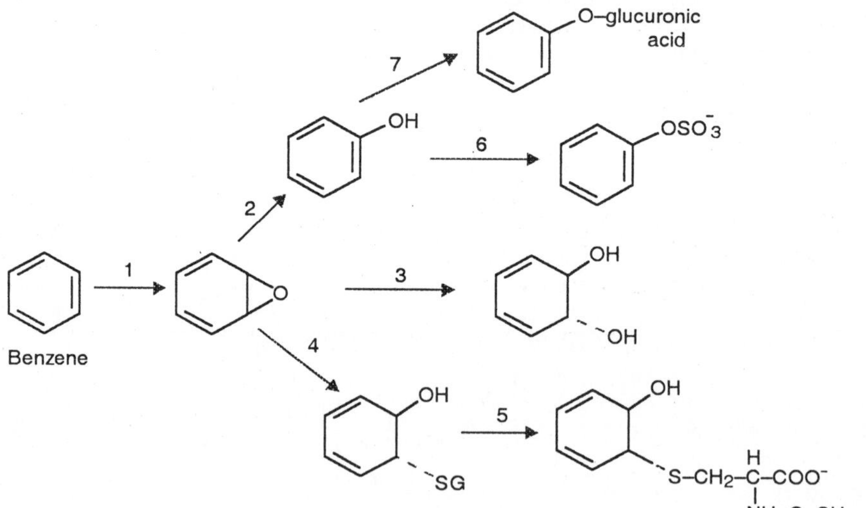

O–glucuronic acid

OH

OSO_3^-

Benzene

O

OH

OH

OH

SG

OH

$S–CH_2–C(H)–COO^-$

$NH–C(=O)–CH_3$

Fig. 5.30. Biotransformation of benzene by phase I and phase II enzyme systems.

1. Benzene is oxidised to benzene oxide by cytochrome P-450 mixed function oxidases (MFOs).
2. Spontaneous rearrangement of benzene oxide to phenol.
3. Conversion to corresponding dihydrodial by the action of epoxide hydratase.
4. Conjugation with glutathione.
5. Glutathione derivative further forms mercapturic acid.
6. Conjugation with sulphate by sulphate transferase.
7. Conjugation with glucuronic acid by glucuronyl transferase.

own metabolism, the phenomenon being called auto-induction or self induction. Since different cytochrome P-450 isoenzymes are involved in the metabolism of different compounds, the enzyme induction by one agent affects metabolism of only those agents which are substrate for the induced isoenzyme. However, some drugs and chemicals like phenobarbitone may affect metabolism of a large number of xenobiotics because they induce isoenzymes which catalyze many compounds.

Microsomal enzyme induction by drugs and chemicals usually require repetitive administration of the inducing agent over a period of several days and the induction, once started, may continue for several days. Metabolising enzyme induction has great clinical importance because it affects the plasma half-life and duration of action of xenobiotics. Toxicants that undergo metabolic inactivation are rapidly metabolised and eliminated, while toxicants that undergo bioactivation become more toxic due to rapid formation of toxic metabolite. Microsomal enzyme induction enhances tolerance and increases chances of xenobiotic interactions.

Inhibition of Metabolising Enzymes

Contrary to metabolising enzyme induction, several drugs and chemicals have the ability to decrease the metabolising activity of certain enzymes called enzyme inhibition. Enzyme inhibition can be either non-specific of microsomal enzymes, or specific of some non-microsomal enzymes (e.g. monoamine oxidase, cholinesterase and aldehyde dehydrogenase). The inhibition of hepatic microsomal enzymes mainly occurs due to administration of hepatotoxic agents, which cause either rise in the rate of enzyme degradation (e.g. carbon tetrachloride and carbon disulphide) or fall in the rate of enzyme synthesis (e.g. puromycin and dactinomycin). Nutritional deficiency, hormonal imbalance or hepatic dysfunction, etc. also inhibit microsomal enzymes indirectly. Inhibition of non-microsomal enzymes with specific function usually results when structurally similar compounds compete for the active site on the enzymes. Such an inhibition is usually rapid (a single dose of inhibitor may be sufficient) and clinically more important than the non-specific microsomal enzyme inhibition.

Enzyme inhibition generally results in depressed metabolism of xenobiotics. As a result, the plasma half-life, duration of action, and efficacy as well toxicity of the object substance (whose metabolism has been inhibited) are significantly enhanced. Enzyme inhibition may also produce undesirable xenobiotic interactions.

BIOACTIVATION AND TISSUE TOXICITY

Formation of harmful or highly reactive metabolites from relatively inert/non-toxic chemical compounds is called bioactivation or toxication. The bioactive metabolites often interact with the body tissues to precipitate one or more forms of toxicities such as carcinogenesis, teratogenesis, tissue necrosis, etc (Table 5.2). The bioactivation reactions are generally catalysed by cytochrome P-450-dependent monooygenase systems, but some other enzymes like those in intestinal flora are also involved in some cases. The reactive metabolites primarily belong to three main categories – electrophiles, free radicals and nucleophiles. The formation of electrophiles and free radicals from relatively harmless xenobiotics account for most toxicities.

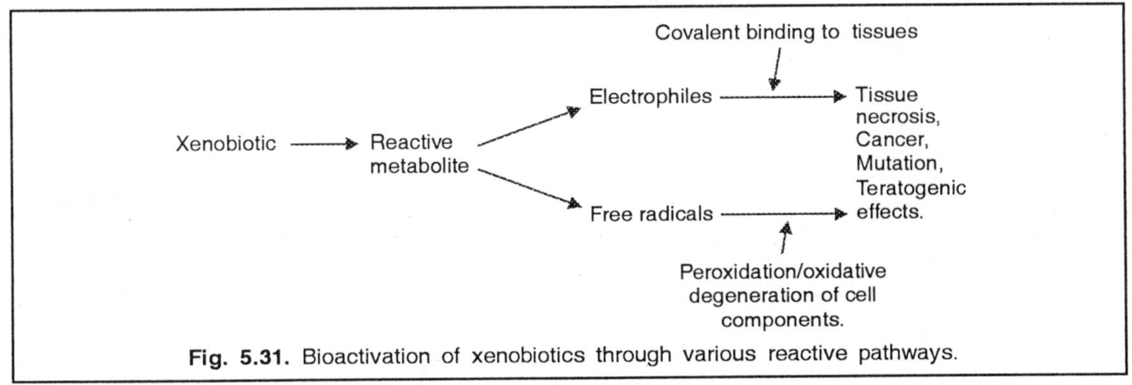

Fig. 5.31. Bioactivation of xenobiotics through various reactive pathways.

a. Electrophiles: Electrophiles are molecules which are deficient in electrons pair with a positive charge that allows them to react by sharing electron pairs with electron-rich atoms in nucleophiles. The enzyme system through which these are generated is cytochrome P-450. Carbon, nitrogen or sulphur containing compounds can be metabolically activated to yield electrophiles. Important electrophiles are epoxides, hydroxylamines, nitroso and azoxy derivatives, nitrenium ions and elemental sulphur. These electrophiles form covalent binding to nucleophilic tissue components such as macromolecules (proteins, nucleic acids and lipids) or low molecular weight cellular constituents to precipitate toxicity. Covalent binding to DNA is responsible for carcinogenicity and tumour formation. For example, epoxides produced by metabolic conversion of benzo(a)pyrene (present in cigarette smoke) causes lung cancer and those produced by aflatoxin B_1 causes liver cancer. Some of the N-hydroxymetabolites, such as those of paracetamol (Figure 5.32), also produce electrophiles that can cause hepatotoxicity or tissue necrosis through covalent binding.

The body's defence against electrophiles is their inactivation by conjugation with glutathione, the most important cellular nucleophile with -SH group. Depletion of glutathione, which occurs in some conditions, exposes to hepatotoxicity and mutagenicity.

b. Free Radicals: Free radicals are molecules which contain one or more unpaired electrons (odd number of electrons) in their outer orbit. Radicals are formed by accepting or losing an electron. They may be positively charged (cation radical), negatively charged (anion radical) or neutral (neutral radical).

$R.^+$	$R^-.$	R.
Cation radical	Anion radical	Neutral radical

Free radicals are generally formed via NADPH cytochrome P-450 reductase or other flavin containing reductases. Xenobiotics that on metabolic activation yield free radicals are quinones, arylamines, nitroaryls and carbon tetrachloride. Most free radicals are organic. They produce toxicity by peroxidation of cellular components. For example, carbon tetrachloride forms trichloromethyl radical, which causes peroxidation of polyunsaturated lipid as well as covalently binds to proteins and unsaturated lipid. An important class of free radicals is inorganic free radicals such as hydrogen peroxide and superoxide anions (O_2^-). These oxidative moieties can cause tremendous tissue damage leading to mutation or cancer. Their potential toxicity is far greater than that of the electrophiles.

Cellular defence mechanisms against free radicals include control imposed by membrane structure, neutralisation by glutathione, and control by non-enzymatic antioxidant scavengers such as Vitamins A, E and C, and enzymatic inactivation by oxygen derived free radicals.

Generation of reactive metabolites is indicated by modification in enzyme activity, formation of glutathione conjugates (or mercapturic acid) and depletion in tissue levels of glutathione. Since the availability of glutathione in body determines the threshold for toxicity, thiols (e.g. N-acetylcysteine) can be used to treat poisoning by drugs such as paracetamol that yield reactive metabolites.

c. Nucleophiles: Nucleophiles are molecules with electron-rich atoms. Formation of nucleophiles is a relatively uncommon mechanism for toxicants. Examples of toxicity induced through nucleophiles

H COCH3 N OH Paracetamol —N-hydroxylation→ HO COCH3 N OH —$-H_2O$→ COCH3 N O Imidoquinone derivative (electrophile) → Conjugation with GSH; → Covalent binding to liver tissues when GSH is depleted

Fig. 5.32. Bioactivation of paracetamol.

include formation of cyanide from amygdalin, acrylonitrile and sodium nitroprusside and generation of carbon monoxide from dihalomethane. Although some nucleophiles like cyanide and carbon monoxide are reactive, many other nucleophiles are activated by conversion to electrophiles.

Nucleophiles are generally detoxified by conjugation at the nucleophilic functional groups. In general, hydroxylated nucleophiles are inactivated by conjugation with sulphate or glucuronic acid, amines and hydrazines with acetyl group, and thiols with glucuronic acid. Detoxification of cyanide occurs through conjugation with thiosulphate.

d. Other pathways: Certain compounds are biotransformed to potentially toxic metabolites by pathways other than those discussed above. These include oxidation of ethanol by non-microsomal dehydrogenase to acetaldehyde, a metabolite responsible for some of the manifestations of alcohol toxicity. Artificial sweetener cyclamate is converted by intestinal bacteria to cyclohexylamine, which is very toxic and can induce teratogenicity and carcinogenicity (urinary bladder tumour). Similarly nitrite, a potent respiratory toxicant, is formed from nitrate by bacterial reduction in the intestine.

Table 5.2: List of important bioactive metabolites of drugs and chemicals.

Compound	Active metabolite(s)	Toxic effect
Drugs		
Carbon tetrachloride	Trichloromethyl radical	Lipid peroxidation
Chloramphenicol	Nitrosochloramphenicol	Aplastic anaemia, leukaemia
Chloroform	Phosgene	Hepatic necrosis
Cyclamate	Cyclohexylamine	Urinary bladder cancer
Diethylstilboestrol	Diethylstilboestrol quinone	Vaginal and mammary cancer
Halothane	Trifluoroacetyl chloride	Immune reaction
Methoxyflurane	Inorganic fluoride	Nephrotoxicity
Nitroprusside	Cyanide	Histotoxic hypoxia
Paracetamol	Imidoquinone derivative	Hepatic necrosis
Chemicals and Toxicants		
Acrylonitrile	Cyanide	Histotoxic hypoxia
Aflatoxin B_1	Epoxides	Liver cancer
Benzene	Muconic aldehyde	Bone marrow injury
Benzo(a)pyrene	Epoxides	Lung cancer
Ethanol	Acetaldehyde	Hepatic fibrosis
Ethylene glycol	Oxalic acid	Nephrotoxicity, hypocalcaemia
Fluoroacetate	Fluorocitrate	Inhibition of Krebs cycle
Hexane	Hexane dione	Axonopathy
Isopropyl alcohol	Acetone	Cardiotoxicity
Methanol	Formaldehyde	Ocular toxicity
Methylene chloride	Carbon monoxide	Hypoxia
Nitrate	Nitrite	Methaemoglobin formation
Nitrite	Nitrosamines	Gastrointestinal cancer

BIBLIOGRAPHY

Anders M (1985) Bioactivation of Foreign Compounds. Academic Press, New York.

Baggot JD (1977) Principles of Drug Disposition in Domestic Animals. W. B. Saunders, Philadelphia.

Beckman DA and Brent RL (1984) Mechanisms of teratogenesis. *Ann. Rev. Pharmacol.* 24 : 483.

Brahmankar DM and Jaiswal SB (1995) Biopharmaceutics and Pharmacokinetics A Treatise. Vallabh Prakashan, Delhi.

Brown SA (2001) Pharmacokinetics: Disposition and fate of drugs in the body. In: Veterinary Pharmacology and Therapeutics. 8th edn. Adams H R (Ed.) p. 15. Iowa State Univ. Press, Iowa.

Caldwell J and Jakoby WB (1983) Biological Basis of Detoxification. Academic press, New York.

Gregus Z and Klaassen CD (1996) Mechanisms of toxicity. In: Casarett and Doull's Toxicology: The Basic science of Poisons. 5th edn. Klaassen CD (Ed.) p 13. McGraw Hill Companies Inc., New York.

Halliwell B (1992) Reactive oxygen species and the central nervous system. *J. Neurochem.* 59 : 1609.

Hughes WW (1996) Essentials of Environmental Toxicology. Taylor & Francis, Washington.

Lu FC and Kacew S (2002) Lu's Basic Toxicology: Fundamentals, Target Organs and Risk Assessment. Taylor & Francis, New York.

Monks TJ and Lau SS (1988) Reactive intermediates and their toxicological significance. *Toxicol.* 52 : 1.

Mudler GJ (1992) Glucuroonidation and its role in regulation of biological activity of drugs. *Ann. Rev. Pharmacol. Toxicol.* 32 : 25.

Nelson SD (1982) Metabolic activation of drug toxicity. *J. Med. Chem.* 25 : 753.

Parkinson A (1996) Biotransformation of xenobiotics. In: Casarett's and Doull's Toxicology: The Basic science of Poisons. 5th edn. Klaassen CD (Ed.) p 113. McGraw Hill Companies Inc., New York.

Radeleff RD (1970) Veterinary Toxicology. 2nd edn. Lea and Febiger, Philadelphia.

Timbrell JA (1995) Biotransformation of xenobiotics. In: General and Applied Toxicology. Ballantyne B, Marrs T and Turner P (Eds.) p 79. Macmillan Press Ltd., London.

Wilkinson GR (2001) Pharmacokinetics: The dynamics of drug absorption, distribution, and elimination. In: Goodman & Gilman's The Pharmacological Basis of Therapeutics. 10th edn. Hardman JG, Limbird LE and Gilman AG (Eds.) p 3. The McGraw-Hill Companies Inc., New York.

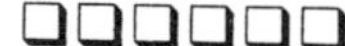

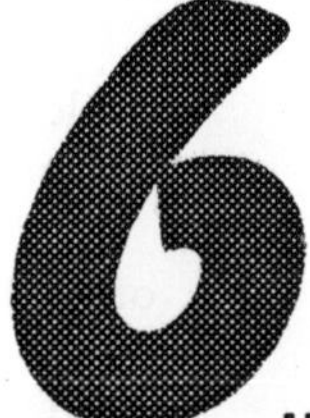

MECHANISMS OF TOXICITY

Specific action of toxicants
Non-specific action of toxicants

The mechanism of action may be defined as the means by which a drug or toxicant produces its effect in the body. Majority of toxic compounds are chemically stable and produce their characteristic effects by interference with biochemical or physiological homeostatic mechanisms. Cellular damage is the basis for most toxicological injury; however, many adverse events are the consequence of disturbance of normal physiology and do not result in cell death. Mechanisms of action of toxicants can be broadly classified into two major groups - specific actions and non-specific actions.

I. SPECIFIC ACTION OF TOXICANTS

Specific action is produced by toxicants that interact with certain specific macromolecular components in the body. These interactions often alter the function of the pertinent component and thereby initiate the biochemical and physiological changes that are characteristic of the response of toxicant. Such interactions are highly specific, often show structure activity relationship (SAR), and can be blocked by specific antagonists. These macromolecules may include receptors, ion-channels, enzymes and carrier molecules.

a. Receptor mediated events: Receptors are specific macromolecular component usually made up of proteins or glycoproteins present on the membrane surface or within the cell to which specific ligand (e.g. hormone, neurotransmitter, drug or toxicant) combines to produce its action. Receptors are the most important targets of drug or toxicant action in the body. Activation of receptors by toxicants results in initiation of toxic effects, whereas inhibition of receptors by blockers stops toxic effects. Some ion-channels, enzymes and carrier-mediated molecules can also be indirectly activated or inhibited by receptor-mediated actions. This type of receptor mediated action is most important for neurotoxins acting within and outside the central nervous system e.g. strychnine, morphine and atropine.

b. Ion-channels mediated events: Ion-channels are spaces or pathways through the cell membrane which allow free movement of certain ions like sodium, potassium, calcium and chloride. Certain toxicants can modulate these ion-channels specifically either directly or indirectly. Direct modulation occurs mainly by binding of toxicants directly to the parts of the channel protein (e.g. barbiturates and chlorinated hydrocarbon insecticides). In this case, the process of channel opening may be inhibited or facilitated by the toxicant. Indirect modulation of ion-channels occurs through interaction of xenobiotics to specific receptors. In this case, ion-channels are linked to a receptor directly (e.g. nicotine) or indirectly involving a G-protein and other intermediaries (e.g. muscarine). Ion-channel modulation by toxicants, acting directly or indirectly, is one of the most important mechanisms by which toxic effects are produced at the cellular level.

c. Enzyme mediated events: Enzymes are the common targets of toxicants. Some toxicants interact directly with specific enzymes, which catalyse some important biochemical and physiological processes. In most cases the toxicants behave as substrate analogues which act as inhibitors of specific enzyme either reversibly (e.g. physostigmine action on cholinesterase enzyme) or irreversibly (e.g. organophosphates action on cholinesterase enzyme). Hydrocyanic acid (HCN) binds to the cytochrome oxidase enzyme and blocks the redox function, thereby inhibiting the aerobic respiration. In some other cases, toxicants behave as false substrates and undergo chemical transformation by enzymes to form abnormal products, which subvert the normal metabolic pathways. For example, fluoroacetate, a known rodenticide, condenses with acetyl CoA in the Krebs cycle to form fluorocitrate, which inhibits the enzyme aconitase and consequently the energy metabolism. In some what similar manner, amino acid antagonists (e.g. azaserine and fluorophenylalanine) can interfere with the utilization of specific amino acid in the synthesis of proteins.

d. Carrier molecule mediated events: Carriers are generally protein molecules that transport ions and small organic molecules across the cell membranes. They are highly selective for the type of molecules or ions that are allowed to cross the membrane. The carrier molecules are targets for certain toxicants, which interact with specific recognition sites on the macromolecule and block the entire transport system. This occurs, for example, with cocaine which blocks reuptake of noradrenaline into adrenergic presynaptic nerve terminals. Similarly, hemicholinium blocks choline carrier and inhibits synthesis of acetylcholine.

II. NON-SPECIFIC ACTION OF TOXICANTS

a. Physical toxicants: Certain toxicants act by their physical disposition in body tissues and organs. Their mechanism of action is entirely due to their physical properties. For example, toxic action produced by industrial and heavy metals dust, silicon and asbestos is entirely due their physical properties. Similarly, CNS depression produced by inhalant anaesthetics like diethyl ether, halothane and chloroform can be correlated well with the physical properties of their oil: water partition coefficients.

b. Direct chemical injury: Toxic actions produced by certain agents are entirely due to their chemical properties, which react extracellularly with endogenous substances. Direct chemical injury to tissues either causes protoplasmic precipitation or alters the membrane dependent homeostatic control of cell functions. Such damages are usually immediate, localised and non-specific. Direct cellular damage usually occurs when cell membranes contact strong corrosives, caustics or compounds that coagulate proteins or damage lipids (e.g. acids, bases, phenols, aldehydes, alcohols, petroleum distillates and some salts of heavy metals). Germicidal actions of oxidising (e.g. potassium permanganate) and reducing (e.g. formaldehyde) agents, and chelating action of some antidotes (e.g. penicillamine and dimercaprol) are also produced by chemical actions.

c. Interference with body metabolism or synthesis : Some toxicants cause interference in the body metabolism or energy synthesis leading to loss of products used for energy, structural components and growth. This may take place in following ways:

i. Uncoupling of oxidative phosphorylation: Some agents (e.g. dinitrophenol and chlorophenol fungicides, and arsenates), called 'uncoupling agents or uncouplers of oxidative phosphorylation', interfere with the synthesis of energy-rich phosphates by blocking phosphorylation of adenosine diphosphate (ADP) to adenosine triphosphate (ATP). As a result, the energy that is normally stored in the form of high-energy phosphates is liberated as heat and there is rise in body temperature.

ii. Inhibition of oxidative phosphorylation : Some agents can result in limited oxygen uptake with lower ATP formation due to inhibition of oxidative phosphorylation. In such toxicities, the effects of fatigue and weakness are similar to that of oxidative uncouplers but there is no fever.

iii. Inhibition of nucleic acid and protein synthesis: Some toxicants (e.g. nitrogen mustards) bind covalently to the replicating DNA and RNA and can cause toxic effects like cancer, mutation and teratogenesis. Inhibition of nucleic acid and protein synthesis can also occur by toxicants that injure DNA or that bind to ribosomes during transcription or translocation (e.g. aflatoxins, organomercurials and trichothecenes).

iv. Interference with fat metabolism: This occurs when toxins affect the rough endoplasmic reticulum resulting in reduced synthesis of lipid acceptor proteins or reduced incorporation of phospholipids and triglycerides into transport lipoproteins. Such interference in fat metabolism by toxicants (e.g. carbon tetrachloride, ethionine, yellow phosphorous and puromycin) leads to fat accumulation in the body cells. Peroxidation of polyenoic fatty acid has been suggested as a mechanism of the necrotizing action of some toxicants like carbon tetrachloride.

d. Impairment of oxygen transport: Certain toxicants impair the oxygen transport mechanism by various modes causing hypoxia. Carbon monoxide binds to haemoglobin at the site where oxygen binds normally and thus causes manifestations of oxygen deficiency in tissues. Some other toxicants like nitrites and aromatic amines enhance formation of methaemoglobin and overwhelm the normal process of its reduction to haemoglobin.

e. Injury to blood and vascular system: Certain agents cause hypoplasia or aplasia of cellular components of blood as a result of their direct toxic effects on bone marrow precursor cells. Inhibitions of vitamin K synthesis by certain agents (e.g. warfarin and brodifacoum) results in spontaneous haemorrhages. Lead ion can increase the fragility of erythrocytes and result in haemolysis.

f. Altered calcium homeostasis: Calcium ions have critical roles in cellular function whose concentration is tightly controlled by a variety of processes and transport mechanisms. Some toxicants (e.g. free radicals, quinones and peroxides) can disrupt the calcium homeostasis with marked deleterious effects on the cell i.e. changes in cytoskeleton, leakage from plasma membrane, impaired mitochondrial function and activation of calcium dependent degradative enzymes (proteases, phospholipases, endonucleases).

g. Immunomodulation: Toxicants can affect both humoral and cell-mediated immunities. Reduced antibody synthesis, interference with complement, altered neutrophil function and reduced lymphoblastogenesis are all toxic effects mediated by various agents e.g. heavy metals, mycotoxins, drugs, and insecticides.

g. Developmental defects: These defects occur primarily *in utero* as a result of toxicants affecting susceptible cells during organogenesis. Most teratogenic effects altering the morphology of the foetus occur in the first trimester of pregnancy. Exposure to toxicants in the third trimester of pregnancy mostly results in reduced growth of the foetus e.g. thalidomide, heavy metals and quinine.

i. Carcinogenesis: Promotion of carcinogenesis is caused by chemicals that produce tissue irritation or damage to macromolecules resulting in expression of the cancer process. This is mainly due to DNA damage e.g. insecticides (DDT), hormones (oestrogen) and saccharin.

j. Deficiency of nutrients and co-factors: Certain toxicants produce deficiency of essential nutrients and co-factors in the body and produce adverse effects. For example, molybdenum produces toxicity due to deficiency of copper (produces secondary hypocupraemia) and oxalate causes toxicity due to chelation of Ca^{++} in the rumen and blood (produces hypocalcaemia). Pyrithiamine inhibits synthesis of essential coenzyme thiamine pyrophosphate and carbon tetrachloride induced release of free radicals destroys NADPH.

k. Non-specific action on enzymes and proteins: Certain toxicants non-specifically inhibit or destroy certain enzymes or structural proteins to produce their toxic effects. For example, rubratoxins inhibit cytochrome P-450 mixed function oxidases besides certain ATP-ases. Arsenic and paraquat damages some intracellular structural proteins like cytoskeleton. Bone cartilages and joints in growing pups are affected by fluoroquinolones.

l. Deposition in tissues/organs: Certain toxicants have special affinity for some organ and tissue, thus producing their toxicity. For example, fluoride deposition in bones and teeth produces exostosis of bones and mottling of teeth; and sulphonamide and oxalate crystals deposition in kidneys produces nephrotoxicity.

BIBLIOGRAPHY

Baggot JD (1982) Mechanisms of drug action. In: John's Veterinary Pharmacology and Therapeutics. 5th edn. Booth NH and McDonald LE (Eds.) p 23. Kalyani Publishers, Ludhiana-New Delhi.

Bartik M and Piskac A (1981) Veterinary Toxicology. Elsevier Scientific Publishing Company, Amsterdam.

Caldwell J (1995) Biochemical basis of toxicity. In: General and Applied Toxicology. Ballantyne B, Marrs T and Turner P (Eds.) p 155. Macmillan Press Ltd., London.

Clarke ECG and Clarke ML (1967) Garner's Veterinary Toxicology. 3rd edn. Williams and Wilkins, Baltimore.

Gregus Z and Klaassen (1996) Mechanisms of toxicity. In: Casarett's and Doull's Toxicology: The Basic Science of Poisons. 5th edn. Klaassen CD (Ed.) p 13. McGraw Hill Companies Inc., New York.

Gupta PK and Salunkhe DK (1984) Modern Toxicology Vol. II. The Adverse Effects of Xenobiotics. Metropolitan Publishing Company, New Delhi.

Hodgson E, Bend JR and Philpot RM (1979) Reviews in Biochemical Toxicology. Elsevier North Holland Inc., New York.

Lu FC and Kacew S (2002) Lu's Basic Toxicology: Fundamentals, Target Organs and Risk Assessment. Taylor & Francis, New York.

Osweiler GD (1996) Toxicology. Williams and Wilkins, Philadelphia.

Ross EM and Kenakin TP (2001) Pharmacodynamics: Mechanisms of drug action and the relationship between drug concentration and effect. In: Goodman & Gilman's The Pharmacological Basis of Therapeutics. 10th edn. Hardman JG, Limbird LE and Gilman AG (Eds.) p 31. The McGraw-Hill Companies Inc., New York.

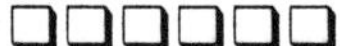

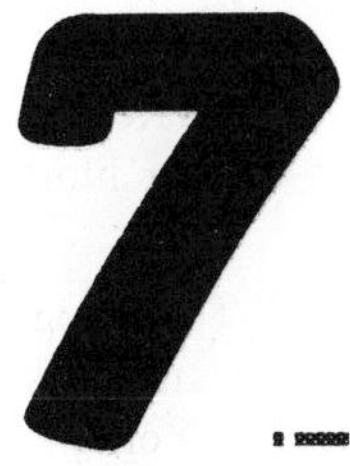

FUNDAMENTALS OF TOXICOLOGY

DOSE-RESPONSE RELATIONSHIP

The relationship between the dose of a compound and the magnitude of response (effect) it produces is called the dose-response relationship (in case of concentration, the term concentration-response relationship may be used). Usually by increasing or decreasing the dose, the response also increases or decreases, respectively and such a relationship becomes the dose-response relationship. If such data are plotted on a graph, then the curve obtained is called dose- response curve.

TYPES OF DOSE-RESPONSE RELATIONSHIP

The dose-response relationship is broadly of following two types:

1. Graded or Gradual dose-response relationship.
2. Quantal or All-or-none dose-response relationship.

1. Graded or Gradual Dose-response Relationship

The graded or gradual response is one involving a continual change in the effect with changing dosages. Most toxicant responses fall in this category. This type of relationship is useful in measuring the incremental responses of a compound and can be seen in an individual organism e.g. contraction of small intestine produced by carbachol, convulsions produced by strychnine, and inhibition of cholinesterase enzyme produced by organophosphorus insecticides. This type of relationship is useful in studying efficacy of therapeutic drugs or toxic symptoms with toxicants.

The graded dose-response relationship is based on following presumptions:

a. The pharmacological/toxicological effect is a result of the known drug/toxicant.

b. There is a molecular or receptor site(s) with which the drug/toxicant interacts to produce the response.

c. The production of a response and the degree of response are related to the concentration of the drug/toxicant at the molecular or receptor site.

d. The concentration of the drug/toxicant at the molecular or receptor site, in turn, is related to the administered dose of the agent.

e. The effect of drug/toxicant is proportional to the fractions of molecular or receptor site occupied by the agent; therefore by increasing or decreasing the dose, the response also increases or decreases, respectively. The maximal effect occurs when the drug/toxicant occupies all molecular or receptor sites.

A simple plot of response against dose will be a parabola with its origin at zero on both axes (Fig. 7.2). From a dose-response curve, some valuable parameters can be obtained such as:

a. Threshold dose: It is the minimal dose which produces the desired observable/recordable response.

b. Ceiling dose/Effective dose-100 (ED_{100}): If is the minimal dose which produces the maximal (100%) response (E_{max}). Beyond ceiling dose, there will be no increase in response even if the dose is increased many fold because no more spare receptors are available to the compound

c. Maximal response/ Maximal effect (E_{max})/ Ceiling effect : It is the maximal response which is produced by the compound under specified conditions. Capability to produce the maximal

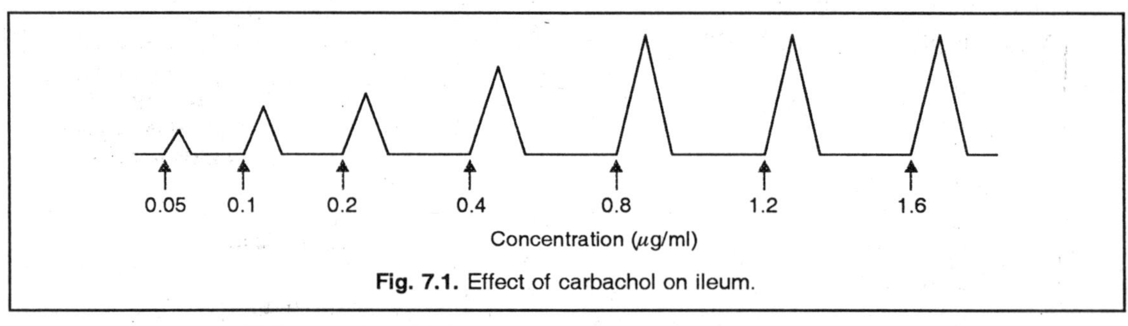

Fig. 7.1. Effect of carbachol on ileum.

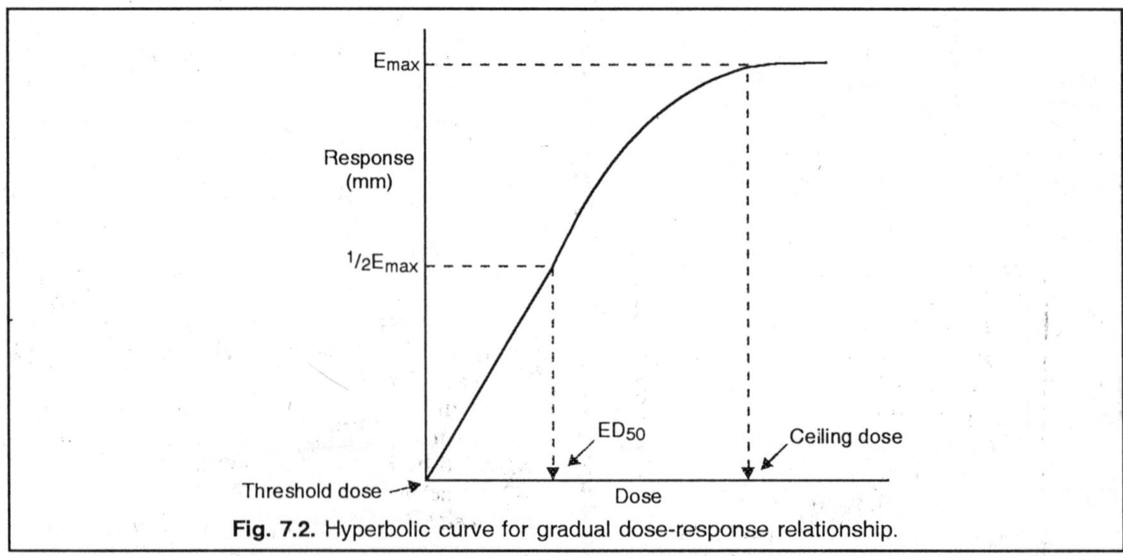

Fig. 7.2. Hyperbolic curve for gradual dose-response relationship.

response indicates maximal efficacy, and is characteristic of a compound.

d. Effective dose-50 (ED_{50}) / Median effective dose (MED): It is the dose which produces half (50%) of the maximal response.

If the response is expressed as per cent of maximal response and plotted against logarithm of the dose (log dose on abscissa and % of maximal response on ordinate), we get a sigmoid curve instead of hyperbolic graded dose-response curve (Fig. 7.3).

The logarithmic transformation of dosage is often employed for the dose-response relationship because :

i. It permits display of a wide range of doses on a single graph.

ii. It facilitates visual and mathematical comparisons between dose-response curves for different agents or for different responses to a single agent.

iii. Log-dose plots usually provide a more linear representation of data.

2. Quantal or All-or-None Dose-response Relationship

Quantal dose-response relationship is one involving an all-or-none response i.e. on increasing the dose of a compound, the response is either produced or not. This relationship is seen with certain responses that follow all or none phenomenon and cannot be graded e.g. death. In toxicology, quantal dose-response relationship is extensively used for the calculation of lethal dose because in it we see only mortality and not the toxic signs. The quantal dose-response relationship is always seen in a population because the assumption is made that individual responds to maximal possible or not at all. The graph of a quantal dose-response relationship does not show the intensity of effect, but rather the frequency with which any dose produces the all-or-none phenomenon.

In quantal dose-response, the log-dose response curve is sigmoid in character (Figure 7.4). The sigmoid curve has a relatively linear portion between 16 and 84 per cent, which is used to determine the slope of the curve. A small proportion of population at left and right sides of the curve respond to low and high doses and constitute hyper-reactive (hypersensitive) and hypo-reactive (hypo-sensitive) groups, respectively. If a compound produces its effect at very low dosage, the individual is said to be hyper-reactive or hypersensitive; if the same effect is produced by the compound at unusually large dosage, the individual is said to be hypo-reactive or hyposensitive.

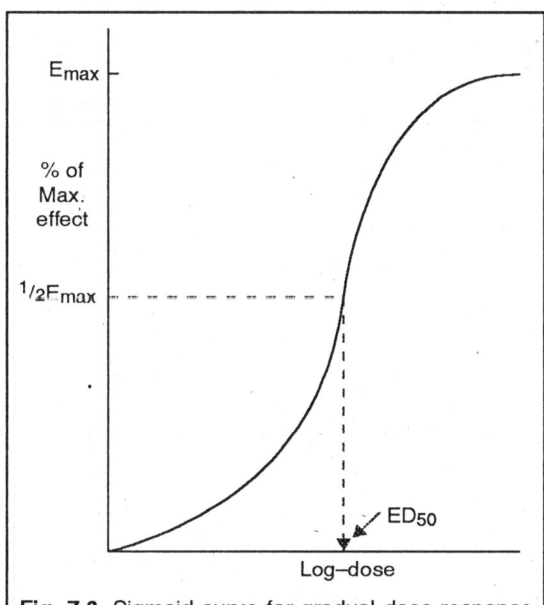

Fig. 7.3. Sigmoid curve for gradual dose-response relationship.

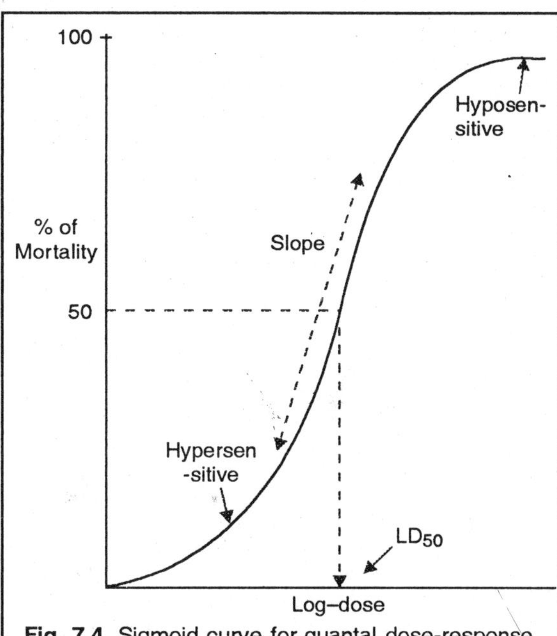

Fig. 7.4. Sigmoid curve for quantal dose-response.

Lethal dose-50 (LD_{50}) / Median lethal dose (MLD) : Lethal dose-50 (LD_{50}), also called median lethal dose (MLD), is the dose that is lethal to 50 per cent of animals exposed to a given toxicant under defined conditions. The LD_{50} value does not pertain to the severity of clinical signs observed or the characteristic changes caused by the toxicant but depends only on the lethality produced by the toxicant. Though recently some toxicological organisations and government regulatory agencies have greatly reduced reliance on the LD_{50} in order to reduce the number of animals needed for study, yet it is still considered an important index to assess the toxicity of chemicals. The calculation of LD_{50} has certain advantages and disadvantages.

Advantages

a. It represents the mid-point of the doses range about which majority of deaths occur.

b. The majority ot animals responding to a toxicant do so symmetrically about the mid-point.

c. The mid-point of the dose-response curve (50 per cent response point) is a convenient description of average response.

d. The 95% confidence limits are narrowest at LD_{50} point i.e. there is least variability at 50% level of response.

Disadvantages

a. Calculation of LD_{50} essentially requires mortality of large number of animals.

b. LD_{50} tells nothing about the shape or slope of the dose-response curve. So it is not possible to know the minimal lethal (LD_1) and maximal lethal (LD_{99}) doses.

c. LD_{50} bears no relationship to long term toxic effects.

Other descriptions: The quantal dose-response data can also be plotted as a frequency distribution curve. This is done by plotting the percentage response at a given dose minus the percentage response at the immediate lower dose. This procedure usually results in a normal gaussian distribution. In such a normal frequency distribution curve, the mean ±1 SD (Standard deviation) represents 68.3 per cent, mean ±2 SD represents 95.5 per cent, and mean ±3 SD represents 99.7 per cent of the population. In it only few animals respond at the lowest dose (hypersensitive) and at the highest dose (hyposensitive). Large number of animals responds to doses intermediate between the two extremes with maximum frequency of response occurring at middle portion (LD_{50} point).

Since quantal dose-response phenomenon is distributed normally, one can convert the per cent to units of deviation from the mean or normal equivalent distribution (NED). Thus NED for a 50% response is zero; and NED of +1 is equated with 84.1% and –1 with 15.9 % response. The units of NED can be further converted to probit units by addition of 5 to them to avoid negative numbers. In this way a 50% response becomes a

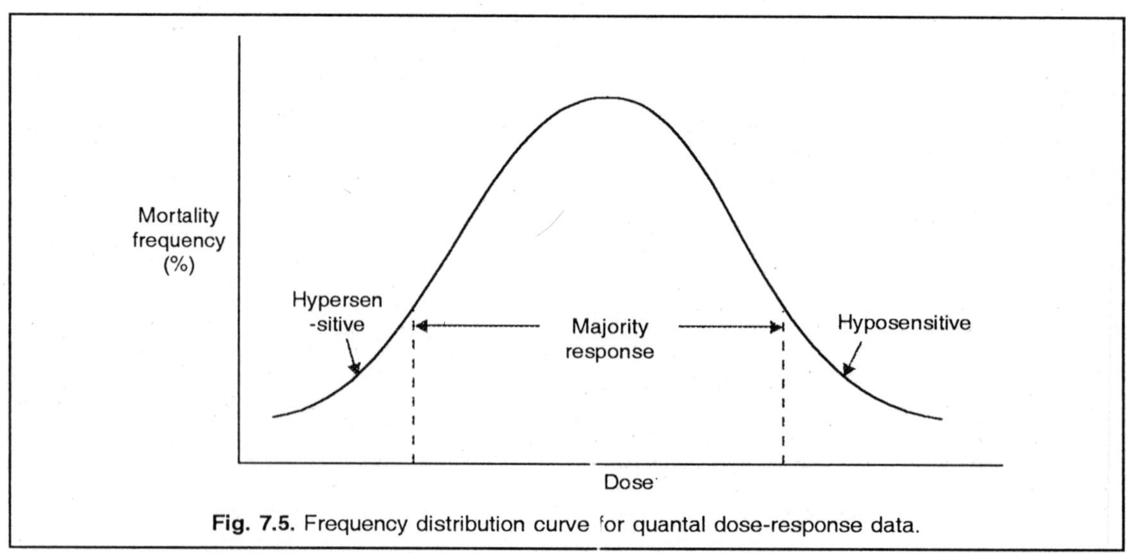

Fig. 7.5. Frequency distribution curve for quantal dose-response data.

probit of 5, and each standard deviation above and below the mean can be expressed as a positive whole number i.e. +1 SD becomes a probit of 6 and −1 a probit of 4.

Per cent Response	Normal equivalent deviation (NED)	Probit
0.1	−3	2
2.3	−2	3
15.9	−1	4
50.0	0	5
84.1	1	6
97.7	2	7
99.9	3	8

The same data from sigmoid curve or a bell shaped curve (normal gaussian distribution) will form a straight line when transformed into probit units (Fig. 7.6).

Plotting data by taking probit units has some advantages like:

a. The curve is obtained as a straight line which gives the slope of the dose-response curve.

b. The LD_{50} is obtained by drawing a horizontal line from the probit unit 5, which is the 50% mortality point, to the dose-response line. At the point of intersection, a vertical line is drawn and this line intersects abscissa at the LD_{50} point.

c. In addition to LD_{50} value, other values like LD_{90}, LD_{10}, etc. can be easily obtained.

d. Comparison of two curves can be done accurately due to the straight line representing data.

Interpretation of acute lethal toxicity information: Depending on the observable response selected for the toxicity test, dosages may be characterised as being effective, toxic, or lethal. The effective dose (ED) represents when the desirable therapeutic/pharmacological response is observed at the dose tested. A toxic dose (TD) represents the dose at which toxicity is evident and a lethal dose (LD) represents the dose at which death of the animal occurs. A numerical subscript is added to the dose selected to denote the cumulative percentage of test organisms that exhibit the pre-determined response. Although 50%

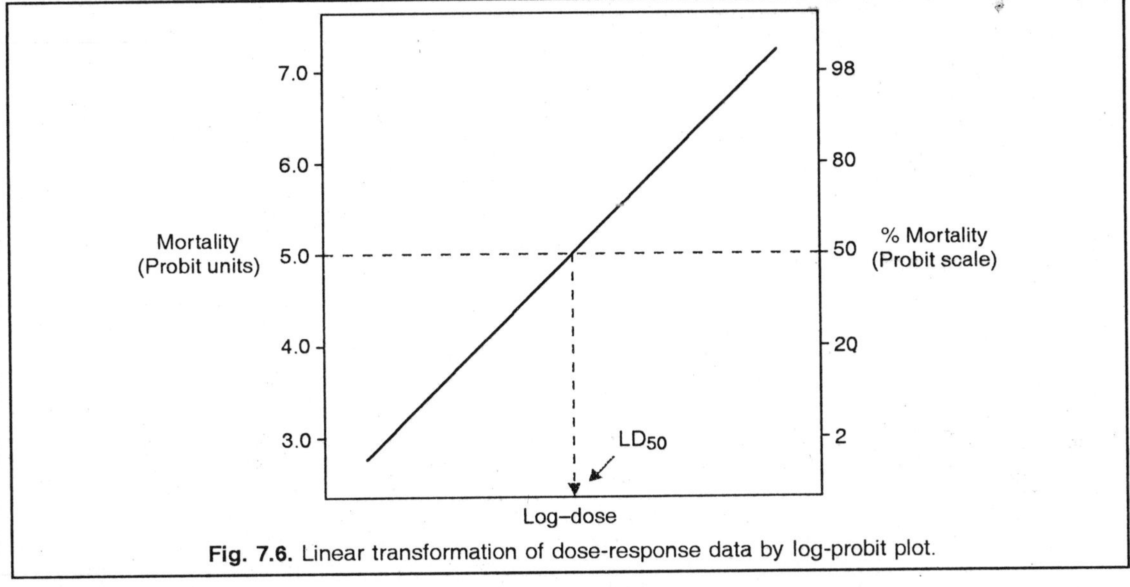

Fig. 7.6. Linear transformation of dose-response data by log-probit plot.

(LD_{50}, TD_{50} or ED_{50}) is often used for comparing toxicity, other cumulative percentages are also used such as ED_{99}, LD_{10}, LD_{01}, etc. The LD_{50} by itself is an insufficient index of lethal toxicity particularly if comparisons are to be made between different toxicants. For complete information, whole of the dose-response information should be examined including the slope of dose-response curve and 95% confidence limits. This is because:

a. If two compounds have same LD_{50} value but different slopes of dose-response curves, then two agents may not have the same or similar toxicity. Figure 7.7 demonstrates two dose-response curves for mortality to two compounds A and B. The LD_{50} for two compounds is same (8 mg/kg), but the slopes of dose-response curves are different. At half of the LD_{50} (4 mg/kg) less than 1 per cent of the animals exposed to compound B die, but at the same dose rate about 20 per cent of animals exposed to compound A would die. So compound A is more toxic than compound B at low doses.

b. If two compounds have different LD_{50} values but overlapping 95% confidence limits, then they are not regarded to have significantly different lethal toxicity. This

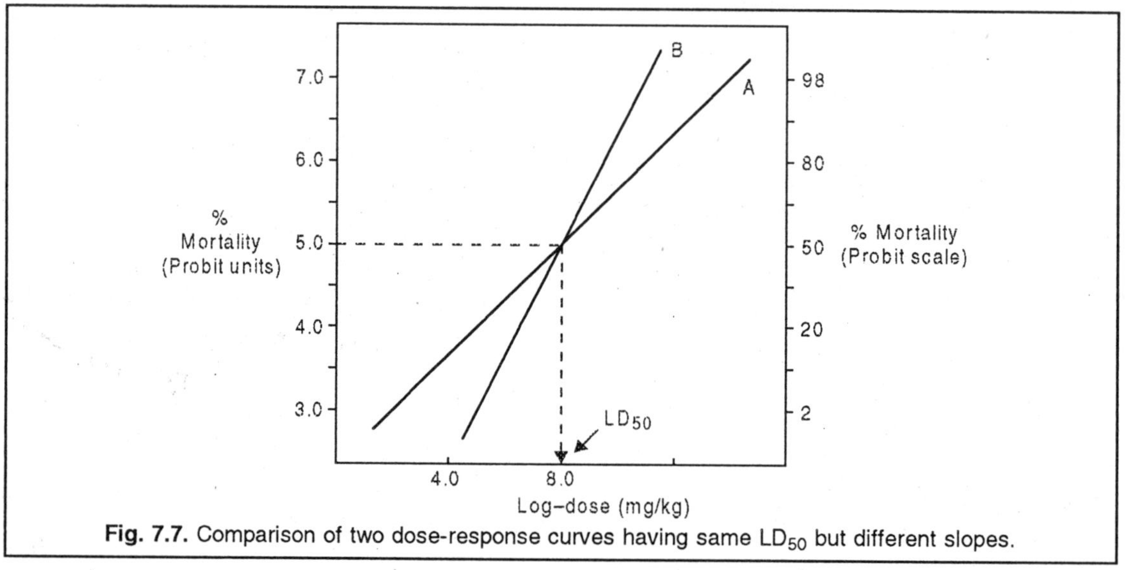

Fig. 7.7. Comparison of two dose-response curves having same LD_{50} but different slopes.

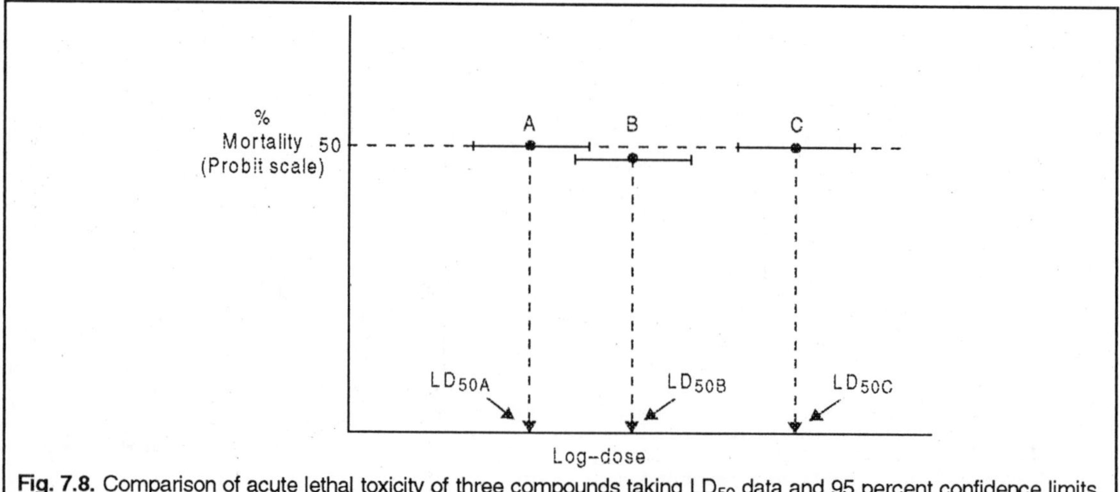

Fig. 7.8. Comparison of acute lethal toxicity of three compounds taking LD_{50} data and 95 percent confidence limits.

is because there is statistical probability that LD_{50} of one compound will be within 95% confidence limits of the other (Figure 7.8, compounds A and B). However, when there is no overlap of 95% confidence limits, then the compounds are considered to have significantly different lethal toxicity at the LD_{50} level. (Figure 7.8, compounds A and C).

c. If two compounds with different LD_{50} values have overlapping 95 per cent confidence limits and identical slopes on the dosage-response lines (and therefore, statistically similar LD_{10} and LD_{90} values), they are lethally equitoxic over a wide range (A and B, Figure 7.9). However, compounds having same/similar LD_{50} values but differing slopes (and hence significantly different LD_{90} and LD_{10} values) may not be considered to be lethally equitoxic over a wide doses range (A and C, Figure 7.9). Acute overdose may be a more serious problem affecting the majority of population for compounds with steeper slope, as a large population is affected by incremental increases in dose (Figure 7.9, compound A). In contrast, compounds having shallower slope (Compound C, Figure 7.9), may represent problems for the hypersensitive groups).

So a proper interpretation of acute lethal toxicity information should include the LD_{50} value, 95% confidence limits, slope and extremes (LD_{90} and LD_{10}) of the dose-response curve.

VARIABLES OF DOSE-RESPONSE CURVE

Irrespective of the shape (linear, sigmoid, hyperbolic), the dose-response curve has 4 characteristic variables: efficacy, potency, slope and biological variations.

a. Efficacy: The maximal effect or response produced by an agent is called its maximal efficacy or efficacy. Efficacy of a compound may be determined by its inherent properties and is indicated by the height (maximal response possible for the compound) of the dose-response curve. Efficacy is independent of the slope or position (potency) of the dose-response curve. In pharmacology and toxicology, efficacy is

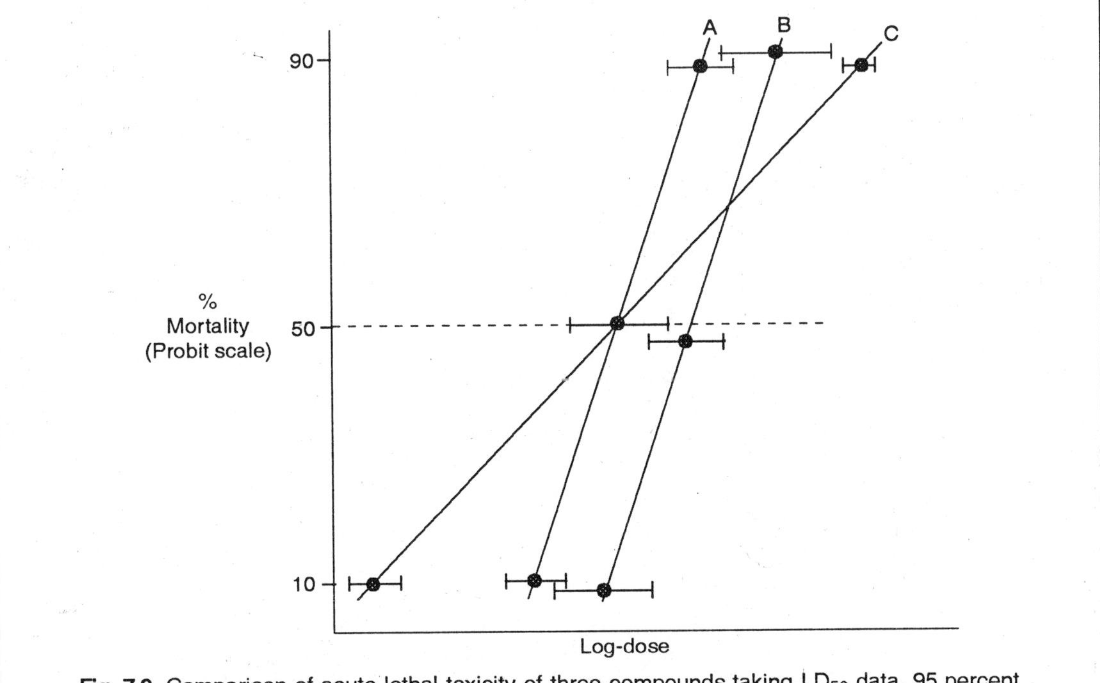

Fig. 7.9. Comparison of acute lethal toxicity of three compounds taking LD_{50} data, 95 percent confidence limits and slope of the dose-response curves.

considered more important than potency because it determines the type or intensity of response. In figure 7.10a, compound A and compound B have equal efficacies as they have same maximal effect (E_{max}). However in Figure 7.10b, compound A is more efficacious than compound C.

b. Potency: Potency is a comparative measure that refers to the different doses of two agents needed to produce the same effect. Potency of a compound depends on its affinity for the receptor or target site and efficiency of xenobiotic-receptor interaction. Therefore, the position of dose-response curve on dose axis is taken as the index of potency. The parameter that determines potency is the ED_{50} or LD_{50}. In figure 7.10a, compound A is more potent than compound B because compound A is required in a smaller dose to produce the same effect as produced by the compound B. So smaller the dose, greater is the potency. Comparisons of potency between two agents can be meaningful only when the agents being compared have log-dose response curves of the same slope. Potency is independent of the efficacy and is important only for selecting dosage and not clinical action. In toxicology, extremely potent agents require special handling due to their low LD_{50} values. Low potency agents are usually considered safe.

Often the terms, potency and efficacy are used interchangeably, but they are not synonymous. Both refer to different characteristics of a compound and should not be confused.

c. Slope: The slope of a dose-response curve gives the relationship between the receptor/target site and the agent. The slope of curve describes the binding of the agent to the receptor site. Steep slope of a curve indicates more binding (affinity) of agent with receptor i.e. more response in comparison to variation in doses. On the other hand, a flat curve indicates lesser binding between drug and receptor, so that little increase in response occurs over a wide range of doses. In a population, the slope is important indicating the range of doses over which the population is affected. In considering lethality, a steep slope indicates that a large proportion of population will be at risk over a small range of doses. Steeper curve also suggests that response of a compound in a population is more uniform. The shallow dose-response curve, in contrast, suggests that response of a toxicant in a population is more difficult to predict due to greater variation in the response. Shallow slope also puts hypersensitive individuals to greater risk than general population. In toxicology, slope of a dose-response curve of a compound should neither be too steep nor too shallow. Slope of curve also facilitates comparison of toxicities of two agents (See Interpretation of acute lethal toxicity information).

d. Biological variations: Variation or variance can be defined as the appearance of differences in the magnitude of response among individuals in the same population given the same dose of a compound. The intersecting brackets in figure 7.10a indicate that biological variations of the dose-

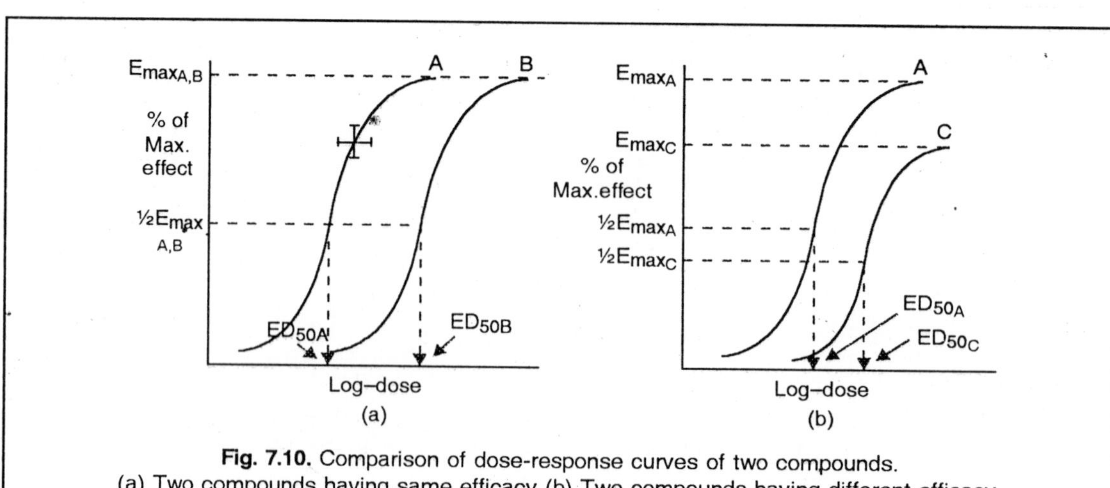

Fig. 7.10. Comparison of dose-response curves of two compounds.
(a) Two compounds having same efficacy (b) Two compounds having different efficacy.

response relationship can be visualised in either of the two ways. The vertical bracket expresses the fact that a range of effects will be produced by a given dose in a population. Alternately, the horizontal bracket expresses the fact that a range of doses is required to produce a specified intensity of effect in all individuals.

Measures of Toxicity

The margin of safety of a compound is determined from the results of two studies, such as an ED study and a LD study. A ratio between selected ED and LD values is then used to express the margin of safety. The larger the ratio, the greater is the margin of safety.

a. Therapeutic Index: Therapeutic index may be defined as the ratio of the lethal dose-50 (LD_{50}) and the effective dose-50 (ED_{50}).

$$\text{Therapeutic index (T.I.)} = \frac{LD_{50}}{ED_{50}}$$

Where, LD_{50} = Dose that is lethal for 50% of the population.

ED_{50} = Dose that is effective for 50% of the population.

Therapeutic index measure is commonly used for evaluating the safety and usefulness of therapeutic agents. The higher the index, the safer is the drug. But it is valid for comparison only if the ED_{50} curve (therapeutic dose-response curve) and LD_{50} curve (lethality dose-response curve) are parallel (Figure 7.11 a). If the two curves are not parallel then therapeutic index is not considered useful for evaluating safety. When the dose-response curve for lethality is shallower than that for the therapeutic response (Figure 7.11 b), then there will be decreasing safety at the lower dose and the hypersensitive groups will be at greater risk. The drug will be much more toxic at 1% or 10% levels and the therapeutic index would be misleading. In such cases (when curves are not parallel), the therapeutic ratio or standard safety margin may be used. In clinical situations also therapeutic index has certain limitations e.g. when a therapeutic agent has have more than one ED_{50} values, one for each of its desired effects, then there may be more than one therapeutic indices. In toxicology, toxic symptoms are more relevant than lethality; therefore, the therapeutic index is sometimes taken as the ratio of the toxic dose-50 (TD_{50}) to the effective dose-50 (ED_{50}).

b. Therapeutic Ratio: Therapeutic ratio may be defined as the ratio of the lethal dose-25 (LD_{25}) and the effective dose-75 (ED_{75}).

$$\text{Therapeutic ratio (T.R.)} = \frac{LD_{25}}{ED_{75}}$$

Where, LD_{25} = Dose that is lethal for 25% of the population.

ED_{75} = Dose that is effective for 75% of the population.

Therapeutic ratio is considered a better index of safety of a compound as it includes steepness of curve also. In toxicity cases, a flatter curve is

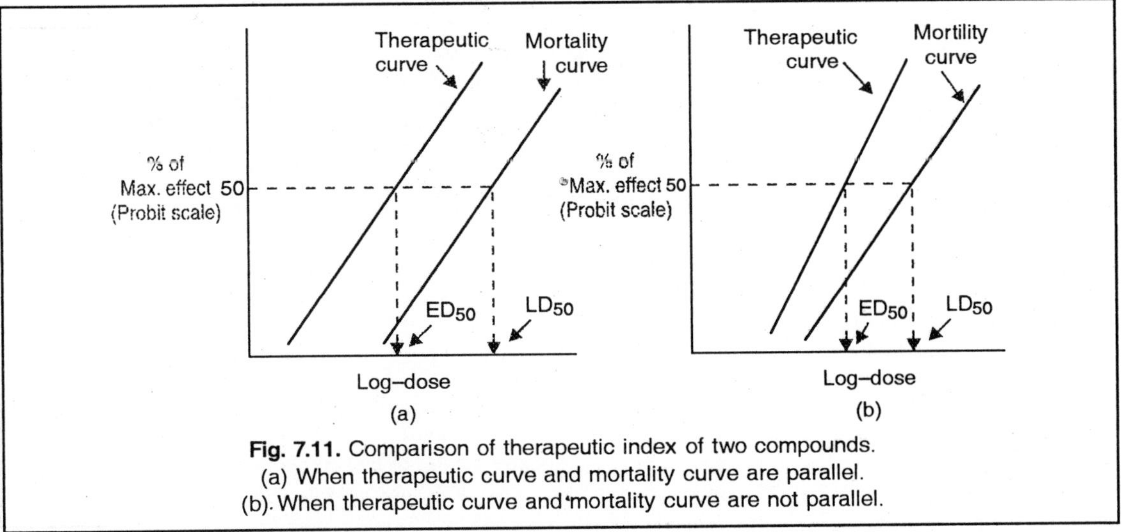

Fig. 7.11. Comparison of therapeutic index of two compounds.
(a) When therapeutic curve and mortality curve are parallel.
(b). When therapeutic curve and mortality curve are not parallel.

considered more toxic as hyper-reactive groups are at a much more risk than hypo-reactive or normal group. Shallower curves usually have low therapeutic ratios. In figure 7.12, computation of therapeutic ratio values reveals that compound A is safer than compound B as B has a flatter curve.

c. Standard Safety Margin: Standard safety margin may be defined as the ratio of the lethal dose-1 (LD_1) and the effective dose-99 (ED_{99}).

$$\text{Standard safety margin (SSM)} = \frac{LD_1}{ED_{99}}$$

Standard safety margin is a more conservative estimate than therapeutic index as values are derived from extremes of the respective dose-response curves. However, values of minimum toxic (LD_1) and maximum therapeutic (ED_{99}) are less precise than the median doses and the difficulty of determining such values with accuracy excludes this possibility.

Note: In quantal dose-response relationship, a normally distributed sigmoid curve approaches a response of 0 per cent as the dose is decreased and approaches 100 percent as the dose is increased, but theoretically never passes through 0 and 100 per cent values. So 1% and 99% are taken as minimum and maximum response, respectively.

d. Chronicity Factor: Chronicity factor is the ratio of the acute LD_{50} (one-dose) to chronic LD_{50} doses.

$$\text{Chronicity factor} = \frac{\text{Acute } LD_{50}}{\text{Chronic } LD_{50}}$$

Chronicity factor is used to assess the cumulative action of a toxicant. Compounds with cumulative effects have a higher chronicity factor. A chronicity factor greater than 2.0 indicates a relative cumulative toxicant. The table 7.1 compares the chronicity factor of some toxicants in rats. Data in the Table 7.1 suggest that mirex is a cumulative toxicant with chronicity factor of 60.8, but sodium chloride is a non-cumulative compound (chronicity factor 1.4). Some toxicants in repeated low doses induce a degree of tolerance in animals and hence have very low chronicity factor. For example, acute LD_{50} of potassium cyanide is 10 mg/kg, but the pre-exposed animals can tolerate even up to 250 mg/kg, thus having chronicity factor of 0.04.

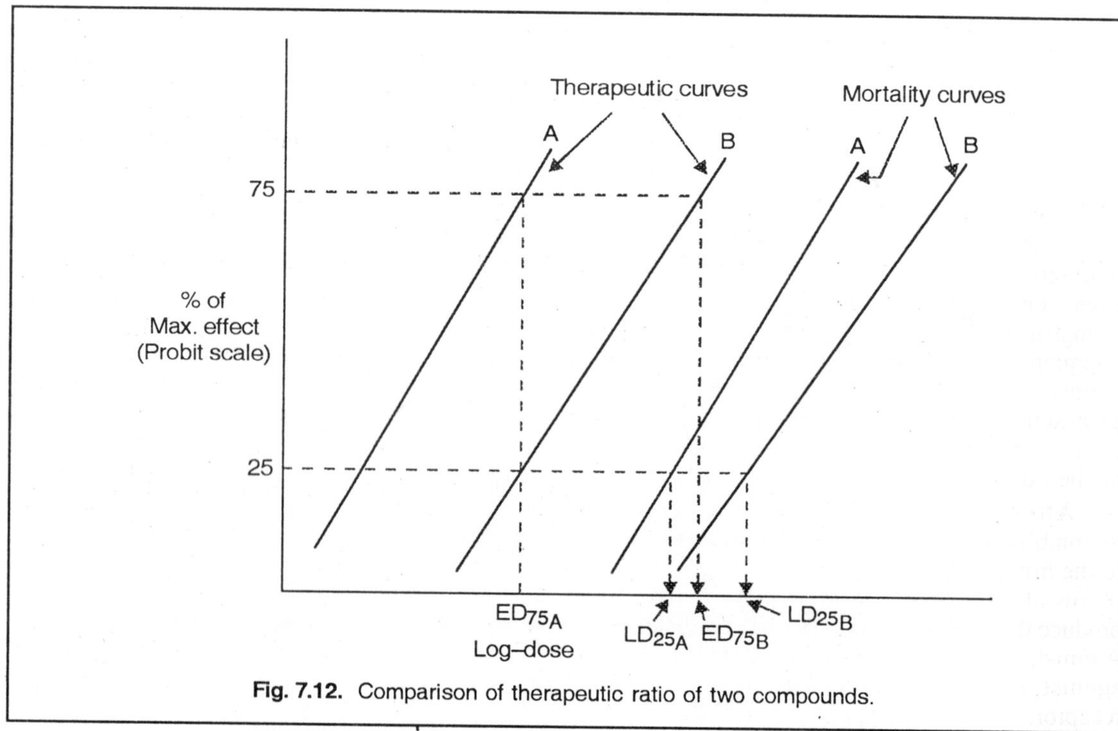

Fig. 7.12. Comparison of therapeutic ratio of two compounds.

Table 7.1 : Chronicity factors for some toxicants.

Compound	Acute LD_{50} (mg/kg)	90-days LD_{50} (mg/kg/day)	Chronicity Factor
Mirex	365	6	60.8
Warfarin	1.6	0.077	20.8
Sodium chloride	3,750	2,690	1.4
EPN	7.7	12	0.64
Potassium cyanide	10	250	0.04

e. Risk Ratio : The ratio between the inherent toxicity and the exposure level gives the risk ratio. Risk ratio indicates the risk of a compound. Substances of higher inherent toxicity may pose little risk as access or exposure of animals to such agents is limited. Compounds of low toxicity may be dangerous if used extensively. For example, Table 7.2 compares risk ratio of the two substances monensin and urea, which are used in cattle feed. Monensin is much more toxic than urea; however, the rate of monensin use (exposure) is much lower than urea. The risk ratios of two compounds suggest that risk of urea toxicosis would be much higher due to its frequent use than the risk of monensin toxicosis.

Table 7.2 : Comparison of risk (hazard).

Compound	Toxicity	Use-level	Risk Ratio
Urea	300 mg/kg	100 mg/kg	3 : 1
Monensin	20 mg/kg	1 mg/kg	20 : 1

XENOBIOTIC-RECEPTOR INTERACTION

Many xenobiotics exert their effects by interacting with specific receptors in the body. This xenobiotic-receptor interaction leads to a change in the macromolecule, which in turn triggers a sequence of events resulting in a response of the tissue or organ. The intensity of response produced by a xenobiotic depends on its intrinsic activity, which in turn depends on the chemical structure of the compound.

Affinity: Affinity is the ability of a xenobiotic to combine with its receptors and is proportional to the binding equilibrium constant K_D. A ligand of low affinity requires a higher concentration to produce the same effect than ligand of high affinity. Agonist, partial agonist, antagonist and inverse agonist have same or similar affinity for the receptor.

Intrinsic activity: It is defined as a proportionality constant of the ability of the agonist to activate the receptor as compared to the maximally active compound in the series being studied. It is maximum of unity for full agonist and minimum of zero for antagonist.

1. Types of Xenobiotic

a. Agonist: Agonist (full agonist) is an agent that interacts with a specific cellular constituent (i.e. receptor) and elicits an observable positive response. The agonist may be an endogenous physiological substance like a neurotransmitter or hormone, or it can be a xenobiotic. Agonist has both affinity for receptor and intrinsic activity (Table 7.3). For an agonist, the intrinsic activity (IA) is equal to unity or 1. Examples of agonist include morphine interaction with opioid receptor, strychnine interaction with glycine receptor and barbiturates interaction with GABA receptor.

b. Partial agonist: Partial agonist (PA) is an agent that acts on the same receptor as other agonists in a group of endogenous ligands or xenobiotics, but regardless of its dose, it cannot produce the same maximal biological response as a full agonist. The partial agonist has affinity for the receptor but very low intrinsic activity. For a partial agonist, the intrinsic activity is always less than 1 (IA between 0 to 1). Thus, PA alone acts as an agonist to produce a response (lower than full agonist) but in presence of an agonist, it acts as an antagonist (decreases effect of full agonist as it occupies receptors and decreases their

Table 7.3. : Mechanism of action of xenobiotics.

Activity	Type of xenobiotic			
	Agonist	Partial agonist	Antagonist	Inverse agonist
Affinity	+++	+++	+++	+++
Efficacy	+++	+	0	
With agonist	Addition or Synergism	Antagonism	Antagonism	Antagonism

availability to agonist). For example, both morphine and codeine act on opioid receptors to produce analgesia, but the analgesic efficacy of codeine is much lower than morphine.

c. Antagonist: Antagonist is an agent that interacts with the receptor or any other part of the effector mechanism to inhibit the action of an agonist. Antagonist has no activity of its own. It may compete with the agonist to occupy the receptor site or may act on allosteric site (site other than receptor's active site) and distorts the structure of receptor so that agonist can not bind. Thus antagonist has affinity for the receptor, but it possesses no intrinsic activity (IA = 0). For example, atropine antagonises action of acetylcholine on muscarinic receptors and naloxone antagonises action of morphine on opioid receptors. Depending on the type of interaction with the receptors, antagonists may be further classified as competitive antagonists and non-competitive antagonists (see for detail, antagonism). Receptor antagonists are often termed as blockers.

d. Inverse agonist: Inverse agonist is a compound that interacts with the same receptor as the agonist, but it produces a response just opposite to that of the agonist. Inverse agonist has affinity but it possesses intrinsic activity with a minus sign (IA = 0 to –1). For example, the β-carbolines (inverse agonist) like dimethoxyethyl carbomethoxy-β-carboline (DMCM) binds with the benzodiazepine receptor, but produces stimulation, anxiety, increased muscle tone, etc. (benzodiazepines have anxiolytic, muscle relaxant and CNS depressant actions).

2. Xenobiotic-Receptor Interaction

Currently it is believed that for most drugs, the drug (D) combines reversibly (as receptors reappear after some time) with the receptor (R) to form a drug-receptor complex (DR) which by sequence of events produces an effect (E).

$$\text{Drug (D)+Receptor (R)} \underset{k_2}{\overset{k_1}{\rightleftharpoons}} \text{Drug-receptor complex (DR)} \xrightarrow{k_3} \text{Effect (E)} \quad (i)$$

Where k_1, k_2 and k_3 are the rate constants of the respective partial reactions.

The above reaction sequence (*i*) is analogous to the interaction of substrate with enzyme. Therefore, the magnitude of effect can be analysed in a manner similar to that for enzymatic product formation. So we get an equation equivalent to Michaelis-Menton equation.

$$E = \frac{E_{max}(D)}{K_D + (D)} \quad (ii)$$

Where E_{max} = Maximal effect produced by drug

(D) = Free drug concentration

K_D = Dissociation constant for drug-receptor complex. K_D can also be defined as drug concentration where effect is ½ E_{max}.

In the equation (*ii*), there are two constants i.e. K_D and E_{max} for a given drug. If we plot two variables of the equation i.e. E and (D), we get a dose-response curve (hyperbolic or sigmoid). If (D) is known, then effect (E) can be plotted. Reciprocal of dissociation constant (K_D) also gives the affinity (association) i.e. more the K_D, less would be the affinity and vice-versa.

Line-Weaver Burk plot : Data analysis can be further facilitated if a linear form of equation (instead of hyperbolic or sigmoid) is taken. This is obtained by taking reciprocal on both sides called double reciprocal plot or Line-Weaver Burk plot.

$$E = \frac{E_{max}(D)}{K_D + (D)}$$

Taking reciprocal on both sides

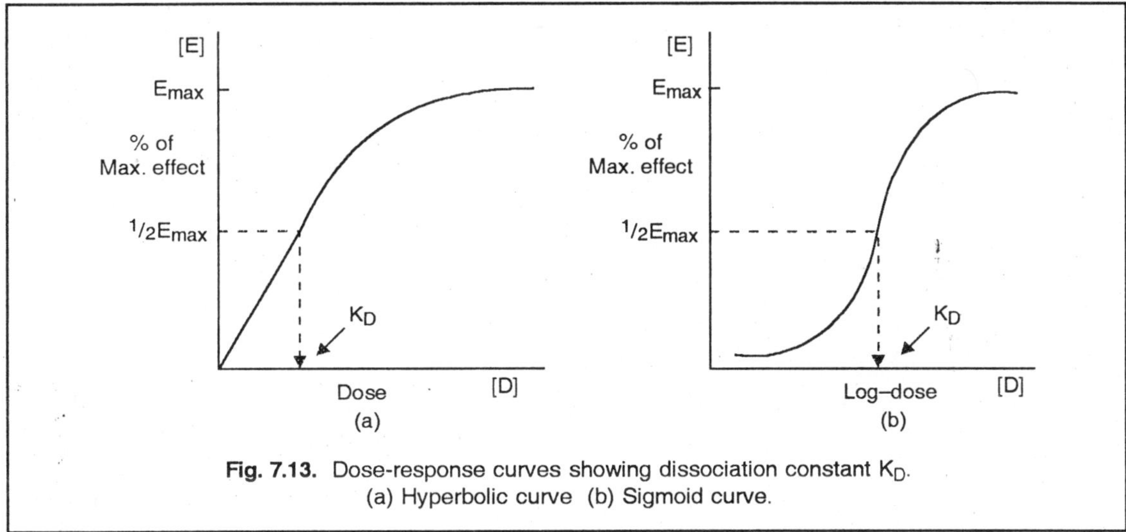

Fig. 7.13. Dose-response curves showing dissociation constant K_D. (a) Hyperbolic curve (b) Sigmoid curve.

$$\frac{1}{E} = \frac{K_D}{E_{max}(D)} + \frac{(D)}{E_{max}(D)}$$

$$\frac{1}{E} = \frac{K_D}{E_{max}(D)} + \frac{1}{E_{max}} \qquad (iii)$$

A plot of 1/E versus 1/D yields a straight line that intersects the Y-axis at $1/E_{max}$ and this has a slope equal to K_D/E_{max} (Figure 7.14). Extrapolation of this line to the X- axis yields the value of intercept shown to by $-1/K_D$. Thus, value of K_D and the maximal effect can be readily calculated from such a plot. This representation is particularly useful for the analysis of drug antagonism.

XENOBIOTIC/DRUG INTERACTIONS

When two or more xenobiotics are used together, the pharmacological/toxicological response is not necessarily the sum of two agents used individually. This is because one agent may interfere with the action of another agent called xenobiotic interactions.

a. Addition/Additive effect: When the combined effect of two compounds given together

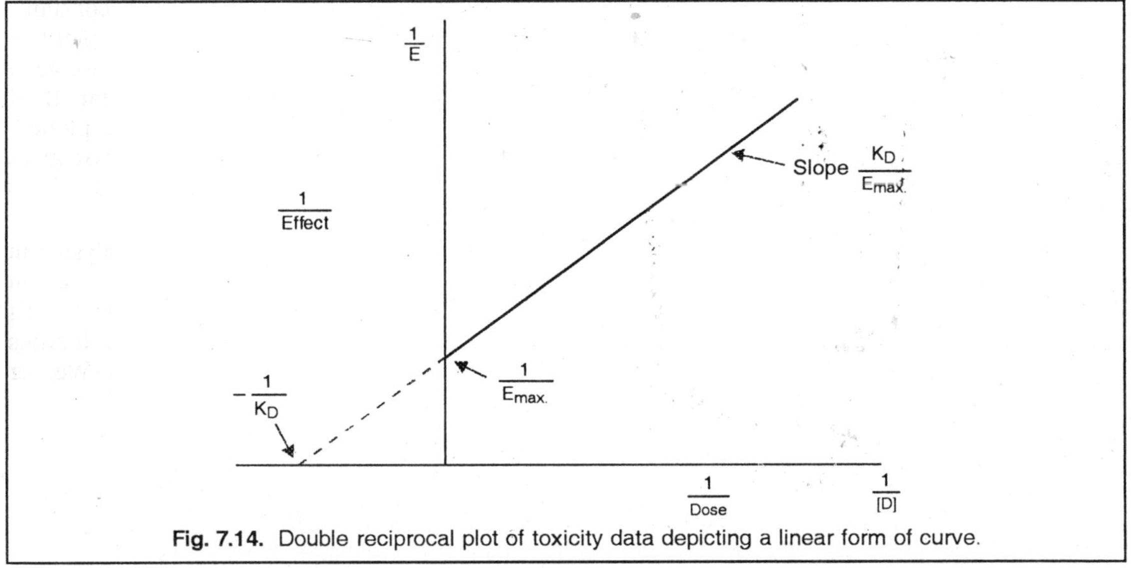

Fig. 7.14. Double reciprocal plot of toxicity data depicting a linear form of curve.

is equal in magnitude to sum of the effects of each compound given alone, the interaction is called addition and the effect produced is called additive effect.

$E_{AB} = E_A + E_B$ or $1+1 = 2$

where E_{AB} = Combined effect of two compounds A and B

E_A = Effect produced by compound A alone.

E_B = Effect produced by compound B alone.

The additive effect is produced mainly when two agents administered together have same/similar mechanism of action and effects are additive. For example, combination of two organophosphorus insecticides produces additive cholinesterase inhibition.

b. Potentiation/Potentiative effect: When one compound having no effect of its own increases the effect of another compound, the interaction is called potentiation and the effect produced is called potentiative effect.

$E_{AB} > E_A + E_B$ or $1 + 0 > 1$

The potentiative effect is seen mainly when one compound lacking the effect of its own enhances the concentration of other compound at its site of action by altering its pharmacokinetics/toxicokinetics. For example, probenecid enhances effect of penicillins by decreasing their renal excretion, and MAO inhibitors (e.g., tranyl cypromine) enhance antihypertensive effect of catecholamines.

c. Synergism/Synergistic effect: When the combined effect of two compounds is greater in magnitude than sum of the effects of each compound given alone, the interaction is called synergism and the effect produced is called synergistic effect.

$E_{AB} > E_A + E_B$ or $1 + 1 > 2$

The synergistic effect is produced mainly when two compounds used together have same or similar effects and they increase each others action at the target site. For example, both carbon tetrachloride and ethanol are hepatotoxicants, but together they produce much more injury to the liver than expected from the mathematical sum of their individual effects.

d. Antagonism/Antagonistic effect: When the combined effect of two compounds is lesser in magnitude than sum of the effects of each compound given alone, or when one compound having no effect of its own decreases or inhibits the effect of other compound, the interaction is called antagonism and the effect produced is called antagonistic effect.

(*i*) $E_{AB} < E_A + E_B$ or $2 + 1 < 3$

(*ii*) $E_{AB} < E_A$ or $2 + 0 < 2$ (True antagonism)

The antagonistic effect is produced mainly when a partial agonist is combined with a full agonist (condition i) or when an antagonist and an agonist are combined together (condition ii, true antagonism). Examples of true antagonism include combination of morphine (opioid receptor agonist) and naloxone (opioid receptor antagonist), and muscarine (muscarinic receptor agonist) and atropine (muscarinic receptor antagonist).

When two agents are given together, then there are 3 possibilities.

(*i*) Both agents are equally active.

(*ii*) One agent is less active than other.

(*iii*) One agent is active, while other has no activity of its own.

(*i*) When both agents A and B are equally active then their combined effect is simply the sum of the effects of two agents given individually (i.e. addition). In such cases the shape of the dose-response curves would be as given in Figure 7.15.

where α = Efficacy of agent A

β = Efficacy of agent B

E_{AB} = Combined effect of agents A and B

[A] = Concentration/dose of agent A

[B] = Concentration/dose of agent B

In such cases the combined effect will be addition

$$E_{AB} = E_A + E_B$$

(*ii*) When one agent B is less active than the other agent A then the curves intersect at one point (b in Figure 17.16) at which $E_{AB} = E_A$ regardless of the concentration of B. At this concentration of agent A, the combined effect of both agents (E_{AB}) is equal to that of A (E_A) alone. To left of the intersecting point (point a in Figure 7.16), at low concentration of A, the same additive effect is seen as observed in the first possibility (*i*) (i.e. $\alpha = \beta$). To the right of the intersecting point (c in figure 7.16), at higher concentration of A, agent B antagonises the effect of agent A, so the

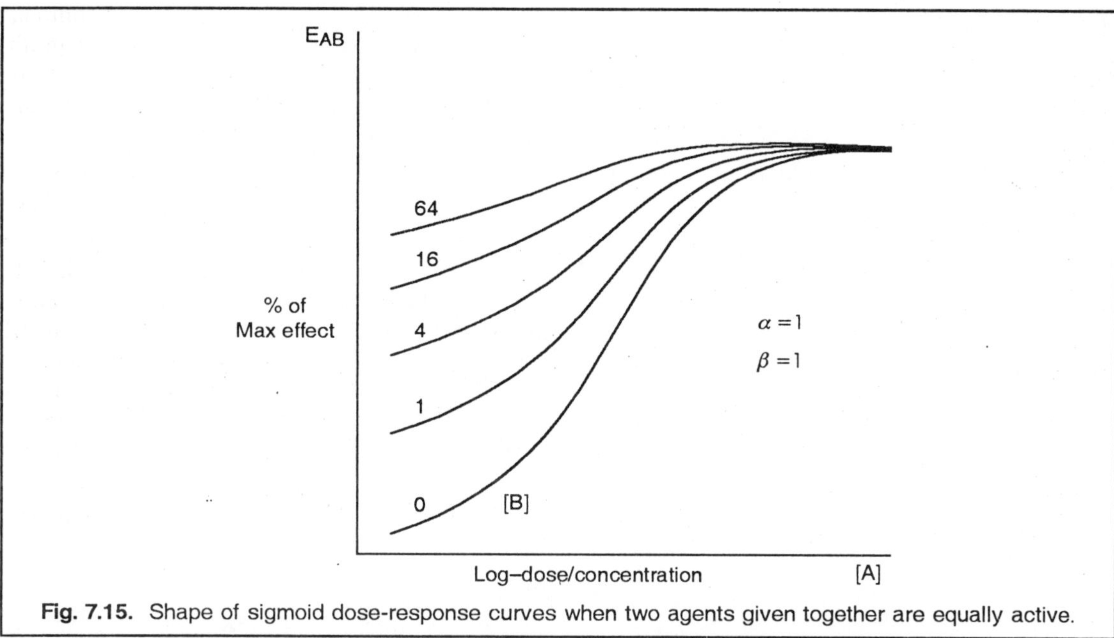

Fig. 7.15. Shape of sigmoid dose-response curves when two agents given together are equally active.

combined effect of A and B will be less than the sum of the effects of two agents. Accordingly in this possibility, the agent B is acting as a partial agonist.

where α = Efficacy of agent A

β = Efficacy of agent B

E_{AB} = Combined effect of agents A and B

[A] = Concentration/dose of agent A

[B] = Concentration/dose of agent B

At '*a*' (left of intersecting point) $E_{AB} = E_A + E_B$

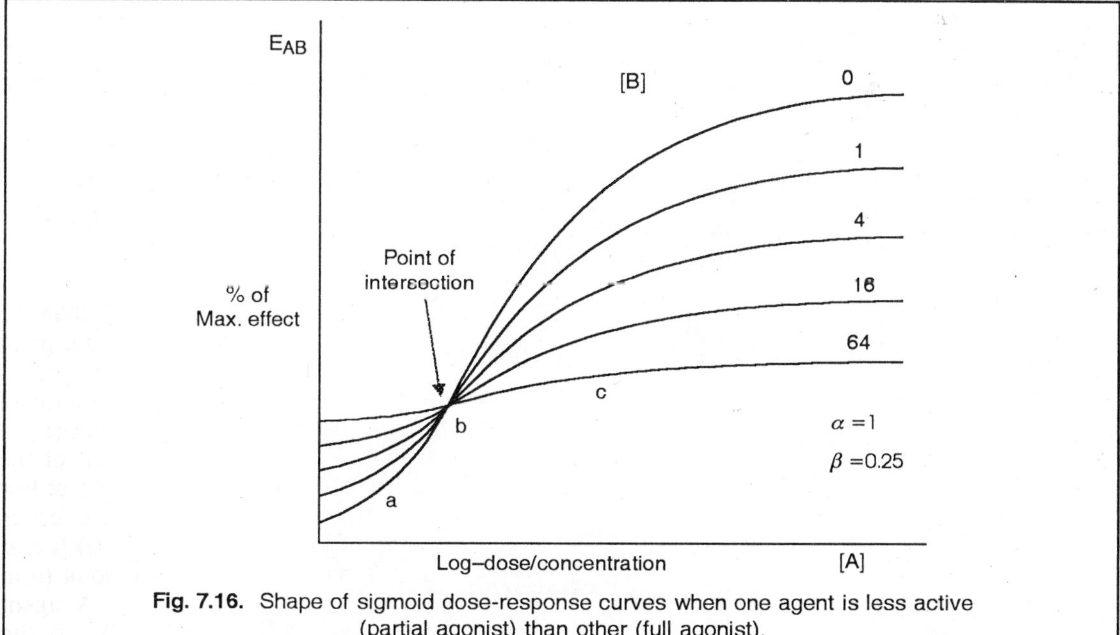

Fig. 7.16. Shape of sigmoid dose-response curves when one agent is less active (partial agonist) than other (full agonist).

'*b*' (point of intersection) $E_{AB} = E_A$

'*c*' (right of intersecting point) $E_{AB} < E_A + E_B$

(*iii*) When one agent A is active and the other agent B has no activity of its own ($\beta = 0$), the point of intersection of curves is entirely out of the diagramme (on the left) and the combined effect of both agents (E_{AB}) is always less than the effect of active agent A alone (E_A). Here, the agent B is acting as an antagonist of the agent A and the curves are parallel to each other.

where α = Efficacy of agent A

β = Efficacy of agent B

E_{AB} = Combined effect of agents A and B

[A] = Concentration/dose of agent A

[B] = Concentration/dose of agent B

In such cases the combined effect will be antagonism.

$$E_{AB} < E_A.$$

ANTAGONISM

Xenobiotics antagonism is broadly of three types: chemical antagonism, physiological antagonism and pharmacological antagonism.

a. Chemical antagonism: Chemical antagonism (inactivation antagonism) occurs when two or more compounds react chemically and form an inactive product. This type of antagonism occurs primarily when two agents have opposite chemical properties, which neutralize each other i.e. acid and base, cations and anions. For example, sodium bicarbonate neutralises acidic compounds and protamine (basic and cationic drug) neutralises anticoagulant effect of heparin (acidic and anionic drug). Chemical inactivation also occurs when dimercaprol (BAL) chelates metal ions such as arsenic, mercury and lead and decreases their toxic effects.

b. Physiological/Functional antagonism: Physiological or Functional antagonism occurs when two agents counterbalance (neutralise) each other by producing opposite effects on the same physiological system. Here two compounds act on two different sites or receptors and produce response in opposite directions. For example, acetylcholine and adrenaline act on muscarinic and adrenergic receptors on heart to produce bradycardia and tachycardia, respectively. In clinical practice, fall in blood pressure produced by severe barbiturate intoxication can be effectively antagonised by vasopressor agents like noradrenaline or metaraminol, and strychnine induced convulsions can be controlled by systemic administration of CNS depressants like pentobarbitone sodium.

c. Pharmacological antagonism: Pharmacological antagonism occurs when two agents act on the same receptor or system to produce less of an effect. Agonist increases the effect and antagonist decreases or abolishes it. Both agonist and antagonist are specific to the receptor or target site. Pharmacological antagonism is of two sub-types: competitive and non-competitive.

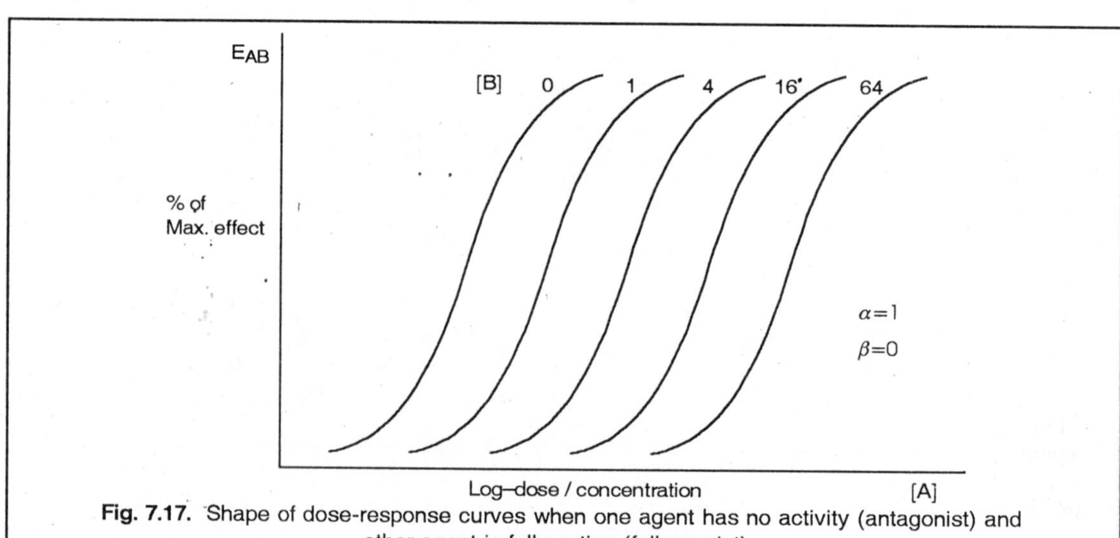

Fig. 7.17. Shape of dose-response curves when one agent has no activity (antagonist) and other agent is fully active (full agonist).

i. Competitive or Reversible antagonism: In competitive (reversible, surmountable) antagonism, the antagonist and agonist compete with each other for occupancy of the same receptor. The interaction between the compound (agonist or antagonist) and the receptor is due to formation of weak bonds, so increasing the concentration of one compound can reverse action of the other compound. Both agonist and antagonist have affinity for the receptor, but compound in higher concentration occupies the receptor. In dose-response relationship, the competitive antagonist causes a parallel shift of the log dose-response curve to the right, but there is no change in its shape, slope or maximal response. In Figure 7.18, the potency (affinity) of agonist decreases in presence of antagonist, but efficacy (E_{max}) remains the same as it can be achieved at a higher dose. In Line-Weaver Burk or double reciprocal plot, the lines meet at 1/E axis, which gives the same E_{max}. The lines diverge at higher agonist concentration indicating that apparent affinity of agonist for the receptor is lowered (reciprocal of dissociation constant i.e. $1/K_D$ is affinity constant). Competitive receptor antagonism is seen when atropine blocks action of acetylcholine on muscarinic receptors and naloxone blocks action of morphine on opioid receptors.

ii. Non-competitive or Irreversible antagonism : In non-competitive (irreversible, unsurmountable) antagonism, the antagonist forms strong bonds (e.g. covalent bond) with its receptor and irreversibly blocks it. Here, antagonist is not

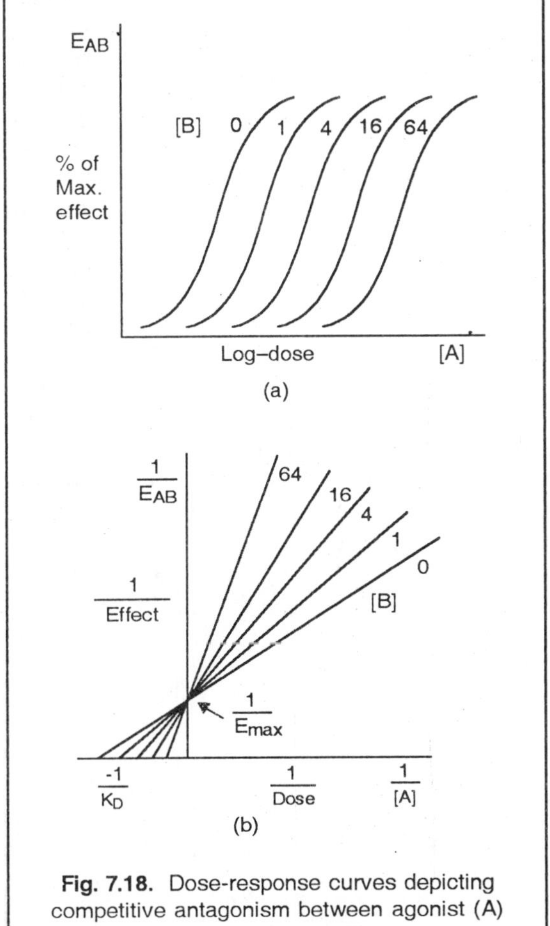

Fig. 7.18. Dose-response curves depicting competitive antagonism between agonist (A) and antagonist (B).
(a) Sigmoid curves (b) Double reciprocal plot.

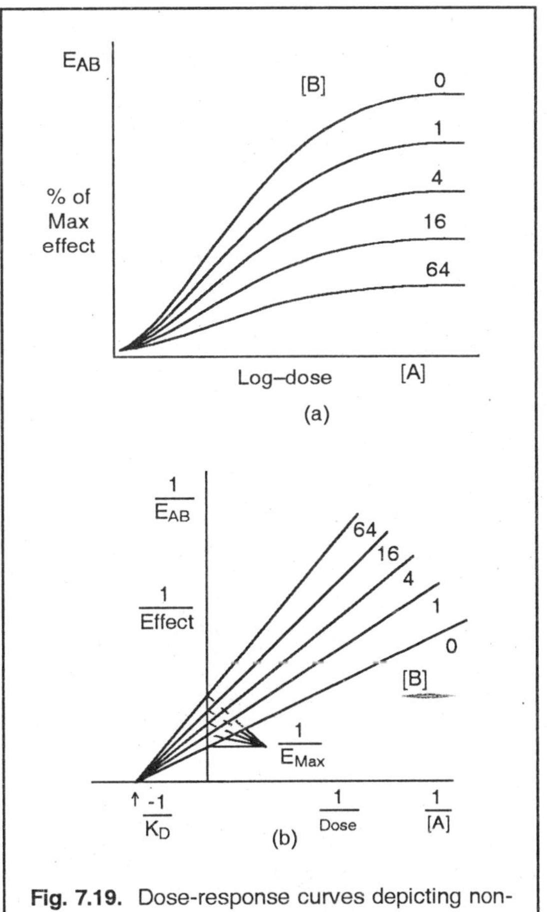

Fig. 7.19. Dose-response curves depicting non-competitive antagonism between compounds A (agonist) and B (antagonist).
(a) Sigmoid-curves (b) Double-reciprocal plot.

displaced by a high concentration of the agonist. Agonist can act only on receptor sites not influenced by the antagonist. The affinity of the agonist for receptor is thus unaltered but its efficacy is reduced as it cannot produce the maximal response (E_{max}) irrespective of its dose. The log dose-response relationship shows flatter curves with reduced efficacy (Figure 7.19). The double reciprocal plot shows meeting of lines at $-1/K_D$ on the 1/Dose axis. The plot shows unaltered affinity ($-1/K_D$ is same) but decreased efficacy (altered $1/E_{max}$). For example, phenoxybenzamine irreversible blocks action of noradrenaline on α-adrenoceptors. Interaction of phenoxybenzamine (antagonist) is initially reversible with α-adrenoceptors, but after some time it becomes irreversible due to formation of strong bonds between them.

BIBLIOGRAPHY

Alarie Y (1981) Dose response analysis in animal studies. Prediction of human responses. *Environ. Hlth. Prespect.* 42 : 9.

Atterwill CK and Steele CE (1987) *In vitro* Methods in Toxicology. Cambridge University Press, Cambridge.

Baggot JD (1982) Mechanisms of drug action. In: John's Veterinary Pharmacology and Therapeutics. 5th edn. Booth NH and McDonald LE (Eds.) p 23. Kalyani Publishers, Ludhiana-New Delhi.

Ballantyne B, Marrs T and Turner P (1995) Fundamentals of toxicology. In: General and Applied Toxicology. Ballantyne B, Marrs T and Turner P (Eds.) p 3. Macmillan Press Ltd., London.

Blodgett DJ (2002) How to evaluate toxicant exposure. *Vet. Clin. North Am: Small Anim Pract.* 32 : 341.

Eaton DL and Klaassen CD (1996) Principles of Toxicology. In: Casarett and Doull's Toxicology: The Basic science of Poisons. 5th edn. Klaassen CD (Ed.) p 13. McGraw Hill Companies Inc., New York.

Farmer J (1974) Comparison of probit and logit models for estimation of LD_{01}. *Fed. Proc.* 33 : 220.

Goldenthal EI (1971) A compilation of LD_{50} values in newborn and adult animals. *Toxicol. Appl. Pharmacol.* 18: 185.

Griffith JF (1964) Interlaboratory variations and the determination of acute oral LD_{50}. *Toxicol. Appl. Pharmacol.* 6: 726.

Gupta PK and Salunkhe DK (1984) Modern Toxicology Vol. II. The Adverse Effects of Xenobiotics. Metropolitan Publishing Company, New Delhi.

Hart JG and Timbrell JA (1979) The effect of age on paracetamol hepatotoxicity in mice. *Biochemical. Pharmacol.* 28 : 3015.

Hughes WW (1996) Essentials of Environmental Toxicology. Taylor & Francis, Washington.

Lu FC and Kacew S (2002) Lu's Basic Toxicology: Fundamentals, Target Organs and Risk Assessment. Taylor & Francis, New York.

Osweiler GD (1996) Toxicology. Williams and Wilkins, Philadelphia.

Osweiler GD (1999) Introduction to toxicology. In: Veterinary Toxicology. Beasley V (Ed.) p. 2. International Veterinary Information Service, Ithaca NY (www.ivis.org).

Paget GE (1970) Methods in Toxicology. Blackwell, Oxford.

Ross EM and Kenakin TP (2001) Pharmacodynamics: Mechanisms of drug action and the relationship between drug concentration and effect. In: Goodman & Gilman's The Pharmacological Basis of Therapeutics. 10th edn. Hardman JG, Limbird LE and Gilman AG (Eds.) p 31. The McGraw-Hill Companies Inc., New York.

Sirover MA and Loeb LA (1976) Infidelity of DNA synthesis *in vitro*: Screening for potential metal mutagens or carcinogens. *Science* 194 : 1434.

Witthaus RA (1955) Manual of Toxicology. 2nd edn. Bailliere Tindall and Cox, London.

Zbinden G and Flury-Roversi M (1981) Significance of the LD_{50} test for the toxicological evaluation of chemical substances. *Arch. Toxicol.* 47 : 77.

□□□□□□

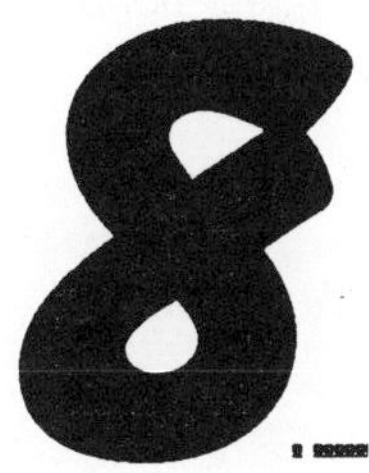

FACTORS INFLUENCING TOXICITY

Factors related to toxicant
Factors related to exposure conditions
Factors related to subject
Factors related to environmental conditions

For a toxic effect to occur, the toxic agent or its active metabolite must reach the target site of action at a sufficient high concentration and for sufficient time duration to initiate a toxic change. While toxicity is an inherent property of a substance, the nature and extent of toxic manifestations in an animal that is exposed to the substance depend on a variety of factors. These factors can be divided into 4 groups.

I. Factors related to toxicant.
II. Factors related to exposure conditions.
III. Factors related to subject.
IV. Factors related to environmental conditions.

I. FACTORS RELATED TO TOXICANT

a. Type of salt form: The nature and type of salt formation of a toxicant influence its solubility, rate of dissolution, absorption and bioavailability. For example, barium sulphate is poorly soluble, less absorbed and hence less toxic than the barium chloride, which is more soluble, readily absorbed and very toxic. Similarly, red phosphorus is non-toxic because it is insoluble, non-volatile and readily eliminated from the body as compared to yellow phosphorus, which is more soluble and toxic.

b. Nature and type of dosage form: Apart from the toxicant itself, toxicity often depends to a great extent on the dosage form of the toxicant. The more complex a dosage form, the greater is the number of rate-limiting steps. As a general rule, the bioavailability of a toxicant from various dosage forms is in the following order: solutions > emulsions > suspensions > capsules > tablets > sustained released products.

c. Composition of sample: Impurities or contaminants present in commercial products can modify the response of biological system to the toxicant. For example, herbicide 2, 4, 5-T use has declined because of contamination by dioxins produced during its manufacturing which are highly hazardous.

d. Formulation and vehicle effects: Toxicity of a compound is markedly influenced by the formulation which can either increase or decrease toxicity by altering the chemical nature of the agent or by affecting the solubility which influences absorption of the toxic agent into biological system. Formulations of wettable powders, suspensions and emulsions can affect the retention rate on hair and skin or the absorption rate from GIT. For example, plant pesticide formulations may be more toxic if used on animals because of the retention properties of the pesticide, which allows excessive pesticide accumulation on animal hair or skin. Organochlorine insecticides (e.g. BHC, DDT) are more toxic if given in oily vehicle due to quick absorption.

e. Physico-chemical properties of toxicant:

i. Lipid solubility: Chemicals with high lipid solubility are more readily absorbed through the lipid-protein matrix of the cell membrane, so are more toxic than those which are water soluble. For example, thiopentone, a derivative of barbituric acid, has high oil: water partition coefficient, so it is rapidly absorbed and rapidly produces CNS depression and general anaesthesia. On the other hand, barbituric acid has low lipid solubility and is inefficient as CNS depressant.

ii. Degree of ionization: Compounds containing groups ionized at physiological pH are usually more water soluble and less likely to be absorbed across membranes (e.g. amines, carboxyls, phosphates and sulphates). Ammonium ion (NH_4^+) is absorbed less across rumen wall than ammonia (NH_3).

iii. Polarity: Non-polar compounds are more readily absorbed across membranes than polar compounds.

iv. Molecular weight: Compounds of low molecular weight are more readily absorbed than large complex molecules. For example, smaller particles may more readily reach the lungs when inhaled than the larger particles that may cling to hair and get deposited in the upper respiratory tract.

v. Proteins binding: Binding of toxicants to physiological proteins (e.g. albumin) can restrict the availability of active drug by limiting its passage across membranes. Such binding may also retard excretion of the toxicant by reducing the glomerular filtration rate.

II. FACTORS RELATED TO EXPOSURE CONDITIONS

a. Dose/Amount of toxicant : The occurrence and magnitude of toxic effect depends on the amount of substance absorbed into blood stream that further depends on the dose or amount of toxicant ingested. Normally, response of a toxicant increases with increase in the dose, but within a limit. Control of dose/dosage is the basis of safety measures in the use of chemicals. A sufficiently large dose of an ordinarily harmless drug (e.g. sodium chloride) may prove fatal, but a small dose of a potent poison is without any effect and even some are used as therapeutic agents (e.g. arsenical compounds and atropine).

b. Route and site of exposure: Major routes by which toxicants gain access to the body are through GIT (oral), lungs (inhalation), skin (topical) and through parental administration. Compounds are usually more toxic by oral route than dermal route. However, some organophosphrus insecticides are quickly absorbed by dermal route and less by intestine. Elemental mercury is virtually non-toxic by oral route, but highly toxic when its vapour is inhaled. DDT is almost equally toxic to insects and mammals when given parenterally, but when applied externally it is much more toxic to insects as the chitinous exoskeleton of insects is more permeable to the DDT than the mammalian skin.

c. Rate of administration: Rate of administration or exposure governs the speed and intensity of toxic response. With few exceptions, rapid intravenous administration of drugs is more toxic than when given by slow infusion. For example, diacetylmonoxime administration by rapid I.V. injection produces severe side effects, but same when given slowly is well tolerated. Urea can be highly toxic when consumed rapidly in sufficient quantity to produce high rise in rumen ammonia concentration.

d. Volume and concentration: Toxicity of agents given by oral route tends to be more when given in dilute solutions. But opposite situation occurs with agents whose toxic effects are due to local irritation. Parenteral administration of hypo- or hyper-tonic solutions is more toxic than isotonic solutions. For example, LD_{50} of normal saline (isotonic) by I.V. route is 68 ml/kg in rats, whereas the same of hypotonic solution is 1 ml/kg. Problems associated with large volume are excessive hydration, impaired renal clearance or vehicle toxicity.

e. Time of administration/exposure: Changes in the susceptibility of biological systems to toxic agents may be related to the time of administration or diurnal factors. Most of the diurnal variations are related to the eating and sleeping habits of the test species. For example, in nocturnal animals such as rats, there is more food in the stomach in the morning than in the afternoon. So absorption of toxic agent is variable depending on the time of its exposure. In human beings, hypnotics are more effective if taken in the evening, as darkness itself has sedative action.

f. Schedule of dosage: Schedule of dosage may have an important influence on the response of a toxicant. Generally, a single large dose produces more response than the same amount given in divided doses. However for a toxicant that is cumulative in nature, divided doses may produce more toxic effect. An oral dose when given empty stomach is usually absorbed over a brief period to produce more toxicity than the same dose administered in full stomach. However, some toxicants like cyanogenetic glycosides are more toxic in full stomach.

g. Duration and frequency of exposure: The toxic response of few substances varies with the duration and frequency of exposure. For some agents, toxic effects of single administration are quite different from those produced by repeated administration. For example, some organophosphorus insecticides (e.g. monocrotophos) in acute toxicity produce characteristic anti-cholinesterase manifestations like salivation, muscle tremors, dyspnoea and convulsions, but they on repeated exposure produce delayed neuropathy (e.g. paralysis of limbs). Some agents are more toxic on repeated administration due to their cumulative toxic effect (e.g. copper) than after the single exposure.

h. Interaction of compounds: The toxicity of a substance may be increased or decreased by a simultaneous or consecutive exposure to another substance. Presence of contaminants like natural toxins (e.g. aflatoxin), feed additives and pesticides etc. in feed or food products may alter the response of any toxicant by interaction.

i. Potentiation: This occurs when toxicity of a substance is increased by another substance that alone has no toxic effect. For example, isopropanol has no effect on the liver, but it can considerably increase the hepatotoxic effect of carbon tetrachloride.

ii. Addition: This occurs when two toxicants having same mechanism of action are given together and they produce an additive toxic effect. For example, simultaneous use of two or more organophosphorus insecticides produces an additive toxic effect due to their combined effect on cholinesterase enzyme.

iii. Synergism: This occurs when two toxicants used together produce a toxic effect that is more than their individual effects. For example, both carbon tetrachloride and ethanol are hepatotoxicants, but together they produce much more injury to the liver than expected from the mathematical sum of their individual effects.

iv. Antagonism: This occurs when two agents neutralise one another's action. For example, there are less chances of OP insecticides toxicity, if atropine is already present in the animal's body. Similarly, tannins and proteins in the GI tract can complex with toxicants and reduce their absorption.

i. Palatability: Palatability may increase voluntary intake of toxicants and thus their toxicity. For example, flavoured and paraffin-embedded rodenticides are used to enhance palatability. This increases toxicant uptake by rodents and thus their mortality.

III. FACTORS RELATED TO SUBJECT

a. Species: There is wide biological diversity among different species in the rate and pattern of metabolism to detoxify a compound. In addition, differences in absorption, excretion, plasma protein binding, tissue distribution and response at the receptor sites have been postulated. For example, belladonna or atropine is toxic to most species, but not to rabbits due to presence of liver enzyme atropinase which hydrolyses it. Dogs vomit after taking red squill and escape from mortality, but rodents cannot vomit (due to absence of vomiting mechanism) and die. Glucuronide conjugation is less developed in cat, so is highly susceptible to poisoning by agents such as phenol. Species differences (insects vs. mammals) are responsible for observed variations in toxic responses to insecticides.

b. Breed: Breed differences exist in toxicant effect, although they have not been well described. These differences have been attributed mainly to variation in the xenobiotic disposition. For example, ivermectin is more toxic to Collies breed of dogs as it readily crosses blood-brain barrier in this species. Greyhounds are more susceptible to the toxic effects of thiobarbiturates because their lean body weight provides little fat for drug re-distribution.

c. Strains: Different strains of same species may show variations in drug response. For example, different strains of mice vary widely in their ability to metabolise barbiturates and consequently the magnitude of pharmacological or toxicological response. Albino Norway rats are more susceptible to norbormide (oral LD_{50}, 4-3 mg/kg) than the wild strain of Norway rats (oral LD_{50}, 12 mg/kg) while the same toxicant is non-toxic to dogs, cats, sheep, and monkeys.

d. Sex : Male and female animals of the same strain and species usually exhibit only slight differences in susceptibility to toxic agents. But there are some exceptions. For example, female rats are 2 times more susceptible to the toxic effect of red squill than the male rats. Male mice are highly susceptible to nephrotoxic effect of chloroform but females show virtually no effect. Sex related differences in toxicity to agents are mostly seen where enzymatic biotransformation of agent is influenced by sex hormones.

e. Pregnancy: Pregnancy causes marked hormonal and metabolic changes, thus affecting toxicity of some agents. High progesterone levels during pregnancy may increase hepatic microsomal enzymes that may cause increase metabolism of some drugs and toxicants. Similarly, development of placenta enhances metabolism of some xenobiotics. In general, pregnancy has been shown to increase the susceptibility of mice to some pesticides. Anticoagulant rodenticides are more toxic to pregnant than non-pregnant animals.

f. Lactation: Similar to pregnancy, lactation alters toxicokinetics of certain poisons. Lactation may enhance excretion of some lipophilic toxicants (e.g., DDT, polychlorinated biphenyls) in the milk. Toxicants in milk may have their own unwanted effects on the suckling young ones and consumers.

g. Age: Young animals are often more susceptible to toxicants than adults. This is mainly due to less development of drug metabolising enzymes and increased membrane permeability. Older animals are also more susceptible to toxicants mainly due to loss of structural proteins and drug metabolising enzymes. For example, calves and lambs are markedly more susceptible than adult cattle or sheep to sprays or dips of chlordane, dieldrin and lindane. Neonates are highly susceptible to carbon monoxide toxicity mainly due to increased CO binding to neonate haemoglobin.

h. Body weight and composition: In toxicological studies, it is customary to adjust the dose on the basis of body weight. However, use of body weight may not always be correct. Differences between body weight and true lean body weight should be taken when dealing with conditions like obesity, starvation, ascites, generalised oedema, starvation, old age, etc. In obese animals, water soluble agents generally do not distribute into increased body fat which may result in higher than expected plasma toxicant concentration and hence adverse effects. On the other hand, highly lipid soluble agents (e.g. anaesthetics) are required in higher dosage in obese animals or species like pigs due to their higher storage in body fat. This increases susceptibility of obese animals or pigs to anaesthetics.

i. Emotional status: Toxicity of a substance may be affected by the emotional status and temperament of animal. This is particularly applicable to centrally acting agents. For example, an excited animal may require higher dose of a CNS depressant than the animal which is already depressed. Anything that emotionally disturbs the animal may influence its physiological reaction and, thus, possible change in reactions to foreign chemicals.

j. Genetic status: Genetic makeup of the subject often markedly influences the response to a toxicant. This may be related to gene-related alterations in xenobiotic metabolism or alterations in tissue-receptor sensitivity. These variations may lead to genetic tolerance, intolerance or idiosyncratic reactions in susceptible individuals. Several genetic factors have been elucidated in man, but they are less studied in animals. For example, individuals having low level of pseudocholinesterase show prolonged muscular relaxation and apnoea produced by suxamethonium. Individuals with Glucose-6-phosphate dehydrogenase deficiency are more susceptible to the haemolytic effect of drugs like sulphonamides, aspirin and acetanilide.

k. Hormonal status : In addition to pregnancy and sex, there are number of other hormonally dependent situations that may influence the toxicity of various agents. For example, hyperthyroidism and hyperinsulinism may alter the susceptibility of animals to toxic agents. In human beings, the elevated thyroid hormones activate some cytochrome P-450 enzymes (e.g. hydroxylation), while activities of others (e.g. N-demethylation) are decreased. Adrenalectomised rats are generally more susceptible to toxicants due to absence of stress fighting hormone adrenaline.

l. Nutritional status : Nutritional status of animal at the time of exposure is an important factor determining the toxic response as a well-nourished animal easily copes with the disposition of toxicants. In animals suffering from protein-caloric malnutrition, absorption, distribution, metabolism and excretion processes may all be impaired. Protein deficiency for longer period results in reduced metabolic activity of microsomal enzyme and lesser availability of endogenous substrates like glutathione. For example, paracetamol is more hepatotoxic in protein deficient animals, possibly due to decreased hepatic glutathione levels. The acute toxicity of captan (fungicide) is many times more in rats maintained on protein deficient diet (oral LD_{50} = 480 mg/kg) as compared to those maintained on normal protein diet (oral LD_{50} = 12,500 mg/kg). Starvation for few hours increases susceptibility of ruminants to urea poisoning due to carbohydrate deficiency and may produce deleterious changes in the conjugative activity of glucuronic acid. Starvation also increases tendency to ingest toxic amounts of poisonous plants and may increase susceptibility to some mycotoxins. Deficiency of vitamins, especially antioxidant vitamins E and C can result in increased damage from free radicals. Dietary deficiency of vitamins (e.g. vitamins A, B_2, B_3, C and E) and minerals (e.g., Fe, Ca, Mg, Cu, and Zn) retard metabolic activity of several enzymes.

m. Tolerance: Failure of an animal to react to the ordinary dose of an agent may be seen after continuous intake of that agent in small doses over long period. Tolerance has been related to the changes either in the disposition of xenobiotic that reduces its effective concentration in the system or in the target system that render the system least responsive. Acquired tolerance can develop to opium, alcohol and some OP insecticides.

n. Individual differences: Individual variations are common in all types of toxicological tests. Within a population, some animals are hypersensitive and some are hyposensitive to toxicants. These individual variations are unrelated to the toxicant and are not attributable to genetic or other biological factors. For example, acute oral toxicity of some pesticides shows great variation in their lethal dose for rats of the same strain in a population.

o. Disease and Pathological states: Pathological conditions, particularly those affecting major organ systems or altering fluid pH and electrolytes, can substantially alter both the disposition and the toxic action of many agents.

i. Liver diseases: Liver diseases may reduce activity of microsomal enzymes, thus altering the biotransformation and action of several drugs and toxicants. Liver diseases can also reduce synthesis of protective binding molecules (e.g. glutathione) allowing increased adverse effect of toxicants. Reduced synthesis of plasma proteins, particularly albumin, may alter the xenobiotic binding capacity. For example, hepatitis impairs biotransformation and prolongs action of injectable anaesthetics as a result of which ultra-short acting barbiturates become toxic. Impaired biotransformation due to acute and chronic hepatitis, cirrhosis of liver and hepatic necrosis also leads to enhanced activity of several pesticides.

ii. Kidney diseases: Kidney diseases often result in decreased drug clearance and, thus, slower removal of toxicants from the body. Drug induced toxicity in renal insufficiency may also result from either derangement of acid-base balance or increased sensitivity to the agent due to uraemia-induced alterations in tissue receptors. For example, in renal patients with impaired function, aminoglycosides and heavy metals (e.g. mercury) accumulate to toxic levels in body.

iii. Other diseases: Several other pathological states may influence the toxic response of a number of agents. Cardiovascular insufficiency due to either cardiac failure or circulatory shock potentially affects disposition of toxicants by altering their distribution and elimination. Neurological disturbances may influence animal's response to several CNS acting toxicants like morphine. Respiratory diseases like asthma render the animals more susceptible to pollutants like SO_2. Constipation increases the toxicity of orally ingested substances due to enhanced absorption as the passage of toxicant is delayed.

IV. FACTORS RELATED TO ENVIRONMENTAL CONDITIONS

a. Temperature: Environmental temperature has been demonstrated to influence toxic response in animals by affecting absorption, storage, metabolism and elimination. Such changes are apparently related to the temperature dependent biochemical reactions responsible for the effect and disposition of chemicals. Low environmental temperature enhances biotransformation of xenobiotics possibly because the metabolic activity increases to keep the body warm. Oxidative uncouplers increase body temperature and, thus, their toxic effect is more significant in hot weathers.

Organochlorine and pyrethroid insecticides show negative correlation with environmental temperature (more toxic in low temperature and vice-versa).

b. Atmospheric pressure and altitude: Atmospheric pressure and altitude can affect the toxic response of some agents. Such changes in response to drugs and poisons are generally associated with changes in environmental oxygen tension. High altitude with low atmospheric pressure reduces the potential of body to oxidise xenobiotics, as low oxygen is available to the body. Similarly, low oxygen concentration resulting from high altitude may be a factor in the toxicity of compounds that primarily affects cardiovascular functions. For example, carbon monoxide, barbiturates and cyanide are more toxic in low oxygen conditions. Greater toxicities of digitalis, red squill and strychnine are observed at high altitude as compared to low altitudes.

c. Light and other radiations: Light factors affect biological rhythms in some animals and influence susceptibility to toxicants. In rat and mouse, the activities of cytochrome P-450 are greatest at the beginning of the dark phase. Certain drugs (e.g. phenothiazine, demeclocycline and tar products) show photosensitization reactions when the individual is exposed to sunlight or UV radiations. Toxicity of atropine generally increases if the intoxicated animal is exposed to direct sunlight because of its mydriatic and cycloplegic effects on eyes. Similar to light, radiation exposure also alters response to a toxicant by modifying enzyme systems and normal disposition of toxicants. Whole body irradiation increases the toxicity of CNS stimulants but decreases that of CNS depressants.

d. Relative humidity: Relative humidity might influence the reaction of an animal to a toxicant especially those exposed by dermal route. For example, dermal absorption of some ectoparasiticides (e.g. organophosphorus insecticides) increases in hot and humid environment because more blood is diverted to skin (so rapid absorption) to affect cooling.

e. Environmental pollution: Chemicals in the environment are capable of influencing toxic responses in a variety of ways by altering biotransformation (induction or inhibition of hepatic microsomal enzymes), affinity for receptors, absorption, distribution and excretion of toxicants. For example, exposure to insecticides (e.g. DDT) and tobacco smoke are well known to induce drug metabolism. Chronic exposure to air pollutants (e.g. sulphur oxide gases) causes thickening of respiratory tract mucous membranes that may impair absorption and action of some respiratory poisons. Inhalation of dusts containing minerals and organic matter for long periods may produce pulmonary diseases in humans and animals.

f. Ventilation: Poor air circulation in sheds and barns may aggravate toxicity of some agents. For example, silo gases accumulate in confined spaces and settle to low spots causing toxicity. Malfunctioning of heating or ventilation equipment in poorly ventilated shed may set the stage for toxicosis from poisonous gases such as carbon monoxide or natural gases which contain methane.

g. Management and social factors: Animal husbandry practices and social factors can modify the toxicity of some chemicals. These include handling of animals, housing (single or in groups), size and type of cages, visitors, bedding material, etc. For example, toxicity of drugs like amphetamine and other CNS stimulants is enhanced by crowding (more number of animals per cage) and handling of animals. External disturbances like sound and visitors generally aggravate poisoning of convulsants like strychnine.

BIBLIOGRAPHY

Ballantyne B, Marrs T and Turner P (1995) General and Applied Toxicology. (Eds.). Macmillan Press Ltd., London.

Brahmankar DM and Jaiswal SB (1995) Biopharmaceutics and Pharmacokinetics A Treatise. Vallabh Prakashan, Delhi.

Clarke ECG and Clarke ML (1967) Garner's Veterinary Toxicology. 3rd edn. Williams and Wilkins, Baltimore.

Eaton DL and Klaassen (1996) Principles of Toxicology. In: Casarett's and Doull's Toxicology: The Basic science of Poisons.

5th edn. Klaassen CD (Ed.) p 13. McGraw Hill Companies Inc., New York.

Garg SK (2000) Veterinary Toxicology. CBS Publishers & Distributors, New Delhi.

Hatch RC (1982) Veterinary toxicology: Introduction. In: John's Veterinary Pharmacology and Therapeutics. 5th edn. Booth NH and McDonald LE (Eds.) p 927. Kalyani Publishers, Ludhiana-New Delhi.

Lu FC and Kacew S (2002) Lu's Basic Toxicology: Fundamentals, Target Organs and Risk Assessment. Taylor & Francis, New York.

Osweiler GD (1996) Toxicology. Williams and Wilkins, Philadelphia.

Osweiler GD (1999) Introduction to toxicology. In: Veterinary Toxicology. Beasley V (Ed.) International Veterinary Information Service, Ithaca NY (www.ivis.org).

Novotny MA (2001) Pharmacodynamics: Mechanisms of drug action. In: Veterinary Pharmacology and Therapeutics. 8th edn. Adams HR (Ed.) p. 9. Iowa State Univ. Press, Iowa.

Rozman KK, Doull and Wyaland JH (2001) Dose, time, and other factors influencing toxicity. In: Handbook of Pesticide Toxicology. 2nd edn. Vol. I: Principles. Krieger RI (Ed.). p 1. Academic Press, San Diego.

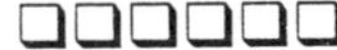

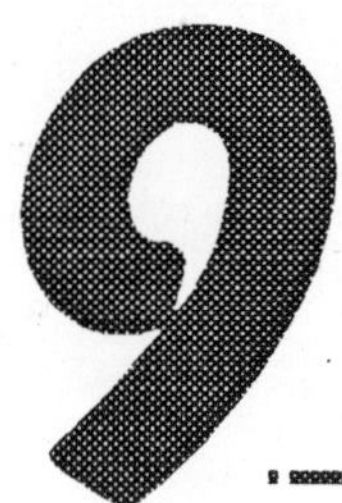

DIAGNOSIS OF POISONING

History
Circumstantial evidence
Clinical signs
Pathological evidence
Analytical evidence
Experimental evidence
Response to treatment

Diagnosis is the evaluation of a patient and the signs and symptoms of a disease or dysfunction to arrive at a cause. It allows application of safety measures to correct the effects of poisoning or to arrive at a conclusion to ascertain the cause of poisoning. Under field conditions, any disease or ailment, if not diagnosed properly, may be suspected for poisoning, particularly when there is sudden death. Diagnosis of poisoning is a difficult task and can not be based on a single observation. A confirmed toxicological diagnosis often rests upon appropriate findings and should take into account the following points:

1. History
2. Circumstantial evidence
3. Clinical signs
4. Pathological evidence
5. Analytical evidence
6. Experimental evidence
7. Response to treatment

1. History

History often gives important clues about the suspected poisoning. Though one should not blindly rely on the history (as it may be corroborated), yet the owner or attendant of the animal should be thoroughly questioned about the nature and type of clinical signs and any other observation made by him as it may give some points or clues. The owner (client) should be questioned about following points that may contribute to the diagnosis of poisoning:

a. Health history:

i. Illness of animal in past 6 months – An animal suffering frequently is less likely to be poisoned (except some chronic toxicity) than that has become ill recently.

ii. Vaccination done in recent past – Rule out non-toxicological problems by knowing the vaccination status of the animal. Recent vaccination, if not done properly, is likely to produce some adverse reaction.

iii. Type and nature of medication given to animal – Recent administration/application of some drug, spray, dip, or anthelmintic, if not carried out properly (e.g. improper dose or improper route), is likely to produce adverse effects. In case of recent medication, try to obtain the sample of the drug and also find out if the drug is given only to one animal or the whole heard.

b. Current clinical history:

i. Number of animals affected in herd/flock – Several animals acutely afflicted at the same time is more suggestive of toxicosis than infectious disease. History of neighbourhood problems with animals inexplicably dying may also be explored.

ii. Animals purchased or home raised – A recently purchased animal may have doubtful history than a home-raised animal.

iii. Persistence of problem in herd/ flock – Persistence of disease in the herd is more suggestive of nutritional or management origin than a toxicological problem.

c. Diet/Food:

i. Type of feed/fodder – Animals often prefer good food. Grazing animals generally do not eat toxic plants, unless good forage is available. Recent application of pesticide on the forage crop may likely to harm animals.

ii. Recent changes in diet – Change in the diet may suggest sudden alteration in nutritional value. Illness with change in diet is also suggestive of the contamination of diet with some harmful substance. Correlate timing of any change in feed with onset of problem.

iii. Source of drinking water – Presence of algae growth or water from nearby industry may be suggestive of its contamination with toxic substances. Pesticides recently applied to the grass, grazing land, or areas through which water might run off and pass through may contaminate water source and make it unfit for consumption.

iv. Presence of spoiled or mouldy feed/food – Spoiled or mouldy food are source of mycotoxins and hence a source of poisoning.

d. Onset of action:

i. Sudden onset of action or signs develop gradually – If animal becomes acutely ill in 3-4 hours, it is more likely to be poisoned than an animal that has been gradually suffering for past few days or weeks. Sudden onset of acute signs is generally more characteristic of toxicosis or trauma than of nutritional or infectious disease.

ii. Occurrence of vomiting or diarrhoea before onset of systemic signs – Occurrence of nausea, vomiting, or diarrhoea before onset of systemic signs is often indicative of a systemic substance. Many toxicants possess irritant properties and are likely to induce nausea/vomiting by GI irritation before they are absorbed in sufficient amount.

e. Clinical signs:

i. Types of clinical signs seen – Type and nature of clinical signs observed are important indicator of poisoning in animals. Type of signs observed like ataxia, salivation, excitation, seizures, vomiting, diarrhoea, depression, etc. should be correlated with the suspected poison.

2. Circumstantial Evidence

Circumstantial evidence is an important factor and provides rapid and simple step for diagnosis of poisoning. Toxicologist should analyse and correlate the circumstances with the available information. Again, no opinion on the circumstantial proof should be made. Toxicologist should certify the cause of death from facts only.

a. Housing:

i. Recently painted house – Recently painted house or furnisher/equipment may expose animals, particularly pets, to the lead and other harmful chemicals in the paint. Ingestion of varnish, solvents, cleaners, spot removers and other materials used during painting and polishing of room/ furnishers also expose pets to their deleterious effects.

ii. Inadequate ventilation – Inadequate ventilation is an important precipitating factor to toxic effect of certain gases like carbon monoxide. Incomplete combustion of fossil fuels used to warm sheds during winter, particularly in poorly ventilated rooms, is a source of toxic gases.

iii. Overcrowding of animals – Overcrowding of animals aggravate effects of CNS stimulants like amphetamine. Overcrowding also disturbs animals and may change their physiological response to external stimuli.

iv. Location of shed/house – Location of animal shed/house near some industry or drainage often exposes animals to various contaminants through air, water and soil. Contamination of water reservoir and herbage by industrial effluents and wastes often leads to poisonings among animals.

v. Recently sprayed shed/pillars – Animals have a tendency to lick or rub their back against pillars/posts. Licking of sheds/pillars that are recently sprayed with pesticides is an important source of poisoning in domestic animals. The present and previous use of pesticides in the premises should be carefully seen.

vi. Roaming – Dogs and cats that run free have more risk of exposure to chemicals than those which are house bound.

b. Food and water:

i. Storage conditions – Faulty storage of food/feed often leads to contamination of food with mycotoxins and bacteriotoxins. The condition of the food should be carefully observed to rule out presence of mycotoxins. Where the food is stored or what is stored with it, should also be taken into account.

ii. Water – Observe carefully the sanitary/condition of drinking water source. Also observe if the pond has been recently sprayed by pesticides for public health purposes.

c. Environment:

i. Atmospheric pollution – Industrial gases, vapours, and dusts often produce adverse effects on the health of animals. Chronic exposure to air pollutants may impair normal respiratory functions and produce respiratory disease.

ii. Poisonous plants or animals – Presence of poisonous plants in the surroundings or movement of snakes around the premises are important source of poisoning. These may be taken into consideration while arriving at any diagnosis in cases of poisoning.

iii. Type of soil – Some soils are rich in some elements and may lead to poisoning through water or fodder grown on it. High level of nitrate/nitrite, arsenic, molybdenum or other heavy metals in water or soil may be responsible for poisoning of animals or birds.

d. Other clues:

i. Smell from surroundings – A peculiar smell from the animal's surrounding may also help in cases of poisoning. Use of pesticides in the vicinity of animals or industrial contamination of water source may be judged from the smell.

ii. Colour of urine – Some poisons impart colour to urine and may be diagnosed from it. Pink colour of urine is seen in phenothiazine poisoning, yellow colour in picric acid, phenacetin or furazolidone poisoning, and dark green colour in phenols and cresols poisoning.

iii. Consistency of faeces – Loose consistency of faeces is observed in poisons that induce diarrhoea. Constipated consistency of faeces may be observed in some poisons like oxalate.

3. Clinical Signs

In this, diagnosis is based on the signs/symptoms shown by the living animal or history given by the owner, if animal is dead. Clinical signs must be used to initiate a search for poisons and should not used alone for the diagnosis. The clinical signs and symptoms although not conclusive are often indicative of specific poisonings (Table 9.1) and speed of onset and duration of signs may identify some of the toxicants and rule out others. Similarly, morbidity and mortality rates may also give clues to the type of toxicant.

Table 9.1: List of toxic signs associated with some important poisons in animals.

I. Central Nervous System
1. *Convulsions:* Ammonium salts, cyanide, lead, nitrate, phenols, strychnine, ethylene glycol, picrotoxin, camphor, theophylline, organophosphorus, carbamate and organochlorine insecticides, and many plants.
2. *Coma:* Bromide, carbon monoxide, chloral hydrate, zinc phosphide, nicotine, barbiturates and other anaesthetics, atropine, alcohols, phenols, turpentine, benzene, morphine and derivatives, and hydrogen sulphide.
Contd..

3. *Ataxia:* Bromide, alcohol, hypnotics/sedatives, organophosphorus and carbamate insecticides and thallium.

II. Digestive system

1. *Nausea, vomiting and diarrhoea:* Heavy metals (antimony, arsenic, barium, chromium, copper, iron, mercury, thallium, zinc), strong acids and alkalis, chlorates, fluoride (acute poisoning), yellow phosphorus, selenium (acute poisoning), alcohols, phenols, paraffin, muscarine, organophosphorus compounds and many plants.
2. *Constipation:* Lead, opioids, thallium and oxalate.
3. *Hypersalivation:* Organophosphorus and carbamate insecticides.
4. *Dry mouth:* Atropine, opioids and phenothiazines.
5. *Gastrointestinal bleeding:* Aspirin, caustics (strong acid or base) and oral anticoagulants.

III. Respiratory system

1. *Dyspnoea:* Alcohols, hypnotics/sedatives, opioids, organophosphorus and carbamate insecticides, carbon monoxide, cyanide, hydrogen sulphide, nitrate and nitrite, sulphur dioxide, zinc phosphide and strychnine.
2. *Hyperpnoea:* Aspirin, ethylene glycol, isoniazid, methanol, pentachlorophenol, hydroxybenzonitrile herbicides, ammonium salts, urea, nicotine, atropine (early stages) and apomorphine.
3. *Slow respiration:* Selenium and atropine (late stages).
4. *Pulmonary oedema:* Aspirin, chlorophenoxy herbicides, irritant gases, organic solvents, paraquat and alpha-naphthylthiourea.

IV. Skin, hair and nails

1. *Cyanosis (methaemoglobin):* Nitrite, aniline and dyes, nitrobenzene and chlorates.
2. *Photosensitization:* Phenothiazine, *lantana camara* and many plants.
3. *Alopecia:* Thallium, alkali sulphide, x-radiation, radium and arsenic (chronic).
4. *Staining of skin:* Iodine (black), bromide (deep brown), picric acid (yellow) and silver nitrate (blue black).

V. Eyes

1. *Dilation of pupils:* Belladonna and derivatives (atropine, hyoscyamine), nicotine (later stages), aconite, stramonium, cocaine, amphetamine, ephedrine, ether, chloroform, hydrogen sulphide, iodine and tricyclic antidepressants.
2. *Constriction of pupil:* Opium derivatives (morphine), nicotine (initial stages) physostgimine and other parasympathomimetic drugs (pilocarpine, muscarine), and organophosphorus and carbamate insecticides.

VI. Urogenital tract

1. *Urinary retention:* Opioids, atropine and tricyclic antidepressants.
2. *Frequent micturition and incontinence:* Organophosphorus and carbamate insecticides.
3. *Haemoglobinurea:* Chlorate and copper (chronic).
4. *Colouring of urine:* Phenol and resorcinol (dark green), picric acid (yellow) and pyrogallol (brown or black).

VII. Body temperature

1. *Hyperthermia:* Organochlorine insecticides, dinitrophenol pesticides, hydroxybenzonitrile herbicides, pentachlorophenol and quinidine.
2. *Hypothermia:* Alcohol, opioids, carbon monoxide, sedatives/hypnotics and phenothiazines.

VIII. Musculo-skeletal system

1. *Muscular inco-ordination:* Ammonium salts, carbon monoxide, cyanide, lead, nitrate and nitrite, nicotine, turpentine, oxalate and some plants.
2. *Lameness:* Fluoride (chronic), selenium (chronic) and ergot.

Limitations

The evidence of toxic signs may not be helpful in all types of poisoning cases, particularly when they are associated with following conditions:

a. Different toxicants produce same type of signs or toxicants of same group produce different signs. For example, BHC and aldrin produce CNS stimulation and depression, respectively, though both belong to organochlorine group of insecticides.

b. One toxicant is neutralised or potentiated by another toxicant. For example, alcohol potentiates CNS depressant effect of barbiturates.

c. Same toxicant produces different signs in different species of animals. For example, morphine produces CNS depression in most mammals but CNS stimulation in cats.

d. Some signs of poisoning (e.g. vomiting, seizures) can also be produced by infectious diseases or metabolic and endocrine disorders.

e. The clinician sees only one phase of the progression of the disease. In such cases owner should be asked if he has seen other signs.

4. Pathological Evidence

If the animal dies, a thorough necropsy should be performed and appropriate specimens collected. Lesions of poisoning are usually less characteristic as many toxicants cause neither gross nor microscopic lesions. However, necropsy findings may provide definite clues to the nature of toxicant in some cases.

***a.* Lesions:** Presence and lack of lesions should be closely observed.

External examination:

i. Odour: A characteristic odour emanating from the carcass (stomach or rumen content on opening the carcass) may be the first indication of poisoning when animal arrives for necropsy. For example, bitter almond smell is given by cyanide or benzaldehyde, garlic smell by phosphorus, and ammoniacal smell by ammonia or urea (Table 9.2). However, a large number of individuals do not have 'gifted' olfactory apparatus to detect all types of smell; therefore, the absence of a classic odour does not exclude the presence of toxicant.

ii. Skin and mucous membranes: The skin and mucous membrane appearance may be important indication for some types of poisonings. For example, skin and mucosa may be jaundiced (pale) in phosphorus, naphthalene and arsine gas intoxication, cyanotic (blue or brownish-blue colour) in carbon monoxide, nitrite/nitrate,

Table 9.2: Characteristic smells associated with some important poisons.

Smell	Possible poison
Ammoniacal	Ammonia and urea
Bitter almond	Cyanide and benzaldehyde
Formaldehyde	Formaldehyde and methanol
Fruity	Alcohols (including ethanol) and esters
Garlic	Arsenic and phosphorus
Mothballs	Camphor and naphthalene
Pears	Chloral hydrate and paraldehyde
Petrol	Petroleum distillate
Phenolic	Phenol and phenolic disinfectants
Rotten egg	Hydrogen sulphide and disulfiram
Stale tobacco	Nicotine
Shoe polish	Nitrobenzene
Sweet	Chloroform and other halogenated hydrocarbons

phenacetin and carbon disulphide poisoning, flushed (red or pink) in alcohol and cyanide poisoning, and yellow in acute copper poisoning. Presence of burns on skin may be observed in case of caustics (strong alkalis and acids) or phenol poisoning and alopecia may be observed in molybdenosis and whole body irradiation.

iii. Condition of carcass: The condition of carcass is suggestive of some types of poisoning. For example, carcass is usually lacerated in cases of extensive convulsive seizures produced by poisons like organochlorine insecticides. Laceration and wound on head or face or broken teeth may be encountered in poisonings which produce agitated and violent behavioural changes e.g. acute lead and organochlorine insecticides poisoning.

Internal examination: Gross examination of tissues/organs on opening the carcass occasionally aids in diagnosis of some of the poisoning cases. Although the lesions of poisoning may not be of pathognomonic importance, they may provide clue to some poisonings.

i. GI tract: The gastrointestinal tract should be examined for signs of irritant and corrosive toxicants which are likely to be found in the oesophagus, stomach and intestine. Severe gastroenteritis indicates that poisoning may be due to corrosive acid or alkali, salts of heavy metals or irritant plants. Stomach and intestinal contents should be examined for abnormal colour (greenish-blue colour in copper and black colour in sulphuric acid poisoning) and presence of plant materials, foreign objects, tablets or capsules, etc.

ii. Respiratory tract: Lesions in the respiratory tract indicates inhalation of irritant gases or volatile liquids. Frothing in the lungs may occur due to excessive exudation and struggling as seen in poisons like ANTU. Other lesions observed in some poisonings may include hydrothorax, pulmonary oedema, pneumonia, etc.

iii. Liver and kidneys: Hepatic and renal lesions indicate that toxicant is irritant in nature, metabolised in liver and excreted via kidney. Fatty liver, centrilobular hepatic necrosis, pale swollen renal cortex, etc. may be observed in some poisonings, but they are generally non-specific and non-characteristic.

iv. Other tissues/organs: Common lesions observed in other body tissues include cardiac dilatation and necrosis, cerebral oedema and haemorrhage, meningitis, bony exostoses, changes in glands, etc. Generalised haemorrhages in body may indicate sweet clover poisoning.

***b.* Histopathology:** Appropriate organs and tissues should be saved in 10% neutral buffered formalin for microscopic examination by a pathologist. Some intoxication can be confirmed by microscopic examination e.g. renal oxalate crystals appear in ethylene glycol poisoning; hepatic lipidosis and bile duct proliferation occur in aflatoxicosis.

5. Analytical Evidence

The important proof of poisoning lies in the detection of a significant amount of the toxic material in the body of animal. Detection of toxicant in the excreta (vomitus, urine, etc.) and blood during life and in the gastrointestinal contents and tissues of the body after death may be done by various methods available including the chemical methods. Samples for toxicological analysis are taken during the post-mortem examination. It is possible to test a group of toxicants or a single toxicant but is not feasible to test all toxicants in an ordinary laboratory. Chemical analysis for toxicants is very important for the diagnosis of poisoning, but it should not be used alone to make a final and conclusive diagnosis due to following reasons:

- *a.* It is possible that the animal might have died from the effects of a toxicant, and yet none may be found in the body after death because whole of the toxicant might have excreted from the body or has been detoxified into inactive metabolite and then eliminated from the body.
- *b.* Some chemicals produce toxicosis but are present at very low levels (below detection levels) in tissues.
- *c.* Some toxicants may not be detected in the viscera, as they have no reliable analytical procedure e.g. organophosphates.
- *d.* Some chemicals can accumulate to high levels in certain tissues without causing toxicosis e.g. organochlorine insecticides residues in body fat.
- *e.* Interactions with other agents or nutrients can inactivate a toxicant stored in the tissues, e.g. mercury can form a complex with selenium and protein, resulting in a non-toxic storage form.

6. Experimental Evidence

Experimental feeding of suspected bait or feed may be useful when other approaches are inadequate. Experimental animals may be fed with the suspected food or the toxicant after it is separated from the viscera and signs exhibited are closely observed. However, the evidence derived in this manner has limited diagnostic applications and can not be relied upon in all cases because of relatively high uncertainty of reproducing field conditions and the poor susceptibility of some experimental species to some groups of toxicants (e.g. rabbits to belladonna leaves and pigeons to opium).

7. Response to Treatment

Response to a test dose of specific antidote in an intoxicated animal may confirm a clinical diagnosis. For example, clinical improvement (reduced salivation, dyspnoea, convulsions, etc.) after administration of atropine is an evidence of anticholinesterase (organophosphorus and carbamate insecticides) poisoning.

BIBLIOGRAPHY

Bartik M and Piskac A (1981) Veterinary Toxicology. Elsevier Scientific Publishing Company, Amsterdam.

Beasley V (1999) Diagnosis and management of toxicoses. In: Veterinary Toxicology. Beasley V (Ed.) p. 36. International Veterinary Information Service, Ithaca NY (www.ivis.org).

Brar R S, Sandhu H S and Singh A (2000) Veterinary Clinical Diagnosis by Laboratory Methods. Kalyani Publishers, Ludhiana-New Delhi.

Brooks VJ and Jacob MB (1958) Poisons. 2nd edn. D Van Nostrand Comp. Inc., Princeton, New Jersey.

Camps FE, Cameron JM and Lanham D (1971) Collectanea of poisons. In: Practical Forensic Medicine. P 343. Hutchinson Medical Publication, London.

Cargill J and Thorpe-Vargas S (2005) Poisoned. Working Dogs Health Articles. (http://www.workingdogs.com/doc0175.htm)

Clarke ECG and Clarke ML (1967) Garner's Veterinary Toxicology. 3rd edn. Williams and Wilkins, Baltimore.

Coles EH (1986) Veterinary Clinical Pathology. WB Saunders Comp., Philadelphia.

Dahlke J (1996) Poison guide. Information page – Poison Guide for Birds and Pets. (http://www.robharvey.com/information/poison.html).

Dorman DC (1997) Diagnosing and treating toxicosis in dogs and cats. *Vet. Med.* 92 : 273.

Franklin CA (1988) Modi's Textbook of Medical Jurisprudence and Toxicology. 21st edn. NM Tripathi Private Ltd., Bombay.

Garg SK (2000) Veterinary Toxicology. CBS Publishers & Distributors, New Delhi.

Hatch RC (1982) Veterinary toxicology: Introduction. In: John's Veterinary Pharmacology and Therapeutics. 5th edn. Booth NH and McDonald LE (Eds.) p 927. Kalyani Publishers, Ludhiana-New Delhi.

Kaye S (1970) Bedside toxicology. *Paed. Clin. North Am.* 17.

Levine A (1993) Forensic toxicology. *J. Anal. Chem.* 65 : 272.

Mofenson HC (1998) Differential diagnosis of poisoning. In: Emergency Toxicology. 2nd edn. Viccellio P (ed.) p 1103. Lippincott-Raven Publishers, Philadelhia.

Olson KR (1992) Poisoning. In: Current Medical Diagnosis and Treatment. Schroeder SA, Knipp MA, Tierneg Lm and Mephce C (Eds.) p 1218. Appleton & Lange, Connecticut.

Osweiler GD (1996) Toxicology. Williams and Wilkins, Philadelphia.

Poppenga RH (1990) Effective use of analytical laboratories for the diagnosis of toxicologic problems in small animal practice. *Vet. Clin. North Am: Small Anim Pract.* 20 : 293.

Radeleff RD (1970) Veterinary Toxicology. 2nd edn. Lea and Febiger, Philadelphia.

Singhal SK (1999) Toxicology at a Glance. 4th edn. MESH Publishing House Pvt. Ltd., Mumbai.

❑❑❑❑❑❑

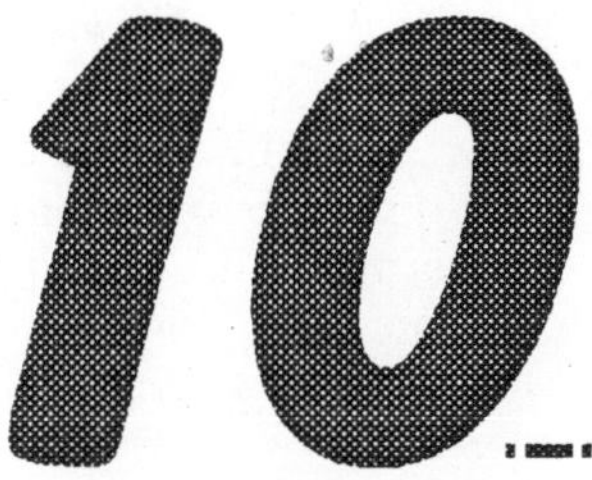

TREATMENT OF POISONING

Preventing continued absorption of toxicant
- Emesis
- Gastric lavage
- Adsorption therapy
- Purgation/Catharsis
- Enema
- Cleansing of skin or hair
- Cleansing of eyes
- Gastrotomy or rumenotomy
- Dilution
- Complex formation

Preventing distribution of toxicant to target site
- Ion-trapping
- Alternate binding site
- Complex formation

Increasing threshold level of toxicity
- Treatment of respiratory depression
- Monitoring of cardiac disturbances
- Control of shock
- Control of acid-base disturbance and electrolyte imbalance
- Treatment of CNS dysfunction
- Treatment of hypothermia or hyperthermia
- Maintenance of uresis
- Specific therapy

Hastening elimination of absorbed toxicant
- Ion-trapping
- Dialysis
- Diuresis
- Specific treatment

Enhancing metabolic conversion of absorbed toxicant

Management of poisoning

Poisoning occurs infrequently, but it is often life-threatening. So treatment and management of poisoning is very important to save the life of the poisoned animals. The treatment should be started as soon as possible because any delay may cause irreparable damage to the animal. Treatment of poisoning differs from treatment of other diseases, being all the cases as emergency cases. The first priority in poisoning is to establish and maintain the vital functions. Specific antidotes like receptor antagonists or chelating agents are available for few poisons and drugs, however for vast majority of drugs and chemicals there is no specific treatment and symptomatic therapy that supports vital functions is the only approach.

The intensity and outcome of *in vivo* toxicity cases depends on many factors including the dose of the toxicant and its concentration at the target site. The delivery of the toxicant to its site of action and its concentration above the threshold level mainly depends on processes of absorption from site of administration into general circulation and distribution via blood to body tissues. The concentration present at the site of action and duration of exposure of a toxicant further depend on the rate of its elimination from the body.

When a toxicant gains access into body by oral, pulmonary or extravascular (IM, SC, etc.) route, it slowly enters the systemic circulation and plasma drug concentration gradually rises to a maximum (peak level). In the time-drug concentration curve (Figure 10.1), the ascending portion of curve to left of peak represents the absorption phase and the descending section of curve to right of peak generally represents the elimination phase. The toxic response is produced only if the toxicant is present above its threshold level at the site of action. The time-drug concentration curve is obtained by measuring the concentration of toxicant in plasma at different time intervals after plotting the concentration of toxicant in plasma (Y-axis) versus the corresponding time at which the plasma samples were collected (X-axis). The time-drug concentration curve is useful in understanding various toxicological parameters and also in the treatment of poisoning.

The major goals in the treatment of poisoned animal include prevention of further absorption of toxicant, removal of unabsorbed toxicant, reduction in distribution of toxicant, use of specific antidote, elimination of absorbed toxicant, support of vital body functions, and symptomatic treatment. The treatment of poisoning can be better explained on the basis of time-drug concentration curve aimed at following points:

I. To decrease slope of ascending portion of curve.
II. To increase threshold level of toxicity.
III. To increase slope of descending portion of curve.

TO DECREASE SLOPE OF ASCENDING PORTION OF CURVE

The slope of ascending curve in the time-concentration profile may be decreased mainly by removing the source of poison. The decrease in the slope of ascending curve leads to slow or no onset of action as the toxicant requires more time to reach the threshold level (Figure 10.2). This may be practically achieved by preventing the continued absorption of toxicant from its exposure site. Decreasing the distribution of toxicant to its target site also delays the onset of action, but the approach involved is of minor importance.

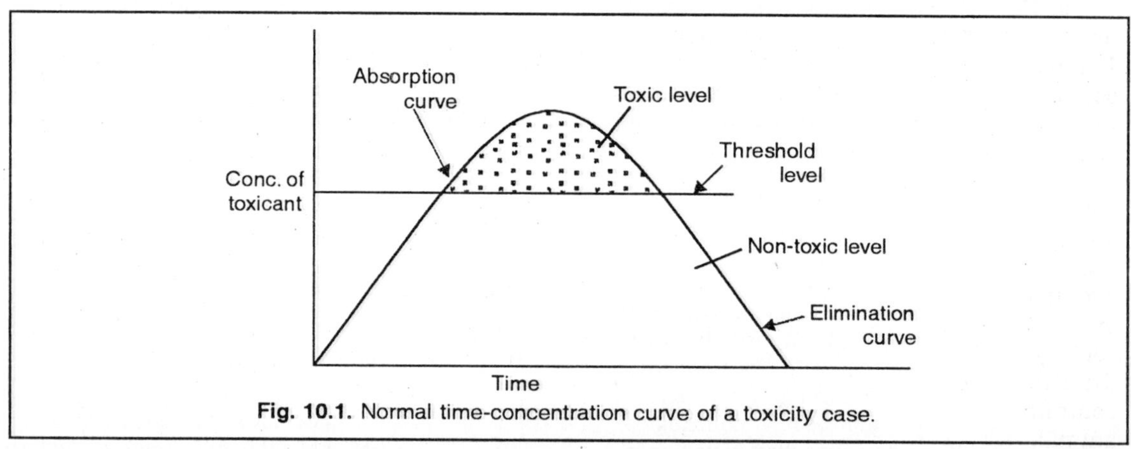

Fig. 10.1. Normal time-concentration curve of a toxicity case.

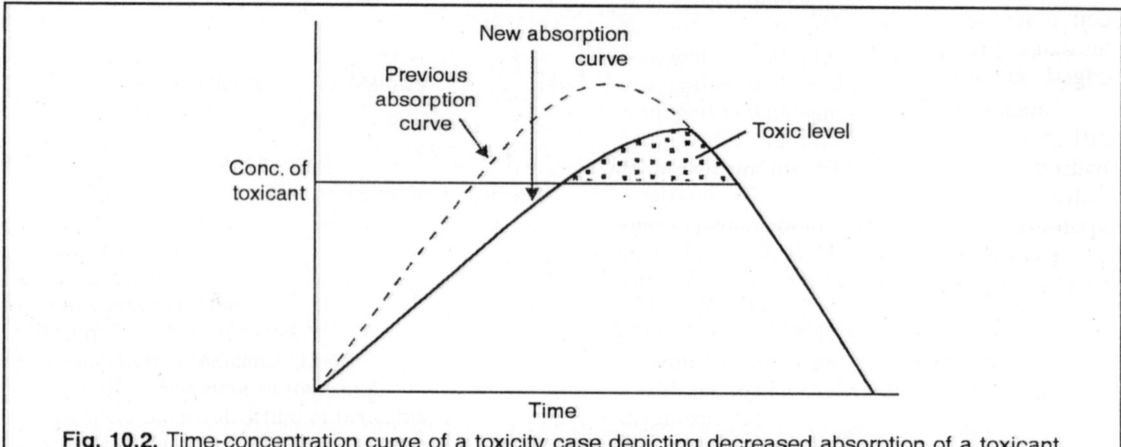

Fig. 10.2. Time-concentration curve of a toxicity case depicting decreased absorption of a toxicant.

Absorption and distribution of a toxicant in the body can be altered in following ways:

A. Preventing Continued Absorption of Toxicant

Continued absorption of toxicant from the exposure site may be prevented or delayed by using several non-specific and specific agents/ measures. These agents/measures either do not allow absorption of toxicant from the site of exposure or cause their elimination before absorption into blood.

I. Non-specific Treatment

Non-specific agents/measures are commonly used in the treatment of poisonings in both human and veterinary practices. These agents/measures are generally considered safe, but their usefulness depends on the route of exposure, type of toxicant and species involved.

a. Emesis : Emesis or vomiting empties the stomach and decreases further absorption of poison. The use of emetics in emergency treatment of poisoning requires good clinical judgement because various toxicants are absorbed at different rates and in different parts of GI tract. Emesis is useful only in recently ingested toxicant in monogastric animals like dogs, cats and pigs. Emetics are more useful in first 2 hours after ingestion of a toxicant and are of limited importance more than 4 hours after ingestion. Emesis is indicated after poisoning by ingestion of many drugs and poisons, but it is contraindicated if a corrosive poison or a petroleum distillate has been ingested. It is also contraindicated in unconscious and comatose animal, severe respiratory distress or severe convulsive seizures (unless controlled) or where animal has ingested some foreign bodies or sharp-edged objects.

Emesis can be induced in animals by using either locally acting (e.g. ipecacuanha syrup, hydrogen peroxide solution and hypertonic sodium chloride solution) or centrally acting (e.g. apomorphine and xylazine) emetics.

Locally acting emetics:

i. Ipecacuanha (Ipecac) syrup
Dogs: 1-2 ml/kg, orally. Total dose should not exceed 15 ml.

ii. Hydrogen peroxide (3%)
Dogs: 1-5 ml/kg, orally. Total dose should not exceed 50 ml.

iii. Hypertonic sodium chloride solution (25%)
Dogs: 30 – 60 ml depending on size of animal, orally

iv. Copper sulphate solution (1%)
Dogs: 10 – 30 ml depending on size of animal, orally.

v. Zinc sulphate solution (1%)
Dogs: 10 – 30 ml depending on size of animal, orally.

Centrally acting emetics:

i. Apomorphine hydrochloride
Dogs: 0.04 mg/kg, I.V. or I.M.; 0.08 mg/kg, S.C.; 0.3 mg/kg topically in conjunctival sac.

ii. Xylazine
Cats: 0.4 – 1 mg/kg, I.M.

Contraindications to induction of emesis

Emetics should not be used to induce vomiting in following conditions:

i. In poisoning by extremely volatile compounds (e.g. gasoline, kerosene, turpentine, paint thinner, xylene, toluene, furnish polish and solvents) because the low viscosity and high volatility of these compounds may lead to inhalation of their fumes or aspiration.

ii. In poisoning by compounds with caustic or corrosive properties (e.g. strong acids and alkalis) because their corrosive action may cause perforation in already damaged oesophagus and stomach.

iii. In poisoning by convulsants or CNS stimulants, or during convulsive seizures because emetics aggravate seizures and convulsions.

iv. Ingestion of sharp objects like nails and metallic wires because forceful contraction of stomach walls during vomiting may lead to injury or rupture of GI tract from these objects.

v. In comatose, unconscious or sedated patients because lack of normal pharyngeal reflex in these animals leads to aspiration.

vi. In cardio-respiratory distress due to chances of heart failure.

vii. In pregnancy due to chances of abortion.

viii. In dehydrated and weak animals or that already have vomited profusely because excessive loss of fluid in such conditions further aggravates poisoning.

ix. In rodents, rabbits, horses and ruminants. Rodents, ruminants and horses are incapable of vomiting and rabbits do not have a stomach wall strong enough to safely tolerate emesis.

b. Gastric lavage : Gastric lavage is performed by inserting a large diameter tube into the stomach and washing it (stomach) with water or a solution. The tube is inserted to a length equivalent to distance from the tip of nose to the last rib. After the stomach tube is put in place, the head is lowered to 30° angle and the lavage fluid is first flushed into stomach at rate of 10 ml/kg body weight and then removed. Administration of lavage fluid must be gentle, preferably by gravity flow, to avoid injury to stomach. The process of pumping out of stomach fluid should preferably be done by suction pressure. The whole process is repeated several times (15-20) until the recovered fluid is clear. Large amount of fluid should be avoided as it may force the toxicant into the duodenum. Attempts should be made to recover as much fluid as administered. A thicker activated charcoal suspension is generally instilled after the gastric lavage.

Gastric lavage is a rapid and useful way of removing the ingested poison from the stomach and is preferred when emesis is refused, contraindicated or when collection of gastric material is required. Lavage may also be indicated in the ingestion of agents in which delayed gastric emptying is anticipated. Lavage is useful in small animals for as long as 4 to 6 hours after ingestion of a poison. The contraindications to this procedure are the same as for emesis, but unlike emesis gastric lavage can be performed in an unconscious, comatose or lightly anaesthetised animal. An endotracheal tube must be placed to prevent aspiration of stomach contents. The choice of the agent used for gastric lavage depends on the condition of patient and the type of poison.

Gastric lavage can be performed in animals by using following agents:

i. Tepid water or saline solution: 10 ml/kg body weight.

ii. Potassium permanganate solution : (1 : 2000)

iii. Tincture iodine (1 : 250 of 5% solution.)

iv. Tannic acid solution.

v. Sodium bicarbonate solution.

In ruminants, the rumen lavage follows similar guidelines. A large hose inserted in the rumen is used to introduce water gently until the abdomen expands slightly. The stomach tube is then lowered and allowed to discharge as much fluid as possible. This can be repeated several times.

Enterogastric lavage: Enterogastric lavage (also called 'through and through enema') is a combination of gastric lavage and a retrograde high enema given with gastric tube and entrotracheal tube still in place. Enema fluid is administered gently until fluid from the gastric fluid flows, indicating nearly complete evacuation of the gastrointestinal tract. As enema fluid reaches the upper intestines, spontaneous vomiting may occur. The enterogastric lavage is not regarded as practical, effective and safe for animals having highly modified, high volume digestive tracts such as ruminants, horses, rabbits and swine (spiral colon).

c. Adsorption therapy : Adsorption is the physical binding of a toxicant to an unabsorbable carrier which is eliminated in the faeces. Activated charcoal is the most effective adsorbent for a wide variety of toxicants, especially large non-polar molecules, and is generally considered the adsorbent of choice when poisoning is suspected. It effectively adsorbs a wide variety of drugs and chemicals (Table 10.1) and prevents their absorption and toxicity. Activated charcoal can also interrupt the enterohepatic circulation of toxicants and enhance the net rate of diffusion of the chemical from systemic circulation/bile into the gastrointestinal tract. Activated charcoal, however, poorly adsorbs some toxicants including caustics, corrosives and mineral acids. Ionized substances are also less firmly bound to activated charcoal than non-polar substances. Activated charcoal can be administered following emesis or gastric lavage or administered when these procedures are contraindicated.

Activated charcoal should be of vegetable source and not be mineral or bone origin. The activated charcoal is prepared by pyrolysis and oxidation. The initial processing of charcoal produces a product with large pore size and further activation increases pores number and surface area. The number of drug or toxin molecules that can be adsorbed varies but is mostly proportional to the molecular size. Activated charcoal can be given via stomach tube or orally at a dose rate of 2.5 g/kg body weight in a water slurry in which 1 g is suspended in 5 ml of water. Charcoal is usually administered with a cathartic such as sodium sulphate (250 mg/kg, orally) or 70% sorbitol (3 ml/kg, orally). This combination hastens removal of the toxicant-charcoal complex and helps to prevent the constipation that can occur from the charcoal. The effectiveness of charcoal is dependent on the time since ingestion and on the dose of charcoal (suitable adsorption is attained if charcoal: toxicant ratio is about 10 : 1). Activated charcoal is usually most effective when administered as soon as possible after exposure to the toxicant and its usefulness is doubtful if administered more than 2 hours of an exposure. In cats and some fractious dogs, charcoal tablets may be easier to administer, but they are approximately 25% less adsorptive than powdered charcoal.

Universal antidote, a formulation initially synthesised for treatment of most poisonings, consists of 2 parts activated charcoal/burnt bread (for adsorption), 1 part tannic acid/strong tea (for precipitation), and 1 part magnesium oxide/milk of magnesia (for catharsis). Universal antidote is rarely used nowadays because neither it is universal nor an antidote to toxicants. It is considered very less effective than the activated charcoal as different ingredients present in it interfere with each others action and neutralise the overall efficacy. Egg white, milk and other demulcents also act as adsorbents but their efficacy is much lower than activated charcoal. Cholestyramine has also been tried, but it has been found effective against only a limited number of toxicants like cardiac glycosides. Kaolin-pectin is occasionally used as a demulcent and adsorbent in the treatment of some toxicoses, but its adsorbent capacity is inferior to activated charcoal.

Table 10.1: List of important compounds adsorbed by activated charcoal*.

Type/Group of compound	Example(s)
Alkaloids	Atropine, cocaine, ergotamine, muscarine and nicotine.
Anticonvulsants	Carbamazepine and phenytoin.
Antidepressants	Tricyclic antidepressants (e.g. imipramine, nortriptyline).
Antimalarials	Quinine and chloroquine.
Antiseptics and disinfectants	Iodine, mercuric chloride, phenol and potassium permanganate.
Cardiac stimulants	Digitalis (e.g. digitoxin).
Chemotherapeutic agents	Hexachlorophene, penicillin, probenecid and sulphonamides.
CNS depressants	Alcohol, barbiturates (e.g. barbital), ethchlorvinol, diazepam, glutethimide, meprobamate and phenothiazines.
CNS stimulants and convulsants	Amphetamine and strychnine.
Emetics	Ipecacuanha.
Laxatives and purgatives	Phenolphthalein.
Metals	Antimony, arsenic, lead, mercury, selenium, silver and tin.
Narcotics/Opioids	Opium, morphine and propoxyphene.
Non-steroidal anti-inflammatory drugs.	Aspirin, antipyrine, mefenamic acid, methyl salicylate, paracetamol, phenylbutazone and salicylates.
Pesticides	Organochlorine insecticides, organophosphorus insecticides (e.g. malathion, parathion), bromethalin, and 2,4-D.
Other poisons	Cyanide, camphor, chlordane, kerosene, methylene blue, oxalate and phosphorus.

* The adsorbent capacity of activated charcoal varies with the type of compound.

d. Purgation/Catharsis : Catharsis is indicated for removal of unabsorbed toxicants especially those that have passed into intestine. Use of cathartics in the management of orally ingested poisons is only of minor importance as they produce loss of fluid and electrolyte and, thus, may cause dehydration and electrolyte imbalance. Preferred agents for most poisonings are osmotic saline purgatives (e.g. magnesium sulphate and sodium sulphate) and sorbitol. Magnesium based cathartics may cause hypermagnesemia under some conditions and should not be administered in poisoning with substances that decrease GI transit time or in case of renal insufficiency. These agents may be used with or without activated charcoal. If used with charcoal, then cathartic may be given 30 min after administration of activated charcoal. Bulk purgatives that do not contain sugar are preferred for toxicants or physical agents (e.g. lead objects or fibre glass insulation) that need safe passage through GI tract. Use of oily cathartics including mineral oil (except in phosphorus intoxication), vegetable oils and irritant purgatives are not recommended in poisoning as they often increase the absorption of toxicant. Cathartic is not recommended if animal has diarrhoea.

i. Sodium sulphate

Dogs: 0.5 – 2 g (total), orally.

Cats: 0.3 – 0.6 g (total), orally.

Cattle: 60 – 120 g (total), orally.

Horses: 30 – 60 g (total), orally.

ii. Magnesium sulphate

Dogs: 5 – 25 g (total), orally.

Cats: 2 – 5 g (total), orally.

Horses: 30 – 100 g (total), orally.

Cattle: 250 – 500 g (total), orally.

iii. Sorbitol (70%)

Dogs & cats: 1 - 3 ml/kg, orally.

e. Enema : Enema may be occasionally indicated in cases where absorption of toxicant has not been completed in the upper GI tract. Enema is also practiced along with cathartics for complete evacuation of lower intestine. In enema, a solution of warm water or soap solution is gently administered into rectum. Enema is performed with help of an enema can or enema pump in horses and cattle, and a human enema syringe in smaller animals.

f. Cleansing of skin or hair : If a toxicant has been spilled or applied over skin or hair, then animal should be gently washed (avoid rubbing) several times using water, mild shampoo or liquid dishwashing detergent. Greasy topical medication or solvent should be avoided as it may do more harm than good either by acting as vehicle to enhance absorption or by dispersing the toxicant and increasing surface area for absorption. Epidermal structures like wings, nails, claws, feathers, or fur should be cleaned thoroughly, paying particular attention to areas such as ears, between toes, etc. The cleaning should be undertaken quickly to avoid licking and ingestion of the toxicant and to limit cutaneous absorption. Long and matted hair may be clipped, if necessary, for complete removal of toxicant residues. Person washing the poisoned animal should wear gloves and other protective garments to avoid exposure to the toxicant.

g. Cleansing of eyes : For toxic ocular exposure, immediate flushing of eyes is advised. The eyes with lids wide open are gently flushed numerous times (20-30) with body temperature tap water, lactated Ringer's solution or normal saline solution to enhance the decontamination. Following adequate irrigation, the animal should be examined for chemical burns to eye and, if found, treated with lubricant ointments to protect the damaged area.

h. Gastrotomy or Rumenotomy : Gastrotomy or Rumenotomy may be necessary in situations that are refractory to emesis, lavage or activated charcoal. Foreign bodies, especially those containing toxic metals such as lead or zinc are indications for surgical intervention. An abdominal radiograph may be useful in detecting retained toxic metals. Persistent materials such as toxic oils and tars also require surgical evacuation.

i. Dilution : Dilution of toxicant with water or milk is often practiced in poisonings; however, dilution is controversial for many toxicants as it can increase absorption. Dilution with water or milk should be recommended in conjunction with a demulcent only for treating poisonings with agents that are capable of causing ulceration of GI tract such as strong acids or alkalis or cationic detergents. Demulcents including egg white, milk, and kaolin-pectin dilute the irritant/corrosive in the GI tract and protect the damaged mucosa. To be effective, demulcents must be used soon after ingestion of poison.

II. Specific Treatment

Some agents specifically interact with or neutralise the toxicants at the site of exposure, thus decreasing their absorption. Relatively few toxicants are neutralised in this way.

a. Complex formation : Specific antidotes can interact with some toxicants in GI tract or other exposure sites to form a stable complex or product which is not toxic (Table 10.2). This complex or product is then excreted unabsorbed from the body.

B. Preventing Distribution of Toxicant to Target Site

I. Non-specific Treatment

a. Ion-trapping : The basic principle of ion-trapping is that ionized compounds do not readily traverse cell membranes and are, therefore, not distributed to target site and subsequently not re-absorbed by the renal tubules. The ion-trapping is more useful for enhancing the excretion of toxicants then altering their distribution because the urine pH can be changed more easily as compared to the blood pH.

b. Alternate binding site : Distribution can also be affected by providing an alternate binding site to the toxicant. For example, infusion of albumin provides an alternate binding site to some toxicants, which then fail to interact with the target site.

II. Specific Treatment

a. Complex formation : Some antidotes can form complex with the specific toxicants in the body making them unavailable to cross the cell membrane or to interact with susceptible receptors (Table 10.3). To be effective, the complex formed must be both inactive and stable until excreted.

TO INCREASE THRESHOLD OF TOXICITY

By using various agents, the threshold level of toxicity can be increased so that more concentration of toxicant is required to produce intoxication. This can be achieved by using specific antidote or appropriate emergency supportive and symptomatic therapy. In the time-concentration curve of a toxicity case, there is elevation in the threshold level of toxicity. Thus more concentration of toxicant is required to produce the toxic effect (Figure 10.3).

I. Non-specific Treatment

Appropriate emergency supportive therapy is often the most valuable part of early treatment for toxicosis. Stabilization of vital functions preserves the life of animal regardless of the etiology,

Table 10.2: List of selected antidotes affecting the absorption of toxicants from exposure sites.

Sr. No.	Toxicant	Antidote/Agent	Product/Complex
1	Iron	Desferrioxamine Sodium bicarbonate	Iron-desferrioxamine complex Ferrous carbonate
2	Silver nitrate	Sodium chloride	Silver chloride
3	Strychnine, nicotine, morphine	Potassium permanganate	Oxidised product
4	Fluoride	Calcium lactate	Calcium fluoride

Table 10.3: List of selected antidotes affecting the distribution of toxicants.

Sr. No.	Toxicant	Antidote/Agent	Product/Mechanism of action
1.	Methanol	Ethanol	Competitive inhibition
2.	Fluoroacetate	Acetate or monoacetin	Competitive inhibition
3.	Heparin	Protamine	Complex formation
4.	Venoms	Antivenin	Complex formation
5.	Digoxin	Digoxin immune Fab	Complex formation

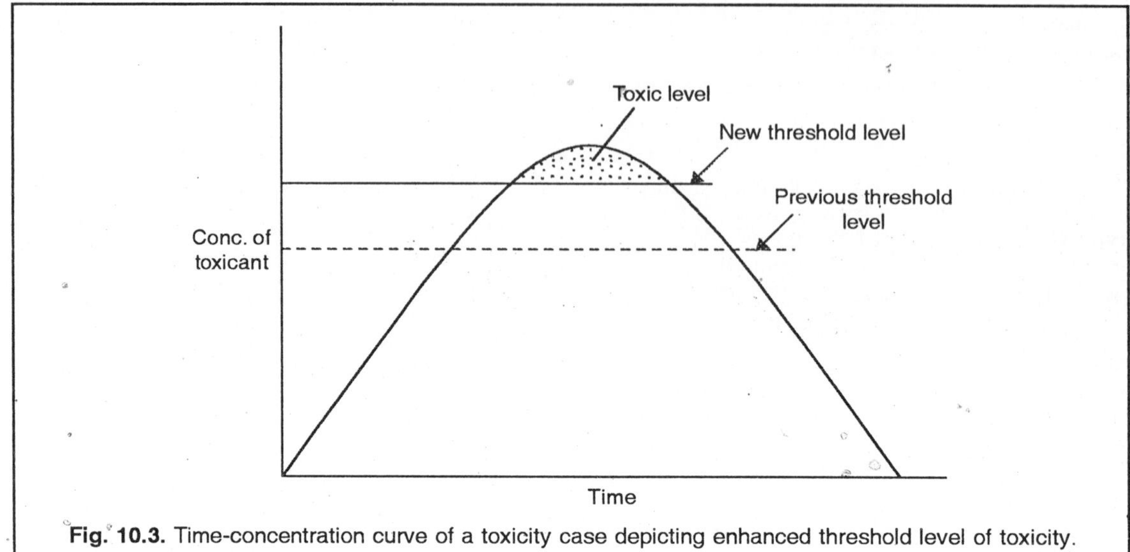

Fig. 10.3. Time-concentration curve of a toxicity case depicting enhanced threshold level of toxicity.

obtaining time for detoxification to occur and for specific antidotes to produce their action. Therefore, major life threatening effects of toxicants need to be assessed and appropriate therapy started at the earliest.

a. Treatment of respiratory depression : Maintenance of normal respiration is very important in poisoning cases. In case of respiratory depression or failure, following measures are helpful:

i. A patent airway should be established with a cuffed endotracheal tube to prevent aspiration of vomitus in a comatose or anaesthetised animal.

ii. Mechanical ventilation or oxygen should be used, if needed, for apnoea, anoxia or severe anaemia.

iii. Respiratory stimulants i.e. doxapram (1-2 mg/kg, I.V.), should be used only if necessary.

b. Monitoring of cardiac disturbances : Continuous cardiac monitoring for arrhythmias is essential in comatose patients and patients with cardiotoxic drug exposure. In case of cardiac arrhythmia, appropriate antiarrhythmic drugs should be employed. When antiarrhythmic drugs are used, the therapy should be specific for the type of arrhythmia present and the species involved.

c. Control of shock : Shock may occur due to toxicants that cause excessive fluid loss, vomiting, diarrhoea, blood loss or cadiomyopathy. In poisonings, adequate circulation and perfusion must be ensured. Use of plasma volume expander, fluid therapy or whole blood administration may be followed. Use of excess fluid should be avoided once shock and hypovolaemia are stabilized, especially in conditions susceptible to pulmonary oedema or cerebral oedema.

d. Control of acid-base disturbance and electrolytes imbalance : Provision of adequate hydration, acid-base, and electrolyte balance are all necessary for normal cardiovascular functions. These should be monitored closely and appropriate fluid and electrolyte therapy administered. Metabolic acidosis is the most common toxicant associated acid-base imbalance. It can initially be treated with either sodium bicarbonate (0.5-2.0 mEq/kg, every 4 hour by I.V. route) or sodium lactate (0.17 molar concentration given at 16-32 mg/kg, I.V.).

e. Treatment of CNS dysfunctions : Central nervous system convulsions or depression is a common result of toxicoses. Use of appropriate drug to counteract it may be helpful.

i. CNS seizures: Seizures can be controlled by using diazepam (0.5 mg/kg, I.V., repeated after 20 minutes for 3-4 times, if required). Diazepam is the drug of choice for acute seizures of unknown aetiology.

Phenobarbitone (6 mg/kg, I.V.) is used if diazepam is ineffective or prolonged seizure control is needed. Pentobarbitone and other CNS depressants can also be used.

ii. CNS depression: Analeptics such as doxapram (1-2 mg/kg, I.V.) have been used to treat CNS depression, especially when respiratory depression is more severe.

f. Treatment of hypothermia or hyperthermia : Hypothermia or hyperthermia may occur during poisoning and should be treated promptly.

i. Hyperthermia : Hyperthermia often occurs with persistent seizures. Hyperthermia may also be a problem with toxicosis caused by uncouplers of oxidative phosphorylation (e.g. pentachlorophenol). Hyperthermia is treated with cold baths, ice packs or cooled intravenous fluids. Exercise or high ambient temperature generally aggravates hyperthermia, so efforts should be made to keep the animal calm and surroundings cool. Antipyretics are generally of little help in hyperthermia induced by toxicants.

ii. Hypothermia : Hypothermia may occur during anaesthesia, heavy sedation or coma. Vital physiological processes are generally depressed when body temperature is sub-normal. Hypothermia may be prevented through use of blankets, warm water bottles and heating pads. Warming the surroundings of the animal is safer than directly applying heat to the body.

g. Maintenance of uresis : To maintain adequate renal flow and to reduce cerebral oedema, osmotic diuretics like mannitol (1-2 g/kg, I.V.) may be used.

II. Specific Treatment

Use of specific pharmacological antidotes to toxicants is most effective in some poisoning cases. Antidotes produce their effect in a variety of ways including chelation, enzyme inhibition or receptor antagonism. Antidotes are generally administered after exposure to toxicants often in response to clinical toxicoses. Some antidotes may be toxic, particularly when used in higher dose or for long duration. As many antidotes are specific to toxicants, so if given in the absence of the particular toxicant they may produce their own adverse effects. Therefore, correct diagnosis is important prior to the use of antidote. General decontamination and use of supportive therapy often help in the effectiveness of antidotal treatment. As the details of antidotal treatment are given in the respective chapters, the present section provides only a brief summary of their action in Table 10.4.

Table 10.4: List of common poisons and their recommended antidotes.

Sr. No.	Toxicant	Antidote or Drug therapy	Product/Mechanism of action
1.	Antimony	Dimercaprol, penicillamine	Chelation
2.	Arsenic	Dimercaprol, penicillamine	Chelation
3.	Atropine	Physostigmine	Receptor antagonism
4.	Benzodiazepines (e.g. diazepam)	Flumazenil	Receptor antagonism
5.	Carbamate insecticides	Atropine	Receptor antagonism
6.	Curare	Neostigmine	Antagonism
7.	Cyanide	Sodium nitrite, sodium thiosulphate	Alternate pathway
8.	Ethylene glycol	Ethanol	Alternate pathway
9.	5-Fluorouracil	Thymidine	Alternate pathway
10.	Iron	Desferrioxamine	Chelation
11.	Lead	Dimercaprol, calcium disodium EDTA	Chelation
12.	Nitrite	Methylene blue	Alternate pathway
13.	Opioids (e.g. morphine)	Naloxone	Receptor antagonism
14.	Organophosphorus insecticides	Atropine	Receptor antagonism
15.	Paracetamol	N-Acetylcysteine	Alternate pathway
14.	Warfarin	Vitamin K	Antagonism

TO INCREASE SLOPE OF DESCENDING PORTION OF CURVE

The slope of descending curve in the time-concentration profile may be increased by facilitating the removal of absorbed toxicant from the body. This may be practically achieved by using certain therapeutic agents which make the toxicant readily excretable via the kidneys or lungs or by other physiological mechanisms. Enhancing metabolism of toxicants to less toxic forms is also possible, but is of minor importance in emergency cases.

A. Hastening Elimination of Absorbed Toxicant

I. Non-specific Treatment

a. Ion-trapping : Alteration of urine pH is a convenient and useful method of preventing renal reabsorption of poisons that undergo glomerular filtration and passive tubular reabsorption. The ion-trapping is carried out with the help of an appropriate urinary acidifier or alkalizer and is clinically useful for enhancing the excretion of many weakly acidic or basic compounds from body. The Henderson-Hasselbalch equation provides the basis for ion-trapping of ionised compounds. Generally, acidic agents (e.g. aspirin, paracetamol, barbiturates and phenoxy herbicides) are more effectively ionised and excreted in alkaline urine, whereas basic agents (e.g. amphetamine and most alkaloids) are more effectively ionised and more readily excreted in acidified urine. Ion-trapping therapy is most suitable in acid-base imbalance conditions.

Urinary acidifier

i. Ammonium chloride

Dogs: 100-200 mg/kg, given in 3 divided doses daily by oral route.

Cats: 20 mg/kg, 2 times daily by oral route.

Cattle: 15 g (total), orally.

ii. Ascorbic acid

Dogs: 100-500 mg (total), 3 times daily by oral route.

All species: 40 mg/kg, by IV route.

iii. Sodium acid phosphate

Dogs: 150-300 mg (total), 3 times daily by oral route.

iv. Arginine chloride

Large animals: 7 – 10 g (total), by IV or IM route.

Small animals: 0.1 – 0.2 g/kg, by IV or IM route.

Urinary alkaliniser

i. Sodium bicarbonate

Dogs & cats: 10-20 mg/kg, 2 to 3 times daily by oral route.

Dogs: 0.5 – 2 mEq/kg, every 4 hours by I.V. route.

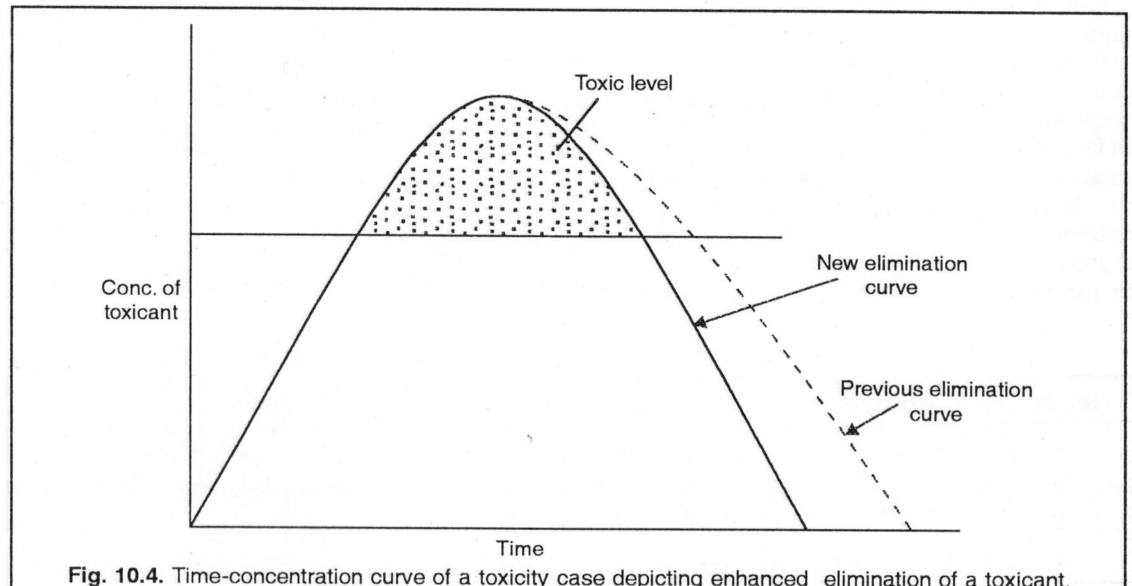

Fig. 10.4. Time-concentration curve of a toxicity case depicting enhanced elimination of a toxicant.

b. Dialysis : Dialysis may be described as the movement of an agent across a semi-permeable membrane. Haemodialysis, peritoneal dialysis and haemoperfusion are important types of dialysis, but these are possible only in sophisticated hospitals. Haemodialysis involves passage of blood from an artery through dialysis membrane which is then returned to body via a vein. In peritoneal dialysis, an essentially isotonic solution is introduced into the peritoneal cavity and later withdrawn. Here, the peritoneum itself serves as the dialysis membrane. Haemoperfusion involves passage through charcoal or some other chambers. Dialysis is useful when patient is in comatose condition, or in situations of renal failure, anuria, hypotension, fluid and electrolytes imbalance, and hepatic failure. Dialysis should also be considered if large amount of toxicant is present in the body. Peritoneal dialysis procedure has limited value for the management of some poisonings as fluid needs frequent change. Dialysis is useful in intoxication by digitoxin, methanol, lithium, phenobarbitone, etc.

c. Diuresis : Forced diuresis may be defined as the promotion of rapid renal filtration of a compound by using certain therapeutic agents. Forced diuresis may be useful for some, but not all toxicants because for it a compound must have to be present in high concentration in an unbound form. Moreover, a substantial portion of filtered toxicant is often reabsorbed by the renal tubules. Forced diuresis may considered useful in certain conditions such as in toxicosis with serious clinical signs (e.g. severe hypotension, coma and arrhythmia), when potentially lethal dose of a compound has been ingested, or when there is progressive deterioration of the condition of animal in face of intensive therapy. Forced diuresis is also useful in oedema due to complications of poisoning i.e. heart failure, ascites from liver failure, pulmonary oedema, acute renal failure, etc. Forced diuresis in most toxicity cases is achieved either by use of diuretics (e.g. mannitol and frusemide) or by intravenous administration of parenteral fluids (e.g. 5%, 10% or 50% dextrose). In large animals, it can be more practical to pump large volumes of water or non-sterile electrolyte solution into the rumen or stomach, often in conjunction with a diuretic. Excessive administration of I.V. fluid should be avoided as it may result in complications including cerebral oedema, pulmonary oedema and disturbance in acid-base or electrolytes status.

i. Mannitol (20-25%)

Dogs: 500 – 1000 mg/kg, by slow IV injection over 15 to 20 minutes.

Cats: 250 – 500 mg/kg, by slow IV injection.

Cattle, sheep, goats and swine: 1000 – 2000 mg/kg, by slow IV injection.

Horses: 250 – 1000 mg/kg, by slow IV injection or IV infusion

ii. Frusemide

Dogs & cats: 2 – 4 mg/kg, 1 to 2 times daily by oral, IV, or IM route.

Cattle: 2 – 5 mg/kg, by oral route.

: 0.5 – 1 mg/kg, by IM or IV route.

Pigs: 5 mg/kg, by IM or IV route.

Horses: 0.5 – 1 mg/kg, 1 to 2 times daily by oral, IM or IV route.

II. Specific Treatment

Some specific antidotes enhance the excretion of toxicants or form a complex with them (Table 10.5) which is less toxic and rapidly excreted from the body.

B. Enhancing Metabolic Conversion of Absorbed Toxicant

Some agents enhance metabolic conversion i.e. detoxification of the toxicant to a less toxic product. For example, drugs like phenobarbitone have been recommended for use in reducing

Table 10.5: List of selected antidotes affecting excretion of toxicants.

Sr. No.	Toxicant	Antidote	Product/Mechanism of action
1.	Bromide	Chloride	Enhance renal excretion
2.	Copper	D-penicillamine	Chelation
3	Lead	Calcium disodium EDTA	Chelation
4.	Molybdenum	Copper	Enhance renal excretion

residues of persistent toxicants in tissues by causing induction of mixed function oxidase enzyme. However, such a practice is not useful for most acutely poisoned animals as the induction of microsomal enzymes takes a few days to become fully effective.

MANAGEMENT OF POISONING

In addition to the treatment of poisoning as discussed above, certain management practices also help in the therapy.

a. When toxicosis has occurred or is occurring, further exposure to the toxicant should be avoided. In case of livestock, changing pastures or feedlots may prevent further exposure. Shifting of pets from area of exposure to another site may also be helpful. Changing of feed and water source prevents further potential ingestion of toxicant.

b. Intoxicated animal should be kept at a place which is free from excessive noise and other disturbances. Convulsive seizures usually aggravate with external stimuli.

c. If animal has been fastened with a chain or rope, its removal is required otherwise the animal may strangulate itself or may get hurt.

d. Vicinity of intoxicated animal should be free of sharp objects and obstacles. This helps in decreasing injury to the animal.

e. Head of a recumbent animal should be kept at a lower level than rest of its body. This will prevent aspiration of the regurgitated material.

BIBLIOGRAPHY

Adams L G and Polzin D J (1989) Mixed acid-base disorders. *Vet. Clin. North Am. Small Anim. Prac.* 19: 307-326.

Albert A (1973) Selective toxicity. The Physico-chemical Basis of Therapy. 5th edn. Chapman and Hall, London.

Barragry TB (1994) Veterinary Drug Therapy. Lea and Febiger, Philadelphia.

Bartik M and Piskac A (1981) Veterinary Toxicology. Elsevier Scientific Publishing Company, Amsterdam.

Beasley VR (1990) Management of toxicoses. *Vet. Clin. North Am: Small Anim Pract.* 20 : 307.

Beasley V (1999) Diagnosis and management of toxicoses. In: Veterinary Toxicology. Beasley V (Ed.) p. 36. International Veterinary Information Service, Ithaca NY (www.ivis.org).

Cargill J and Thorpe-Vargas S (2005) Poisoned. Working Dogs Health Articles. (http://www.workingdogs.com/doc0175.htm)

Clarke ECG and Clarke ML (1967) Garner's Veterinary Toxicology. 3rd edn. Williams and Wilkins, Baltimore.

Dahlke J (1996) Poison guide. Information page – Poison Guide for Birds and Pets. (http://www.robharvey.com/information/poison.html).

Dorman DC (1997) Diagnosing and treating toxicosis in dogs and cats. *Vet. Med.* 92 : 273.

Drobatz KJ (1994) Clinical approach to toxicities. *Vet. Clin. North Am.: Small Anim. Pract.* 24 : 1123.

Franklin CA (1988) Modi's Textbook of Medical Jurisprudence and Toxicology. 21st edn. NM Tripathi Private Ltd., Bombay.

Gale FD and Hall JO (1990) Field investigations of small animal toxicoses. *Vet. Clin. North Am: Small Anim Pract.* 20 : 283.

Garg SK (2000) Veterinary Toxicology. CBS Publishers & Distributors, New Delhi.

Gwatlney-Brant SM and Rumbeiha WK (2002) Newer antidotal therapies. *Vet. Clin. North Am: Small Anim Pract.* 32 : 323.

Homan CS and Ryan JG (1998) Enhancement of elimination. In: Emergency Toxicology. 2nd edn. Viccellio P (ed.) p 165. Lippincott-Raven Publishers, Philadelhia.

Kaye S (1970) Bedside toxicology. *Paed. Clin. North Am*. 17.

Klaassen CD (2001) Principles of toxicology and treatment of poisoning. In: Goodman & Gilman's The Pharmacological Basis of Therapeutics. 10th edn. Hardman JG, Limbird LE and Gilman AG (Eds.). p 67. The McGraw-Hill Companies Inc., New York.

Lorgue G, Lechenet J and Riviere A (1996) Clinical Veterinary Toxicology. Blackwell Science Ltd., United Kingdom.

Marrs TC and Bateman DN (1995) Antidotal studies. In: General and Applied Toxicology. Ballantyne B, Marrs T and Turner P (Eds.) p 277. Macmillan Press Ltd., London.

Mofenson HC, Caraccio TR and Gerald MB (1998) Initial evaluation and management of the poisoned patient. In: Emergency Toxicology. 2nd edn. Viccellio P (ed.) p 63. Lippincott-Raven Publishers, Philadelhia.

Olson KR (1992) Poisoning. In: Current Medical Diagnosis and Treatment. Schroeder SA, Knipp MA, Tierneg Lm and Mephce C (Eds.) p 1218. Appleton & Lange, Connecticut.

Osweiler GD (1996) Toxicology. Williams and Wilkins, Philadelphia.

Porter RS (2007) The Merck Manuals Online Medical Library – Section: Accidents and Injuries. (http://www.merck.com/mmhe/sec24.html).

Radeleff RD (1970) Veterinary Toxicology. 2nd edn. Lea and Febiger, Philadelphia.

Rosendale ME (2002) Decontamination therapy. *Vet. Clin. North Am: Small Anim Pract*. 32 : 311.

World Health Organization (2005) Guidelines for poison control. The International Programme on Chemical safety, WHO, Geneva. (http://www.who.int/ipcs/publications/training_poisons/guidelines_poison_control/en/index.html).

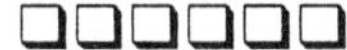

SECTION-II

CLINICAL TOXICOLOGY

11 METALS

Arsenic
Mercury
Lead
Copper
Molybdenum
Cadmium
Iron
Zinc
Thallium

Metals are a unique class of toxicants that occur and persist in nature, mainly dispersed in rocks, ores, soil, water and air. Metals can assume different chemical forms because of their physicochemical, biological and anthropogenic activities. Most of them are widely used in industry, agriculture and medicine. Some metals are essential elements, while others only pose health hazards to humans and animals.

1. Arsenic

Arsenic (As) is an irritant and cumulative poison that is found mainly in soil, water and air as a common environmental toxicant. Arsenic was described and used more than 2400 years ago in Greece and Rome as a therapeutic agent and a poison and its preparations are found in Paracelsus writings (1520 A.D.). The element is usually not mined as such but is recovered as a by-product from the smelting of copper, lead, zinc and other ores. Arsenic poisoning is caused by different types of inorganic and organic arsenical compounds.

Properties: Arsenic is a metalloid which belongs to the group V of the periodic chart of elements and has some properties similar to phosphorus, antimony and bismuth. The arsenic atom exists in three oxidation forms i.e. elemental (As^3), trivalent (As^{3+} or arsenite) and pentavalent (As^{5+} or arsenate). The organic arsenical compounds contain arsenic linked to a carbon atom by a covalent bond, where it exists in the trivalent or pentavalent states. Trivalent arsenic compounds, known as arsenites, are more soluble and, therefore, more toxic (5-10 times) than pentavalent or arsenate compounds.

Inorganic forms of arsenic (i.e. arsenic trioxide) and pentavalent and trivalent forms of sodium, potassium and calcium salts (arsenates and arsenites, respectively) are more toxic than the organic forms e.g. trivalent monosodium methanearsonate (MSMA), disodium methanearsonate (DSMA), thiacetarsamide, and pentavalent arsanilic acid and sodium arsanilate. Arsine (arsenic hydride) gas, which may come from charging of storage batteries or by the action of water on pyritic ores, is most toxic arsenic compound. In general, toxicity increases in the sequence of organic arsenicals $< As^{5+} < As^{3+} <$ Arsine (AsH_3).

Sources of toxicity: Arsenic was a common poison used for homicidal or suicidal purposes in ancient times. Accidental arsenic poisoning was also common a few years ago because it was often used in ant and roach baits. Arsenic is less common cause of poisoning in livestock nowadays because of its displacement from almost all phases of farming activity. Still arsenic is an important poison and its toxicosis in animals may occur from following sources:

a. Indiscriminate use of arsenic as a drug in ruminatoric preparations, skin tonics and for control of ectoparasites (e.g. lead arsenate as dip) and blood parasites (e.g. sodium thiacetarsamide).

b. Excessive use or accidental ingestion of arsenical pesticides i.e. insecticides (e.g. copper acetoarsenite or Paris green), defoliants/herbicides (e.g. sodium or potassium arsenite or arsenate, monosodium methanearsonate), rodenticides (e.g. arsenic trioxide), wood preservatives (e.g. arsenic pentoxide) and ant baits (e.g. sodium or potassium arsenate).

c. Arsenic-contaminated soils or burn piles, which are often licked by animals that crave for salt or minerals.

d. Contaminated drinking water especially well water containing high concentrations of arsenic. Underground water having high arsenic may result in widespread poisoning in human beings and livestock.

e. Overdosage or extended use of organic arsenical feed additives in poultry or swine as growth promoters (e.g. arsanilic acid and sodium arsanilate).

f. Burning of wood products treated with arsenical preservatives or coals which have variable concentration of arsenic. Arsenic is released into the environment during combustion.

g. Smelting of copper, zinc, lead and other ores can release arsenic as a by-product into the environment.

h. Arsine gas and arsenic trioxide used in the manufacture of most computer chips using silicon-based technology. These may cause occupational toxicosis.

i. Litter from poultry fed phenylarsonic compounds.

j. Pastures and crops near smelters contaminated with arsenic.

k. Dyes and paints containing arsenic (much rarer, now).

l. Malicious poisoning with arsenic trioxide (very common).

Factors affecting toxicity: Toxicity of arsenic in animals varies with several factors such as species, oxidation state, solubility and duration of exposure.

a. *Species*: Herbivores are commonly poisoned due to ingestion of contaminated forages. Cats and dogs are poisoned less, while fowl and swine are rarely effected due to their limited exposure to arsenic.

b. *Oxidation state*: Inorganic arsenic in the trivalent state is more toxic (up to ten times) than the inorganic pentavalent form (as pentavalent form has less affinity for thiol group), which in turn is more toxic than organic form. Toxicity of pentavalent arsenicals is largely due to their conversion *in vivo* to trivalent state.

c. *Solubility / Form*: Finely divided soluble arsenic compounds are more toxic than coarse and poorly soluble ones because the insoluble compounds are poorly absorbed.

d. *Status / Health of animal*: Dehydrated, weak, ill and poor conditioned animals are more susceptible to arsenic toxicity due to slow renal excretion of arsenic.

e. *Tolerance:* Constant exposure to arsenic may confer some degree of tolerance to its toxicity.

Toxicity: All species are susceptible to arsenic poisoning, but it is most commonly observed in bovine and feline animals followed by horses and sheep. Incidence of arsenic poisoning is less common in dogs and rare in swine and poultry. The single dose lethal toxicity of sodium arsenite for most species is in range of 1-25 mg/kg body wt. with arsenic trioxide being 3-10 times less toxic. The average total lethal dose of arsenic trioxide and sodium arsenite, respectively is: horses 10-45 g and 1-3 g ; cattle 15-45 g and 1-4 g ; sheep and goats 3-10 g and 200-500 mg ; dogs 100-150 mg and 50-150 mg; and fowls 50-300 mg and 10-100 mg. Cats are highly susceptible to arsenicals and may succumb to sodium arsenite at a dose rate of 20 mg/kg. Chronic poisoning is not often seen and not well described in domestic animals as arsenic is rapidly excreted from the body.

Toxicokinetics: Soluble arsenicals (both trivalent and pentavalent) are readily absorbed from all body surfaces including GI tract and skin. Percutaneous toxic dose, however, is much lower (probably one-tenth of) than the oral toxic dose. The absorption is more if the animals are dipped in hot weather, if the fleece is long and if they are crowded too tightly in draining yard. Absorption of poorly water-soluble arsenicals such as As_2O_3 greatly depends on the physical state of the compound; coarsely powdered material is eliminated in faeces before it dissolves. After absorption, arsenic is distributed throughout the body but tends to reach higher concentration in liver, kidneys, heart and lungs. Because of high sulphydryl contents in keratin, high concentrations of arsenic are found in hair and nails where it stays for months. Because of its chemical similarity to phosphorus, arsenic is deposited in bone and teeth and retained there for long period. Deposition in the keratinised tissues primarily occurs after the continuous intake of arsenic.

In domestic animals, arsenic does not stay in tissues for very long and is partly methylated (detoxification) in the liver and rapidly excreted in the urine, faeces, bile, milk, saliva and sweat. Some portion of pentavalent arsenic (arsenate) is reduced to the more toxic trivalent arsenic. In this process, the pentavalent arsenic is coupled to the oxidation of glutathione (GSH) to its disulphide (GSSG) to form trivalent arsenic (arsenite) which is further methylated to form monomethyl arsenite and then dimethylarsenite (Figure 11.1) which is readily eliminated from the body. This conversion from pentavalent arsenic to trivalent arsenic in the kidneys may also account for nephrotoxicity Arsenic crosses placental barrier in significant amount but its passage to CNS through blood brain barrier is limited. Excretion of arsenic in domestic animals is rapid and nearly complete within a few days.

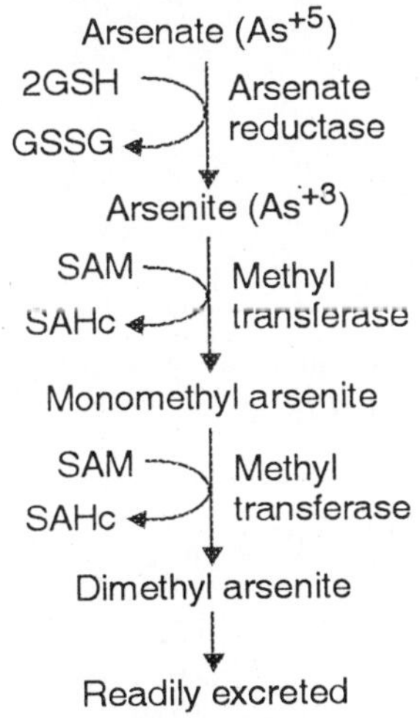

Arsenate (As^{+5})
2GSH → GSSG — Arsenate reductase
Arsenite (As^{+3})
SAM → SAHc — Methyl transferase
Monomethyl arsenite
SAM → SAHc — Methyl transferase
Dimethyl arsenite
↓
Readily excreted

Fig. 11.1. Biotransformation of pentavalent arsenic (arsenate).

Mechanism of action: Regardless of the form of arsenic entering the body (pentavalent or tivalent), the major effects are believed to be attributable to the trivalent form.

a. *Trivalent arsenic:*

   i. Trivalent arsenic binds primarily to sulphydryl compounds especially lipoic (thioctic) acid to form stable compounds that subsequently disrupt enzymes involved in cellular respiration (Figure 11.2). As such, trivalent arsenicals inhibit many proteins and enzymes by reacting with biological ligands containing available -SH groups. The pyruvate dehydrogenase system is especially sensitive because interaction of arsenic with two sulphydryl groups of lipoic acid results in a stable six-membered ring. Lipoic acid is an essential cofactor for the enzymatic decarboxylation of keto acids such as pyruvate, ketoglutarate and ketobutyrate. By inactivating lipoic acid, arsenic inhibits formation of acetyl, succinyl, and propionyl coenzymes-A. Other oxidative decarboxylations that use lipoic acid are probably also inhibited. The major effect of lipoic acid inhibition is slowing or inhibition of glycolysis and TCA cycle. Inhibition of mitochondrial enzymes and impairment of tissue respiration seems to be related to the cellular toxicity of arsenic. Tissues with high oxidative energy requirement (e.g. actively dividing cells such as intestinal epithelium, kidneys, liver, skin, lungs etc.) are most affected.

   ii. Trivalent arsenic affects capillary integrity by an unknown mechanism. Although all capillary beds are affected, the splanchnic area in the GI tract is the most sensitive. Loss of capillary integrity and dilation in GI tract allows transudation of plasma fluids into the intestinal mucosa and lumen with

CH_2-SH
|
CH_2
|
$CH-SH$ + $R-As=O$ ⟶ Arsenic–lipoic acid complex (CH_2, CH_2, CH bound through S, S to $As-R$; $(CH_2)_4$; $COOH$) + H_2O
|
$(CH_2)_4$
|
$COOH$

∝ – Lipoic acid | Trivalent arsenic | Arsenic–lipoic acid complex

Fig. 11.2. Inhibition of -SH containing lipoic acid by trivalent arsenic.

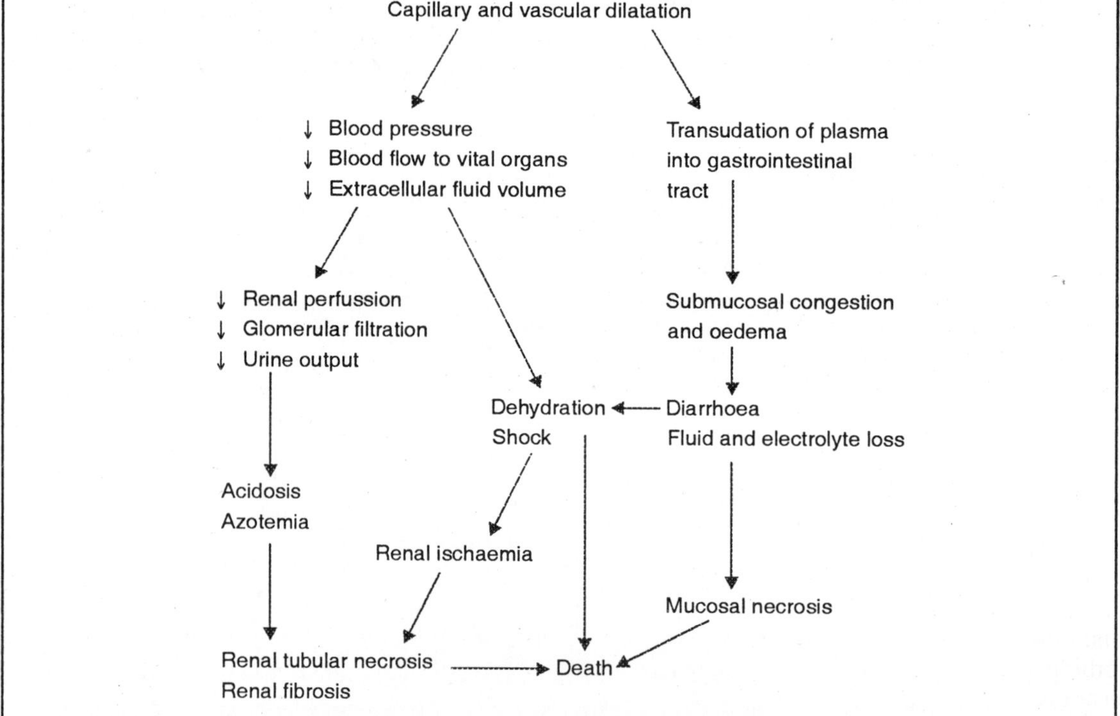

Fig. 11.3. Pathogenesis of toxicosis from trivalent arsenicals. The decreased renal perfusion and renal damage (necrosis of renal tubules) is also caused by arsenical inhibition of energy metabolism.

reduced blood volume, hypotension, shock and circulatory loss. Oedema, vesiculation and eventual loss of GI mucosa also occur that further aggravate fluid loss and shock. Dilatation and swelling of glomerular capillaries in kidneys accompanied by hypotension and hypovolaemia lead to decreased renal perfusion, nephrosis and oliguria (Figure 11.3). Following percutaneous absorption, capillary dilation and degeneration cause vesiculation, blistering and oedema of skin.

b. *Pentavalent inorganic arsenicals:* The arsenate (pentavalent) ion appears to substitute for phosphate in oxidative phosphorylation. Arsenate is a well-known uncoupler of mitochondrial oxidative phosphorylation. There is competitive substitution of arsenate for inorganic phosphate in the formation of adenosine triphosphate, with subsequent formation of an unstable arsenate ester that is rapidly hydrolysed. This process is called arsenolysis. However, elevated body temperature is not a characteristic of arsenate as seen with other oxidative uncouplers (e.g. nitrophenols).

c. *Pentavalent organic arsenicals (feed additives):* They act by an unknown mechanism. They produce demyelination and axonal degeneration, which perhaps is due to interference with the B vitamins required for maintenance of nervous tissue. This effect of arsenic has been associated with peripheral nerve and spinal cord dysfunction in man.

d. *Arsine gas (AsH_3):* Arsine is a gaseous hydride of trivalent arsenic. Arsine does not cause typical signs of arsenic poisoning. It causes haemolysis and pulmonary oedema by mechanisms which are not clearly understood. Rapid and fatal haemolysis results probably from arsine combining with haemoglobin and then reacting with oxygen to cause haemolysis. This effect of arsenic does not apparently depend on sulphydryl inhibition and hence dimercaprol has no effect on the haemolysis.

Clinical signs :

a. Trivalent inorganic or organic arsenicals

Acute and Peracute toxicity: Acute or peracute poisoning with arsenic is common with high morbidity and mortality. Major action of acute or peracute toxicosis is on the GI tract and cardiovascular system. In peracute cases, there are no signs and the animal is found dead. Alternately, there may be sudden and severe colic, staggering gaït, collapse, paralysis and death.

In acute cases, the signs include severe gastroenteritis, colic, staggering gait, extreme weakness, trembling, salivation, vomiting (in dogs, cats and pigs), increased thirst, projectile watery diarrhoea, possible blood in fäeces, fast and weak pulse, hypotension, dehydration, oliguria or anuria, rumen atony, hind limbs paralysis, prostration, normal or subnormal temperature, coma and death in 1-3 days. Severity of clinical signs in cattle correlates with haemoconcentration as indicated by the PCV. Animals inadvertently sprayed with soluble arsenites may exhibit vesicles, pustules, ulcers and skin necrosis.

Subacute toxicity: In subacute cases, the animal may live several days with same clinical signs as mentioned for acute toxicity, but generally less pronounced. The important signs include colic, anorexia, depression, staggering, weakness, diarrhoea with blood and/or mucous discharge, polyuria and then anuria, dehydration, polydipsia, partial paralysis of rear limbs, cold extremities, and hypothermia. Convulsions rarely occur. Acidosis and azotemia may cause death. Percutaneous absorption of arsenic may cause oedema of skin, skin eruptions and secondary skin infections.

Chronic toxicity: Chronic cases are rarely seen in domestic animals, but are well documented in man. Chronic arsenic poisoning in animals is characterised by wasting, poor condition, thirst, brick red discolouration of visible mucous membranes, normal temperature and weak irregular pulse. Swelling of the joints, joint pains with stiffness and paralysis have also been reported. Following percutaneous absorption, the skin becomes dry, papery, and may crack, bleed and develop secondary infection. Disorders of reproduction (sterility, abortion) have been associated with chronic arsenic exposure. Chronic arsenic poisoning in animals is generally encountered in industrial regions following ingestion of forage contaminated by industrial pollutants. Deliberate or criminal poisoning is often referred to but is rarely seen in veterinary medicine.

In human medicine, arsenicosis is recognized by the skin blotches that arise all over face and body with hyper-pigmentation of the chest and upper arms, hard patches on palms and soles, inability to walk accompanied with debilitating pain and watery eyes. Arsenic is carcinogenic and its chronic exposure can result in skin, pulmonary and bladder cancers.

b. Pentavalent organic arsenical feed additives: Early signs are apparent after 2-4 days and include nervous derangement such as ataxia, incoordination and blindness. Affected animals (mostly swine) become weak, assume a sitting dog posture, and eventually become paralysed in lateral recumbency. Appetite remains normal and animal is alert. Blindness is characteristic of arsinilic acid poisoning and not of other arsenicals.

Post-mortem findings: In peracute arsenic toxicosis, no lesions may be seen. Necropsy lesions in acute poisoning include inflammation of GI tract, oedema, rupture of blood vessels, and necrosis of epithelial and subepithelial tissues. The necrosis may progress to perforation of the gastric or intestinal wall. Contents of the gut are fluid, often foul smelling and blood tinged and may contain shreds of epithelial tissue. There may be diffuse inflammation of the liver and other abdominal viscera. Occasionally haemorrhages may occur on all surfaces of the heart. Skin is dry, leathery and peeling following cutaneous exposure. In subacute cases, there are pale swollen kidneys, pale liver, petechial haemorrhages of intestinal serosa and mucosa.

Microscopic lesions in the GI tract include intestinal capillary dilatation, mucosal and submucosal oedema, and necrosis and sloughing of mucosa. In kidneys, all portions of nephron are affected with glomerular sclerosis and severe renal tubular necrosis. Hepatic fatty degeneration and necrosis may be observed in liver. Capillary degeneration is observed in various organs including gut, skin, lungs and kidneys.

Diagnosis: Diagnosis is made from history, circumstantial evidences, clinical signs and lesions. A sudden onset of severe colic, bloody or watery diarrhoea containing mucosal shreds, and post-mortem findings of haemorrhagic gastroenteritis and degenerative changes in liver and kidneys should always be interpreted as possible arsenic poisoning. No other metal or metalloid, with the possible exception of thallium, causes such a speedy onset of severe GI damage. Chemical determination of arsenic in tissues and ingesta provides confirmation. Antemortem samples include urine, vomitus, faeces and hair. After death, hepatic, renal and nervous tissues (organic pentavalent toxicosis) may be taken. Analysis of feed, plant, soil should also be done. Liver and kidney tissues of healthy animal rarely contain > 1 ppm arsenic (wet wt.), whereas toxicity is associated with concentrations > 3 ppm. Urinalysis reveals high arsenic content for many days, proteinuria, increased specific gravity and casts.

Arsenic poisoning has to be differentiated from:

a. *Lead poisoning:* Lead poisoning, if severe enough, can mimic various aspects of arsenic poisoning but with lead there are nervous and behavioural signs.
b. *Caustics, irritants, urea:* These also show GI signs like diarrhoea and colic and require careful identification. The nervous syndrome in pigs poisoned by organic arsenicals may be confused with organic mercury poisoning, salt poisoning and encephalitis, but the mildness of signs, lack of effect on appetite and absence of fever differentiate it from others.

Treatment and management :

Specific therapy: Specific therapy is aimed at the known affinity of arsenic for sulphydryl groups, particularly dithiols.

a. *Dimercaprol/British Anti-Lewisite (BAL)* : It is a dithiol-containing chelating agent that can form a relatively non-toxic and easily excretable complex with arsenic. However, it is relatively ineffective unless given prior to a set of clinical signs as enzymes that have been inhibited for long time are not easily regenerated by dimercaprol. Further, if arsenic is present in large excess, neither dimercaprol nor any other chelator can be expected to work very well to regenerate enzyme activity. Dimercaprol also has toxic effects (vomiting, tremors, and convulsions) which limit its dosage and frequency of administration.

   Large animals: 3 mg/kg (5% sol. in 10% sol. of benzyl benzoate in arachis oil) by deep I.M. injection. The injection should be repeated every 4 hours for the first 2 days, every 6 hours the 3rd day and twice a day for next 10 days until recovery. Renal function should be monitored during therapy.

   Small animals: 2.5-5 mg/kg (10% sol. in oil). Dose intervals are same as in large animals.

   Dosage and frequency of BAL is highly specific i.e. if administered too late or in insufficient doses at infrequent intervals the animal may die of arsenic poisoning, and if administered in excess or at too frequent intervals the animal may die of BAL poisoning. This is also true for other specific chelating agents used in metal toxicosis.

b. *Thioctic acid*: Thioctic acid (α-Lipoic acid) is considered more effective than dimercaprol for arsenic poisoned cattle, however, it is not available in a commercial dosage form. Thioctic acid is used alone or in combination with dimercaprol.

Cattle: 50 mg/kg body wt., I.M., thrice a day as 20% solution (50 g of dl -6, 8-thioctic acid dissolved in 100 ml of warm 5N NaOH, cooled, then adjusted to pH neutrality with 1N HCl and brought to volume with distilled water).

c. *Sodium thiosulphate:* Sodium thiosulphate is a safe antidote to arsenic poisoning. The sulphur of thiosulphate probably reacts with arsenic and immobilises it.

Horses and cattle: 8-10 g (total dose) I.V. as 10-20% solution plus 20-30 g orally in about 300 ml water.

Sheep and goats: One fourth of above dose.

d. *Mesodimercaptosuccinic acid (MDSA) and Dimercaptosuccinic acid (DMSA, succimer)*: These are water soluble derivatives of dimercaprol and said to be superior to dimercaprol, but efficacy is not well tested against arsenic poisoning.

Supportive therapy and maintenance

a. Emetics, gastric lavage and activated charcoal may be employed if the arsenic ingestion is recent. Emesis and vigorous lavage is contraindicated after clinical signs have developed, due to possibility of increasing the likelihood of perforation and shock.
b. Correction of shock, dehydration and acidosis with extracellular electrolyte solutions may be done. Blood may be given, if necessary.
c. Renal function should be monitored and urinary flow may be promoted using 10% dextrose solution.
d. Animal should be kept warm and comfortable.
e. Sufficient vitamins, antibiotics, analgesics and other symptomatic care may be instituted.
f. A high protein diet is recommended during the post-exposure period.

Prognosis: The prognosis of arsenic poisoning is grave if the animal is not treated promptly or if there has been extensive organ damage and animal is prostrate. The mortality rate is high among acutely poisoned animals with inorganic trivalent arsenicals. With organic pentavalent arsenicals, the mortality is low but morbidity is high and recovery may take 2-4 weeks with good nursing and supportive care.

Public health concerns: All arsenicals should be treated as poison. Their containers must bear a warning label 'poison' and must be kept out of general reach. These may be used only by trained workers and any use must be strictly recorded. In domestic animals, arsenic does not stay in tissues for very long. Milk from poisoned cows can be toxic for humans, but the flesh of surviving animals is said to be safe for human consumption.

Some important compounds of arsenic:

Inorganic arsenic compounds

a. *Hydrogen arsenide (Arsine):* Hydrogen arsenide (AsH_3 or arsine) is a colourless gas with garlic odour. It is generated under the effect of hydrogen on arsenic compounds. It is a very strong poison (10 to 20 times as toxic as CO); 10 ppm is toxic within a min. It has MAC of 0.05 ppm.
b. *Arsenic trioxide:* Arsenic trioxide (Arsenious oxide, As_2O_3, *Sankhya*) is commonly called white arsenic or simply arsenic. It is white amorphous, vitreous or crystalline matter, slightly soluble in cold water (1-2 mg/ml) but highly soluble on boiling (0.2 - 0.3 g/ml). The solution formed is acidic and is called arsenious acid. Arsenic trioxide has a property of floating on water as a white film. It is largely used as principal ingredient of fly papers, rodenticides, anthelmintic, etc.
c. *Potassium arsenite and Sodium arsenite:* Potassium arsenite (K_3AsO_3) and sodium arsenite (Na_2AsO_3) are white powders, soluble in water. Both are poisonous and are used in manufacturing of fly papers, insecticides, herbicides, sheep dips, rodenticides, etc.
d. *Sodium arsenate and Potassium arsenate:* Arsenic acid (H_3AsO_4, obtained by warming arsenious oxide with nitric acid) combines with metals to form salts called arsenates. The arsenates of the alkali-

metals are soluble in water. Both sodium arsenate (Na_2AsO_4) and Potassium arsenate (K_3AsO_4) are poisonous and are used for homicidal and malicious poisoning of cattle.

Organic arsenic compounds

e. *Acetarsone:* Acetarsone (3-acetylamino-4-hydroxy phenyl arsonic acid, acetarsol) is an organic compound of arsenic used in veterinary medicine as antihistomonad in turkeys and spirochetocide in poultry. It has also been used as a tonic. It occurs as colourless crystals and contains 27% of arsenic.

f. *Thiacetarsamide:* Thiacetarsamide (Arsenamide) is an organic arsenic compound used in the treatment of heartworm infection in dogs, especially the adult stages.

g. *Copper acetoarsenite:* Copper acetoarsenite (Paris green) is an insecticide, but is less used nowadays due to high toxicity.

2. Mercury

Mercury (Hg) is a heavy metal that exists in liquid form at room temperature. It possesses significant toxicological importance with several incidents of mercury poisoning reported throughout the recorded history. Mercury also possesses therapeutic values and remained an important constituent of drugs for centuries, but now it has been replaced by better drugs. Mercury as an environmental pollutant is a major concern today because of increased usage of fossil fuels and agrochemicals, which contain mercury. Acute toxicosis in animals is not common because of limited availability of toxic amounts of mercury.

Properties: Mercury is a liquid metal having a bright silvery lustre which is volatile even at room temperature. Mercury is found both in inorganic and organic forms. The inorganic form consists of elemental mercury and mercury salts. The elemental mercury (Hg^o; metallic mercury or mercury vapour) is the most volatile of various forms of the metal and its main concern is exposure to industrial occupational workers. Mercury salts, commonly called inorganic mercury, exist in two oxidation states : monovalent mercurous salts and divalent mercuric salts. Mercuric salts are more irritating and are acutely toxic. Elemental mercury may become inorganic compounds by oxidation and revert back to elemental form by reduction. Organic mercury, called organomercurials, can be found in 2 forms - aryl (e.g. phenyl) and short and long chain alkyl (e.g. ethyl, methyl, propyl and dimethyl) compounds. As compared to aryl organic mercury compounds, alkyl organomercurials tend to be more toxic, especially after repeated exposure. Although all forms of mercury are toxic, the organic mercurials are considered more toxic than inorganic mercury compounds.

Sources of Toxicity: Mercury poisoning was common throughout the 19th century and early 20th century because of its wide spread use in drugs, agricultural and household products, and industry. Now a majority of mercurial products have been substituted and incidence of mercury toxicity has declined. Still mercury is an important toxicant and its toxicosis in man and animals may occur from following sources:

a. Ingestion of grains and seeds treated with organomercurial fungicides (e.g. ethyl mercuric-chloride and -hydroxide).

b. Occupational exposure in industries where mercury is used in the manufacture of electrical equipments, anti-foul paints, small batteries, thermometers, mirrors, semiconductor cells, fingerprinting products, fluorescent and mercury lamps, infrared detectors, chloroalkali (e.g. bleach), plastics, dental amalgams, etc. (See also Table 11.1).

c. Ingestion of fish contaminated with organomercurials such as methyl mercury. Several aquatic organisms including fish accumulate methyl mercury from pullulated watersheds, bays, etc.

d. Due to volatile nature, there is a constant emission of the mercury vapour from underground deposits, fossil fuels (coals), volcanic action and sea water evaporation. These vapour return to earth via rainfall and may contaminate soil and water.

e. Inadvertent and indiscriminate use of some mercury containing drugs such as ointments (e.g. red mercuric iodide), antiseptics (e.g. mercurochrome and phenylmercuric nitrate) and diuretics (e.g. mersalyl).

f. Use of thimerosal, an organomercurial, as additive preservative in some vaccines

Table 11.1: List of important sources of mercury toxicity.

Elemental Mercury
Barometers, batteries, bronzing, calibration instruments, chlor-alki production, dental amalgams, electroplating, fingerprinting products, fluorescent and mercury lamps, fossil fuels, infrared detectors, jewellery industry, manometers, neon lamps, paints, paper pulp production, photography, semiconductor cells, silver and gold production, thermometers, underground and sea-water evaporation, and volcanic eruptions.
Inorganic mercury
Acetaldehyde production, chemical laboratory work, cosmetics, drugs (antiseptics, disinfectants, cathartics, caustics, counter-irritants, vesicants), explosives, embalming, fur hat processing, ink manufacturing, mercury vapour lamps, mirror silvering, perfume industry, photography, spermicidal jellies, tattooing inks, taxidermy production, vinyl chloride production, and wood preservatives.
Organic mercury
Drugs (antibacterials, antifungals, antiseptics, diuretics), embalming agents, farming industry, fungicides, germicidal agents, insecticidal products, laundry products, paper manufacturing, pathology products, histology products, seed preservatives, vaccines, and wood preservatives.

(e.g. DTP vaccine, inactivated influenza vaccine, and hepatitis B vaccine) to prevent bacterial contamination.

g. Contamination of water with sewage sludge containing industrial waste.

h. Chronic exposure to mercury in ambient air after inadvertent mercury spills in poorly ventilated rooms, scientific laboratories, etc.

i. Dental amalgams used for filling teeth.

Factors affecting toxicity:

a. *Species:* Ruminants, particularly calves and cows, show the highest sensitivity to mercury. Horses, pigs and fowls are relatively less susceptible.

b. *Chemical form*: Organic mercury compounds are more lipid soluble, more absorbable and uniformly distributed in body. So organomercurials are more toxic than inorganic mercury compounds.

c. *Solubility*: Insoluble inorganic mercury salts (mercurous chloride or monovalents) are less toxic than soluble inorganic salts (mercuric chloride or divalents) as they are slowly absorbed.

d. *Route of exposure*: Elemental mercury is virtually non-toxic after oral administration but highly toxic after inhalation.

e. *Dietary factors*: Interacting substances in diet like selenium and vitamin E decrease toxicity of organic mercurials.

f. *Duration of exposure*: Short term exposure to elemental mercury produces corrosive and pulmonary lesions due to its irritant action, whereas long-term exposure produces mainly neurological signs.

g. *Bioaccumulation*: Organic mercurials like methyl mercury are continuously taken in small amounts by fishes from marine water and accumulate them in very high concentration. This becomes a source of potential toxicity in fish eating animals and human beings.

Toxicity: Mercury in any form is toxic. The difference lies in the chemical form, solubility, route of exposure, and species involved. Mercury poisoning can result from vapour inhalation, ingestion, injection, or absorption through skin. Overall, alkyl mercury compounds are the most toxic forms of mercury, followed by aryl organomercurials, inorganic mercuric salts, and elemental mercury (except vapour inhalation that is highly toxic).

The oral LD_{50} of different organomercurials in swine is about 13.4 mg Hg/kg. Feeding of methylmercury dicyaniamide to pigs at the rate of 2.5 mg/kg causes no apparent illness, 5-15 mg/kg causes illness and levels of 20 mg/kg are fatal. It is toxic to pigs when fed daily at a rate of 0.2-0.75 mg of mercury per kg for 60-90 days. In rabbits, dogs and cats, the toxic dosage of methylmercury is 0.4-1 mg Hg/kg/day for 10-90 days. In calves, the toxic dose of methylmercury is about 0.4 mg Hg/kg/day for 35 days or a total dose of 12 mg/kg.

In general, methyl mercury toxicosis results from continued exposure to dosages of 0.2-5.0 mg/kg body weight. The oral LD_{50} of phenylmercury acetate is about 25 mg/kg in rats. In cats, 2-3 mg Hg/kg/day of ethylmercury compounds produces clinical signs in 2-3 weeks and death in 4 weeks.

Toxic dose of inorganic mercury in horses is 8-10 grams. Chronic toxicity of inorganic mercury has been observed by ingestion of 0.4 mg/kg/day over a several-week period of time.

Toxicokinetics: Soluble salts of mercury are absorbed and distributed better than insoluble or less soluble salts hence toxicokinetics depends primarily on the chemical form of the mercury.

a. *Elemental Mercury*: Elemental (liquid) mercury remains practically unabsorbed after ingestion and, therefore, cannot cause acute poisoning. However, elemental mercury may be volatilised to mercury vapour at room temperature, which is lipid-soluble and can be absorbed by inhalation (70-90%). Once in blood (after alveolar penetration of the mercury vapour), elemental mercury (Hg°) is rapidly oxidised to inorganic divalent mercuric ions (Hg^{+2}) within 15-20 min. The Hg^{+2} ions mainly combine with the blood plasma proteins. This inorganic form has similar properties to inorganic mercurials (e.g. poor lipid solubility, limited permeability to blood brain barrier, and excretion in faeces). Some mercury vapours, which remain unoxidised, continue to persist and penetrate the blood brain-barrier. In the brain, elemental mercury get ionized and trapped, attributing to its storage and severe lesions in the CNS.

b. *Inorganic mercury:* Inorganic mercury salts are poorly absorbed from skin and GI tract, usually not exceeding 10% of the ingested amount. Soluble mercury salts (mercuric, Hg^{+2}) after oral administration are mainly stored in the alimentary tract, particularly in the mucous membrane of colon. Insoluble mercury salts (mercurous; Hg^{+}) may undergo some oxidisation to soluble salts and are then absorbed to limited extent. After absorption the soluble mercury combines with blood and tissue proteins depending largely on the affinity of Hg^{2+} for proteins. Overall, the inorganic mercury has a non-uniform mode of distribution secondary to poor lipid solubility and accumulates mostly in the kidneys, causing significant renal damage. Although their poor lipid solubility characteristics limit CNS penetration, the slow elimination and chronic exposure may allow for significant CNS accumulation of mercuric ions and subsequent toxicity. Long-term dermal exposure to inorganic mercury may also lead to toxicity.

c. *Organic mercurials:* In contrast to elemental or inorganic mercury salts, organic mercurials are absorbed via all routes of exposure including dermal. Intestinal absorption of organic mercurials after oral administration may be as high as 90% of the dose in some species. After absorption, the aryl and long chain alkyl compounds are largely converted to their inorganic forms and possess similar toxic properties to inorganic mercury. The short chain alkyl mercurials such as methyl or ethyl mercury generally remain stable in their initial forms. Alkyl organic mercury has high lipid solubility and is distributed uniformly throughout the body, accumulating in the brain, kidneys, liver, muscles, hair, and skin. Organic mercurials also cross the blood brain barrier and placenta and penetrate erythrocytes, attributing to neurological symptoms, teratogenic effects, and high blood to plasma ratio, respectively. Aryl mercurials tend to be somewhat less absorbable via the skin, such that some of these agents are used in topical medications. The alkyl organomercurials are poorly excreted and tend to accumulate in muscles, brain and other tissues. The aryl (phenylmercury) compounds are more readily excreted via the kidneys and less likely to accumulate in brain and muscles.

Mercury is eliminated from the body mainly via intestines and kidneys and in negligible amounts in milk and saliva. Inorganic mercury is eliminated primarily via urine, while organic mercury is eliminated mainly via bile and faeces. The elimination of organic mercury is generally slower than that of inorganic mercury. The hair of animals also store high concentration of mercury and very slowly release them. Half-life of methyl mercury in cats and humans has been reported as 70-74 days and 60 days, respectively. Marine mammals and some other marine animals can bioaccumulate and store mercury at high concentrations for very long time, primarily because of formation of insoluble mercury complexes intracellularly.

Mechanism of action :

a. *Interaction with sulphydryl group:* The biochemical basis of the toxicity of mercury is primarily seen in its interaction with the sulphydryl (-SH, thiol) groups of enzymes and other proteins. Mercury has high affinity for sulphydryl groups and it readily forms covalent bonds with sulphur to produce compounds of the type $R–S–Hg^+$, R–S–Hg–S–R and $R(S_2)Hg$. Living systems have many sulphydryl groups, where divalent mercury replaces the hydrogen atom to form mercaptides such as X–Hg–R and $Hg–(SR)_2$ (Mercaptides are derivatives of mercaptanes in which hydrogen from the SH-group is replaced with a metal atom). Even in low concentration, Hg^{+2} ions dysfunction many sulphydryl containing enzymes, especially those present in mitochondria and microsomes. Inhibition of sulphydryl groups in essential enzymes and proteins blocks several metabolic processes.

   Organic mercurial compounds, due to their high affinity for sulphydryl groups, combine with several membrane and intracellular proteins. They interfere with metabolic activity and prevent synthesis of essential proteins, leading to cellular degeneration and necrosis. Their most important target is brain. Organic mercury targets specific sites in the brain, including the cerebral cortex (especially visual cortex), motor and sensory centres, auditory centre (temporal cortex), and cerebellum. They also produce dysfunction of blood-brain-barrier, increase permeability of membranes and interfere with substrate utilisation. One important enzyme that is inhibited by methyl mercury is choline acetyltransferase, which is involved in the final step of acetylcholine production. This inhibition may lead to acetylcholine deficiency, contributing to the signs and symptoms of motor dysfunction.

b. *Corrosive and irritant action:* Inorganic mercurial salts cause direct tissue necrosis and renal tubular necrosis. Soluble inorganic salts precipitate proteins and produce strong corrosive action on GI mucosa. They intensively damage the membranes of renal canaliculi. The glomerular filter membranes become more permeable to plasma proteins which enter the urine. So the blood levels of plasma proteins are reduced. Inorganic salts also have hepatotoxic action.

c. *Other actions:*

   i. Mercury in addition to sulphydryl groups has affinity (less than -SH groups) for other functional groups in the following sequence: SH > $CONH_2$ > NH_2 > COOH > PO_4. Mercury interacts with these groups and blocks activity of several essential enzymes including alkaline phosphatase, G-6-phosphatase, adenosine triphosphatase, succinic dehydrogenase and amino-levulinic acid dehydrogenase. This leads to blocking of active glucose transport into cells and altered membrane permeability.

   ii. Mercury disturbs the immune function and is responsible for some adverse effects on kidneys. Glomerular nephritis and proteinuria are associated with antigen-antibody and complement deposition on epithelial surface of glomerular basement.

   iii. Both Hg^{+2} and methyl mercury can disrupt ion exchange across voltage-gated and ligand-gated channels. Mercury may irreversibly inhibit voltage gated K^+ out-current in the early developing nervous system, which may help explain neurological teratogenicity.

   iv. Methyl mercury is believed to increase production of reactive oxygen species through disruption of the mitochondrial electron transport chain. This increase in free radicals in turn disrupts glutathione and mediates neuronal injury.

v. Methyl mercury inhibits production of ATP and causes release of Ca^{++} from mitochondria. The enhanced intracellular Ca^{++} concentration leads to spontaneous depolarization and release of acetylcholine.

vi. Methyl mercury decreases uptake of choline by cholinergic nerve terminals. The reduced choline uptake disrupts synthesis of acetylcholine and hence cholinergic transmission.

vii. *In vitro*, methyl mercury has shown to disrupt microtubule assembly and cellular migration.

Clinical signs: The clinical presentation of mercury toxicity can manifest in a variety of ways, depending on the route of exposure, intensity of exposure, chemical form, and species involved. Acute toxicity usually is related to the inhalation of elemental mercury or ingestion of inorganic mercury. Exposure to organic mercury leads to chronic toxicity and, occasionally, acute toxicity.

Elemental mercury: Short term exposure to the vapour of elemental mercury may produce signs within several hours which include weakness, chills, nausea, vomiting, diarrhoea, dyspnoea and cough. Acute exposure caused by inhaled elemental mercury can lead to pulmonary signs, which may progress to an interstitial pneumonitis with severe compromise of respiratory function. Recovery is usually without sequelae, but pulmonary complications of inhaled toxicity may include interstitial emphysema, pneumatocele, pneumothorax, pneumomediastinum, and interstitial fibrosis.

Chronic exposure of elemental mercury mainly causes neurological signs like depression, irritability, excessive shyness, vasomotor disturbances (such as excessive perspiration, uncontrolled flushing), salivation, gingivitis and tremors.

Inorganic salts of mercury: Inorganic mercury salt exposure mainly occurs through the oral and GI tract. The corrosive properties of inorganic mercury or mercuric salt account for most of the acute signs and symptoms of toxicity. The most pronounced lesions in acute oral exposure are severe corrosion of the mucous membranes of mouth, pharynx and intestine which produces intense pain, colic, vomiting, bloody diarrhoea, fluid and electrolyte loss and hypovolaemic shock. The mucous membranes are ashen-grey secondary to precipitation of mercuric salts. Systemic effects usually begin several hours post-ingestion and may last several days. These effects include stomatitis, gingival irritation, foul breath, loosening of teeth, and renal tubular necrosis leading to oliguria or anuria. The death of poisoned animals may occur as early as 2-4 days. The divalent mercuric salts are more corrosive and more toxic than the monovalent mercurous salts.

Subacute or chronic exposure of inorganic mercury salts produces GI, neurological, and renal dysfunctions.

Organic mercurials: Organic mercury poisoning in animals usually results from ingestion of contaminated food and feed and is more common in species like swine. The time within which the signs develop depends on the size of daily dose and on the type of compound. The long chain and aryl forms of organic mercury have similar characteristics of inorganic mercury toxicity, whereas short chain organic mercury (e.g. methyl mercury) affects the CNS and produces neurological signs. The onset of signs usually is delayed (days to weeks) after exposure because organic mercury targets enzymes and depletion of these enzymes must occur before the onset of signs. Early signs are erythema of skin, conjunctivitis, lachrymation and stomatitis. Neurological signs related to toxicity include visual disturbance (occasional blindness), disorientation, ataxia, paresthesias (early signs), hearing loss, dysarthria, muscle tremor, movement disorders and, with severe exposure, paralysis, coma and death. Other effects in animals may include oral mucosal ulcers, skin oedema, alopecia, hyperthermia, depression, epistaxis, convulsions and haematuria. Maternal exposure to organic mercurials can lead to spontaneous abortion in pregnant animals or produce retardation or malformation in foetus.

Chronic poisoning with organomercurials is relatively non-specific and difficult to diagnose. The clinical signs may include anorexia, weight loss, and fall in milk production. Several episodes of trembling and shaking, persistent convulsions, deterioration in health, leading to death in several weeks to several months may suggest chronic organic mercury poisoning. Reduced hatchability and eggs without shell have been observed in birds.

Post-mortem findings: Gross gastrointestinal lesions include gastric ulcers, necrotic enteritis, colitis, etc. There is focal congestion of lungs and GI mucosa. Liver is pale and reduced in size. Renal lesions include pale, swollen kidneys with renal tubular necrosis, especially affecting the proximal tubular epithelium. Glomerulonephritis is possible with chronic exposure due to antigen-antibody complex deposition. Inhalation of mercury vapour may produce acute, corrosive bronchitis and interstitial pneumonia. In elemental mercury and organomercurials toxicosis, degenerative lesions in the brain may be seen. In contrast to inorganic mercury salts, organomercurials have no corrosive action on the mucous membranes.

Microscopic lesions include fibrinoid degeneration of cerebral arterioles, neuronal necrosis, neuronophagia, cortical vacuolation, axon swelling and gliosis in the CNS. The cerebrum is the most severely affected region of the central nervous system. In peripheral nerves, myelin and axonal degeneration may be observed. In inorganic salts toxicosis, heart and liver may show fatty degeneration and kidneys show tubular necrosis.

Diagnosis: Diagnosis of mercury poisoning on the basis of clinical signs and lesions is difficult because multiple organ systems are affected (e.g. CNS, kidneys and mucous membranes) and the manifestations can mimic a variety of other diseases. So the diagnosis mainly depends on analytical evidences. Laboratory analysis should differentiate between the normal concentration of mercury in tissues and feed (< 1 ppm) and the concentration associated with acute poisoning. Concentrations of mercury in acute poisoning may be elevated in the kidneys (> 10-15 ppm), liver and brain.

Mercury poisoning should be differentiated from other poisonings like lead, thallium, phenylarsonic feed additives and ethylene glycol. Certain diseases like hog cholera, erysipelas, gastroenteritis, polioencephalomalacia and dermatitis (exfoliative) also mimic signs of mercury toxicosis.

Treatment and management: Treatment of mercury poisoning is essential and should be instituted early, but the neurological damage, if occurs, may be permanent. Treatment involves both specific and supportive therapies.

Specific therapy: The specific therapy includes chelation of mercury with dimercaprol, D-Penicillamine or succimer. The chelators are effective mainly against the inorganic mercury salts and less against organic mercurials. The short-chain organic mercurials (e.g. methyl mercury) are difficult to mobilise from the body by chelators.

a. *Dimercaprol*: The dimercaprol (British anti-lewisite) is an effective chelator of mercury for high-level exposure or symptomatic patients. It is effective in increasing urinary excretion of inorganic

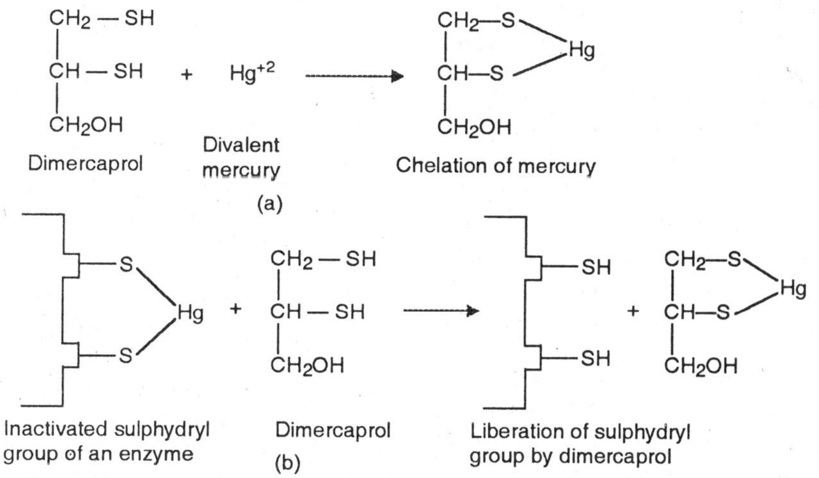

$CH_2—SH$ / $CH—SH$ / CH_2OH (Dimercaprol) + Hg^{+2} (Divalent mercury) → $CH_2—S$ / $CH—S$ (Hg) / CH_2OH (Chelation of mercury)

(a)

Inactivated sulphydryl group of an enzyme (–S–Hg–S–) + Dimercaprol ($CH_2—SH$ / $CH—SH$ / CH_2OH) → Liberation of sulphydryl group by dimercaprol (–SH, –SH) + $CH_2—S$ / $CH—S$ (Hg) / CH_2OH

(b)

Fig. 11.4. Mechanism of action of dimercaprol.
(a) Chelation of free mercury (b) Regeneration of inactivated sulphydryl group.

mercurials, but the chelation therapy with dimercaprol is not much useful with the organic mercurials as only a small fraction of organic mercury is in plasma and hence is not readily available for excretion. Rather, dimercaprol is contraindicated with organic mercurials as by causing release of mercury from other tissues, it may increase the brain concentration. Dimercaprol is also contraindicated with pre-existing liver or kidney damage.

Large animals: 3 mg/kg (5% sol. in 10% sol. of benzyl benzoate in arachis oil) by deep I.M. route every 4 hourly for first 2 days, 6 hourly on 3rd day and 12 hourly for next 10 days or until recovery is seen.

b. *D-Penicillamine:* D-Penicillamine is an effective chelator of some metals including mercury. It should be used only after the intestine is cleared of mercury and only if renal function is present, otherwise is dangerous.

All species: 15-50 mg/kg daily by oral route.

c. *Mesodimercaptosuccinic acid (DMSA) and Dimercaptopropane sulphonate (DMPS):* The DMSA (Succimer) and DMPS are water soluble analogues of dimercaprol, which are less lipid soluble and less toxic than the dimercaprol. The DMSA is considered more effective than the DMPS in reducing the methyl mercury contents of kidneys, brain and liver. The efficacy of DMSA and DMPS at increasing the urinary excretion of inorganic mercury salts is in the following order: DMSA > Dimercaprol > DMPS. Both DMSA and DMPS are used orally.

DMSA: 10 mg/kg, orally, three times daily.

d. *Sodium thiosulphate*: Sodium thiosulphate may be used in mercury poisoning in combination with dimercaprol. Sodium thiosulphate binds the mercury and helps in its excretion.

Sodium thiosulphate (20% sol.): 10 ml/45 kg body wt. by I.V. route, 4 doses at 8 hour intervals.

Supportive and detoxification therapy

a. Gastric lavage with sodium formaldehyde sulphoxalate (100-250 ml, 5% solution) is useful. This reduces divalent mercury to the less toxic monovalent form.

b. Egg white or activated charcoal may be administered orally to adsorb ingested mercury.

c. A saline cathartic or sorbitol promotes clearance of mercury from the intestinal tract.

d. Supplemental selenium and vitamin E are somewhat protective against organomercurials like methyl mercury toxicosis.

e. Short-term respiratory support in elemental mercury vapour poisoning is helpful.

f. Fluids and electrolytes may be used for corrosive GI syndrome.

g. Seizures, if present, may be controlled with CNS depressants like diazepam or barbiturates (phenobarbitone or, if it fails, pentobarbitone).

Prognosis: Prognosis is grave once the neurological signs develop in elemental and organic mercury compounds toxicosis.

Public health concern: Organic mercurials can accumulate in edible organs and muscles; therefore, mercury intoxicated animals should not be used as food. Presence of mercury in some industrial wastes pose widespread environmental problems and methyl mercury is formed by some aquatic microorganisms which is taken by fish and then by fish eating animals and human beings.

Some important compounds of mercury:

Inorganic compounds

a. *Mercuric oxide:* Mercuric oxide (HgO) is a brick red crystalline powder but forms an amorphous yellow powder when the mercuric salt is acted upon by caustic soda or potash. Both the red and yellow varieties are insoluble in water. The red variety is known as red iodide of mercury (Hydrargyri oxidum rubrum) and is used in the preparation of red ointment.

b. *Mercuric chloride:* Mercuric chloride (Perchloride of mercury/$HgCl_2$) exists in the form of heavy, colourless mass of prismatic crystals or as white crystalline powder. It is used as pesticide, wood preservative and preservative of anatomical preparations. It is also used as caustic, antiseptic and disinfectant.

c. *Mercuric iodide:* Mercuric iodide (HgI_2), also called red iodide of mercury or biniodide of mercury, is a scarlet red powder obtained by the action of a watery solution of mercuric chloride on potassium iodide. It has been used as a topical antiseptic, counterirritant and vesicant.

d. *Mercuric sulphide:* Mercuric sulphide (HgS) occurs as the chief ore of mercury and is artificially prepared as a red, crystalline powder, which is then known as the pigment vermillion. It is regarded as non-poisonous, but its vapours are poisonous.

e. *Mercurous chloride:* Mercurous chloride (Calomel, Hg_2Cl_2) is a heavy amorphous, white and tasteless powder, which is insoluble in water, alcohol and other organic solvents. When heated, it sublimes without fusing. It has been used orally as a cathartic and locally as an antiseptic and desiccant.

Organic compounds

f. *Ethyl mercuric chloride:* Ethyl mercuric chloride (CH_3CH_2HgCl) is an alkyl organic mercurial, used mainly as fungicide for seed and grain dressings. It is highly toxic and its chronic exposure leads to permanent injury to brain. Percutaneous absorption causes skin burn.

g. *Mersalyl:* Mersalyl (Mersalin) is an aryl organic mercurial used occasionally as a diuretic. Its excessive use may produce systemic mercury toxicity and attenuate kidney damage.

h. *Thimerosal:* Thimerosal (Merthiolate) is an aryl organic mercurial used occasionally as topical antibacterial and antifungal agent. It is also added to certain vaccines as a preservative.

i. *Phenylmercuric nitrate:* Phenylmercuric nitrate (Merphenyl nitrate, $C_{12}H_{11}Hg_2NO_4$) is an aryl organomercurial used mainly as topical antiseptic, antibacterial and antifungal agent. It possesses potential risk of toxicity, if used indiscriminately or at high concentration.

3. Lead

Lead (Pb) is a metal of toxicological importance since ancient times and is presently recognized as a major environmental health risk throughout the world. Lead intoxication is one of the most frequently diagnosed poisoning in veterinary medicine world-wide and has been reported in all domestic and several zoo species. The historical use of lead acetate (also known as sugar of lead) by the Roman Empire as a sweetener of wine is considered by some to be the cause of dementia which affected many of the Roman Emperors.

Properties: Lead is a true metal which belongs to the group VI of the periodic chart of elements. Lead is very soft, highly malleable, bluish-white metal that has poor electrical conductivity. It exists in elemental, inorganic and organic forms. Lead is present in trace amounts in all soils, water and foods. It is more ubiquitous than most other toxic metals as a result of its natural occurrence and industrial use.

Sources of toxicity :

a. Accidental ingestion of lead objects such as batteries, gun shots, lead solders and candy bar wrappers carelessly thrown near animal farms are important source of poisoning in animals. Junk piles of farm machinery in pastures are another common source of poisoning in cattle.

b. Ingestion or licking of lead-based paints (freshly painted walls, dry pealing paints) and related products (lead primers, putty of caulking materials) cause poisoning in many animals. Lead based paints are less used now, but crumbling of old painted surfaces continues to be one of the most frequent causes of plumbism in cattle, particularly in young calves with pica.

c. Grass near busy highways may contain toxic amounts of lead from auto exhausts. The contamination of grass or land by lead is more in the immediate vicinity of motorways, busy roads and junctions. Increased use of lead-free petrol, however, has reduced the amount of lead from this source.

d. Pastures and vegetation contaminated by atmospheric fallout from smelters and mining operations contain significant amount of lead. Vegetables and fodders that have been grown in soils saturated with lead (e.g. land around the site of old lead mines) may contain toxic amounts of lead. Animals particularly sheep are reported to acquire a taste for lead and frequently graze in high contamination areas.

e. Vapours, fumes and powder generated from lead based industries such as lead smelting, lead refining and battery manufacturing constitute major environmental source of lead poisoning. All types of mining industries, especially strip mining can cause lead and other minerals to leech into ground water, soil and even release into the air as dust particles. Steel industry or any other industry that uses steel in production can contribute to the bioaccumulation of lead in soil, water and air.

f. Lead is used as a colouring element in ceramic glazes, notably in colours red and yellow. Improper glazing of enamelled or ceramic pots and dishware can leech lead into foods, especially if used for acidic foods or liquids.

g. Accidental consumption or licking of used engine oil filters, motor oil spilt, grease, or other farm products that are contaminated with gasoline.

h. Natural sources of lead such as galena or soils are not particularly toxic but can add to the total body burden. Ingestion of lead contaminated soil may be a major problem in animals with pica.

i. Agricultural use of fertilizers, fungicides and herbicides that contain appreciable amounts of lead (e.g. lead arsenate) also result in lead poisoning in animals.

j. Lead parasiticide sprays, particularly those containing lead arsenate, may cause toxicity in cattle grazing in recently sprayed orchards or vegetable crops.

k. Drinking water from old lead pipes or glazed crockery pots may contain toxic amounts of lead. Industrial effluents in streams may also contaminate drinking water.

l. Milk secreted from lead-poisoned animals can be dangerous for the young animals.

Factors affecting toxicity :

a. Age: Young animals are more susceptible because they absorb greater fraction of ingested lead than the adults.

b. Species: Dogs, cattle, horses and water fowl are more susceptible to lead and are all poisoned relatively often. Cats and sheep are probably of intermediate sensitivity, and goats, swine and chickens are comparatively tolerant.

c. Pregnancy: Pregnant ewes are more sensitive to lead poisoning than are non-pregnant ewes.

d. Rate of ingestion: Large amounts of lead ingested in 1 or 2 days may be fatal, but smaller amounts ingested over a period of several weeks may not be.

e. Form: Soluble salts (e.g. lead acetate) are more readily absorbed so are more toxic than insoluble salts (e.g. lead oxide).

f. General status: Poorly nourished, weak and emaciated animals are more susceptible to lead toxicity than healthy animals.

g. Past exposure: Previous chronic low-level exposure may impart a degree of tolerance to some of the biochemical effects of lead. However, previous acute exposure may reduce the subsequent amount required to produce a lethal effect.

h. Condition of GI tract: Presence of ingesta in GI tract may delay or reduce absorption of lead. Absorption of lead from the damaged intestinal mucosa is relatively more.

Toxicity: Cattle, horses and dogs are more susceptible to lead poisoning and are exposed to a greater extent than other species because of their habit of licking, chewing, or eating foreign objects such as soil and flakes of old paints from the wall. Lead poisoning is rare in cats, probably because of their fastidious eating habits. Lead poisoning can occur in both free-flying birds and poorly managed companion or commercialized birds. Though pigs can be poisoned with very high levels of lead, yet they are quite resistant and field cases of lead toxicity in pigs are rare.

Lead toxicosis is usually due to acute exposure, but can result from repeated exposure with a gradually increased build-up of lead in body. Toxicity of lead varies with different lead salts. The acute oral lethal dose of lead acetate in various species is: calves = 200-400 mg/kg; cattle = 600-800 mg/kg; horses = 400-600 mg/kg; dogs and pigs = 800-1000 mg/kg; and poultry = 200-600mg/kg. In chronic toxicity, ingestion of lead over a period of days, weeks or months is required. The chronic oral lethal dose in different species is: cattle 6-7 mg/kg/day of lead acetate for 6-8 weeks, horses 1-7 mg lead/kg/day; sheep (non-pregnant) 8 mg lead acetate/kg/day, sheep (pregnant)1 mg lead acetate/kg/day, and dogs 0.32 mg lead/kg/day for 6 months. Ingestion of 1-3 lead shotgun pellets can be lethal to water fowl; ingested lead shot tends to remain in gizzard, from where the lead is progressively dissolved and absorbed.

Toxicokinetics: Most common route of lead exposure is oral ingestion. Irrespective of the chemical form of ingested lead, only a small proportion (< 10%) is absorbed because of the formation of insoluble lead complexes which are excreted in faeces. Absorption depends in part on the surface area; therefore, finely divided lead as that occurs in used motor oil is more toxic. In cattle and birds, ingested lead objects are lodged in reticulum and gizzard, respectively allowing absorption of lead over an extended period of time. Lead absorption rates may increase with iron, zinc and calcium deficiencies. After inhalation, lead is absorbed to good extent (up to 90% depending on the form). The inhaled lead particles are also cleared by mucociliary action and then swallowed. Airborne lead particles that are less than 0.5-1 microns in diameter are generally completely absorbed by the alveoli. Inorganic lead cannot easily penetrate skin, but organic lead (e.g. tetraethyl lead in regular petrol) can penetrate intact skin readily.

Once lead is absorbed, 85-90% of it binds to haemoglobin in erythrocytes. The remainder is bound to serum albumin. Only <1% of the circulating lead is free and available to tissues and is responsible for the toxic effects. Inorganic lead is distributed initially in the soft tissues, particularly the tubular epithelium of kidney and liver as diphosphate and triphosphate. With time, lead is redistributed and deposited in bone, teeth and hair. About 95% of the body burden of lead is found in bone (bone acts as a sink of lead). However, lead in the bone does not contribute to poisoning except in chronic toxicity. The body may mobilize its lead stores during periods of stress, fever, hyperthyroidism, prolonged immobilization, pregnancy and lactation. Only small quantities of inorganic lead accumulate in the brain, with most of it in grey matter and basal ganglia. The presence of lead in bone marrow suppresses haematopoiesis. This trapping action of bone does not occur after single acute exposure rather it is a slower process entailing redistribution of lead from the soft tissues of the body.

Lead readily passes membrane barriers such as the blood-brain barrier and placenta. Lead is slowly excreted in animals, predominantly via the bile. High blood levels also result in some urinary excretion; urine excretion is more when chelation therapy is administered. Lead is excreted in milk in ratio that equals approximately 5% of the blood concentration. The half-life of lead is 1 to 2 months and a steady state is achieved in about 6 months. Clinical signs of toxicosis may suddenly appear when bones get saturated. This occurs due to rising blood and soft tissue lead concentrations during exposure to the metal.

Mechanism of action: Lead affects multiple tissues, especially the nervous system, gastrointestinal tract and haematopoietic system. The exact mechanism of lead toxicosis at a molecular level is not fully known, but mainly comes from its ability to mimic other biologically important metals such as calcium, zinc and iron. Lead may compete with or replace these metals in some important enzymes and molecules, as a result of which such molecules function differently and fail to carry out biological reactions. Lead, like a number of other metals, inhibits sulphydryl groups of essential enzymes of cellular metabolism. Lead also interferes with Na^+/K^+-ATPase and alters cellular and mitochondrial membranes, thereby increasing cellular fragility.

a. *Neurotoxicity:* Lead affects the nervous system by multiple different mechanisms, most of which are unexplored. Lead causes cerebral oedema and neuronal damage centrally and demyelination and reduced nerve conduction peripherally.

   i. After entry into the brain cells (neurons, glia), lead probably disturbs the function of cellular calcium, which is needed to activate protein kinase C in brain capillaries. This causes damage to capillary endothelium and inactivates blood brain barrier with resulting cerebral oedema and haemorrhage. The leakage of proteinaceous fluid and brain oedema affects almost all parts of the CNS. In growing rats, brain capillary endothelial buds (angioblasts) appear to be primary target. Death of these buds may lead to encephalopathy. Damage to other kinds of cells could be secondary to endothelial damage and circulatory deficiency. This may also lead to neuronal necrosis in the CNS.

ii. Lead affects action of several neurotransmitters in the CNS. It interferes with γ-aminobutyric acid (GABA) and dopamine uptake by synaptosomes. At high concentrations, lead inhibits the inhibitory interneuron junctions in the CNS, possibly due to interference with GABA mediation. In humans, inhibition of N-methyl-D-aspartate (NMDA) receptor by lead and its interference with excitatory neurotransmission by glutamate has been associated with disruption in neuronal development and cognition.

iii. In the peripheral nervous system, lead causes segmental demyelination of motor neurons and destruction of Schwann's cells, resulting in reduced conduction velocity and motor neuron dysfunction. Interference with cholinergic function is also associated with reduced extra-cellular calcium.

b. *Gastrointestinal toxicity:* Specific mechanisms for the gastro-intestinal effects of lead (e.g. anorexia, vomiting and colic) are not described, but could be secondary to neurological mechanisms. Lead causes contractions of the smooth muscle lining of intestinal walls, leading to severe, excruciating, colicky abdominal pain. Gastroenteritis is also produced by the caustic action of lead salts on the GI mucosa.

c. *Haematopoietic toxicity:* The haematopoietic system is extremely sensitive to the adverse effects of lead. A common haematological result of chronic lead poisoning is depression of bone marrow and hypochromic microcytic anaemia. These effects result from two important factors - inhibition of heme synthesis and decreased life span of erythrocytes.

i. Very low concentrations of lead can influence the synthesis of heme by inhibiting certain key enzymes. Among various enzymes involved in the synthesis of heme, five are susceptible to the inhibitory effects of lead. Delta-aminolevulinic acid dehydratase (δ-ALAD) and heme synthetase (ferrochelatase), which are important sulphydryl containing enzymes, are the most susceptible, whereas delta-aminolevulinic acid synthetase (δ-ALAS), uroporphyrinogen decarboxylase (UROD) and coproporphyrinogen oxidase (COPROD) are less sensitive to inhibition by lead (Figure 11.5). Inhibition of these enzymes reduces heme synthesis and causes accumulation of heme precursors (e.g. $\delta-$aminolevulinic acid, coproporphyrins, zinc protoporphyrin) in the blood. In addition to its effect on heme synthesis, lead also inhibits union of heme with globin. Because heme is important for the function of cytochrome system and cellular respiration, lead poisoning has tremendous impact on the entire organism. Other heavy metals like Zn, Cu and Hg also depress haemoglobin synthesis activity in circulating blood, but not to the same degree as lead. Alcohol and possibly ethylene glycol can also depress this activity.

ii. Inhibition of enzyme pyrimidine -5'-nucleotidase by lead is thought to be responsible for basophilic stippling (the aggregation of ribonucleic acid) and increased fragility of erythrocytes. Basophilic stippling is not pathognomonic of lead poisoning, but is usually an indication of bone marrow response to anaemia. The basophilic stippling occurs most often in dogs.

iii. Failure of heme synthetase to incorporate iron atoms into the heme molecule causes protoporphyrin to

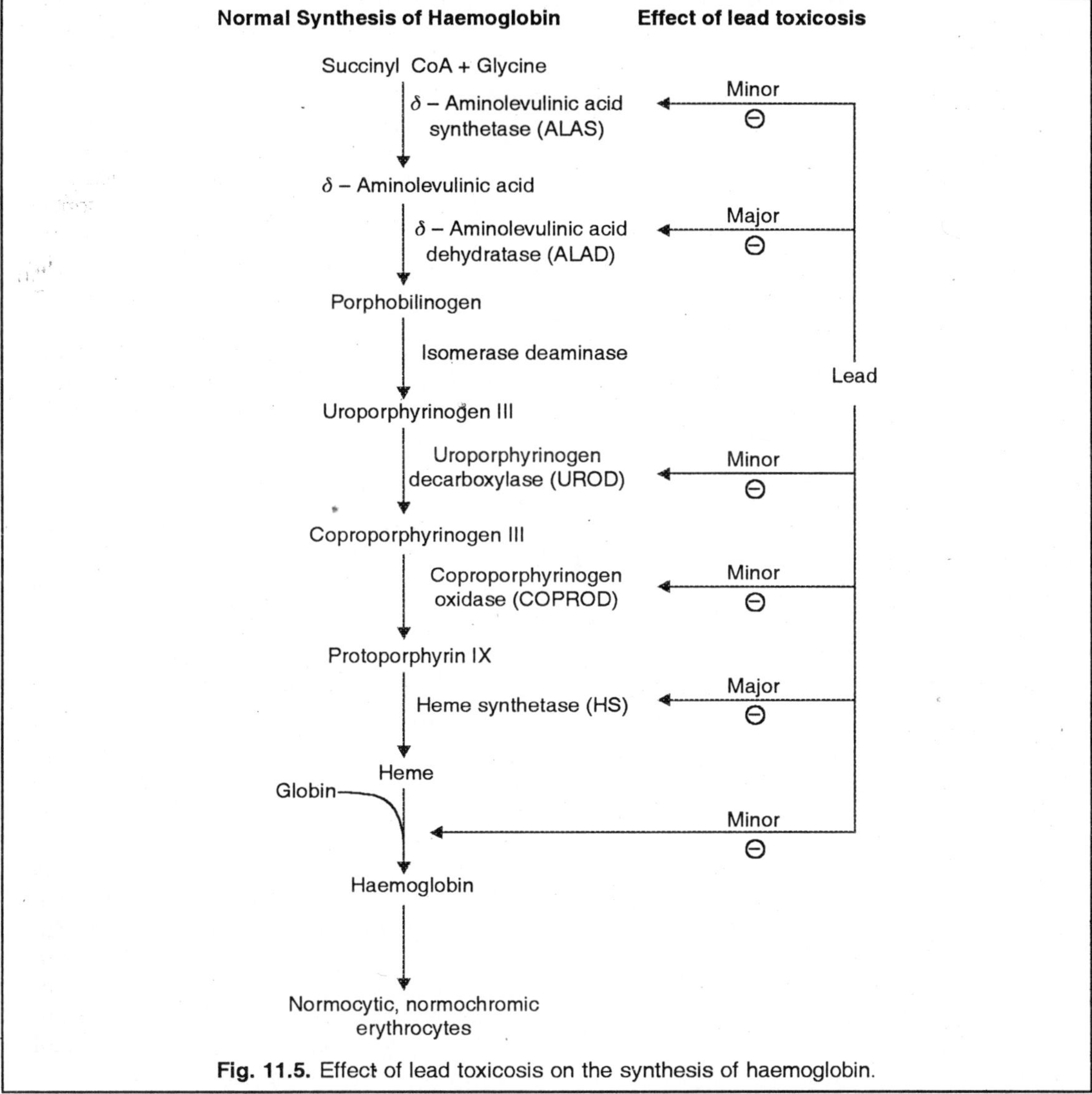

Fig. 11.5. Effect of lead toxicosis on the synthesis of haemoglobin.

chelate endogenous zinc atoms. The newly formed RBCs thus have zinc protoporphyrin. This indicates a chronic metabolic effect of lead on erythrocytes.

iv. Lead inhibits Na^+/K^+-ATP pump and attaches to RBC membrane, leading to their lysis.

d. Immunotoxicity: Lead can suppress production of antibodies to certain viral and bacterial agents. The mechanism of this effect is not known, but implications with regard to infectious diseases are obvious.

e. Nephrotoxicity: Lead nephropathy develops because of the inhibitory effects of lead on cellular respiration. Lead causes a generalized dysfunction of renal tubular and energy dependent functions. The proximal tubule appears to be the main target of lead toxicity. One characteristic of lead poisoning is the presence of lead 'inclusion bodies' in the nucleus of tubular cells.

f. Endocrine toxicity: Lead is reported to impair the release of growth hormone and insulin growth factor and interferes with skeletal calcium resulting in abnormalities in bone growth. Chronic exposure to lead may also result in reduced thyroid functions.

g. Reproductive toxicity: Lead adversely affects reproductive functions, mainly through its gametotoxicity in both male and female animals. It causes low sperm count and abnormal sperm morphology in males and infertility, spontaneous abortion and stillbirths in females.

Clinical signs: Clinical lead toxicosis is commonly observed in cattle and dogs, occasionally encountered in horses, rarely seen in cats, and almost unheard of in pigs. Clinical signs manifested by different species do have some differences, but the overall impression is of an encephalopathy, preceded or accompanied by GI malfunction. Onset of clinical signs of lead poisoning may take few hours, days or weeks depending upon the amount ingested, species involved and other factors.

Cattle: Clinical signs in cattle usually commence 2-3 days following ingestion of a fatal dose of lead. Neurological effects predominate, but vary in their presentation. The animals may bellow, stagger, show maniacal excitement, crash into objects and appear blind. Death may occur within 2 hours or convulsive episodes may be interspersed with periods of depression, ataxia and erratic behaviour i.e. circling and leaning, pacing and pushing on objects (due to cerebral oedema). Shaking, irritability, muscle twitching, twitching of ears, 'snapping' of eyelids and grinding of teeth are common. In some cases, dullness and anorexia along with signs of colic predominate. Often constipation persists for several days. In older cattle, usually there is diarrhoea. Gastrointestinal signs are common but occur less frequently than nervous signs. Abortion (in mid to late gestation), opisthotonos, salivation, lachrymation, nasal discharge and paralysis may also be observed. Death may occur within several hours to several days.

Chronic ingestion of lead for weeks or months, during which cattle are asymptomatic, may suddenly culminate in a seizure and death. The chronic toxicity is relatively uncommon in animals, particularly in cattle, or more correctly more difficult to identify and diagnose accurately.

Dogs: The gastrointestinal signs appear earlier and generally predominate. The initial signs of lead poisoning in dogs may consist of anorexia, emesis, colic and diarrhoea or constipation. The occurrence of neurological signs may be expressed as either depression or excitation. Excitatory signs include hyperesthesia, hysterical barking, muscular spasms and seizures. These signs are intermittent with periods of nearly normal behaviour. Other neurological signs may include opisthotonos, blindness, lassitude and apathy, leading to paralysis. Death may occur and is relatively slow in onset (several days). The presence of many nucleated erythrocytes without severe anaemia is nearly pathognomonic for lead poisoning.

Horses: A chronic lead syndrome is characteristic in horses with a peripheral neuropathy leading to respiratory signs. The important signs include anorexia, weight loss, depression, weakness, stiffness, knuckling of fetlocks and often anaemia. Paresis of lower lip, laryngeal paresis and pharyngeal paresis are characterised by roaring (stertorous sound caused by paralysis of recurrent laryngeal nerve) and regurgitation of water from nose when horse drinks. More severe signs can occur following massive exposure to lead. Death in horses can occur from respiratory paralysis during convulsions.

Birds (Swans and waterfowl): Clinical signs of lead poisoning in birds are often vague and may include non-specific gastrointestinal, renal and neurological dysfunctions. Important clinical signs are depression, weakness, anorexia, regurgitation, polyuria, greenish-black diarrhoea, weight loss and ruffled dull feather. Abnormal stance or posture (e.g. head on the ground), ataxia, blindness, circling, immobility with intermittent periods of collapse and falling to ground, and convulsions are also reported. Death is rapid, generally occurring within few hours of lead exposure.

Post-mortem findings: Gross lesions in most species are mild and non-specific. Animals may die with no observable gross lesions. Ingested lead-containing material (paint chips, used motor oil, etc.) may be found in the GI tract. There may be gastritis or enteritis, hyperaemia, petechiae or ecchymoses in various organs. Oesophageal dilatation may be found in some dogs. Liver and muscle may appear pale and kidneys may be acutely hyperaemic or hemorrhagic. Oedema, swelling and increased prominence of vessels may be observed in the brain. In chronic poisoning, plasma may fluoresce under ultraviolet light because of the presence of excess porphyrins. Horses sometimes die as a result of aspiration pneumonia secondary to laryngeal paralysis. There might be lead lines in the metaphyses of long bones.

Microscopically, cerebral cortical necrosis and poliomalacia may occur in cattle. Capillary damage and collapse of small arterioles may also be observed in brain. Liver of cattle and calves may manifest centrilobular necrosis. Hepatocytes and renal tubular epithelium may contain eosinophilic acid-fast intranuclear inclusions. Neutrophilic leucocytosis, moderate anaemia, and basophilic stippling of RBCs are frequently observed in dogs. Although both basophilic stippling of erythrocytes and acid-fast intranuclear eosinopilic inclusions in kidney or liver cells are highly suggestive of lead poisoning, these lesions are not pathognomonic (also found in autoimmune haemolytic anaemia).

Diagnosis: Diagnosis of lead poisoning can be made from history, circumstantial evidences, clinical signs and lesions. Liver, kidneys, urine, faeces, bones and suspected materials (fodder, feed-stuffs and drinking water) should be analysed for lead. The concentration of lead in renal cortex (>4 ppm), liver (4 ppm) or whole blood (0.6 ppm) provides definitive confirmation of lead exposure. The lead concentration of 0.35 ppm with signs and especially with confirmatory tests (e.g. δ-ALA) is also diagnostic. As lead is carried on the RBCs (90% of circulating blood concentration), the serum blood is not routinely used and is not readily interpretable. Measurements of blood δ-aminolevulinic acid dehydratase and/or free erythrocyte protoporphyrin also are useful in the diagnosis of lead intoxication. Increase in nucleated red blood cells in greater proportion than the degree of anaemia indicates lead toxicosis. In young dogs, radiograms may have lead lines in images of long bones.

Lead poisoning should be differentiated from following conditions:

a. Encephalitic diseases and brain disturbances induced by tumour, trauma, haemorrhage or abscess can cause signs like those of lead poisoning. These should be ruled out from history, observations, and pathological or microbiological testing.

b. *Organochlorine Insecticides*: Organochlorine insecticides (OP) cause marked increase in body temperature, marked neuromuscular signs, abnormal posturing and severe convulsive activity with postictal depression. However, there is no blindness in OC insecticides poisoning.

c. *Urea*: Urea causes abnormal posturing, blindness, head pressing or compulsive hypermotility. Colic is prominent but diarrhoea is not prominent. Convulsions are strychnine like and followed by postictal rigidity instead of depression.

d. *Organophosphorus and carbamate insecticides*: They produce market parasympathetic signs, marked neuromuscular signs and little or no behavioural changes. Response to atropine in OP and carbamate insecticides is remarkable, but little (only dry mouth) in lead toxicosis.

e. *Other toxicants and conditions* : Certain toxicants like metaldehyde, salt, strychnine, fluoroacetate, nicotine, mouldy feed, arsenic and mercury and diseases like hypovitaminosis A, meningitis, rabies, listeriosis, hepatoencephalopathy, hypomagnesaemic tetany and nervous acetonemia produce clinical signs resembling to those of lead toxicosis. However, details of history, clinical signs, haematological findings and lesions produced by these agents or diseases do not fit well in lead poisoning.

Treatment and management: Treatment of lead toxicity involves both specific and supportive therapies.

Specific therapy: Specific treatment of lead intoxication involves use of chelating agents. The chelating agent preferentially binds the ions of metal to form a non-ionised soluble complex (chelate) that is less toxic and rapidly excreted in urine. Prior to metabolism, lead in organic compounds (e.g. tetraethyl lead) is non-ionic and therefore not accessible to chelation therapy. Orally administered chelating agents generally enhance absorption of metals when present at elevated concentrations in the GI tract, therefore, they are used by this route (orally) only after the metal has left the GI tract. Whenever chelating agents are used, water intake and urine output should be monitored closely.

a. *Calcium disodium edetate:* Calcium disodium edetate (Disodium calcium ethylenediamine tetraacetate, Ca-Na_2-

EDTA) has high affinity for lead and some other metals such as zinc, cadmium, manganese and copper. In animals, Ca-EDTA (not EDTA-acid or sodium EDTA because they chelate blood calcium and produce hypocalcaemia) is the most commonly used chelating agent for lead toxicity as it chelates lead that is stored in bone. Lead is also mobilised from renal intra-nuclear inclusion bodies, but Ca-EDTA has less ability to chelate lead in soft tissues or erythrocytes. Injudicious use of calcium disodium edetate should be avoided as it may cause gastrointestinal and renal toxicosis with clinical signs of anorexia, depression, diarrhoea and vomiting. This occurs largely due to large mobilisation of lead from bones that increases its concentration in blood and soft tissues (so toxic signs are also aggravated) and kidneys may not be capable of excreting a large amount of chelated lead quickly. Zinc supplementation may reduce the GI upsets associated with Ca-EDTA therapy.

Horses & cattle: 110 mg/kg (as 1-2% solution in 5% dextrose), IM, IP, or slow IV, 2 times daily for 4 to 5 days. Drug may be repeated after a gap of 2 days (no therapy for 2 days) for another 4 to 5 days, if required. During second or subsequent courses of Ca-EDTA, it is better to monitor urine lead concentration before and after drug treatment to know the status of lead in body. Animals suffering from acute or subacute toxicosis may not respond much as they do not have much lead in their bones.

Dogs & cats: 25 mg/kg (as 1% solution in 5% dextrose), SC, 4 times daily for 5 days. The total dose should not exceed 2 g/day.

Birds: 35 – 50 mg/kg, IM or slow IV, 1 to 3 times daily for 5 days. Drug may be repeated after 5-7 days of waiting period, if required.

b. *D-penicillamine.* It is an oral sulphydryl-containing chelating agent that can be used in dogs. This drug may produce unpleasant side-effects like anorexia, listlessness and vomiting. The adverse effects are less if smaller doses are given more frequently or if 5-7 days rest periods are alternated with 5-7 days treatment regime. The drug should be given on an empty stomach. It should not be used in cattle, horses or sheep. It is contraindicated when lead is still present in the GI tract.

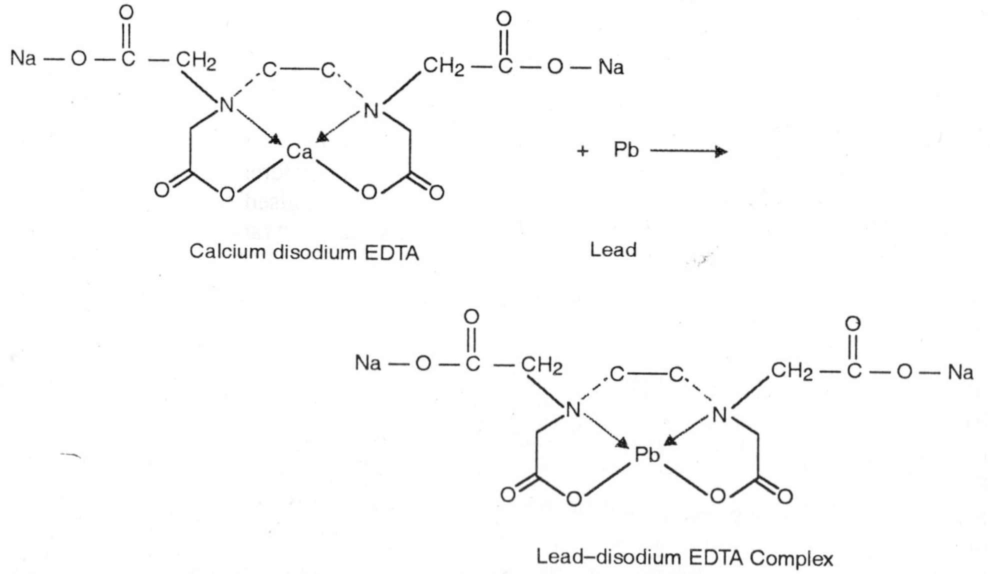

Calcium disodium EDTA + Pb → (Lead)

Lead–disodium EDTA Complex

Fig. 11.6. Chelation of lead by calcium disodium EDTA.

Dogs: 110 mg/kg, PO, daily in 3 to 4 divided doses for 2 weeks given on an empty stomach. If vomiting, anorexia, or depression occurs, the dose may be reduced to 33-55 mg/kg, daily in 3 to 4 divided doses.

c. *Dimercaprol/BAL*: Administration of dimercaprol prior to initiation of calcium EDTA therapy may help alleviate acute neurological signs because it crosses the blood-brain-barrier. This combination is considered more useful in humans, but has limited value in veterinary science except in small animals where severe CNS signs are present.

Supportive therapy:

a. *Thiamine*: Thiamine helps symptomatically and gives good result in cattle. Thiamine alleviates clinical manifestations and reduces deposition of lead. Combined Ca-EDTA and thiamine may produce more beneficial effects. Even without chelation therapy, some improvement may be seen.

Cattle: 2-4 mg/kg by I.M. or S.C. twice a day for 5 days.

b. Corticosteroids (e.g. dexamethasone) and osmotic diuretic (e.g. mannitol) may be used either in combination or alone to reduce cerebral oedema in cattle and horses.

Cattle & horses: Dexamethasone 0.1 mg/kg, I.V., S.C. or I.M. and/or Mannitol (20%) 1-2 g/kg, slow IV.

c. Zinc supplements may alleviate the severity of epiphyseal enlargement in colts.

d. Diazepam or barbiturates may be used to control seizures.

e. An osmotic cathartic (e.g. sodium or magnesium sulphate) promotes GI evacuation and precipitates lead to form insoluble complex of lead sulphate.

f. Ruminants with rumen stasis and heavy lead contamination may require rumenotomy.

g. Supplement feeding and administration of oral or parenteral fluids may be necessary to counteract anorexia, which may be prolonged.

h. Reinoculation of the rumen with active ruminal contents promotes return of normal rumen function.

i. Since lead may be immunosuppressive, broad-spectrum antibiotics may be indicated to control secondary bacterial infections.

j. Optimization of stores of calcium, copper and zinc in body reduces lead absorption from the GI tract.

Prevention: Lead poisoning can be easily avoided by following good management practices in the animal farms. Prevention is easier, cheaper and more effective than the treatment. The farmers may be advised to adopt following waste management practices on the farms to minimize risk of lead poisoning:

a. Do not leave petroleum products lying around or stored in open containers. Place used motor oil in sealed containers.

b. Keep trash out of pastures and other sites that are used by animals. Fence the dump sites and bury trash. A single dump site is safer than several sites.

c. Dispose of used batteries without spilling their contents. Do not leave batteries in barns, pastures, or farmyard.

d. Use lead-free paint on barns, fences or other structures used by livestock. Always keep paint cans closed and keep them away from animals.

e. Do not park farm machinery in the barn or near areas used by livestock. Service farm machinery in an area that is completely separate from animals.

f. Immobilize lead in soil with $Ca(H_2PO_4)$. The lead immobilization practice is somewhat effective, but this treatment tends to mobilize arsenic in soil.

g. Add organic material in soil. Organic material tends to bind metals including lead in the soil. This practice, however, is not much effective because the organic materials tend to degrade over time in the environment.

Prognosis: The prognosis is grave in acute lead toxicosis and whenever nervous and behavioural signs are severe. Lead encephalopathy carries a far worse prognosis than other conditions.

Effectiveness of therapy depends on the extent of injury to tissues, especially the nervous tissues.

Public health concerns: Sources of lead are similar for humans and animals. Lead toxicosis in dogs or cats should call attention to review of potential lead exposure to children in a household. Food animals that have recovered from plumbism store lead mainly in bones; therefore, meat products containing scraps of bone or ground bone should be avoided. Milk samples from lead toxicosis recovered animals should be thoroughly evaluated before consumption.

Some important compounds of lead:

Inorganic compounds

a. *Lead arsenate:* Lead arsenate ($PbHAsO_4$) is a white heavy powder. It has been used as a taenicide and insecticide.
b. *Lead sulphide:* Lead sulphide (PbS) is naturally found in the form of cubic crystals, but is sold in a powder form as *"Surma"* in place of sulphide of antimony which is used as a collyrium for the eyes (Antimony trisulphide is actual *surma*).
c. *Lead tetroxide:* Lead tetroxide (Pb_3O_4) is red lead or *"Sindur"*. It is a scarlet, crystalline powder, varying in colour, according to its mode of preparation and is employed as a pigment. It is insoluble in water, but partially soluble in nitric acid.

Organic compounds

d. *Tetraethyl lead:* Tetraethyl lead ($Pb(C_2H_4)_4$) is highly toxic organic lead compound that is liquid and somewhat volatile at ordinary temperature. It is added as admixture usually in motor petrol to prevent 'knocking' and is known as ethyl petrol or ethyl gasoline. Tetraethyl lead is absorbed both by inhalation and through intact skin and acts as a dangerous poison to persons engaged in the manufacture of tetraethyl lead.
e. *Lead acetate:* Lead acetate ($Pb(C_2H_3O_2)_2.3H_2O$) is commonly called sugar of lead or salt of Saturn. It occurs in white masses of acicular crystals, having a sweet, astringent taste. It was used in ancient times to sweeten wine and to sweeten and preserve fruits. Nowadays, it is medicinally used as astringent (usually in lotions) for bruises and superficial inflammation.

4. Copper

Copper is an essential trace element that catalyses various processes in heme synthesis and iron absorption. It acts as co-factor in the function of cellular enzymes such as tyrosinase, cytochrome oxidase, dopamine-β-hydroxylase, lysyl oxidase, and peroxidases. It is also involved in nerve conduction, connective tissue, cardiovascular system and immune system. Copper is widely distributed in nature and, like other heavy metals, is toxic in higher concentrations. Copper has complex interrelationship with some elements such as molybdenum and sulphur. Among animals, acute copper toxicosis is not common.

Properties: Copper (Cu) occupies a position between nickel and zinc in group 1B of the periodic table and is a noble metal like gold and silver. Copper exists in three oxidation states: metallic copper (0), cuprous ion (+1, monovalent) and cupric ion (+2, divalent). Cuprous ions dissociate rapidly in aqueous solution to cupric and metallic copper. Cupric compounds are blue or green in colour and are usually very soluble in aqueous solution. Copper is a strong oxidizing agent.

Sources of toxicity: Acute toxicity of copper is not common in animals, but it may occur from the contamination of food and water or excessive use of copper in agricultural and veterinary practices. Chronic copper toxicity apparently results from a combination of genetic susceptibility and continuous copper intake.

a. Copper is routinely used as a livestock dietary supplement. Acute toxicosis may result after accidental administration of excessive amounts of soluble copper salts in mineral mixtures, rations, etc. In particular, feeding to sheep of complete feed intended for cattle, horses or poultry can provide copper levels toxic to sheep.
b. Animals may ingest copper from sprayed foliage or pasture grass which may accumulate up to 200 ppm of copper from the soil. Copper containing pesticides such as bordeaux mixture (contains 1-3% copper sulphate) is sometimes used in orchards.
c. Copper sulphate is used as foot bath, fungicide and anthelmintic in veterinary and public health practices. Its indiscriminate use for a longer time or in excessive amount may produce toxicity.

d. Consumption of water from ponds treated with copper containing algicide can cause toxicosis in animals.

e. Contamination of forages, pastures or soil in the vicinity of mines or smelters may cause poisoning. Contamination of forages, soil or water may also occur from effluents from industries using copper like dye manufacturing, petroleum refining, and electrical appliances units.

f. Soils and plants fertilized with used poultry litter or swine manure, which may be rich in copper, are also possible sources of poisoning.

g. Copper can be released into the environment by natural sources such as decaying vegetation, forest fires and sea spray. Copper may also enter the air during combustion of fossil fuels. Copper in air slowly settles down when it starts to rain and ends up mainly in soil. Copper from these sources rarely cause toxicosis.

Factors affecting toxicity: Toxicity of copper varies with factors such as species, solubility of compounds, presence of other minerals, etc.

a. *Species:* There are marked differences among species in their ability to tolerate high levels of copper. Although all species are susceptible to copper toxicity, sheep are affected most often because they accumulate copper in the liver more readily than other farm animals. Goats are 3-4 times more tolerant to copper than sheep. Horses and swine are relatively tolerant to copper. Dogs are more susceptible to copper overload as a result of differences in copper metabolism. Poultry are more resistant to copper poisoning than most mammals.

b. *Interaction:* Low levels of dietary molybdenum and sulphate increase toxicity of copper (ratio of copper to molybdenum is the most important dietary factor affecting copper toxicity in sheep). Elevated levels of zinc block copper absorption from GIT by formation of complexes with epithelial proteins responsible for transport of copper. High levels of ascorbic acid may also reduce the amount of copper absorbed from the diet and hence its toxicity. Deficiencies of manganese, iron, and B-vitamins can cause copper to accumulate in body.

c. *Breeds:* Some breeds of dogs like Bedlington Terrier breed are highly sensitive to copper toxicosis. Genetic defects in Bedlington Terrier and some other breeds of dog cause excessive storage of copper in the liver eventually resulting in liver damage.

d. *Solubility:* Toxicity from soluble copper compounds is comparatively more due to better bioavailability than from the insoluble salts. Insoluble or slightly water soluble compounds are relatively less absorbed, so are less toxic.

e. *Stress*: Stress from any cause contributes to copper imbalance. Stresses such as adverse weather, polluted environment, poor nutrition, fear, transportation and handling can also cause the liver cells to die and release the stored copper into bloodstream. Stress also stimulates adrenal glands and lowers the zinc level in the body. Whenever zinc becomes deficient, copper tends to accumulate.

f. *Soil:* Sandy soils with low pH possess the greatest potential for leaching copper. However, copper is less affected by soil pH than other metals.

g. Hepatotoxic substances, if administered with copper, precipitate copper toxicosis. Hepatogenous plants (which contain hepatotoxic alkaloids) such as *Heliotropium* or *Senecio* spp. result in excessive Cu retention in liver.

h. Accumulation of copper may occur secondary to any cholestatic liver disease that alters hepatic copper excretion.

Toxicity: Acute or chronic copper poisoning is encountered in most parts of the world. A minimum safe concentration for copper in diet and that required for toxicity cannot be given with great accuracy, since copper absorption and utilization in the animal can be markedly affected by several mineral elements and other dietary factors and also it varies with the species (Table 11.2) and the type of copper compound. Sheep accumulate copper in the liver more readily than other farm animals and are hence most susceptible to copper toxicity. In sheep and young calves, the toxic oral dose of copper sulphate is 20 mg Cu/kg (less for lambs) and in cows it is about 200 mg Cu/kg. As little as 50 ppm copper in feed pellets, 10-15 ppm in total diet or 12 ppm in clover pasture can poison a sheep, if taken daily. In pigs, oral intake of 250-400 ppm of copper is toxic and 1000 ppm is considered lethal. Copper sulphate added to diets at 125 ppm or higher may be lethal to rabbits. Chronic copper poisoning may either be primary (long-term administration of copper in feed or fodder) or secondary (ingestion of hepatogenous plants which either produce mineral imbalance and retention of copper or produce liver damage which causes copper retention).

Copper distribution after absorption occurs in two stages - transport from intestinal mucosa to liver and transport from liver to peripheral tissues for utilization. In the first stage, copper in portal blood loosely binds to albumin and a copper transport protein transcuprein and is taken to liver. Transcuprein has a higher affinity for copper than albumin, but is much less abundant. In the liver, copper combines with a hepatic protein metallothionein and is stored for further utilization. The copper is largely incorporated into the mitochondria, endoplasmic reticulum, nuclei and cytosol of hepatocytes. The hepatic storage is normally meant for short-term needs, but it may increase with accumulation of copper in disease states. In the second stage, copper is transported from hepatocyte to peripheral tissues for use. This transport occurs via ceruloplasmin, an α_2-globulin produced in the liver. Copper associated with ceruloplasmin constitutes about 90% of the copper that circulates in plasma. The concentration of copper in liver varies with the species of animal. The liver cells of ruminants especially sheep and calves have very high affinity for copper. Low molybdenum and sulphate in the diet increases copper absorption and its retention in liver, and vice-versa.

Table 11.2: Minimum safe and toxic concentrations of copper in diet of different species.

Class of Animal	Copper Requirement in Total Diet (ppm)	Toxic Level in Total Diet (ppm)
Dairy Cattle	12-16	40
Beef Cattle	10 (4-15)	100
Sheep	7-11	25
Swine	5-6	>250
Poultry	6-8	250-800
Horses	9	Not known

Toxicokinetics: The absorption of copper from GI tract largely depends on a number of factors including the chemical form of copper, interaction with other metals (e.g. zinc, selenium, molybdenum, cadmium) and dietary components. The amount of copper stored in body, however, does not affect the absorption of copper from GI tract. In general, absorption of most copper compounds from GI tract is relatively low and most of the ingested element is eliminated in faeces. Copper administered as sulphate is absorbed (~5%) mainly from the small intestine whereas copper given in the form of sulphide enters body via the large intestine (~2%). Metallic copper is insoluble and, therefore, its absorption from the GI tract is small. Copper is probably absorbed as low molecular weight, soluble complexes formed with both the products of food digestion and gastrointestinal secretion. In the intestine copper is absorbed into the epithelial cells primarily by passive diffusion, with a small amount absorbed by energy-dependent processes. Within the epithelial cell, the copper then binds to epithelial cell metallothionein, a cysteine-rich protein. Metallothionein also binds zinc and cadmium.

Copper homeostasis is regulated primarily by excretion. Usually about 80% of copper absorbed from the diet is excreted in bile, which is mainly responsible for maintenance of copper balance in body. Biliary excretion varies in response to liver copper load and therefore to copper intake. Intestinal absorption of copper is negligible because of its binding to bile and amino acids. Most of the copper excreted through biliary route is eliminated in the faeces. Copper is also eliminated from the

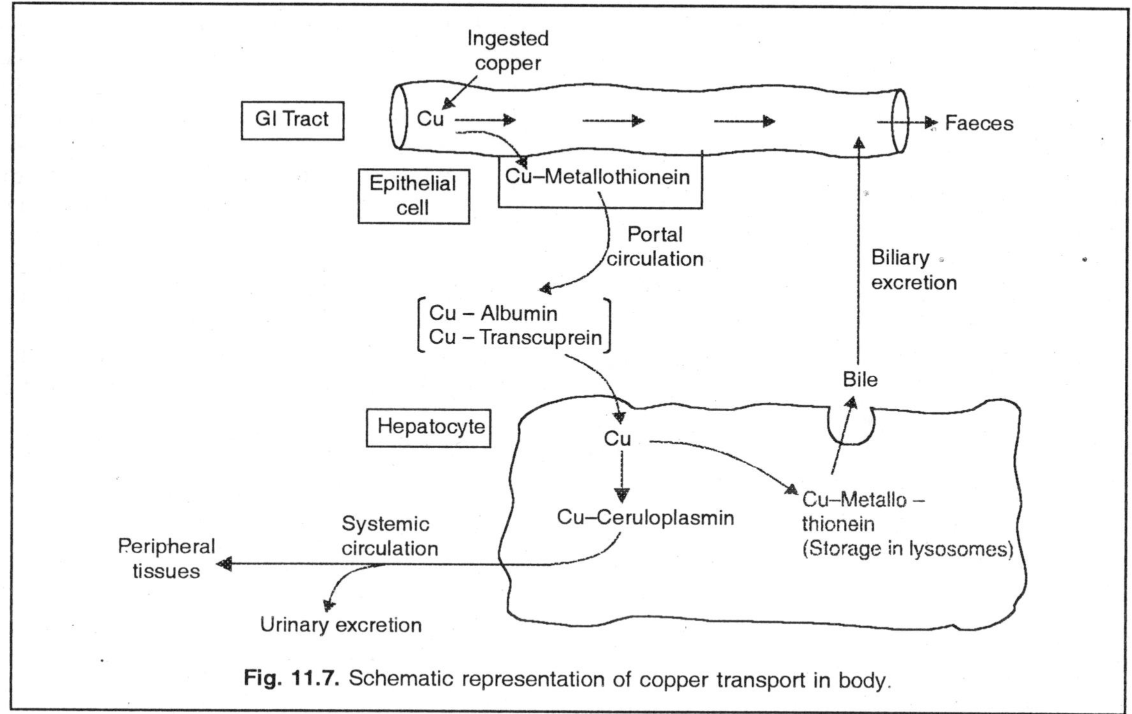

Fig. 11.7. Schematic representation of copper transport in body.

body via urine and through intestine. The amount of copper excreted in the milk is low, thus milk is a low copper body fluid.

Influence of molybdenum and sulphate on copper disposition: The molybdenum and sulphate influences the disposition of copper in body. The liver metabolises considerable copper without ill effects provided that molybdenum and sulphate are present in sufficient amounts. *In vivo*, copper forms a complex with molybdenum and copper in this complex is biologically unavailable. The copper-molybdenum complex thus reduces copper accumulation in liver and hastens its excretion in urine and bile. The molybdenum also forms an insoluble complex, $CuMoO_4$, with copper in the gastrointestinal tract, which reduces copper absorption. Similar to molybdenum, increased dietary concentration of sulphate increases urinary and biliary excretion of copper and also reduces GI absorption of copper by forming a complex with it.

Mechanism of action: Abnormal copper accumulation in liver is primarily responsible for toxicity in animals. Copper accumulation in liver may occur from any of the three processes: abnormal absorption, abnormal storage and defective excretion. Though the exact biochemical mechanisms by which copper causes various signs and lesions are not clear, yet the interaction of copper with cellular or molecular sulphydryl, carboxyl or amino groups and subsequent interference with their structure or function are important.

a. Ruminants:

i. In ruminants (also other species) excessive accumulation of copper occurs in hepatic mitochondria and lysosomes. Excessive copper affects integrity of plasma membranes. Copper damages lysosomal membrane, which causes leakage of copper and enzymes into the cytosol where further destruction occurs. Overall, excessive copper accumulation causes progressive hepatocyte organelle damage and cellular degeneration or necrosis. Profound morphological changes in mitochondria and peroxisomes have been observed following copper toxicity.

ii. Excessive accumulation of copper inhibits essential metabolic enzymes. Inhibition of vital enzymes may lead to liver malfunction, which also initiates necrosis and inability of the liver to excrete and store more copper. Main enzyme inhibition is thought to be dihydrolipoyl dehydrogenase which leads to inhibition of pyruvate (and also α-ketoglutarate) dehydrogenase system. This results in disturbance in the energy metabolism of cells.

iii. Liver damage and necrosis release large amounts of copper and other oxidative substances from the liver into the blood stream. Excess copper in blood oxidises erythrocyte membranes and increases their fragility resulting in sudden and massive erythrocytes lysis, freeing haemoglobin and causing a haemolytic crisis. Excess haemoglobin causes clogging of renal tubules leading to renal tubular and glomerular necrosis and production of darkened (gun metal grey) kidneys and subsequent death. There is also oxidation of haemoglobin by copper to form methaemoglobin which can not transport oxygen and may aggravate the acute haemolytic crisis. The haemolytic crisis is precipitated by many factors, including transportation, lactation, strenuous exercise, or malnutrition.

iv. Cupric sulphate is a gastrointestinal irritant that produces erosion of the lining of gastrointestinal tract with possible coagulative necrosis of gastrointestinal mucosa. Copper is also a respiratory irritant that produces mucosal irritation of the mouth, eyes and nose.

b. Swine: In swine, in addition to above mechanisms causing hepatic necrosis and other lesions due to copper accumulation, copper inhibits absorption of iron from the GI tract leading to iron-deficiency anaemia. Death is due to combination of microcytic hypochromic anaemia (like baby-pig anaemia) and organ-damage but not necessarily haemorrhage.

c. Dogs: In Bedlington Terriers, autosomal recessive defect causes increased copper retention (>1500-2000 ppm) in the liver, which results in hepatic damage. This inherited derangement of copper metabolism in Bedlington Terriers occurs primarily due to abnormal binding of copper with hepatic metallothionein, which sequesters copper in hepatic lysosomes and prevents normal biliary excretion of copper. Death occurs from liver damage and hepatopathy. This syndrome or one very similar to it also occurs in some other breeds (e.g. Doberman Pinschers, Skye Terrier) of dogs.

Clinical Signs :

Acute toxicity: Acute copper poisoning, in which animals ingest large amount of copper salt at one time, is a type of caustic poisoning. There is severe gastroenteritis characterised by rapid onset of salivation, reduced feed consumption, colic, diarrhoea (some times with a greenish tinge), rapid dehydration, melena or haematemesis, shock, collapse and death. Haemolysis and haemoglobinuria occur after 3 days if the animal survives the GI disturbances. Anuria or oliguria may develop, but renal dysfunction is usually mild. Excessive accumulation of copper in liver may cause jaundice and necrosis of liver.

Chronic toxicity: The term chronic is misleading. Ingestion of copper can be chronic but onset of toxicosis is acute because of sudden release of copper from the liver. Clinical signs in sheep, cattle and some other species are usually associated with the haemolytic crisis leading to acute anaemia (a sudden haemolytic crisis may not be observed in some animals, particularly in lambs). Affected animals exhibit depression, sudden onset of weakness and trembling (exhaustion), anorexia, thirst, haemoglobinuria, jaundice but no additional GI disturbances. Signs of respiratory insufficiency (dyspnoea, panting) and shock (tachycardia, weak pulse, cold extremities) may be expected. Death occurs 1-4 days after onset of clinical signs. The copper content of blood is generally within the normal range until 24-48 hours before the onset of clinical signs. Animals that survive the acute episode may die of subsequent renal failure.

With disease of longer duration, coagulation abnormalities may result in petechial or ecchymotic haemorrhages, melena, or epistaxis. In some dogs (generally older dogs), chronic signs may be slow in onset with signs of lethargy, anorexia, weight loss, cachexia, ascites, encephalopathy and death. In lambs, chronic copper poisoning may be manifested as GI haemorrhage, pulmonary oedema, ascites, and liver damage, but generally no haemolytic crisis or jaundice. In laying hens, decreased egg production, diarrhoea, and oral mucosal ulcers and vesicles are important manifestations of chronic poisoning.

Post-mortem findings: Acute copper poisoning produces severe gastroenteritis with erosions and ulcerations in abomasum of ruminants and in stomach of non-ruminants. Jaundice develops in animals that survive >24 hrs. In chronic poisoning, tissues are discoloured by jaundice and methaemoglobin. The lesions include pale-yellow liver, enlarged pulpy spleen (indicative of haemolysis), distended gallbladder with greenish bile, and bluish-black kidneys (known as 'gunmetal kidneys'). Microscopic lesions include swollen and necrotic hepatocytes, hepatocyte vacuolation, periportal fibrosis, occasional bile duct proliferation, renal tubular necrosis, haemoglobin casts in renal tubules and excessive fragmented erythrocytes in spleen. Histopathological severity in dogs with inherited copper hepatotoxicity often correlates with the degree of copper accumulation. The first lesions may be prominent lysosomal granules laden with copper followed by focal hepatitis, later chronic active hepatitis, and finally focal or generalised cirrhosis.

Diagnosis: Diagnosis is made from history, clinical signs, lesions and copper levels in the body fluids, faeces and tissues. Evidence of blue-green ingesta, and elevated faecal (8000-10000 ppm) and kidney (> 15 ppm, wet wt) copper levels are considered significant in acute copper poisoning. In chronic poisoning, blood and liver copper concentrations are elevated during the haemolytic period. Blood level of copper is 5-20 μg/ml as compared to normal levels of ~1μg/ml. Liver concentrations > 150 ppm (wet wt) may be seen in sheep. The urine of animals in haemolytic crisis contains an increased amount of haemoglobin and bile pigments.

Changes in the laboratory parameters include elevated bilirubin levels, haemoglobinaemia, and haemoglobinuria. Elevated levels of certain hepatic enzymes like aspartate aminotransferase (AST), lactate dehydrogenase (LDH), sorbitol dehydrogenase (SDH) and arginase indicate necrosis. Serum or plasma liver enzymes may be elevated 3-6 weeks before haemolytic crisis and can be used to forewarn toxicosis. Exposed but still asymptomatic animals may have elevated liver enzymes but serum copper levels remain within normal limits until about 24-48 hours prior to the onset of clinical signs.

Differential diagnoses include infectious gastroenteritis (acute salmonellosis) and leptospirosis as well as arsenic, mercury or selenium toxicoses and phenothiazine and some other anthelminthic poisonings.

Treatment and management: The treatment of copper poisoning often is not successful and almost all animals acutely or chronically poisoned by copper die, especially when the clinical signs have already set in. Regardless of the cause for hepatic accumulation, the excess copper will cause hepatocellular damage and cellular hepatitis. Measures to prevent further accumulation of copper in the liver may be adopted to arrest further deaths in a flock

Specific therapy: Approach to treatment of copper poisoning is twofold: to decrease any further absorption of copper from GI tract and to enhance excretion of copper from body.

a. *Chelating agents:* Urinary copper excretion may be increased by use of cupretic agent (copper chelators). Metal chelators like penicillamine bind with copper in blood or tissues and promote its removal through the kidneys. Treatment with chelators has produced beneficial effects in sheep and dogs with increased hepatic concentrations.

   D-penicillamine

   Sheep: 50 mg/kg, orally for up to 6 days, alone or in combination with BAL.

   Dogs: 10-15 mg/kg twice daily by oral route.

b. Ascorbic acid given with meals has been found to decrease intestinal absorption of copper in dogs. It may also enhance copper excretion through the urine.

   Dogs: 500-1000 mg (total) per day.

c. Oral doses of ammonium molybdate (0.5 -1 mg/kg/day) and sodium sulphate (6-20 mg/kg/day) may be given to combat chronic copper poisoning. Molybdenum and sulphate are known to decrease copper absorption and augment copper excretion.

d. Ammonium tetrathiomolybdate (1.7-3.4 mg/day) three treatments on alternate days by I.V. or S.C. route aids in rapid binding and excretion of copper.

e. Oral zinc supplementation decreases intestinal absorption of copper by inducing the synthesis of mucosal metallothionein. This results in impeded serosal transfer of copper with eventual loss in the faeces when intestinal cells are shed. However, zinc is slow in action and may require a few weeks to achieve the therapeutic response.

Dogs: 5-10 mg (elemental zinc)/ kg, orally twice daily.

Supportive therapy: Supportive therapy may be instituted in all cases as deemed necessary.

a. Complications from hepatic encephalopathy and ascites should be treated as they occur.
b. Anti-oxidant therapy with Vitamin E (400-500 mg/kg, orally) has shown protective effect against hepatic damage in dogs.
c. Symptomatic therapy should be carried out to alleviate shock and colic pains.
d. Alkalization of urine helps to decrease renal damage from haemoglobin.
e. Supplementation of sheep rations with 2-16 ppm molybdenum is efficacious in reducing incidence of haemolytic crisis and in decreasing liver copper retention.

Prevention: If the area is deficient in molybdenum or high in copper, feed samples should be analyzed routinely to monitor the copper: molybdenum ratio in the diet. Sheep consuming copper/molybdenum rations exceeding 10:1 (normal ratio 6:1), are reported to accumulate excess copper in the hepatocytes. Supplemental feeds which are known to be low in copper should be used whenever possible. In regions where spontaneous chronic poisoning occurs, the soil should be enriched with molybdenum (300 g per hectare). Feeding a properly fortified trace mineralized salt is essential to the health and production of the sheep flock. Steps should be taken to remove the hepatotoxic plants from the pasture and forage.

Prognosis: Prognosis is grave once the haemolytic crisis occurs.

Some important compounds of copper :

Inorganic compounds

a. *Copper sulphate:* Copper sulphate (Cupric sulphate; $CuSO_4.5H_2O$) occurs in large, blue slightly efflorescent crystals, and is freely soluble in water. It is used as an emetic, anthelmintic and fungicide. In higher doses, it acts as an irritant poison.
b. *Cupric carbonate:* A basic cupric carbonate ($Cu_2(OH)_2.CO_3$) occurs native as malachite. It is green to blue amorphous powder or dark-green monoclinic crystals. It is occasionally used as seed treatment fungicide and in poultry and animal feeds.
c. *Cuprous oxide:* Cuprous oxide (Red copper oxide, Cu_2O) exists as cubic crystals of microcryst powder. It is occasionally used as crop and seed treatment fungicide, antiseptic for fishnets, and as red pigment for glass and ceramic glazes.

Organic compounds

d. *Copper glycinate:* Copper glycinate (Cupric glycinate, $C_4H_8CuN_2O_4$) is prepared from glycine and cupric salt. It is used parenterally for copper deficiency in ruminants.

5. Molybdenum

Molybdenum (Mo) is an essential trace element and a component of a number of enzymes, including sulphite oxidase (metabolism of sulphur amino acids), xanthine oxidase (oxidation of purines and pyrimidines and production of uric acid), and aldehyde oxidase (oxidation of aldehydes). Molybdenum is present in the earth's crest largely as molybdenum disulphide (MoS_2) and is a biogenic element of microorganisms, plants and animals. Trace amount of molybdenum is essential for a group of nitrogen fixing bacteria, especially which reside in the root of legumes. Molybdenum toxicosis is most often seen in ruminants and less in other animals.

Properties: Molybdenum is a high-melting silver-grey metal with atomic number 42 and atomic weight 95.94. It occurs in periodic table in the triad of transition elements that includes chromium and tungsten. The transition element molybdenum exists in five oxidation states (II–VI); the predominant states are Mo (IV) and Mo (VI). Molybdenum does not exist naturally in the pure metallic state, but occurs in association with other elements. The predominant form of molybdenum occurring in soil and natural waters is the molybdate anion, MoO_4^{-2}.

Sources of toxicity :

a. Excess molybdenum is found in the soils of certain geographical areas. Acidic soils, poorly drained soils, and those contaminated with mining wastes also contain high levels of molybdenum. Grazing of cattle on pastures with high molybdenum content leads to toxicity in animals.

b. Plants (especially legume plants) can absorb and accumulate water-soluble molybdates from contaminated soils. Ingestion of such plants rich in Mo contents but low in copper contents may result in molybdenosis.

c. Occasional poisoning may be caused by contamination of soil, plants and water by smoke in the proximity of factories such as steel works, bauxite plants, oil refineries or metal alloy production plants.

d. Contamination of soils and forages may occur in the vicinity of certain mining or smelting operations in which molybdenum containing ores are heated to high temperatures.

e. Excessive use of molybdenum containing fertilizers may occasionally result in high molybdenum contents in soils and forages.

f. Calves may be poisoned by milk from cows on high molybdenum diets.

Factors affecting toxicity :

a. *Species*: Cattle are the most susceptible species to excess Mo levels. Horses and pigs are not usually affected by molybdenosis.

b. *Interactions:* Molybdenum has a strong inverse relationship with copper and sulphur. Toxicity of molybdenum increases when intake of copper is less. High dietary sulphate increases Mo toxicosis by decreasing copper absorption. However, on the other hand, low dietary sulphate decreases Mo excretion in the urine thus increasing its toxicity.

c. *Form:* Water soluble form of molybdenum (e.g. tetramolybdate) is more toxic than water insoluble form (e.g. molybdenum disulfide).

d. *Age*: Young animals are more susceptible to molybdenum poisoning than adult animals.

e. *Types of plant* : Legumes take up more of the element than other plant species so are concentrating more of Mo.

f. *Season*: Molybdenum in herbage is less during the winter season, but begins to increase in the spring and reaches maximal concentration in the late summer and early autumn.

Toxicity: Molybdenum is present in all biological fluids and tissues including bones. Molybdenum has a strong inverse interaction with copper and sulphur. Molybdenosis usually results from inadequate Cu : Mo ratio in the soil, fodder and diet. In the diet, Copper : Molybdenum ratio of 6 : 1 is ideal, 2 : 1 to 3 : 1 is borderline, and < 2 : 1 is toxic. Dietary molybdenum of 10 ppm can cause toxicity regardless of copper intake and as little as 1 ppm may be hazardous if copper content is < 5 ppm (dry-weight basis).

Toxicokinetics: Absorption of molybdenum varies over a wide range (25-90%). Soluble molybdenum compounds are readily absorbed, whilst insoluble compounds are not. After oral administration, molybdenum compounds (except sulphides) are absorbed readily from the intestine. In the blood, Mo is bound to plasma proteins and erythrocytes. Molybdenum occurs in low concentrations in all fluids and tissues of the body. The highest concentration of Mo is present in bones and liver, but liver does not store molybdenum. Lower concentrations of Mo may be present in kidneys, spleen, heart and skeletal muscles. Molybdenum is eliminated very rapidly via the kidneys (>80%) and bile hence under normal conditions the element does not accumulate in the body. Normally only small amounts of Mo are excreted in the faeces with exceptions in certain gastrointestinal disorders. High dietary sulphate increases excretion of Mo in the urine because it blocks the reabsorption of molybdenum from the renal tubules. Molybdenum is also excreted in milk and may affect young calves suckling the dams.

Mechanism of action: Molybdenum toxicosis results primarily due to copper deficiency induced by Mo (secondary hypocuprosis). The interaction of copper, molybdenum and sulphate is complex and not completely understood. It appears that the interaction of molybdates and sulphides in the rumen gives rise to thiomolybdates, which decrease the availability of dietary copper and, when absorbed, impede the metabolism of tissue copper. Molybdenum also promotes hepatic copper excretion by forming a copper-molybdate complex that is readily excreted in urine causing a clinical copper deficiency. The deficiency of copper in turn produces following effects:

a. Copper is an important metal component in many enzymes including lysyl oxidase/amine oxidase, tyrosinase, dopamine-β-hydroxylase, ceruloplasmin/ferroxidase, and cytochrome oxidase. Other enzymes affected by copper deficiency include lactase, ascorbic acid oxidase, superoxide dismutase, uricase, monoamine oxidase, and δ-aminolevulinic acid dehydratase. Deficiency of copper may reduce activities of these Cu-dependent enzymes and affect vital functions.

i. Copper is a cofactor for lysyl oxidase, an enzyme that is responsible for the connective tissue integrity by cross-linking elastin. The decreased activity of lysyl oxidase (amine oxidase) leads to decreased stability and strength of collagen in bones and elastin in the major blood vessels like aorta. The tensile strength of aorta and other major vessels is markedly reduced in copper deficiency, which may result in spontaneous ruptures of the major blood vessels.

ii. Decreased synthesis of phospholipids in the myelin sheaths that cover and protect nerves has been related to the diminished activity of some Cu-dependent enzymes such as cytochrome oxidase. The decreased/defective synthesis of myelin in nerves causes nerve damage and demyelination. The nerve damage and demyelination are important aspects of 'enzootic ataxia' and 'sway back' observed in sheep, particularly in lambs.

iii. The decreased activity of tyrosinase, a copper-containing enzyme that converts tyrosine to melanin (skin and hair pigment), interferes with the production of melanin. Diminished melanin production in animals is manifested as achromotrichia and depigmentation of skin (leucoderma).

iv. In ruminants and some other species, osteoporosis and spontaneous fractures may be associated with decreased activity of certain bone enzymes. Reduced bone cytochrome oxidase activity has been demonstrated in copper deficient chicks.

v. Copper deficiency affects the working of superoxide dismutase (SOD), a copper-dependent enzyme that catalyzes the removal of superoxide radicals from the body. Inefficient removal of superoxide radicals by SOD causes damage to cell membranes.

vi. As a part of the enzymes cytochrome c oxidase, dopamine hydroxylase, and Factor IV, copper plays a role in energy production, conversion of dopamine to noradrenaline and blood clotting, respectively. Deficiency of copper is known to affect energy production, nerve transmission and clotting of blood in animals.

b. Copper deficiency produces progressive atrophy of myocardium with replacement of fibrous tissue. The weakened heart may result in sudden death (falling disease in cattle), usually after excitement or exercise. The exact mechanism of this condition in not known.

c. Molybdenum can compete with phosphorus for mineralization of bones. Molybdenum can even cause the displacement of phosphorus. This along with inhibition of certain essential enzymes in bone may explain the occurrence of skeletal lesions.

d. Anaemia characteristic of an iron deficiency (microcytic, hypochromic) is associated with diminished activity of ceruloplasmin, a copper containing protein that transports and utilizes copper. In addition to its role as a transport protein, ceruloplasmin acts as an enzyme (called ferroxidase), catalyzing the oxidation of ferrous iron (Fe^{+2}) to ferric iron (Fe^{+3}). Copper deficiency, due to its effects on ceruloplasmin, thus, impairs iron absorption, transport, and utilization and reduces heme synthesis. Copper deficiency also decreases integrity of red blood cells.

e. Persistent scouring with passage of liquid faeces full of gas bubbles could be due to a complex formation between molybdenum and catechols in the GI tract. The catechols, like other phenols, are bacteriostatic and control the activity of bacteria in the gut. The molybdenum inactivates catechols by formation of a complex, which enhances bacterial activity markedly and then results in scouring diarrhoea (teart). This activity of molybdenum may not be related directly to copper deficiency.

Clinical signs: Molybdenum toxicity in animals is commonly referred to as molybdenosis or teart. Acute toxicity of molybdenum compounds does not occur under normal farming conditions in animals. Clinical signs are prominent in ruminants. In cattle, diarrhoea occurs 8-10 days following access to pastures high in Mo which is characterised by persistent, severe scouring making a parabola (shooting diarrhoea) and watery faeces with unpleasant odour and full of gas bubbles (called peat scours or teart). Other signs of acute toxicity in cattle may include anorexia, excessive salivation, lachrymation, generalised weakness, inability to stand, paresis, and prolapsed third eyelid. Death may occur in extreme cases.

The clinical signs of subacute and chronic molybdenosis in many species are similar in appearance to the disease of copper deficiency. Non-specific signs may include unthriftiness, anaemia (microcytic, hypochromic), emaciation, loss of body weight, slower growth, joints pain, lameness, osteoporosis, stiffness of legs with upright pastern and reluctance to get up. Changes in bones are manifested by hobbling and occasional fractures. Young animals have deformed fore-limbs. Joint and skeletal lesions appear to be due to defects in connective tissue and growth-plate development. The hair coat is rough, dull and depigmented. Depigmentation is most noticeable in black animals and especially around eyes, which gives a spectacled appearance. Focal or generalized depigmentation of skin (Leucoderma) is observed in some species including buffaloes. Reproductive disorders i.e. decreased libido in bulls and infertility in cows and drop in milk production may also occur. Death occurs within few days to several weeks.

Sheep develop pica. Sheep and lambs show stiffness of back and legs with reluctance to rise and paralysis of hind quarters; the condition called 'Enzootic ataxia' in Australia, while the syndrome is called 'Swayback' in U.K. Ewes become anaemic with stringy and depigmented wool, whereas lambs are severely uncoordinated, ataxic and usually blind. In human beings, elevated uric acid levels, which are associated with the onset of gout, are hypothesised to be caused by stimulation of xanthine oxidase by high molybdenum intake. Occupational exposure by inhalation to molybdenum containing dusts has been associated with pneumoconiosis.

Post-mortem findings: Lesions are not specific. Enteritis with flaccid, fluid-filled intestine may be seen. Bone rarefaction (e.g. osteoporosis) and exostosis may be found. There is depigmentation of the skin and hair coat and carcass is usually emaciated. Haemorrhages and breakdown of periosteum may also be observed. Microscopically, degenerative changes are seen in the liver and kidneys. In lambs with enzootic ataxia or swayback, there is lysis of white matter of the cerebrum and degeneration of motor tracts of the spinal cord. The damage in the white matter varies from microscopic foci to massive subcortical destruction. There is often neuronal degeneration and demyelination.

Diagnosis: Diagnosis of molybdenum toxicosis can be made from clinical signs, lesions, circumstantial evidences (soil rich in Mo) and response to therapy (diarrhoea stops within a few days of oral dosing with copper sulphate). Diagnosis is confirmed by demonstrating abnormal concentration of molybdenum and copper in blood (more than 0.1 ppm Mo and less than 0.6 ppm Cu) and liver (more than 5 ppm Mo and less than 10 ppm Cu) and a high dietary intake of molybdenum relative to copper. The specimens for chemical examinations are feed, liver, kidneys, and if considered necessary, altered limbs, bone, urine and hair.

Molybdenosis may be confused with several other enteritides and commonly mistaken for internal parasitism.

Treatment and management :

a. *Copper:* Provision of copper, orally or parenterally, is specific to molybdenum toxicosis. Copper gives good response, but care should be taken with sheep as they are extremely sensitive to copper.

   i. For severe and subacute cases, copper glycinate may be injected subcutaneously. The dose is 60 mg for calves and 120 mg for cattle, given subcutaneously.

   ii. Copper sulphate in diet at the dose rate of 1-2 g/adult cow/day in cattle and 0.25 g/45 kg body weight/day in sheep is given until symptoms disappear. In areas, where for various reasons, cattle do not consume mineral supplements the required copper may be drenched in 100 ml of water.

   iii. Copper sulphate is provided in salt licks at concentrations of 1-5%.

   iv. Pasture treatment with copper sulphate may be done for grazing animals.

Prognosis: In mild to moderate cases, animal responds favourably to the copper therapy.

Some important compounds of molybdenum:

a. *Molybdenum trioxide:* Molybdenum trioxide (MoO_3) exists as a white to slightly yellow to slightly bluish powder or granules. It is chiefly used as a reagent for chemical analysis.

b. *Molybdenum sesquioxide:* Molybdenum sesquioxide (Mo_2O_3) exists as greyish black powder. It is often combined with iron (ferrous sulphate) as 'Mol-Iron' and used as haematinic.

6. Cadmium

Cadmium is a toxic metal that occurs in nature mainly in lead and zinc ores. In recent years, cadmium has become a major environmental contaminant as a result of effluents from plants smelting zinc, copper and lead as well as from its industrial usage. Acute or chronic cadmium poisoning of farm animals does not occur under normal farming conditions, but it has become a cause of concern in animals found in or around industrial work places. In human beings, cadmium rank is close to lead and mercury as a metal of toxicological concern.

Properties: Cadmium (Cd) is a transition metallic element found in Group IIb of the periodic table with atomic number 48. Cadmium is soft, bluish-white metal and is easily cut with a knife. The most common oxidation state of cadmium is +2, though rare examples of +1 can be found. Cadmium is similar to zinc in many of its chemical properties and often mimics action of zinc in the animal body. Cadmium has no biological role in the human or animal body.

Sources of toxicity :

a. Contamination of soil and crops may occur as a result of effluents from plants smelting zinc, copper and lead (as cadmium occurs in nature in association with zinc and lead). Contamination of soils and animal feeds may also take from burning coal and sewage sludge (especially that is used to fertilise soils). Cadmium is an important component of municipal sludge in areas in which the appropriate industries are located. When cadmium concentrations in soils are high they can influence soil processes of microorganisms and threat the whole soil ecosystem.

b. Cadmium is used in industries in the manufacture of plastics, solder alloys, nickel-cadmium batteries, photocells, rubber tires and many other items. Environmental contamination is an important source of poisoning in human beings (mainly) and animals (occasionally).

c. Cadmium oxide and cadmium anthranilate are sometimes used as anthelmintic for treatment of ascariasis in pigs. Cadmium sulphide is used in antiseborrhoeic shampoos. The injudicious use of these drugs may cause toxicosis in animals.

d. Cadmium added to soil strongly adsorbs to organic matters in soils and its uptake through plants may increase. Cadmium accumulates primarily in the leafy portion of plants and may reach toxic concentrations in grains as well. Ingestion of such plants or grains may produce harmful effects in animals.

e. Cadmium containing fungicides (cadmium chloride, cadmium succinate) were once used on turf grass. The practice is not popular now, but could be a source of poisoning.

f. Some foodstuffs that are rich in cadmium can greatly increase the cadmium concentration in human or animal body. Examples of Cd rich food stuffs are liver, mushrooms, shellfish, mussels, cocoa powder and dried seaweed.

g. Excessive use of cadmium chloride as feed supplement produces harmful effects in animals.

h. In human beings, cigarette smoking is a major source of cadmium. One cigarette contains about $1 \mu g$ of cadmium, of which nearly 30 percent goes into the lungs and is absorbed and the remaining 70 percent goes into atmosphere to be inhaled by others or to contaminate the environment.

Factors affecting toxicity :

a. Dietary interactions: Low levels of dietary protein, zinc, calcium or iron enhances cadmium absorption from GI tract and hence its toxicity.

b. Age: Young animals absorb more cadmium from GI tract than the adults. However, cadmium levels tend to increase with age since cadmium is one of the most bioacccumulative poisons.

Toxicity: The toxicity of cadmium in domestic animals depends on various factors such as dose, mode of exposure, length of exposure, other interacting metals and species of animal affected. Cadmium and solutions of its compounds are toxic even in low concentrations because they generally bioaccumulate in organisms and ecosystems. However, the incidence of cadmium toxicosis is low in farm animals mainly because the animals are mostly kept in places away from Cd contaminated environment. In rats, oral LD_{50} of cadmium chloride is 90 mg/kg and that of cadmium succinate is 660 mg/kg. Calves can tolerate 40 ppm of cadmium in diet; 160 ppm of cadmium reduces their growth with loss of appetite, and 2550 ppm Cd produces death in 2-8 days. Dietary zinc and calcium reduces the toxicity of cadmium.

Toxicokinetics: The main routes of cadmium absorption are the alimentary tract (up to 10%) and respiratory tract. Absorption of cadmium from tissues after parenteral administration is very slow. After absorption, most of cadmium is transported in plasma bound to albumin or gamma globulins. A limited amount is carried by erythrocytes. The largest amount of cadmium is stored in liver and kidneys. Cadmium taken up by the liver can combine with glutathione (GSH) and is excreted in bile or can bind to metallothionein (MT), a low molecular weight metal-binding protein having one-third of amino acid residues as cysteine. The formation of cadmium-metallothionein complex protects various organs from high exposure to the metal. However the Cd-metallothionein complex is increasingly taken up by the kidneys, which damages renal tubules, particularly the proximal tubules. Thus, cadmium is first distributed to the liver and then redistributed slowly to the kidneys as cadmium-metallothionein. Normally most of cadmium is excreted in the faeces (up to 90%), but in case of Cd-induced renal damage excess cadmium is excreted in the urine and renal concentration of the metal falls.

Mechanism of action :

a. Cadmium owes its toxic action mainly to its high affinity for proteins. The reaction of cadmium with proteins damages the mucous membranes of GI tract and causes pathological changes in mucous membranes of respiratory tract. Chronic bronchitis, progressive fibrosis of lower airway and rupture of interalveolar septae lead to emphysema.

b. When taken up by the kidney cells, the cadmium-metallothionein (Cd-MT) complex enters the lysosomes. In the lysosomes, the MT is degraded to its component amino acids (aa) and the Cd is released into cytosol which damages kidney tubules (Fig. 11.8). The renal tubular damage results in their inability to absorb small molecular proteins such as β_2-microglobulin, lysozyme, ribonuclease, immunoglobulin light chain and retinol-binding protein. Renal tubular damage also results in aminoaciduria, glycosuria, and phosphaturia. At later stages, there may be hypercalcinuria, which in conjunction with altered bone metabolism may lead to osteomalacia.

c. As cadmium and zinc are similar in structure and function, the Cd competes

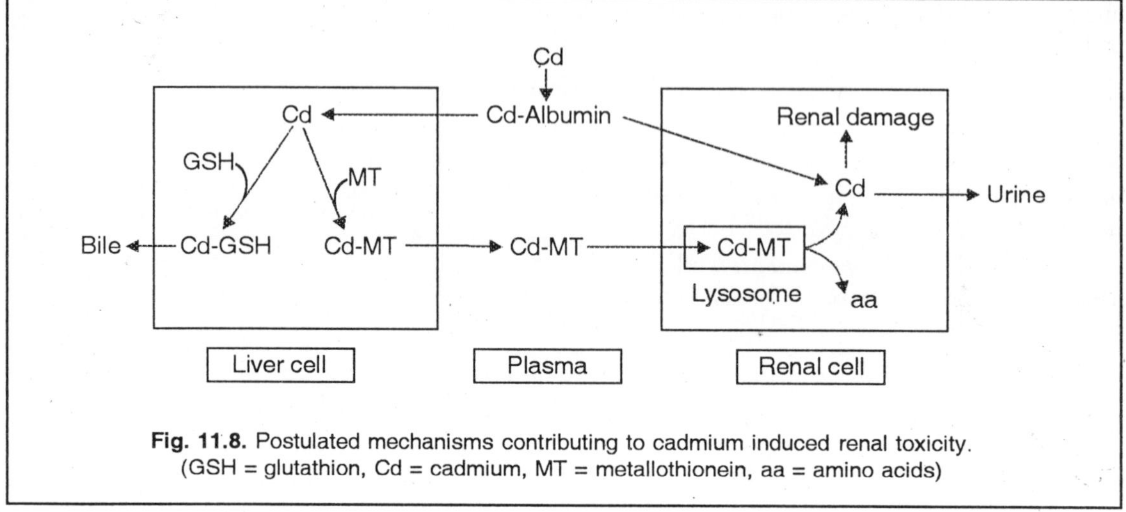

Fig. 11.8. Postulated mechanisms contributing to cadmium induced renal toxicity. (GSH = glutathion, Cd = cadmium, MT = metallothionein, aa = amino acids)

with zinc for binding sites in animal body. It inhibits zinc metallo-enzymes and may even displace zinc in some of its important enzymatic and organ functions. As zinc has an affinity for the testes, cadmium is also stored there in higher concentrations than in other tissues and may produce testicular damage. Cadmium may also compete with other metals such as selenium for inclusion into metallo-enzymes and calcium for binding sites on regulatory proteins such as calmodulin.

d. Cadmium may act as a catalyst to oxidation reactions, which can generate free-radical tissue damage.

Clinical signs :

Acute toxicity: Acute poisoning of cadmium usually results from inhalation of cadmium dust and fumes or ingestion of very high concentration of the metal. Such poisonings are relatively rare but dangerous. Acute oral exposure to high concentration of Cd causes severe gastrointestinal disorders, slobbering, excessive salivation, vomiting, abdominal pain, diarrhoea, spasms, hypotension, ataxia and collapse. If the disease has a protracted course, the liver and kidneys are also damaged. Inhalation causes irritation in the respiratory tract, coughing, laboured breathing and vomiting. Pulmonary oedema develops after 12-36 hours, followed by bronchopneumonia and insufficiency of blood circulation.

Chronic toxicity: Chronic toxicity is more common than acute toxicity. There is pulmonary emphysema, chronic coughing, anaemia and proteinuria. The development of testes is retarded or testes may degenerate. Chronic exposure to high levels of cadmium may also cause retarded growth, anaemia, osteoporosis, osteomalacia, deformed bones and spontaneous fractures with increased mortality rate. Pigs and calves show symptoms of parakeratosis (due to deficiency of zinc). In hens, cadmium damages the ovaries leading to atresia and inhibition of egg laying. Occupational exposure to cadmium in human beings has been implicated in significant increase of lung, prostate and some other cancers.

Post-mortem findings: Morphological changes occur mainly in the liver, lungs and kidneys. There is hepatic damage and nephrosis. Degenerative changes are also seen in testes, ovaries, central nervous system and blood vessels. The organs of chronically poisoned animals may store cadmium without visible morphological changes.

Diagnosis: Diagnosis can be made from history, circumstantial evidences, clinical signs, lesions and chemical analysis of cadmium in feed and body organs. Muscles and visceral organs (kidneys, liver and spleen) may contain cadmium level up to 0.1 ppm and 0.5 ppm, respectively. The elevated concentration of cadmium in kidneys, liver and hair correlates to a greater extent with the amount of cadmium absorbed by the body. Horses tend to have much higher concentration of cadmium (in normal animals) than other domestic species. The normal concentration of cadmium in plants ranges between 0.01 ppm and 1.0 ppm. However, severely contaminated plants may contain more than 400 ppm of Cd. In cadmium poisoning, urinary threonine and serine excretion are increased.

Treatment and management: There is no effective antidote for cadmium poisoning, so therapy is usually supportive and symptomatic.

a. *Chelation therapy:* Metal chelators like disodium-calcium-EDTA ($CaNA_2$ EDTA) may decrease mortality in acute cadmium poisoning, but they are ineffective and may even increase cadmium concentration in kidneys in the chronic toxicity. Sulphur containing agents like dimercaprol and penicillamine are not recommended for cadmium toxicosis because they increase cadmium concentration in the kidneys and therefore are nephrotoxic.

b. Gastric lavage may be done, if ingestion is recent.

c. Administration of selenium forms a selenium-cadmium complex which protects against testicular necrosis.

d. Vitamin D may be used to reduce the effects of osteoporosis.

e. In chronic cadmium toxicosis, supplementation with zinc, copper and iron in more than normally adequate doses is significantly protective. Cadmium and calcium are antagonists, so calcium supplements can help remove cadmium. Vitamin C and cysteine also aid in protection.

Prognosis: Effective therapy for cadmium poisoning has been difficult to achieve. Prognosis is grave once the clinical signs set in.

Some important compounds of cadmium :

Inorganic compounds

a. *Cadmium oxide:* Cadmium oxide (CdO) is insoluble in water, but soluble in dilute acids. It is widely used in manufacture of silver alloys, glass, storage battery electrodes, electroplating and as catalyst for organic reactions. In veterinary medicine, it is occasionally used as an ascaricide in swine. Cadmium oxide fumes are strong pulmonary irritant.

b. *Cadmium sulphide:* Cadmium sulphide (CdS) is used as a pigment and colouring agent for textiles, paper, rubber, in printing inks, ceramic glazes, etc. It is also used in fireworks and in phosphorus and fluorescent screens, semiconductors and photoconductors. In medicine, it is used in medicated shampoos for various dermatological conditions.

Organic compounds

c. *Cadmium succinate:* Cadmium succinate (Cadminate, $C_4H_6CdO_4$) exists as needles or plates. It is used mainly as a plant fungicide.

d. *Cadmium salicylate:* Cadmium salicylate ($C_{14}H_{10}CdO_6$) is slightly soluble in cold water, but freely soluble in boiling water. It is occasionally used as antiseptic.

7. Iron

Iron is a necessary trace element used by all living organisms. Iron-containing enzymes, usually containing heme prosthetic groups, participate in cataysis of oxidation reactions and transport of number of soluble gases. Although iron is an essential mineral for normal cellular physiology, its excess can result in cell injury. Iron toxicosis usually results when the pharmaceutical preparations of iron salts are injected in large doses or less often when iron salts are given orally.

Properties: Iron (Fe) is a group 8 and period 4 metal element with atomic number 26. It is a extracted from iron ore and is almost never found in free elemental state. Iron has an ability of switching back and forth between two ionic states – the ferrous and the ferric irons. In the reduced state iron is known as ferrous iron (Fe^{+2}) and in oxidised state it is called ferric iron (Fe^{+3}). Iron has a unique ability to serve as both an electron donor and an acceptor. Because iron can exist in different ionic states, it can serve as a cofactor to enzymes involved in oxidation-reduction reactions. Many animals incorporate iron into the heme complex, an essential component of cytochromes, and in oxygen carrying proteins haemoglobin and myoglobin.

Sources of toxicity: Iron is used as a mineral supplement and for treatment of anaemia. Main source of iron toxicity is either parenteral use of iron-carbohydrate complexes (iron-dextran, -dextrin, -polysaccharide, -sorbitol) or orally administered salts such as ferrous-sulphate, -chloride, -glutamate, -fumarate or -carbonate. Iron toxicity most often occurs as the result of accidental ingestion of oral supplements or their over dosages. Patients with anaemias that require frequent blood transfusions also are at risk for developing chronic iron toxicity.

Factors affecting toxicity :

a. *Species:* Baby pigs are most susceptible to iron toxicity, although all species are potentially susceptible.

b. *Iron status:* Iron deficient animals are less susceptible to iron poisoning than animals with enough iron in the body.

c. Vitamin E deficiency enhances iron toxicity, probably through generation of excess free radicals. Pigs born to vitamin-E deficient sows are more susceptible to iron toxicosis.

d. *Dose:* Massive dose of iron often leads to toxicosis because excess iron easily breaks the mechanisms controlling GI absorption. Iron given in divided doses over a period is less toxic.

e. *Preparation:* Iron toxicity, in general, is greater with the injectable preparations than with oral salts.

Toxicity: Iron is essential to life, but it can also be potentially toxic. All animals are susceptible to iron toxicity, but the condition is usually seen in piglets. An oral dose of 20-60 mg/kg elemental iron is moderately toxic, > 60 mg/kg elemental iron is severely toxic and > 200 mg/kg elemental iron is lethal. However, toxicity depends on the amount of iron already present in the body as most animals lack a mechanism for excreting iron.

Toxicokinetics: Absorption of iron is under physiological control and depends on the amount of iron already present in the body. In general, absorption of iron from GI tract is poor (<10%). The dietary iron is present mainly in ferric state that has low solubility and, therefore, poor absorption. In stomach, the ferric iron is reduced to the ferrous state by gastric acid that is more soluble and hence more readily absorbed. In the gastric and intestinal mucosal cells, the absorbed ferrous iron is metabolized to ferric (Fe^{+3}) form and is then transported across the cell membrane into blood, where it is bound to transferrin, a β_1-glycoprotein. In this bound form, iron is transported throughout the body. Iron is utilized for synthesis of haemoglobin or is incorporated in iron enzymes (e.g. catalase, peroxidase and various cytochromes). Excess iron absorbed over a period of time is stored as haemosiderin or ferritin and can be re-utilised for erythropoiesis. Excessive quantities of iron are mainly excreted through desquamation of iron bearing cells in the gut. It is also excreted in bile and in traces in urine, nails and sweet. Excess iron in the circulation is not readily eliminated because the rate of excretion is extremely low.

Mechanism of action: Iron toxicity can be broadly classified as corrosive or cellular.

a. *Corrosive toxicity:* Iron is extremely corrosive to the GI tract. It acts on the mucosal tissues and causes direct damage to GI epithelial cells (e.g. gastric mucosa). Damage to GI cells leads to diarrhoea and loss of electrolytes; patients may become hypovolaemic because of fluid and blood loss. Mucosal damage also allows absorption of bacterial toxins, which produces adverse systemic effects.

b. *Cellular toxicity:* In an acute iron overdose, the process of control of iron absorption is damaged, which allows absorption of iron in excess of the body's demand in dose-dependent manner. Large overdose also saturates the transferrin, allowing total serum iron to exceed iron-binding capacity, increasing the free circulatory iron. Large amounts of free iron in the circulation may cause damage to critical cells in the liver, heart and other metabolically active organs like kidneys and lungs. Damage to cells via irritant action (less important), free radical production, and/or destruction of mitochondria results in reduced cellular levels of ATP, lysosomal fragility, impaired cellular calcium homeostasis, and damage to DNA, all of which may contribute to cellular injury and death.

i. The absorption of excessive quantities of ingested iron results in hepatotoxicity as a result of its direct irritant action on liver cells. Hepatic damage interferes with essential liver functions like mobilization of glucose and synthesis of albumin and clotting factors.

ii. Severe overdose causes iron to enter the mitochondria and acts as a mitochondrial poison. Iron inhibits mitochondrial enzymes and impairs oxidative phosphorylation and cellular respirations, resulting in mitochondrial acidosis and cellular death. In hepatocytes, iron overload impairs hepatic mitochondrial respiration primarily through interference in cytochrome C oxidase activity and hepatocellular calcium homeostasis. In cardiac myocytes, mitochondrial respiratory enzymes and plasma membrane enzymes such as sodium-potassium-adenosine triphosphatase (Na^+- K^+-ATPase) may be key targets of damage by non-transferrin-bound iron.

iii. Iron's ability to donate and accept electrons plays a catalytic role in the conversion of hydrogen peroxide into free radicals. The resulting oxyradicals have the potential to cause damage to wide variety of cellular structures including lipids, nucleic acids, proteins, and carbohydrates, resulting in wide-ranging impairment in cellular function and integrity that ultimately kills the cell. The rate of free radical production

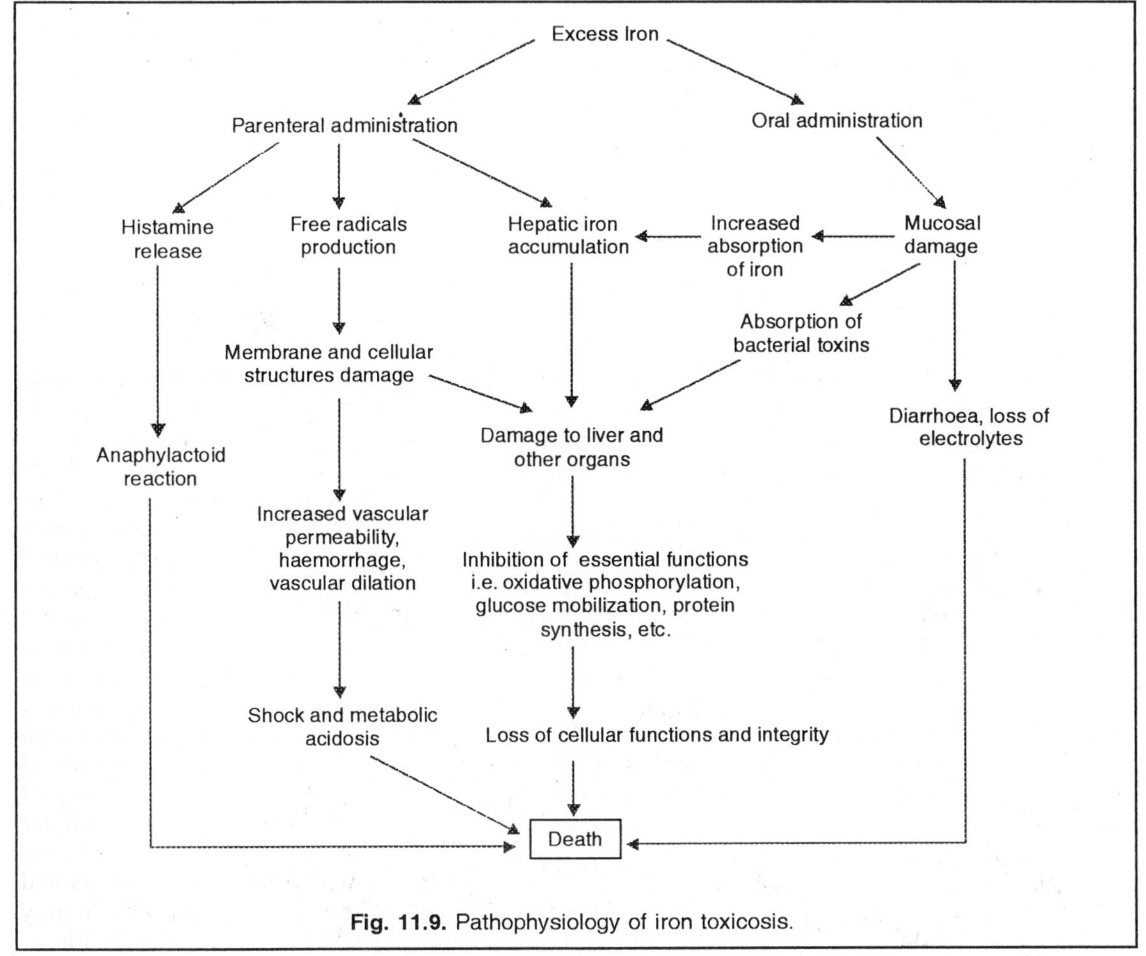

Fig. 11.9. Pathophysiology of iron toxicosis.

must overwhelm the cytoprotective defences of cells before injury occurs. There is also substantial evidence that iron overload can result in oxidative damage to lipids *in vivo*, once the concentration of iron exceeds a threshold level. In the liver, this lipid peroxidation is associated with impairment of membrane-dependent functions of mitochondria and lysosomes. DNA has also been reported to be a target of iron-induced damage, and this may have consequences in regard to malignant transformation.

iv. Excess of iron increases capillary permeability (probably through free radical damage to membranes) and post-arteriolar dilatation leading to hypotension, cardiovascular collapse and shock. There is also interference with blood coagulation leading to haemorrhages. Death mainly occurs due to inadequate perfusion of vital organs with blood.

c. *Anaphylactoid reaction:* Parenteral administration of injectable iron complexes may produce anaphylactoid like reaction due to release of histamine and like substances from the mast cells. This usually happens when drug is given inadvertently by intravenous or intra-arterial route.

Clinical signs :

Oral preparations: Early signs (appearing within 6 hours of ingestion) include drowsiness, depression, vomiting and haemorrhagic diarrhoea. Then apparent improvement may follow for 6-24 hours. After 24 hours, the diarrhoea returns accompanied by dehydration, shock, acidosis and coma. Occasionally, acute haemolytic anaemia, jaundice, haemoglobinaemia and coagulopathy may occur.

Parenteral preparations: Iron toxicity following parenteral injection may occur in various forms. In some animals, particularly piglets, death occurs quickly from 30 min to 6 hours after injection and in others death is delayed for several days.

a. In first acute or peracute form of toxicity, the syndrome mimics an anaphylactic shock reaction and is primarily a vascular collapse followed by rapid death. Damage to muscles around the injection site releases potassium and other substances which interfere with the heart's action. Affected piglets become weak, can not stand, have muscle tremors followed by convulsions. There are signs of cyanosis, dyspnoea and shock.

b. In second less acute or subacute form of toxicity, the animal may be drowsy, exhibit vomiting and diarrhoea, both of which may be bloody. These signs may be followed by a period of apparent improvement. Thereafter cardiovascular collapse and death occur. The excess iron also appears to block the body's defence mechanisms by overwhelming the phagocytic cells which increases likelihood of infection like *Escherichia coli* enteritis. Death occurs after 2-4 days.

c. In third, a more rare form of toxicity, there is massive mobilisation of calcium following injection of iron preparation. Calciphylaxis can occur within several days of iron injection and there is development of hard swellings at injection sites. Death may also occur.

Post-mortem findings :

Oral preparations: Lesions of iron poisoning may include mucosal necrosis or ulceration or both. Usually there is enteritis with intestinal contents fluid to haemorrhagic. Congestion of splanchnic vessels, liver and kidneys and liver necrosis, jaundice and haemoglobinuria may also be found.

Parenteral preparations: Lesions in acute or peracute anaphylactic type of iron toxicosis may include pale skin and muscles, oedema and brownish black discolouration at the injection sites. Waxy degeneration of skeletal muscle, haemorrhages in heart, and necrosis of liver and kidneys may be seen. In less acute form (2nd form) some of the changes seen in first form may occur but usually are less obvious. Enteritis contributes markedly to lesions. In third form, calcification in different parts of body may be seen at necropsy.

Diagnosis: Diagnosis can be made from history of treatment with iron preparations, appearance of shock-like signs and lesions. Total serum iron levels are elevated. Concentrations of iron 50-100% above the normal range (normal

~100-300 $\mu g/dl$) suggest toxicosis. Haemoconcentration, consistent with shock and dehydration is evident. Serum hepatic enzymes and bilirubin levels are increased. Acidosis is detectable and urinalysis reveals haemoglobinuria.

Treatment and management: Iron toxicosis is a severe illness. Its treatment is hindered by the presence of hepatic necrosis, haemorrhages and shock.

Specific therapy

a. Desferrioxamine: Desferrioxamine (Deferoxamine) is a specific iron-chelating agent and is useful in acute and subacute toxicosis. It forms a non-toxic complex with ferric iron, which is excreted in the urine. Excretion of desferrioxamine along with chelated iron gives a 'von rose' (reddish brown) appearance to the urine. Desferrioxamine is useful against both oral and parenteral iron toxicoses. After parenteral administration, it is widely distributed in body and chelates the iron. After oral administration, desferrioxamine is not absorbed itself, but it binds to iron present in gut and prevents its absorption. Potential adverse effects of desferrioxamine may include pain or swelling at injection sites, allergic reactions and GI distress. Rapid IV administration can cause histamine release resulting in fall in blood pressure, itching, urticaria, tachycardia, and shock.

For acute iron-toxicosis

Dogs: 15 mg/kg/hour, IV infusion.

: 40mg/kg, IM, 3 to 6 hours daily, depending on clinical status.

To prevent iron absorption from GI tract

Dogs: 1 – 2 g (total) as 5% solution, by oral route.

b. Oral ascorbic acid administered concurrently with desferrioxamine enhances excretion of iron. However, ascorbic acid should be used only after the gut is thoroughly cleared of iron sources.

Supportive and detoxification therapy

a. Milk of magnesia (MgOH) administered orally precipitates iron in the intestinal tract as insoluble iron hydroxide (FeOH), which is not effectively absorbed. This helps to remove iron from the GI tract. Activated charcoal is not effective for adsorbing iron.

b. Any animal in shock from iron toxicosis should receive IV fluids and other appropriate measures. Supportive measures to control dehydration and acidosis are necessary.

c. Anaphylactoid reaction should be treated by administration of anihistaminics, adrenaline and oxygen.

d. Iron toxicosis can be prevented by raising the levels of Vitamin E (50 I.U./kg of feed) and selenium by feed.

Prognosis: Overall prognosis of iron toxicosis is grave.

Some important compounds of iron :

a. Ferrous sulphate: Ferrous sulphate (FeO_4S) occurs as blue-green, odourless crystals or granules. It is widely used in iron electroplating baths and fertilizers, and as food and feed supplements, weed killer and dye for leather. In medicine, it is used as haematinic and astringent. Ingestion of excess ferrous sulphate produces GI disturbances, haematemesis, hepatic damage and peripheral vascular collapse.

b. Ferric chloride: Ferric chloride (Cl_3Fe) exists as dark leaflets or pallets. It is used in photoengraving, photography, as catalyst in organic reactions, and as mordant in dyeing and printing. Its hexahydrate form is used in human and veterinary medicine as astringent, styptic and diagnostic aid.

c. Ferrous fumarate: Ferrous fumarate ($C_4H_2FeO_4$) is a reddish-orange to reddish-brown, granular powder. It is primarily used as haematinic in iron deficiency anaemia.

8. Zinc

Zinc is an essential element that is important for the normal functioning of several enzymes like carbonic anhydrase, carboxypeptidase, lactic dehydrogenase and alkaline phosphatase. It is essentially required for growth, skeletal development, collagen formation, feathering, dermal health, wound healing, reproductive performance, and synthesis of DNA, RNA, proteins and insulin. The body needs zinc also to metabolize carbohydrates, fats, protein and alcohol and to utilize vitamin A and dispose of carbon dioxide. Although zinc deficiency affecting various biochemical processes has been known for many years, poisoning produced by excess levels of zinc in small animals and birds have been recognized only recently. Poisoning by zinc compounds in large animals has also been described, but is less commonly encountered under normal farming conditions.

Properties: Zinc (Zn) is a chemical element in the periodic table with atomic number 30. Its common oxidation state is +2 (Zn^{++}). Zinc reacts with acids and alkalis and other non-metals and is generally soluble in acids and alkalis, but insoluble in water. The supplemental zinc is available in both organic (e.g. zinc-picolinate, -orotate, -gluconate, and –monomethionine) and inorganic (e.g. zinc-sulphate and –oxide) forms. The supplemental organic zinc is provided mostly in chelated form that enhances its absorption.

Sources of toxicity :

a. Poisoning may arise from consumption of feed mixtures that contain an excessive amount of zinc salt, owing to negligent mixing.

b. Farm animals take excessive zinc by chewing on galvanised bars, pipes, coins, wires and licking zinc coated containers. Ingestion of zinc-containing hardware items like nuts, bolts and wires found on certain types of animal transport cages are important source of zinc toxicosis in small animals. Birds may ingest zinc from zinc coated (galvanised) wire fencing. Drinking rain water collected from galvanised iron roofs or pipes may also produce toxicosis.

c. Food stuffs which produce acidic reaction dissolve zinc from zinc-containers and get contaminated (e.g. formation of zinc lactate induced by the action of lactic acid of fermented milk on zinc containers). The zinc in galvanized bowls can be dissolved by water, fruit juices and acidic foods and can be a source of toxicity in small animals.

d. Excessive and inadvertent use of zinc containing medicines may in some cases expose to harmful effects of zinc. Toxicosis may arise from frequent licking of zinc oxide ointment used to treat skin lesions.

e. Zinc salts are widely used in the cosmetics industry. A mixture of zinc salts of stearic and palmitic acids are used to prepare zinc soaps and some zinc salts are used in bath preparations and hand creams. If ingested accidentally, they can produce zinc toxicosis in small animals.

f. Poisoning may occur due to excessive use of zinc-containing fertilizers and fungicides (e.g. maneb).

g. Chronic poisoning may occur in the proximity of zinc ore roating plants or other zinc processing works.

h. Zinc poisoning may occur by inhalation of industrial fumes which contain ZnO, $ZnCl_2$ and ZnS.

Factors affecting toxicity :

a. *Salt forms:* Soluble salts of zinc (e.g. zinc-chloride, -sulphate, -acetate) are more toxic than slightly soluble salts (e.g. zinc-carbonate, -oxide, and salts of higher fatty acids).

b. *Species:* Ruminants are more susceptible to Zn intoxication than mono-gastric animals. However small animals like dogs are most often affected due to their feeding habits and because the acidic nature of stomach promotes a continued leaching of zinc from the objects ingested by animals. Zinc is extremely toxic to birds.

c. *Age:* Young animals are usually more susceptible to zinc toxicosis than adult animals.

d. *Dietary interactions:* Zinc toxicosis is influenced by other elements and nutrients present in diet. Zinc has strong interaction with copper and iron and can interfere with their absorption.

Toxicity: Although all animals and birds require certain amount of zinc to remain healthy, too much zinc is toxic to them. In general, zinc salts are of low toxicity and very large quantities are required to be ingested to produce clinical toxicosis. The median lethal dose (LD_{50}) of zinc salts (e.g. zinc chloride) is approximately 100 mg/kg body weight. Dietary zinc levels that exceed 2000 ppm cause chronic zinc toxicosis in most domestic animals. A concentration of 50-500 ppm Zn in drinking water is toxic to pigs. Rats, pigs and poultry tolerate dietary levels of 1000-2000 ppm Zn without adverse effects. Zinc at 500-1500 ppm in diets fed to ferrets is lethal.

Toxicokinetics: After ingestion, approximately 10-20% of zinc is absorbed primarily from the duodenum and intestine by a carrier mediated mechanism. The absorption rate may be much higher if the mucous membranes of gut are corroded as in acute poisoning. Absorbed zinc initially binds to plasma albumin and β_2-macroglobulin and is deposited in the liver, kidneys, prostrate, muscle and pancreas. Most of the orally and parenterally administered zinc is then eliminated rapidly in the faeces mainly with pancreatic juices and to a lesser extent with bile. Only a small amount of zinc is eliminated via urine and in milk.

Zinc has strong interactions with some other metals. Cadmium prevents the normal distribution and utilisation of zinc as a component of many enzymes. Increased zinc content in food may reduce copper concentration in various organs.

Mechanism of action: Although nutritional levels of zinc are necessary for normal body functioning, the exact mechanism by which excess zinc produces toxic effects is not clearly understood.

a. Zinc compounds possess corrosive and astringent action and can precipitate proteins with main action on mucosal membranes of digestive tract.

b. Excessive intake of zinc can promote deficiency of other dietary minerals and nutrients. The intake of zinc, even at a low supplementary concentration, has been suggested to interfere with the utilisation of copper and iron and to adversely affect cholesterol concentrations. The antagonistic effects of zinc against copper and iron may result in suppression of haematopoiesis.

c. Zinc ions are reported to inhibit some essential enzymes such as catalase, acid phosphatase, acetylcholinesterase, pepsin, trypsin, and SH-dependent amylase.

Clinical signs :

Acute toxicity: The clinical signs of acute zinc poisoning by soluble salts include painful local irritation and corrosion of GI tract mucosa leading to vomiting and diarrhoea with blood in faeces, abdominal pain and hypotension. Damage to liver in cattle is manifested as icteric colouring of the visible mucous membranes. Death of animals may occur. Clinical signs in birds exposed to a large amount of zinc include ataxia, loss of balance, green diarrhoea and sudden death.

Subacute and Chronic toxicity: Subacute or chronic zinc toxicosis primarily affects the renal, hepatic and haematopoietic tissues. The most important clinical signs in small animals include vomiting, lachrymation, depression, anorexia, haemoglobinuria or myoglobinuria, diarrhoea, weakness and jaundice. Cattle and sheep may manifest anorexia, depression, pica, abdominal distension, polydipsia, polyphagia, fatigue, grinding of teeth, decreased milk production, decreased growth rate, weight loss, exophthalmia, convulsion and death. Pigs may hobble or suffer from paresis of hind legs. In foals, lameness, epiphyseal swelling, stiffness, emaciation, unthriftiness and weight loss are prominent signs. The signs of chronic zinc toxicity in birds may be expressed as anorexia, depression, intermittent lethargy, vomiting or regurgitation, ruffled feathers and neurological signs such as ataxia and seizures. Death may occur as a result of anaemia and damage to internal organs.

Post-mortem findings: Necropsy lesions of zinc poisoning include gastroenteritis, renal tubular necrosis and hepatocyte necrosis. Haematuria, proteinuria, urinary casts and uraemia indicate renal damage. In chronic poisoning in pigs, the findings may include non-specific degenerative arthritis, osteoporotic lesions in bones, damage to kidneys, subcutaneous haemorrhages, gastroenteritis, and haemorrhages in lymph nodes, spleen and cerebral ventricles. Pancreatic and kidney lesions are important findings in birds.

Diagnosis: Diagnosis of zinc toxicosis from clinical signs and lesions is difficult. A tentative diagnosis of zinc poisoning can be made by correlating history of exposure to zinc substances with expected clinical observations. The more reliable diagnosis is based on determination of high zinc contents (many fold) in feed, blood, liver, kidneys, hair and some other tissues. The normal zinc concentration in liver is about 40-60 ppm and in kidneys about half as much. However, the normal zinc concentration in liver, kidneys, and hair largely depend on the content of zinc in diet (high zinc diet may lead to high zinc concentration in body tissues without eliciting clinical signs).

Zinc poisoning has to be differentiated from acute auto-immune haemolytic anaemia.

Treatment and management: Treatment of zinc toxicosis involves eliminating the source of zinc from the animal in conjunction with specific and supportive therapy.

Specific therapy

a. Chelating agents may be used, either by oral or parenteral route. Calcium disodium EDTA (110 mg/kg body weight/day in 3 to 4 divided doses in 5% dextrose, by I.V. (initial dose) and S.C. route thereafter) or D-penicillamine (110 mg/kg for 1-2 weeks by oral route) is the specific therapy to zinc toxicosis. The efficacy of this therapy should be evaluated after 2-5 days to avoid potential nephrotoxicity.

b. Sodium carbonate (1% solution) is administered as an antidote to produce insoluble zinc carbonate. Tannic acid and egg albumin can also be administered for the same purpose.

Detoxification and supportive therapy

a. Emetics and laxatives should be given to clear the GI tract of zinc. Cathartics may aid in the expulsion of small zinc particles.

b. A magnetized instrument may be employed to remove galvanized wire pieces from the digestive tract. Surgical (gastromy or enterotomy) or endoscopic removal may be necessary to remove zinc particles or foreign bodies that are visible radiographically.

c. Intravenous parenteral fluids and bicarbonate (slow IV) is used to help prevent renal failure, if haemolysis is a problem. Blood transfusion may be indicated in severe cases.

d. Symptomatic and supportive therapy may be instituted to treat gastroenteritis and anaemia.

Prevention: Prevention is the best method of dealing with zinc toxicity. Removal of the potential sources of zinc from the vicinity of animals and birds is the safest way of preventing toxicosis.

Some important compounds of zinc :

a. *Zinc chloride:* Zinc chloride (Butter of zinc, $ZnCl_2$) occurs as colourless, opaque, deliquescent rods of masses which are freely soluble in water, alcohol and ether. Zinc chloride is used in medicinal preparations as a caustic and as an astringent. It is also used as an antiseptic in shaving creams, dentifrices and mouthwashes.

b. *Zinc sulphate:* Zinc sulphate (white vitriol, $ZnSO_4 . 7H_2O$) is a colourless crystalline salt which is extremely soluble in water

Table 11.3: Selected zinc compounds used for medicinal and agricultural purposes.

Zinc compounds	Common uses
Zinc acetate	As astringent, styptic, emetic and protective (topical).
Zinc borate	As fungistat.
Zinc bromide	In photography and emulsions.
Zinc carbonate	As astringent, antiseptic and protective (topical). Also used in rations to prevent Zn deficiency.
Zinc chloride	As caustic, astringent and antiseptic. Also used in treatment of ulcers, fistulas and pododermatitis.
Zinc iodide	As topical antiseptic and astringent.
Zinc oleate-stearate	As antiseptic and astringent in cosmetic creams.
Zinc oxide	As antiseptic, astringent and topical protectant.
Zinc peroxide	As disinfectant, antiseptic and deodorant.
Zinc phosphide	As rodenticide.
Zinc propionate	As topical antifungal.
Zinc pyrithione	As bactericide and fungicide used in antidandruff products.
Zinc ricinoleate	As fungicide, emulsifier and stabiliser.
Zinc sulphate	As astringent (ophthalmic) and emetic.

but insoluble in alcohol. It is used as a wood preservative and a mordant for dyes.

c. *Zinc oxide:* Zinc oxide (ZnO) is a soft, white, tasteless, odourless powder commercially known as zinc white (*jasat bhasham*). It is largely used as a pigment in place of "white lead" and in white wall tiles. It is commonly used in pharmacy for making pastes, ointments and lotions. It is also incorporated in face powders, creams and dusting powder.

9. Thallium

Thallium is a heavy metal mainly used in dye and glass industries, for making optical lenses, imitation jewellery, etc. Some insecticides and rodenticides also contain thallium though such compounds are less commonly used nowadays due to high toxicity. Thallium is toxic to all domestic animals, but dogs are most commonly affected.

Properties: Thallium (Tl) is a soft, heavy metal with atomic weight of 203 and a melting point of 303.5°C. It has a tin-white lustrous colour but on exposure to the air, tarnishes upon its surface due to formation of black thallous oxide. It exists in two oxidative states : +3 (thallic) and more common and stable +1 (thallous). It is ubiquitous in nature and occurs especially in sulphide ores of various heavy metals, but normally in low concentrations. Only a few areas contain a naturally very high-thallium concentration. Thallium is very toxic and resembles lead in most of its characters.

Sources of toxicity : Thallium is present in the environment as a result of natural processes and from man-made sources.

a. Thallium is used in some rodenticide or insecticide formulations in the form of syrups, jellies or pastes. The use of thallium in pesticides has been discontinued in advanced countries, but it is still available as rodenticide and ant-killer in other countries.

b. Salts of thallium are used in the manufacture of electronic components, optical lenses, semiconductor materials, alloys, gamma radiation detection equipment, imitation jewellery, artist's paints, low temperature thermometers, and green fireworks and as reagents in analytical chemistry. The dust emitted from various industrial outlets is either inhaled or settled down to contaminate surface water or soil.

c. Thallium exposure may occur from emissions released from coal fired power plants, smelting operations (mainly lead and zinc), cement industries, rodenticide manufacturing plants and refinery (as a by-product of cadmium production).

Factors affecting toxicity :

a. Water-soluble salts (sulphate, carbonate) are easily absorbed from the gut and are more toxic than the less water-soluble (sulphide, iodide) forms.

b. Young animals are more sensitive to thallium poisoning than adult animals.

Toxicity: Thallium poisoning may occur via oral ingestion, inhalation of contaminated dust, or dermal absorption. Toxicity usually occurs with thallous salts (thallous sulphate and thallous acetate) and less with thallic salts. In rats, the acute oral LD_{50} of thallous sulphate is 16-25 mg/kg and in other domestic species it varies from 10-25 mg/kg body weight. The oral lethal dose (LD_{50}) of thallium is different species is: cattle 20 mg/kg, sheep 25 mg/kg, dogs 15-50 mg/kg, chickens 30-40 mg/kg and pigeons 50-100 mg/kg. Chronic poisoning with thallium is not common but may occur due to its accumulation in the body.

Toxicokinetics: Exposure to thallium is possible through oral, inhalation, dermal, eye, parenteral, and other routes. Thallium is readily absorbed from the gut or skin and rapidly distributed intracellularly throughout all body tissues. Its concentration in kidneys is 5-15 times more than other tissues. In human beings, thallium follows a 3-phase toxicokinetics: first intravascular distribution, then CNS distribution, and finally elimination. In the first 4 hours following exposure, thallium is rapidly distributed to blood and well-perfused organs such as the kidneys, liver, and muscles. Over the next 4-48 hours, thallium is distributed into the CNS. The elimination phase begins about 24 hours after ingestion.

Thallium shows bi-phasic elimination in some species. During the first day after exposure, the kidneys are the main route of excretion with high urinary concentration. In the subsequent days, the concentration of metal in faeces is more with excretion mainly in bile. The high concentrations of thallium found in the kidney (>5.5 times more than other tissues) result from renal filtration with approximately 50% undergoing reabsorption in the kidney tubules. Overall, the elimination of thallium is slow with an elimination half-life of 3-8 days, varying with dose and chronicity of the exposure. Because of this prolonged elimination phase, thallium may act as a cumulative poison.

Mechanism of action: The exact mechanism of thallium toxicity is unclear. However following actions may account for most of the toxic effects of thallium:

a. Because of its similarity in charge and ionic radius to potassium, thallium substitutes potassium in various processes including its active transport in muscles and nerves. Thallium enters the cells, inhibits sodium-potassium ATPase and may impede proper functioning of sodium-pump for which thallium has a significantly greater affinity than potassium. This action of thallium interferes with energy production at essential steps in glycolysis, Krebs cycle and oxidative phosphorylation. Furthermore, its similarity to potassium allows it to accumulate in areas rich in potassium including muscular, hepatic and nervous tissues. Its accumulation in muscular tissue is the basis for the use of radioactive thallium in cardiac imaging studies.

b. Thallium has high affinity for sulphydryl groups and its toxicosis could be related to inhibition of sulphur containing macromolecules. Thallium combines with sulphydryl enzymes (e.g. succinic dehydrogenase, monoamine oxidase, cethepsin) and may interfere with formation of disulfide bonds. Inhibition of mitochondrial sulphydryl enzymes causes an interference with oxidative phosphorylation. This action of thallium results in inhibition of aerobic metabolism in some organs like skin, brain and kidneys.

c. A further possible toxic mechanism of thallium is interference in riboflavin homeostasis. Thallium forms insoluble complexes with riboflavin resulting in its intracellular sequestration. Deficiency of this vitamin results in dermatitis, alopecia, and neuropathy, which are the hallmarks of thallium poisoning.

Clinical signs :

Acute toxicity: Onset of clinical signs in acute thallium toxicity may be delayed for 1-3 days. Although all body systems are affected, the most severe signs are related to the alimentary tract, and respiratory, integumentary and nervous systems. Gastrointestinal signs include vomiting, abdominal pain, anorexia, salivation, gastro-enteritis, colic and diarrhoea (occasionally haemorrhagic). Other important manifestations are dyspnoea, blindness, fever, conjunctivitis, gingivitis, hyperaesthesia, tremors or seizures, paresis, stumbling and paralysis of limbs. After an apparent recovery or after repeated small doses, chronic dermatitis characterised by alopecia, erythema and hyperkeratosis may occur. The entire course of thallium poisoning progresses slowly over a period of 3 to 10 days. The animal may die of thallium poisoning, malnutrition, thirst or secondary infections.

Chronic toxicity: Incidence of chronic thallium poisoning is rarely seen in animals. Important clinical signs of chronic toxicity are vomiting, diarrhoea, anorexia, and loss of hair around eyes and on limbs with pustular eruptions, weakness and pain in extremities. Alopecia and drying and scaling of skin can occur over 1-3 weeks post-ingestion.

Post-mortem findings: In acute thallium poisoning, there is haemorrhagic gastroenteritis, ulceration of gastric mucosae, hepatic congestion and inflammation of respiratory mucosa. Necrosis of many tissues is common. There are degenerative changes in heart, kidneys and liver (especially marked in chronic poisoning).

Diagnosis: Diagnosis of thallium intoxication should be based on history, characteristic clinical presentation, lesions and laboratory analysis. Confirmation of the diagnosis, however, is possible only by means of laboratory analysis of thallium in urine, faeces and kidneys. Any thallium level in body may be considered significant.

Treatment and management :

Specific therapy

a. *Prussian blue:* Prussian blue is a non-absorbable lattice of potassium ferric furocyanide. It is not absorbed orally but helps to enhance elimination of thallium from the gut. Mechanical removal of faeces may be necessary before administration of Prussian blue because its efficacy is lost in patients not able to evacuate the bowel due to constipation and/or absence of intestinal motility. Prussian blue has been found useful against thallium toxicity in human beings, but data on its efficacy in domestic animals are lacking.

b. *Diphenylthiocarbazone:* Oral administration of diphenylthiocarbazone has shown efficacy against thallium toxicity in small animals.

   Small animals: 70 mg/kg, orally.

c. *Sodium thiosulphate:* Sodium thiosulphate is an effective antidote against cyanide toxicity and is considered useful in thallium poisoning as well. It provides exogenous sulphur and helps in the excretion of thallium.

   All species: 50-100 mg/kg (as 1.5-2% solution), by intravenous route.

d. *Sodium diethyldithiocarbamate:* Sodium diethyldithiocarbamate has been recommended for thallium toxicity in small animals with variable success.

Detoxification and supportive therapy

a. Emetics and gastric lavage with sodium iodide solution (1%) may be indicated for very recent exposures.

b. Symptomatic treatment of the diarrhoea and convulsions, if required.

d. Correction of fluid and electrolytes imbalance by parenteral fluid therapy.

e. Treatment of skin lesions, as needed.

Important compounds of thallium :

a. *Thallium sulphate:* Thallium sulphate (Thallous sulphate, O_4STl_2) exists as white rhomboid prisms. It is mainly used as a rat poison, rat bait and a reagent in the analytical chemistry. Its oral LD_{50} in rats is approximately 25 mg/kg.

b. *Thallium nitrate:* Thallium nitrate (Thallous nitrate, NO_3Tl) exists as white crystals. It is mainly used as a reagent in analytical chemistry. It is a toxic compound with oral LD_{50} in dogs approximately 45 mg/kg.

BIBLIOGRAPHY

Allen GS (1968) An outbreak of zinc poisoning in cattle. *Vet. Rec.* 83 : 8.

Aronson AL (1972) Lead poisoning in cattle and horses following long-term exposure to lead. *Am. J. Vet. Res.* 33 : 627.

Ballantyne B, Marrs T and Turner P (1995) General and Applied Toxicology. Macmillan, London.

Barceloux DG (1999) Copper. *Clin. Toxicol.* 37 : 217.

Barceloux DG (1999) Selenium. *Clin. Toxicol.* 37 : 145.

Bartik M and Piskac A (1981) Veterinary Toxicology. Elsevier Scientific Publishing Company, Amsterdam.

Beasley V (1999) Veterinary Toxicology. International Veterinary Information Service, Ithaca NY (www.ivis.org).

Berger LL (1991) Copper toxicity in sheep. (http://www.saltinstitute.org/publications/stm/stm-2.html).

Booth NH and McDonald LE (1982) John's Veterinary Pharmacology and Therapeutics. 5th edn. (Eds.). Kalyani Publishers, Ludhiana-New Delhi.

Brar RS (1993) "Studies on clinico-pathological, biochemical and histoenzymological alterations in lead toxicosis in domestic fowl and buffalo calves". Ph.D. Thesis, Punjab Agricultural University, Ludhiana.

Brar RS, Brar KS and Grewal GS (1994) The disposition of lead in blood and tissues of buffalo calves (*Bubalus bubalis*). *Vet. Res. Comm.* 18 : 109.

Campbell JR, Clarkson TW and Omar MD (1986) The therapeutic use of 2, 3-dimercaptone-1-sulphonate in 2 cases of inorganic mercury poisoning. *J. Am. Med. Assoc.* 256 : 3127.

Catchi A and Harmuth-Hoene AE (1979) Pharmacology and therapeutic applications of agents used in heavy metal poisoning. In: The

Chelation of Heavy Metals. Levin WG (Ed.). Pergamon Press, New York.

Clarke ECG and Clarke ML (1967) Garner's Veterinary Toxicology. 3rd edn. Williams and Wilkins, Baltimore.

Clarkson TW (1972) The pharmacology of mercury compounds. *Ann. Rev. Pharmacol.* 12 : 275.

Clarkson TW (1987) Metal toxicity in the central nervous system. *Environ. Hlth. Perspect.* 75 : 59.

Davis G, Steffens TJ, Engle TE, Mallow KL and Cotton SE (2006) Diagnosing selenium toxicity. Colorado State University Extension – Natural Resources. (http://www.ext.colostate.edu/pubs/natres/06109.html)

Dhillon KS, Singh TJ, Gill BS, Sandhu HS and Singh J (1993) Chronic molybdenosis in buffaloes. 2. Cutaneous afflictions. *Ind. J. Anim. Sci.* 63: 740.

Frasher CM, Bergeron JA, Mays A and Aiello SE (1991) The Merck Veterinary Manual: A Handbook of Diagnosis, Therapy and Disease Prevention and Control for the Veterinarians. 7th edn. Merck and Company, Rahway.

Garg SK (2000) Veterinary Toxicology. CBS Publishers & Distributors, New Delhi.

Goyer RA (1996) Toxic effects of metals. In: Casarett & Doull's Toxicology: The Basic Science of Poisons. 5th edn. Klaassen CD (Ed.) p 691. Mcgraw Hill Companies Inc., New York.

Graziano JH, Cuccia D and Friedham E (1978) The Pharmacology of 2,3-dimercaptosuccinic acid and its potential use in arsenic poisoning. *J. Pharmacol. Exp. Therap.* 207: 1051.

Green A (2002) Lead poisoning . (http://www.drgreene.com/21_1132.html).

Gupta PK and Salunkhe DK (1985). Modern Toxicology. Vol. III. Immuno and Clinical Toxicology Metropolitan Publishing Company, New Delhi.

Gwatlney-Brant SM and Rumbeiha WK (2002) Newer antidotal therapies. *Vet. Clin. North Am: Small Anim Pract.* 32 : 323.

Haque I, Advayi EA and Sibanda S (1993) Copper in soil, plants and ruminant animals' nutrition with special reference to Sub-Saharan Africa. *J. Plant. Nutr.* 16 : 2149.

Hintz H (1993) Are high Cu horse feed toxic to goats. *Eq. Pract.* 15 : 6.

Jones MM (1991) New development in therapeutic chelating agents in antidotes for metal poisoning.. *Crit. Rev. Toxicol.* 21 : 209.

Kehoe R (1976) Pharmacology and toxicology of heavy metals: Lead. *Pharmacol. Therap.* 1:161.

Klaassen CD (1996) Casarett & Doull's Toxicology: The Basic Science of Poisons. 5th edn. Mcgraw Hill Companies Inc., New York.

Klaassen CD (2001) Heavy metals and heavy metal antagonists. In: Goodman & Gilman's The Pharmacological Basis of Therapeutics. 10th edn. Hardman JG, Limbird LE and Gilman AG (Eds.) p 1851. The McGraw-Hill Companies Inc., New York.

Lorgue G, Lechenet J and Riviere A (1996) Clinical Veterinary Toxicology. Blackwell Science Ltd., United Kingdom.

Lu FC and Kacew S (2002) Lu's Basic Toxicology: Fundamentals, Target Organs and Risk Assessment. Taylor & Francis, New York.

Martin SJ (1998) Chronic copper poisoning in sheep. Ministry of Agriculture, Food and Rural Affairs, Ontario (http://www.omafra.gov.on.ca/english/livestock/sheep/facts/health-copper.htm).

Mossman BT and Begin RO (1989) Effects of Mineral Dusts on Cells. Springer-Verlag, Berlin Heidelberg.

National Research Council (1976) Selenium - Medical and Biological Effects on Environmental Pollutants. National Academy of Science, Washington.

Oehme GD (1979) Toxicity of Heavy Metals in the Environment. Part 1, 2. Mercel Dekker, Inc., New York.

Osweiler GD (1996) Toxicology. Williams and Wilkins, Philadelphia.

Palmer JS (1963) Mercurial fungicidal seed protectant toxic for sheep and chickens. *J. Am. Vet. Med. Assoc.* 142 : 1385.

Parai TP, Pandey NN and Prashad MC (1993) Pathomorphological changes in mercuric chloride induced nephropathy in cattle. *Ind. J. Anim. Sci.* 63 : 274.

Peoples SA (1964) Arsenic toxicity in cattle. *Ann. New York Acad. Sci.* 111, 2 : 644.

Piper R, Miller VL and Dickinson EO (1971) Toxicity and distribution of mercury in pigs with acute methylmercurialism. *Am. J. Vet. Res.* 32 : 263.

Porter RS (2007) The Merck Manuals Online Medical Library – Section: Accidents and Injuries. (http://www.merck.com/mmhe/sec24.html).

Radeleff RD (1970) Veterinary Toxicology. 2nd edn. Lea and Febiger, Philadelphia.

Robinette CL (1990) Zinc. *Vet. Clin. North Am: Small Anim Pract.* 20 : 539.

Roche B (2005) Lead poisoning in livestock. (http://www2.dpi.qld.gov.au/health/4213.html).

Rodostits O M, Gay C C, Blood D C and Hinchcliff K W (2000) Veterinary Medicine: A Textbook of the Diseases of Cattle, Sheep, Pigs, Goats and Horses. 9th edn. W. B. Saunders, London.

Rofas LX and McDowell LR (1995) Development of acute Cu poisoning in sheep fed organic or inorganic copper. *Ind. J. Am. Sci.* 10 : 41.

Rolfe DS and Twedt DC (1995) Copper associated hepatopathies in dogs. Vet. Clin. North Am: Small Anim Pract. 25 : 399.

Sandhu HS, Singh TJ, Dhillon KS and Sidhu SS (1992) Normal blood levels of molybdenum in farm animals. *Ind. J. Am. Sci.* 62 : 61.

Schoenian S (2000) Copper toxicity in sheep. Maryland Cooperative Extension, University of Maryland.

Smith BP (2001) Large Animal Internal Medicine. 3rd edn. Mosby, St. Louis.

Sugawara N, Li D, Sugawara C and Niyoki H (1995) Response of hepatic function to hepatic Cu deposition in rats fed a diet containing copper. *Biol. Trace Elem. Res.* 49 : 161.

Thomas RL (2007) Plumbism. The Eclectic Practice of Medicine. (http://www.henriettesherbal.com/eclectic/thomas/lead-pois.html).

Vallee BL and Ulmer DD (1972) Biochemical effects of mercury, cadmium and lead. *Ann. Rev. Biochem.* 41 : 91.

Venugopal B and Luckey TD (1978) Metal Toxicity in Mammals. Vol. 2. Plenum Press, New York.

White ME (2005) Cornell Consultant Toxicity Data. Alphabetical Search for the Cornell Consultant for Data on Intoxication, Poisoning or Toxicity in Animals. Cornell University College of Veterinary Medicine (Online service, http://homepage.eircom.net/~progers/consultox.htm).

Yaremcio B (2001) Lead poisoning in cattle. Agriculture, Food and Rural Development, Alberta. (http://www1.agric.gov.ab.ca/$department/deptdocs.nsf/all/agdex791)

Zook BC, Kopito MS and Carpenter JL (1972) Lead poisoning in dogs: Analysis of blood, urine, hair and liver for lead. *Am. J. Vet. Res.* 33 : 903.

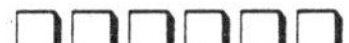

12 NON-METALS

Fluoride
Selenium
Phosphorus
Nitrate and Nitrite
Chlorate
Sulphur

1. Fluoride

Fluorine is a very reactive non-metallic element. It exists in nature mostly as fluoride in a combined form with many minerals/elements like aluminium, iron, calcium, phosphates, etc. and thus is an important constituent of many of the rocks and ores. It is widely distributed in the environment and present in varying amount in soils, water, air, plants, and animal tissues. Fluorosis is a chronic disease caused by continued ingestion of small but toxic amounts of fluorine. Fluorosis is endemic in at least 25 countries across the globe, including India.

Properties: Fluorine (F) is highly reactive halogen with atomic number 9. It does not exist in elemental state in nature but occurs mostly in ionic form as fluoride (F^-). It is the most electronegative of the elements and forms compounds with a variety of other inorganic and organic materials. It has strong affinity for calcium, iron and aluminium. In nature, fluoride may occur as inorganic (e.g. sodium fluoride, calcium fluoride, potassium fluorosilicate, sodium hexafluorosilicate) or organic (e.g. trifluoromethane, barium fluoroacetate) fluorine compounds.

Sources of toxicity :

a. Some feed supplements and mineral mixtures are high in fluoride-containing rock phosphates ($CaHPO_4$) or superphosphates (produced from rock phosphates) and phosphatic limestones. High fluoride in such feeds may cause toxicosis. Normally, feed-grade phosphates should not contain more than 1 part of fluorine to 100 parts of phosphate.

b. Drinking water in fluoride rich soils, usually from deep wells, contains high levels of fluoride and may contribute to a chronic build-up of fluoride in body. In India, fluoride-laden water derived from borewells dug deep into the earth is the most common cause of fluorosis in man and animals.

c. Consumption of forages by livestock that are grown on high fluorine soil may cause toxicosis in animals. The seeds or grains of crops do not accumulate fluoride, but the stem and leaves accumulate fluoride in significant amount. In general, accumulation of fluoride in plants is poor with mean value less than 4 ppm.

d. Factories that manufacture mineral supplements and fertilizers from fluoride-bearing phosphate rock, electrolytically produce aluminium, and prepare bricks from fluorine-bearing clays may contaminate environment through fluorine containing gases or dusts. This form of fluoride is more dangerous as fluoride from these sources is carried in the wind and settles on vegetation, water or feed sources.

e. Industrial effluents or fumes from aluminium-smelting factories, steel works, cement factories, coal-burning power stations, glass manufacturers and glass-itching industries contaminate nearby water sources and fields and cause toxicosis in animals.

f. Accidental ingestion of fluoride pesticides such as sodium fluoride (as acaricide in pigs) and sodium fluorosilicate or fluoroacetate (as rodenticide) may cause toxicosis in animals.

g. Dusts and gases from volcanic eruptions may cause fatal fluorine intoxication in the period immediately after the eruption.

Factors affecting toxicity: Fluoride toxicosis is affected by following factors:

a. *Species*: All species are susceptible to fluoride toxicosis, although the maximal tolerable level varies with species. In general, dogs are more susceptible to acute toxicosis through ingestion of fluoride-containing pesticides, while chronic toxicosis is noted most often in herbivores grazing on contaminated pastures.

b. *Dose:* If level or amount of fluoride in the diet or forage is more than 2-4 ppm, it may become toxic.

c. *Duration of exposure*: If fluoride is taken for a longer period then it accumulates in bones and teeth and produces fluorosis.

d. *Solubility*: More soluble fluoride compounds (e.g. sodium fluoride) are more toxic than less soluble compounds (e.g. calcium fluoride).

e. *Age*: Young growing bones and teeth are more susceptible to fluoride toxicosis than fully grown tissues/organs.

f. *Nutritional status*: Weak and emaciated animals are more susceptible to toxicosis than healthy animals. Malnutrition intensifies fluoride toxicosis.

g. *Stress*: Presence of stress factors such as cold or drought conditions may precipitate fluoride toxicity. Other stressors like simultaneous exposure to other potentially toxic substances also aggravate fluorosis.

Toxicity: Man and animals normally ingest low levels of fluoride throughout their lives, but adverse effects do not accompany such ingestion. Fluorosis can occur only if the amount of fluoride ingested is more or if the accumulation of fluoride in body is affected by other factors. Acute fluoride poisoning, though rare in animals, may occur from ingestion of inorganic fluoride compounds such as hydrogen fluoride, sodium fluoride and sodium fluorosilicate. Chronic poisoning usually occur after continuous ingestion of water, forages and feed supplements high in fluoride contents and is more common among animals.

The maximal tolerable level of fluoride varies with species from 40-50 ppm for cattle to 200 ppm for chickens. In cattle, a mild form of fluorosis can occur if the diet containing 40 ppm fluoride as sodium fluoride or 100 ppm fluoride from rock phosphate is fed for a period of 3-5 years. Ingestion of plant materials having 5 ppm fluorine does not produce dental changes, 14 ppm produces dental changes and 100 ppm causes changes in skeleton and joints within a month in cows and sheep. Chronic intoxication has occurred in sheep and cattle drinking deep well water containing 12-19 ppm fluoride. More serious systemic effects do not occur until the water contains 30 ppm fluoride. Oral acute lethal dose of NaF is about 500 mg/kg.

Toxicokinetics: Soluble fluorides are readily absorbed (75-90%) from the digestive tract and get distributed throughout the body. After passive absorption from intestine, about half of the fluoride is excreted rapidly in urine and the rest is stored in calcified tissues like bone and teeth. Bone is a natural sink for fluoride (like lead) with 96-99% of the absorbed fluoride being incorporated into the hydroxyapatite crystalline structure of bone. Normal adult bones contain about 1000-1500 ppm fluoride. Fluoride is gradually excreted in urine; the unabsorbed fluoride is eliminated in faeces. A small amount gets into the milk. Fluoride has cumulative action only when a constant or increasing amounts are ingested over time, otherwise urinary excretion will tend to maintain body fluoride below toxic levels. In cases of fluorosis, the tissue fluoride concentration may be elevated two to three times than normal.

Mechanism of action :

Acute toxicity: Mechanism of action in acute toxicity depends upon the individual fluoride compound and may include:

a. After ingestion, large amounts of soluble inorganic fluoride form hydrofluoric acid in the acidic medium of stomach, which leads to GI irritation or corrosive effects. Compounds like hydrogen fluoride cause direct irritation to mucous membranes and skin. Following ingestion, the GI tract is the earliest and most commonly affected organ system.

b. Fluoride (Fl^-) binds to several cations such as Ca^{++}, Mn^{++} and Mg^{++} in body and disrupts ionic balance. It interferes with calcium metabolism intracellularly and lowers plasma calcium concentration due to formation of insoluble precipitates of fluoride and calcium. Hypocalcaemia also affects neurotransmission in the CNS. Fluoride inhibits Na^+/K^+-ATPase, which may lead to hyperkalaemia by extracellular release of potassium. Death mainly occurs due to hyperkalaemia and associated changes in heart, and hypocalcaemia. Seizures may result from both hypomagnesaemia and hypocalcaemia

c. Fluoride ion being very reactive has direct cytotoxic effects and interferes with a number of enzyme systems. Fluoride inhibits preglycolytic and phosphatase enzymes and impairs utilisation of glucose. In high concentration, fluoride may cause inhibition of cholinesterase enzyme and increase sensitivity of the body system to acetylcholine. Fluoride also disrupts oxidative phosphorylation, probably through inhibition of some essential enzymes. Central vasomotor depression as well as direct cardiotoxicity may also occur.

d. Fluoride acts as anticoagulant because it precipitates the calcium in the form of calcium fluoride (CaF_2). In acute poisoning, some coagulative defects are seen due to this effect of fluoride, but this action does not account much for chronic toxicity as only mobile form of calcium combines with fluoride.

Chronic toxicity: Excessive fluoride intake for longer time affects primarily the teeth and bones. Deposition of fluoride in bones occurs throughout life, but its deposition in teeth occurs only during the formative stages.

a. *Teeth*: In developing teeth (prior to eruption), excessive amount of fluoride damages ameloblasts and odontoblasts. Matrix laid down by damaged ameloblasts and odontoblasts fails to accept minerals normally as a result of which there is delayed and impaired mineralization of the teeth. The degree of damage varies directly with the level of fluoride exposure. Malformed enamel and dentin produced during tooth eruption allow rapid and excessive wear of molars and incisors in adults. Oxidation of organic material in areas where the enamel is defective also results in brown or black discolouration of the teeth. The dental lesions do not develop in mature teeth as enamel formation does not occur in fully formed teeth. Therefore, dental lesions may be absent even in very severe fluorosis cases, if the exposure to adult animals occur.

b. *Bone*: The exact mechanism relating to fluoride induced bone malformation is not known. It is thought that skeletal fluorosis results in disrupted osteogenesis leading to inadequate matrix formation and defective irregular mineralization. There is accelerated bone resorption (osteoporosis) and remodelling with production of abnormal bones (e.g. exostosis, sclerosis). Bone lesions may result also from the replacement of hydroxyl radicals by fluoride ions in the hydroxyapatite crystal structure of bone substance. There is increased calcification at the sites where muscles are attached to the bones or at bone exostoses. Inhibition of certain enzymes associated with bone and teeth formation is also suspected to be involved in the action of fluoride. There is decrease in production of phosphopyruvate, which is a substrate for bone phosphatase.

In bones, deposition of fluoride is highest on the periosteal surfaces of long bones, where exostoses develop. Bones that are more active metabolically, such as those used in locomotion, chewing or breathing, are more affected than the bones that are primarily protective and less active in function. Also growth areas of bone are more affected than less active areas.

Clinical signs :

Acute toxicity: Acute poisoning is rare and can result from inhalation of fluorine containing gases or ingestion of large amounts of fluoride compounds. Severity of signs depend on the amount of fluoride ingested or inhaled. Inhalation of fluoride containing fumes or gases produces very rapid onset with respiratory signs and pulmonary oedema. After ingestion of fluoride compounds, onset of signs usually occurs within 30 minutes of exposure and includes severe gastroenteritis with complete anorexia, nausea, vomiting, hypersalivation, abdominal pain and diarrhoea. In ruminants there may be ruminal stasis with constipation or diarrhoea. Affected animals are dyspnoeic. Cardiovascular signs include various arrhythmias, cardiac arrest and shock. Nervous signs are characterised by excitability, muscle tremors and weakness. There is pupillary dilatation, a startled expression, hyperesthesia and constant chewing. Tetany and collapse follow, and death occurs within few hours. Death in acute fluoride toxicosis usually results from respiratory paralysis, arrhythmia, or cardiac failure.

***Chronic toxicity*:** Clinical signs in chronic fluorosis may not be apparent until several months or years after initial exposure. Chronic fluorosis is mostly presented in a definite sequence and observed in livestock with signs related to the skeletal and dental lesions.

i. *Skeletal fluorosis:* The skeletal lesions start with sudden onset of lameness, unthriftiness, stiffness, painful gait and posture. Lameness is periodic and intermittent, usually of moving type, i.e. first one leg is involved, then second leg is also involved and then others. There is thickening and enlargement of sternum, mandible, ribs and spine. In severe cases, there is increase in diameter of metacarpals and metatarsals and phallenges. Bony exostoses may be seen or felt on the legs with swelling of limbs. Palpation of affected bones causes severe pain. There is decreased feed intake, anorexia, rough hair-coat, emaciation, weigh loss and decreased milk production. Osteofluorotic (proliferative osteoporosis) lesions may lead to spontaneous fractures. General worsening of skeletal and dental lesions ultimately progress to cachexia and death.

ii. *Dental fluorosis:* Dental lesions are noted only in those animals ingesting toxic amounts of fluoride at the time of permanent teeth development (1-5 years of age). In dental fluorosis, the teeth have a characteristic mottling and patchy loss of dentine. Teeth are lustreless and become pitted. In mild cases, there may be only a few white flecks or small pits on the enamel of teeth. In more severe cases, teeth become stained brown around eroded areas and wear unevenly (show uneven upper lining). The final stage culminates in complete deformation of the dental tables or even there is shedding of teeth in worst affected cases, which leads to significant difficulty in prehending or swallowing food.

Post-mortem findings :

Acute toxicity: There is cyanosis and early rigor mortis. There may be haemorrhagic gastroenteritis and haemorrhages, congestion and oedema in various organs including the brain. Bone and dental lesions are absent.

Chronic toxicity: Mottling, staining and excessive wearing is seen in the teeth that develop during the time of excessive ingestion. The teeth that are fully formed before exposure are largely unaffected. The bones may become chalky white (instead of normal ivory colour), soft, thickened in diameter and in the extreme cases develop exostoses that may be palpated, especially along the long bones and on the mandible. Bone marrow cavity is diminished and shows gelatinous degeneration and aplastic anaemia. Degenerative changes in the kidneys, liver and several endocrine glands, and anaemia have been reported but the lesions are not pathognomonic.

Histopathological changes in chronic fluorosis include cortical thickening, periosteal hyperostosis, uneven mineralization, resorption of endosteal bone and excessive osteoid tissues. There is atrophy of spongia, defective and irregular calcification of newly formed osseous tissue, hypoplasia of enamel and dentine. Degenerative changes are observed in kidneys, liver, adrenal glands, heart muscles and central nervous system. In kidneys, degeneration and disintegration of tubular epithelium, slight glomerular changes, thickened arterioles and fibrosis are also observed. Severe gastroenteritis is absent in chronic poisoning.

Diagnosis: Diagnosis is based on circumstantial evidences (location of factory nearby, fluoride contaminated water, etc.), history of feeding of rock phosphates or derived feed products, clinical signs and bone and tooth lesions. X-ray examination reveals sclerosis, perosis, hyperostosis or a combination of these. Analysis of serum electrolytes shows hyperkalaemia, hypocalcaemia, hypomagnesaemia, and hypoglycaemia. Accurate diagnosis, however, depends on demonstrating elevated fluorine levels in plasma, urine, bones and dental tissues, and ultimately discovering the source of the element. Samples should be taken by either biopsy (living animal) or necropsy (dead animal) from the metatarsals, metacarpals, ribs, pelvis, mandible, etc. Fluorotic cattle may have 3000 ppm or more of fluoride in bones (normal level is 400-1200 ppm on dry weight, fat free basis). Affected sheep have 5000 ppm fluoride or more against 250 ppm in normal sheep. Urine may contain 15-20 ppm of fluoride as compared to 2-6 ppm in normal animal. Where clinical signs of intoxication appear, there is usually up to 2% fluorine in bone ash and 1% in teeth ash.

The signs and lesions of acute fluoride toxicosis can be confused with signs produced by any strong caustic (i.e. inorganic arsenic), anticholinesterase pesticide, metabolic inhibitor (e.g. fluoroacetate) or anticoagulant rodenticide (e.g. warfarin). In chronic toxicosis, the clinical signs may be similar to osteoporosis, or deficiency of calcium, phosphorus or vitamin D. The lameness in advanced cases may be wrongly attributed to an accident.

Treatment and management :

Acute toxicity: There is no specific treatment for acute fluoride toxicity. Symptomatic treatment may save some animals.

a. Calcium compounds (e.g. calcium gluconate), aluminium salts or milk may be administered orally to bind excess fluoride in GI tract before absorption.

b. Gastric aspiration and lavage are most effective when instituted within 1 hour of ingestion. Adsorption therapy with activated charcoal is not helpful because fluoride does not bind to charcoal.

c. Administration of quinidine helps to prevent fluoride induced hyperkalaemia by blocking K^+ efflux.

d. Hypocalcaemia may be corrected with intravenous calcium chloride. Intravenous calcium salt helps to control tetany and hyperesthesia.

e. Dialysis may be performed to remove fluoride and potassium.

Chronic toxicity: No specific treatment exists for chronic toxicity at present.

a. Tolerance to fluoride can be increased by balanced intake of calcium, phosphorus and vitamin D.

b. Aluminium sulphate or chloride, calcium carbonate and defluorinated phosphate can be administered orally to form insoluble compounds with fluoride in the gut. The feed or water containing excess fluoride can be diluted with feed or roughage that is low in fluoride.

c. Supportive therapy might include steroids, antibiotics, analgesics and fluid therapy.

Prevention :

a. Remove intoxicated animals from the contaminated pasture.

b. Change the feed and drinking water. If the drinking water is high in fluoride, feed the animals roughages low in fluoride level.

c. Correct mineral deficiencies in the food rations, notably calcium and phosphorus. Add vitamins A and D to the feed.

Prognosis: In acute fluoride intoxication, prognosis is grave. In chronic poisoning, no drug or chemical has yet been shown to cure the adverse effects of fluorine. Treatment is ineffective once the dental and skeletal lesions have developed.

Some important fluoride compounds :

Inorganic compounds

a. *Sodium fluoride:* Sodium fluoride (NaF) is a crystalline compound which is soluble in water. It is used as anthelmintic, pediculicide, acaricide and insecticide compound for wood impregnation and control of farm pests. It is also used to prevent dental caries.

b. *Ammonium fluoride:* Ammonium fluoride (NH_4F) occurs as deliquescent colourless small crystals, soluble in water. It is mainly used for glass etching. It is highly toxic to animals.

c. *Sodium hexafluorosilicate:* Sodium hexafluorosilicate (Na_2SiF_6) is produced as a by-product in superphosphate production. It is slightly soluble in water.

On evaporation, it produces silicon tetrafluoride (SiF_4) gas which is poisonous. Sodium hexafluorosilicate is mainly used for wood impregnation, for control of farm pests and in disinfection of skin. It is poisonous to most species.

d. *Hydrofluoric acid:* Hydrofluoric acid (HF) is a highly toxic and corrosive solution of hydrogen fluoride in water. It is used in etching of glass and other industrial applications, including integrated circuit manufacturing. Exposure to highly concentrated solutions may lead to acute hypocalcaemia, followed by cardiac arrest and death.

Organic compounds

e. *Sodium fluoroacetate:* Sodium fluoroacetate (FCH_2COONa) is a white powder, which has no taste and odour. It is used as rodenticide and is a very strong poison.

f. *Diflouro-diphenyl trichloromethyl methane :* It is a toxic substance used as insecticide mainly for the control of flies.

g. *Fluoroethyl ester of fluoroacetic acid ($CH_2FCOO.CH_2$-CH_2F)*: It is a highly poisonous gas. A concentration of 92 mg/m^2 (in air) is lethal within 10 min.

2. Selenium

Selenium is a non-metal that functions both as a toxicant and an essential element. Trace amounts of selenium (0.1 - 0.3 ppm) in the diet are required to prevent deficiency diseases such as white muscle disease in cattle, exudative diathesis in chicks and liver necrosis in swine. The element may function in this regard as an intracellular antioxidant. Selenium poisoning occurs when animals ingest excessive amounts of selenium. Selenium was discovered in 1817 by Berzelius who named it after 'Selene', the Greek goddess of the moon, but Marco Polo gave the first account of selenium toxicity that he observed during his travels in western China in the 13th century. He linked sloughing of the hooves of horses to their consumption of certain plants in the regions. The soils of those areas are now known to contain the highest concentrations of selenium in the world.

Properties: Selenium (Se) belongs to group VIa of the periodic chart of elements to which sulphur belongs. The selenium exists in four oxidation states: 0 (elemental selenium), –2 (selenide). +4 (selenite), and +6 (selenate). Elemental selenium is stable, insoluble in water and hence relatively non-toxic. Selenium present in inorganic and organic forms is toxic, although the degree of toxicity varies with the chemical form. Like elemental selenium, the selenide is insoluble in water and less toxic, whereas the selenite and selenate are soluble in water and therefore possess greater bioavailability and toxicity. Inorganic selenite and selenate predominate in water whereas organic selenium compounds (primarily selenomethionine and selenocysteine) are incorporated in plant proteins. The toxicity ranking of selenium in various forms is : natural organoselenium > selenite (+4) = selenate (+6) > selenide (–2) > elemental selenium.

Sources of toxicity: Toxicosis may occur after ingestion of either inorganic selenium or organic selenium. Organic selenium is more soluble in water and plays more important role in livestock intoxication. Selenium intoxication may occur from following sources:

a. *Plants*: Plants are major source of selenium toxicosis in animals. The primary source of selenium in soil is the weathering and leaching of parent bedrock materials. Plants preferentially accumulate selenate because this form is less bound to soil particles. A large number of plants (Table 12.1) are known to easily accumulate selenium (both inorganic and organic forms) from the soil and transform it into organic compounds whose toxicity may be higher. Plant fodder containing more than 5 ppm of selenium should be treated as dangerous for ruminants. Depending upon their ability to accumulate selenium, plants are of following 3 types:

i. *Obligate accumulator or Indicator plants*: The obligate selenium accumulator plants (e.g. Astragalus, Stanleya, Oonopsis and Xylorrhiza) require large amount of selenium for their growth and survival. Therefore their presence and growth indicates relatively high concentration of selenium in the soil. These plants may concentrate as much as 100-15,000 ppm selenium. Such plants when not removed may decay, become incorporated in top soil and become source of selenium for other plants. Fortunately, most of these obligate accumulators are not readily consumed by grazing animals because they are unpalatable and emit a garlic-sulphur odour. Cattle and horses eat obligate Se accumulators only if forced to by overgrazing and near starvation. Sheep, however, may eat these plants more readily.

ii. *Facultative accumulator plants*: Facultative selenium accumulator plants (e.g. species of Aster, Astriplex, Penstemon and Acacia) do not require selenium for their growth, but if selenium is present in soil they accumulate it. These are, therefore, found in both seleniferous and non-seleniferous soils. They can accumulate selenium up to 25-100 ppm. Often these plants cause Se poisoning because some are quite palatable and readily eaten by animals.

iii. *Non-accumulator plants*: Non-accumulator plants include crop and some other plants (e.g. corn, wheat, barley, grass and hay) that when grown on seleniferous soils may accumulate 1-25 ppm of selenium as part of their protein make-up in integral proteins (i.e. seleno-cysteine, selenomethionine and selenocystathionine). Forages and grains from seleniferous areas may be more palatable than those from other sources.

b. *Water:* Selenium is present in water as a result of both wet and dry deposition from the atmosphere and by surface and subsurface drainage. High concentrations of selenium in surface and ground water usually occur in farm areas where irrigation water drains from soils with high selenium content.

c. *Air:* Combustion of fossil fuels and coal, incineration of rubber, municipal waste and paper are important sources of selenium in ambient air. Volcanic gases are major natural source of selenium to the air. Most selenium in ambient air is present in the form of elemental selenium bound to fly ash and particles.

d. *Food:* Food such as meat, fish, poultry, grains and cereal products is the major source of selenium exposure in human beings. Fish and certain organs of animals (liver and kidney) contain the highest concentration of selenium followed by meat and eggs. Sea-foods (e.g. fish and shell fish) accumulate selenium that exists naturally in the ocean, but these are not very important from toxicology point of view. Selenium enriched yeast, wheat, and some other plants contain high concentration of organo-selenium and are more important source of selenium than the animal products. Milk generally contains low level of selenium.

e. Excessive use of feed supplements containing selenium is a rare but important source of selenium poisoning in animals. The feed formulations containing 0.1-0.3 ppm selenium are mostly used in selenium deficient regions.

f. Industrial and commercial practices like rectifiers, xerography, photoelectric cells, glass, ceramics, some electronic instruments, copper and steel industries use selenium. However, these inorganic sources of selenium are not a major industrial hazard if handled with care.

g. Iatrogenic parenteral administration of excessive doses of selenium intended as therapy or prevention of various diseases of calves, foals, lambs and pigs may produce toxicosis in animals.

h. Excessive use of medicated shampoos containing selenium disulphide for treatment of some types of dermatitis and dandruff may result in toxicosis in small animals.

Factors affecting toxicity: Toxicity of selenium in animals varies with factors such as oxidation state (selenide, selenite or selenate), age and species involved.

a. Organic forms of selenium, usually present in plants, are more toxic than inorganic selenium. Selenite is equally or more toxic than selenate. Elemental selenium is relatively non-toxic.

b. High-protein diet and ingestion of other elements (e.g. mercury, copper, cadmium)

Table 12.1 : List of selected selenium accumulator plants.

Common name	Botanical name
Obligate (Primary) selenium accumulators	
Golden weeds	*Oonopsis* spp.
Milk vetches	*Astragalus* spp.
Princes plume	*Stanleya pinnata*
Woody aster	*Xylorrhiza* spp.
Facultative (Secondary) selenium accumulators	
Acacia	*Acacia* spp.
Asters	*Aster* spp.
Beard tongue	*Penstemon* spp.
Paintbrush	*Castilleja* spp.
Sages	*Artimisia* spp
Saltbrush	*Astriplex* spp.

that complex selenium in the gut decrease chances of selenium toxicity. Vitamin E deficiency increases the toxicity as well as the physiological requirement of selenium, thus effectively reducing the margin of safety.

c. Se toxicity is most common in areas that have arid or semi-arid climates (less than 20 inches annual precipitation) and soils with pH levels above 7.0 (above neutral level). A low rainfall predisposes to selenium poisoning because soluble selenium compounds are not leached out of the topsoil and lack of good forage may force animals to eat large quantities of seleniferous plants.

d. Young or small animals are at higher risk from overdosage resulting from the use of an inappropriate parenteral selenium product than adult animals.

e. Selenium-containing indicator plants have strong odour so deter animals, however, plants containing moderate selenium are not as offensive and therefore pose a greater risk.

f. Toxicosis is favoured by large or rapid intake of selenium in Selenium deficiency.

g. Poor health or condition of the animal favours selenium toxicosis.

Toxicity: Selenium is necessary for growth, fertility and prevention of a variety of diseases in animals. It is also toxic at higher concentrations. The maximum tolerable concentrations for cattle, sheep, and horses range from 1 to 5 ppm, while its daily requirement is 0.1-0.3 ppm in diet. Therefore, there is a narrow gap between deficient and toxic Se levels in feed. The selenium concentrations at which toxicity occurs depends on factors like chemical form, quantity ingested, duration of exposure and species involved. Selenious acid is the most toxic from of selenium and ingestion of this compound often causes fatalities. Acute selenosis may be observed after ingestion of obligate indicators (>400 ppm Se). Acute toxicosis in many species is produced at dose of 1 to 5 mg Se/kg orally and 0.2 mg Se/kg parenterally. The acute oral MLD of selenium as sodium selenite in different species is: horses = 3.3 mg/kg; cattle = 10 mg/kg; and pigs = 17 mg/kg. Subacute toxicosis is produced by feeding 3 ppm of selenium in diet for 3 days or more in swine. Chronic poisoning (alkali disease) is produced in cattle, horses and swine after feeding 5-10 ppm of selenium in diet for several weeks. The subcutaneous injection of selenium, as sodium selenite, causes poisoning in sheep at dose of 0.8 mg/kg and is lethal at dose of 1.6 mg/kg.

Toxicokinetics: In high concentrations, naturally occurring selenoamino acids (e.g. selenomethionine and selenocysteine) and soluble selenium salts are readily absorbed from small intestine. Absorption of selenite and selenate is quicker than selenides and elemental selenium but slower than seleno-amino acids (organic selenium).

The absorption of seleno-amino acids occurs via active transport mechanisms shared with amino acids. The absorption of selenium as selenites occurs via passive diffusion and absorption of selenate results from the action of sodium-mediated carrier transport shared with sulphate. Selenium does not cross intact skin but may penetrate abraded or diseased skin.

In blood, the absorbed selenium binds primarily to plasma proteins and is transported and distributed throughout the body, particularly to the liver, kidneys and spleen. Concentrations in the brain and muscles are lowest. Selenium can cross placental barrier of mammals and enter avian eggs causing foetal malformations and embryotoxic effects. In the body, all forms of selenium (selenide, selenate) are converted to the +4 state (selenite) which then substitutes sulphur in the synthesis of amino acids and hence proteins. A significant portion of the total body pool of selenium is incorporated in skeletal muscles as selenomethionine.

Selenium is mainly excreted in the urine after metabolism as inactive trimethylselenonium ion and to lesser extent in the faeces as metal selenide or elemental selenium. It may also be excreted by the lungs as volatile methylated selenium, particularly after very high doses. Normally, a very small amount of selenium is excreted in bile. Nearly 25% to 70% of sub-toxic amount of dietary selenium may be eliminated within 2 days of ingestion.

Mechanism of action: Selenium has number of biochemical effects in the body.

a. Selenium replaces sulphur in amino acids such as cysteine and methionine. This results in synthesis of abnormal structural and enzyme proteins. This may explain hoof and hair defects of chronic selenium toxicosis. However, this mechanism does not fully account for all aspects of selenosis.

b. Selenium causes depletion of glutathione (GSH) probably by direct complexation of two molecules of GSH for every selenite ion, decreased synthesis or regeneration of GSH through inhibition of some sulphydryl enzymes, stimulation of liver and erythrocyte GSH-peroxidase activity (a Se-containing enzyme) or combination of various mechanisms. Lipid peroxidation is another probable factor in toxicosis.

c. The cytotoxic action of selenium perhaps results from the pro-oxidant catalytic activity of selenide (RSe^-) anions, which produce superoxide anions, hydrogen peroxide, and other reactive metabolites (e.g. hydrogen radicals).

d. Chronic selenosis depresses adenosine triphosphate (ATP) formation possibly as a result of inhibition of sulphydryl-containing enzymes such as succinic acid dehydrogenase and other dehydrogenases.

e. Tissue ascorbic acid (Vitamin C) decreases, possibly because of enhanced oxidation by ascorbic oxidases. This contributes to the vascular damage caused by selenosis.

f. Gastrointestinal signs and lesions in acute selenium poisoning are, in part, due to irritant nature of selenium in large concentrations.

Clinical signs: Selenosis occurs in three forms: acute, subacute and chronic.

Acute toxicity: Acute poisoning may occur in all species of animals primarily due to ingestion of obligate indicator plants or iatrogenic toxicosis after parenteral administration of selenium containing drugs. Accidental ingestion of selenious acid may also result in acute toxicosis. Acute selenosis under field conditions, however, is rare because animals usually avoid indicator plants. Poisoning occurs only when pasture is limited and scarcity of fodder forces animals to consume highly seleniferous plants. In ruminants, acute toxicosis is manifested within few hours to few days by signs such as lethargy, unresponsiveness, colic, bloat, dark watery diarrhoea, quickened and weak heart beats, dyspnoea with laboured breathing, frothing (often blood-tinged) from nostrils, polyuria, cyanosis, weakness, uncertain gait, prostration, coma and death in 1-2 days. Death occurs from respiratory failure. In horses, important signs include anorexia, ataxia, colic, diarrhoea, dyspnoea, fever, head pressing, increased respiratory rate, sweating, and sudden death. Animals receiving acutely toxic doses of Se develop a garlicky breath odour, although absence of characteristic odour does not rule out selenium poisoning.

Subacute toxicity (Blind staggers): Subacute selenium toxicity is often called "blind staggers," although the affected livestock may not always be blind or staggering. This develops in large animals and swine consuming moderate amounts of obligate or facultative indicator plants (usually containing > 30 ppm) or sodium selenite in the diet over a period of weeks or months. Daily consumption of selenium at moderate concentration (20-25 ppm) produces focal symmetrical poliomalacia after several weeks. Blind staggers in cattle is manifested in 3 stages:

i. The animal tends to wander or may walk into objects in its path. Body temperature is normal but vision is impaired and appetite is poor.

ii. The wandering increases, front legs become weak and vision becomes further impaired.

iii. The throat and tongue become paralysed, temperature is subnormal and death follows from respiratory failure.

In sheep the 3 stages are less clearly differentiated. In swine, alopecia, ataxia, quadriplegia with flaccid paralysis and sternal recumbency may be seen.

Chronic toxicity (Alkali disease): Initially, it was thought that this condition develops due to drinking of alkaline water. However, it is now known that chronic poisoning in cattle, horses and pigs develops when non-accumulator plants grown on seleniferous soils (5-40 ppm) or grains or forages containing 5-25 ppm Se are consumed over weeks or months. The signs common to these species include cracking of hooves, lameness, stiffness of joints, dullness and loss of vitality, emaciation and loss of hair. In horses, the loss of hair from mane and tail usually is the first clinical sign and is followed by cracking of hoof at the coronary band. In severe poisoning, hooves may be sloughed off or may be retained. If retained, then new growth of the hoof pushes the dead tissue downwards and results in deformed hoof 6-7 inches long and turned upward at the end (more common in cattle). Cracks in the tail and horns also appear and they may be shed off. Sometimes affected animals are unable to walk a short distance even to drinking water and thus may die of thirst and hunger. Gangrene of distal extremities (below tarsus or carpus, tips of ears, muzzle, tip of tail or tongue) occurs occasionally. Pronounced anaemia is also an important sign of selenium poisoning. Pigs show break in the hoof similar to cattle. Sows have lowered conception rate and there is increase in number of piglets born dead. Birds show low hatchability and embryos are usually deformed, without beaks and with "ropy feathers." Teratogenesis in water fowl and poultry may be manifested as underdeveloped feet and legs, missing or underdeveloped lower or upper beak and deformed or missing eyes.

Post-mortem findings: Lesions of acute toxicosis include congestion of organs, gastroenteritis, renal necrosis and haemorrhages, hydrothorax, pulmonary oedema, and pale cardiac muscles. Lesions of subacute toxicosis include congestion and necrosis of liver, congestion of renal medulla, epicardial petechiae, ulceration of abomasum and small intestine, and erosion of articular surfaces (particularly of tibia). In swine, there is focal symmetrical poliomyelomalacia which is most common in the cervical and thoracic spinal cord. Lesions of chronic selenosis almost resemble those of blind staggers. In addition, transverse lines of abnormal growth on hooves, cardiomyopathy and chronic fibrosis or cirrhosis may be observed.

Diagnosis: Diagnosing selenosis is usually easier particularly if grazing stock has access to known seleniferous plants and later develops the typical signs and lesions of selenosis. Suspected feed and internal organs should be examined for the presence and quantity of Se. Adult animals that die of selenosis generally have following concentrations of Se in the tissues: blood 1-4 ppm in chronic cases and up to 25 ppm in acute cases; liver and kidney 4-25 ppm; urine 0.1–8 ppm; and milk 1-3 ppm. In chronic selenosis, bovine hoof and hair may contain selenium at 5-20 and 5-10 ppm, respectively. Blood changes due to excessive selenium in chronic intoxication include decreased fibrinogen and prothrombin activities and elevated serum ALT, AST, and SDH levels. There is increased content of oxidised glutathione with a concomitant decrease of reduced glutathione.

Diseases or conditions that may be confused with acute or subacute (blind staggers) selenosis include anthrax, pneumonia, infectious hepatitis, enterotoxaemia and pasteurellosis. Conditions which mimic aspects of chronic selenosis include freezing, ergotism, molybdenosis, fluorosis and laminitis.

Treatment and management: There is no specific antidote or treatment for selenium toxicosis. Various metal chelators such as dimercaprol, calcium disodium edentate, DMPS or DMSA are either ineffective or aggravate (e.g. dimercaprol) selenium poisoning.

Acute selenosis: In advanced cases, treatment is of limited value. Only supportive and symptomatic treatment is advised which include:

a. Therapy to combat gastroenteritis and shock.

b. Saline purgatives such as magnesium sulphate to eliminate selenium from the gut.

c. Oxygen therapy and treatment of pulmonary oedema.

d. Acetylcysteine as substitute of depleted glutathione at the loading dose of 140 mg/kg body weight by I.V. route followed by 70 mg/kg daily in 4 divided doses.

Subacute and chronic selenosis: Three possibilities exist for the prevention or treatment of selenosis in animals.

a. Treatment of the soil so that Se uptake by plants is reduced. The high seleniferous areas should be identified and removed from production.

b. Treatment of the animals so that selenium absorption is reduced or excretion is increased. But none of the treatment is effective in all conditions.

i. Administration of small amounts of arsenic compounds in drinking water (e.g. water with 5 ppm As in the form of sodium arsenite or 25 ppm As in the form of sodium arsenate). Addition of organic arsenic in diet to increase biliary excretion is suggested for poultry, cattle and pigs, but is not recommended for horses.

ii. A high protein diet especially containing sulphur amino acids (cysteine, methionine, etc.) helps to control chronic Se poisoning.

iii. Stiffness in cattle and horses may be relieved by oral administration of compounds such as naphthalene and bromobenzene which forms mercapturic acid. The usual treatment is 4-5 g of naphthalene daily for 5 days, repeated after a 5-day interval.

iv. Addition of sulphate in diet or its daily oral administration may be helpful in selenosis in buffaloes. Sulphur (S) and Se are Group VI elements, thus S may neutralise Se in soil and in body.

c. Addition of substances in the diet that antagonise or inhibit toxic effects of Se e.g. linseed oil meal, arsenic, silver, copper and cadmium. However, their practical utilities are limited.

Contraindications:

a. Dimercaprol: Dimercaprol (British Anti-lewisite, BAL) inhibits the recovery from selenium poisoning. It alleviates liver damage but worsens kidney damage.

b. Vitamin E: Vitamin E has synergistic action with selenium.

Prognosis: Once the lesions of selenosis are well established, no treatment can completely heal them.

Some important compounds of selenium:

Inorganic compounds

a. Selenious acid: Selenious acid (Monohydrated selenium dioxide, H_2O_3Se) is the most toxic selenium compound. It is mainly used as a reagent and oxidizing agent for alkaloids. Acute ingestion of selenious acid is invariably fatal.

b. Hydrogen selenide: Hydrogen selenide (H_2Se) is a gas prepared by heating selenium and hydrogen in a sealed tube. It possesses disagreeable odour and is irritating to eyes and mucous membranes. Acute inhalation of hydrogen selenide initially causes upper respiratory tract irritation followed by bronchopneumonia and pulmonary oedema.

c. Selenium dioxide: Selenium dioxide (Selenium oxide, O_2Se) exists as lustrous tetragonal needles and is prepared by burning selenium in oxygen. It is used in manufacture of other selenium compounds and as a reagent for alkaloids. Dermal exposure to selenium dioxide may produce dermatitis and skin burns.

d. Selenium disulphide: Selenium disulphide (Selenium sulphide) is primarily used in detergent preparations as topical antiseborrhoeic. It is also useful in conditions like eczemas and dermatomycoses. Toxicity from medicated shampoos containing selenium disulphide is rare, although skin allergy or sensitivity may be occasionally observed.

3. Phosphorus

Phosphorus is universally distributed in soil and plants and plays important functions in biological systems. Phosphorus along with calcium is important in the production and maintenance of teeth and bones. Inorganic phosphorus in the form of phosphate (PO_4^{3-}) plays a major role in biological molecules such as DNA and RNA where it forms part of the structural framework of these molecules. Living cells also utilize phosphate to transport cellular energy via adenosine triphosphate (ATP) and in synthesis of several essential intracellular components, coenzymes and phospholipids. Although deficiency of phosphorus resulting in osteomalacia and rickets is a common syndrome, the toxicity of phosphorus is of less common occurrence. The yellow or white phosphorus is toxic whereas red phosphorus is non-toxic. Accordingly, the toxicity of white or yellow phosphorus is described in detail.

Properties: Phosphorus (P) is a multivalent non-metal of the nitrogen group with atomic number 15. It is commonly found in inorganic phosphate rocks and in all living cells. Inorganic phosphorus exists mainly in three allotropes i.e. white or yellow, red and black. Yellow phosphorus (P_4) is an oil-soluble, waxy solid with a garlic odour, which ordinarily occurs in the form of white, translucent soft cylinders that on exposure to light becomes yellow. It is a strong oxidising agent and is often stored under water. When exposed to air, it emits white fumes of phosphorus trioxide which have garlic like odour and are luminous in the dark (gives greenish light). The yellow phosphorus is a highly toxic variety and is used in chemical industry, manufacture of fire-works, gunpowder, fertilizer, rodenticide and in incendiary ammunition. Red phosphorus is prepared by heating the yellow phosphorus at a temperature of 240°C. It is not luminous in dark and has no taste or odour. Unlike yellow phosphorus, it does not oxidise in air at ordinary temperature and is not poisonous. Commercial preparation of red phosphorus may be poisonous as it contains traces of yellow phosphorus. Red phosphorus is used in the production of many phosphorus compounds, but its main industrial use is in the production of match heads and friction surfaces of match box. Black phosphorus is amorphous and is the least reactive type. It is mostly used for scientific purposes.

Sources of toxicity:

a. Accidental ingestion of phosphate (PO_4^{3-}) fertilizers may cause toxicity in farm animals.

b. Factories that manufacture fireworks, gunpowder, incendiary ammunition, smoke bombs, fertilizers, match sticks, and industrial chemicals containing phosphorus may contaminate environment through effluents and dusts.

c. White phosphorus has been used commonly by the military as an incendiary agent or as an igniter for munitions. It is commonly found in hand grenades, mortar and artillery rounds, and smoke bombs. These weapons are particularly dangerous to exposed people and animals.

d. Phosphorus in finely divided form is occasionally mixed with fats and oils to promote their absorption. Over-consumption of such fats and oils may result into phosphorus poisoning.

e. Phosphorus is occasionally used as rodenticide. Poisoning in animals may result from direct ingestion of phosphorus rodenticide bait or from ingestion of poisoned rodents.

f. Feeding of excess of wheat bran which is very rich in phosphorus and low in calcium causes bran disease in horses. Similarly, meat high in phosphorus and low in calcium causes hyperphosphataemia in dogs.

Toxicity: Red phosphorus is inert and non-toxic, but white or yellow phosphorus is highly toxic and dangerous. The acute oral LD_{50} of yellow phosphorus is 2 mg/kg body weight in dogs. The toxicity potential of phosphates is low and they need to be ingested in considerable quantities before toxicity signs appear. Oral doses of 250 mg/kg per day of phosphates or superphosphates for 30 days do not cause adverse effects in sheep.

Toxicokinetics: White phosphorus is highly lipid soluble and is believed to have rapid absorption from GI tract after ingestion and from skin after dermal exposure. In the body, phosphorus circulates first as element and then is oxidised to phosphate. Some phosphorus is also eliminated by lungs and this provides the exhaled air a smell of phosphorus (garlik-like) and a glow in dark. Similarly, the vomitus of GI tract contents may be luminous and have the same odour. Main excretion of phosphorus is in the urine and expired air.

Mechanism of action: Exact mechanism of phosphorus-induced toxicity in animals is not known.

a. Phosphorus is a strong irritant and corrosive and also has a necrotising effect on the stomach mucosa. After ingestion it causes severe irritation of gastrointestinal mucosa and induces gastroenteritis and diarrhoea.

b. After absorption, phosphorus acts as a protoplasmic poison. It also has direct cardiotoxic effect resulting in cardiovascular collapse. Phosphate formed in body due to oxidation of phosphorus causes hepatic necrosis.

c. On dermal exposure, white phosphorus results in painful chemical burn injuries. The damage is done in part by the heat of flame as phosphorus ignites when comes in contact with air. The resulting compound causes further damage by acid corrosion.

Clinical signs :

Acute toxicity: White phosphorus can cause acute toxicity and death after ingestion and dermal exposure.

Ingestion: The onset of clinical signs after phosphorus ingestion is either almost immediate or delayed for up to several hours. The early signs are referable to gastrointestinal irritation and may include abdominal pain, colic, profuse vomiting (occasionally haematemesis), severe diarrhoea (often haemorrhagic), and a garlic-like odour from the breath. Thereafter, there is apparent recovery of a few hours up to 4 days. Then the abdominal pain and vomiting reoccur, this time accompanied with jaundice and the animal goes into profound depression, shock, coma and death. Massive hepatic failure is followed by convulsions and death. Pathological changes in the kidneys result in development of progressive oliguria and anuria. Alternatively, the animal may make a recovery without neurological signs. Pigs vomit profusely and the vomitus is luminous in dark and gives a characteristic garlic odour. Horses and poultry may exhibit a paralytic-like weakness without other definite signs.

Dermal exposure: Phosphorus, if comes in contact with skin may cause burns which are painful and slow to heal. The resultant burn typically appears as a necrotic area with a yellowish colour and characteristic garlic-like odour. Burns frequently are second and third degree because of rapid ignition and highly lipophilic properties of white phosphorus. Phosphorus burns carry a greater risk of mortality than other forms of burns due to the absorption of phosphorus into body through the burned area, resulting in liver, heart and kidney damage, and in some cases multi-organ failure.

Chronic toxicity : In chronic phosphorus poisoning, the main clinical feature is necrosis of jaw called "phossy jaw". The salient clinical feature of phossy jaw includes first toothache which leads to its extraction. The socket fails to heal and there is an offensive discharge; the bone is exposed and show necrosis with formation of a sequestrum. The condition progresses and animal may die of debility or it may result in gross disfigurement and disability.

Post-mortem findings: Lesions include severe gastroenteritis, fatty degeneration of liver, muscles and endothelium of blood vessels. There may be multiple haemorrhages, haematoma formation, and black tarry blood that fail to clot. Liver is enlarged, pale and yellowish in colour and spleen is small and atrophied. Fatty changes are also observed in kidneys and heart. The carcass may be phosphorescent and the gastric contents have a garlic odour. Lesions of severe hepatitis and renal damage may be present. There are also evidences of jaundice. Inflammation of skin is observed when dermal exposure has occurred.

Diagnosis: In the living animal, diagnosis may be difficult but history, clinical signs, lesions, and odour and luminescence of the breath, vomitus and stomach contents may help. Hepatic enzymes and bilirubin levels may be elevated. Chemical tests must be used for confirmation. The best material for analysis is vomitus. In animals surviving the first day, faeces instead of stomach contents may be preferred.

Treatment and management: Specific antidotes are not available for phosphorus poisoning. Detoxification and supportive therapy are the only alternative.

a. For oral exposure, careful gastric lavage (with potassium permanganate or 0.2% copper sulphate) is preferred to emesis due the corrosive action of phosphorus.

b. Non-absorbable oil (e.g. mineral oil) should be administered orally to solubilise phosphorus and prevent its absorption. Activated charcoal and sorbitol or saline cathartic may be useful. Oils are contraindicated because they facilitate phosphorus absorption.

c. A diet high in cysteine and carbohydrates but low in fat may be given to combat liver damage. High doses of vitamin B and ascorbic acid also tend to lessen the severity of hepatic failure.

d. Hypoprothrombinaemia and haemorrhage is treated with vitamin K_1. In severe cases, whole blood or plasma transfusion may be advised.

e. Dehydration, loss of electrolytes and hypotension may be treated with excess fluid therapy.

Prognosis: Prognosis of phosphorus poisoning is guarded to grave because of vascular dysfunction and severe liver and kidney damage.

4. Nitrate and Nitrite

All living systems need nitrogen to exist since it is used to build many essential components such as proteins, DNA, RNA vitamins, hormones and enzymes. Plants provide the bulk of nitrogen for all living systems mainly in form of nitrate (NO_3^-), which is reduced to nitrite (NO_2^-) for subsequent utilization in body. Nitrate and nitrite poisoning is fairly common among farm animals with large number of ruminants, pigs and fowls affected every year. Nitrate and nitrite toxicoses are usually described together, owing to their joint occurrence and partly to similarity of the clinical course and pathological lesions in poisoned animals. Both nitrate and nitrite are toxic, but it is difficult to differentiate between the two poisonings and to treat them separately as nitrate can be converted to nitrite. Presently, nitrate/ nitrite poisoning has become a potential health threat worldwide due to extensive use of nitrogen fertilizers for crop production.

Properties and occurrence: Nitrate represents the most oxidized chemical form of nitrogen found in natural systems and is one of the most water soluble anions known. In nature, nitrate is normally present in soil, forages, ground water, silages, crops, weeds, animal tissues, decaying organic matter, excreta, etc. due to its participation in the nitrogen cycle : Atmospheric nitrogen ⟶ microbial fixation as nitrate in soil ⟶ assimilation into plant proteins ⟶ animal proteins ⟶ metabolic wastes or decaying of dead plants or animal bodies ⟶ microbial nitrification to nitrate and nitrite ⟶ microbial denitrification to nitrogen ⟶ liberation of nitrogen into the atmosphere. If nitrate reducing bacteria are present in soil or water, nitrite may be formed from nitrate (either before or after ingestion of nitrate), which is much more toxic than nitrate. In the rumen of cattle and sheep, nitrate is reduced to nitrite, which in turn is reduced to ammonia and then incorporated into bacterial proteins (Figure 12.1).

Sources of Toxicity: Anything which increases nitrate concentration in the soil and water may lead to toxicosis through crops and water. Nitrate/Nitrite toxicosis also occurs through use of therapeutic agents or chemicals.

a. Heavy use of nitrogen fertilizers (e.g. ammonium nitrate, potassium nitrate and urea) and herbicides (e.g. 2, 4-D) increases nitrate contents in plants. Poisoning may also occur when nitrogen fertilizer is eaten directly from bags or spray containers.

b. Nitrate containing plants are the important source of poisoning in ruminants and occasionally some other species. Soils naturally high in nitrogen tend to increase nitrate contents in forages. Though any plant may be suspected for taking large concentration of nitrate, some plants like cereal grasses (especially oats, millets and rye), corn (maize), sunflower and sorghum readily accumulate nitrate. Some specific weeds like red root, Russian thistle, white rag weed, variegated thistle are known as nitrate accumulators. More than 80 specific crop and weed plants are known to cause nitrate/nitrite poisoning, some of which are listed in Table 12.2.

c. Nitrogen in water tends to occur in nitrate (NO_3^-) oxidation state. Nitrate accumulates in ponds and wells due to increased water run off from nitrate rich soil, decaying manure in barnlots, silo pits, and freshly fertilized fields or due to direct contamination with nitrate and nitrite. Deep wells filled by seepage from highly fertile soil may contain nitrate levels as high as 1700-3000 ppm. Consumption of water rich in nitrate concentration is an important source of poisoning.

d. Animal wastes, sewage, decaying organic matter, industrial effluents and geologic sources such as lime-stone, calcites, etc. increase soil and water nitrate concentration.

e. Hay made from crops especially those grown under draught conditions and cut while sappy can develop toxic nitrite level when they heat up. The nitrate content of hay may even increase during storage due to moisture loss. In contrast, fermentation during the ensiling process (silage preparation) results in loss of much of nitrate and greatly reduces the risk of toxicity.

f. Nitrate and/or nitrite is used in pickling and curing brines for preserving meats. Water contamination from butcher's shop and meat processors may cause toxicosis.

g. In medicine, organic nitrates such as glyceryl trinitrate, isosorbide mononitrate (ISMN) and isosorbide dinitrate (ISDN) are used as vasodilator-antihypertensive agents and are particularly useful for prevention and treatment of angina pectoris. Sodium nitrite is used as therapeutic agent against cyanide toxicosis. Excessive use of such drugs may be harmful.

h. Potassium nitrate is used for the manufacture of gun powder and ammonium nitrate for dyanamite production.

Table 12.2: List of important nitrate-accumulating plants.

Crop plants	Weeds
Alfalfa *(Medicago sativa)*	Canada Thistle (*Cirsium arvense*)
Barley (*Hordeum vulgare*)	Cheeseweed (*Malva parviflora*)
Blackberry *(Rubus fruticosus)*	Dock (*Rumex crispus*)
Fescue (*Festuca* spp.)	Fat hen/Lambsquarters (*Chenopodium album)*
Linseed (*Linum usitatissimum*)	Fireweed (*Kochia*)*
Maize/Corn (Zea mays)*	Jimson weed *(Datura*)
Oats (*Avena sativa*)	Johnson Grass (*Sorghum* helepense)*
Rape (*Brassica napus*)*	Marshmallow (*Althaea officinalis)*
Rye (*Secale cereale*)	Mintweed (*Salvia reflexa*)
Sorghum (*Sorghum* spp.)*	Nightshade (*Solanum* spp.)
Soybeans (*Glycine max*)	Red root or Pigweed (*Amaranthus retroflexus*)*
Sudan Grass (*Sorghum* sudanense)*	Russian thistle/Tumbleweed (*Salsola*)
Sugar beat (*Beta vulgaris*)*	Smartweed (*Polygonum hydropiperoides*)
Sweet Clover (*Melilotus officinalis*)	Variegated thistle *(Silybum marianum)**
Turnip tops (*Brassica rapa*)	White ragweed (*Franseria discolour*)*
Wheat (*Triticum* spp.)	Wild sunflower (*Helianthus*)

* = Plants of high risk

Factors affecting toxicity :

a. *Species:* Many species are susceptible to nitrate/nitrite poisoning, but there is considerable difference in their susceptibility. Ruminants are much more susceptible to nitrate poisoning than monogastric animals.

   i. Cattle are affected most frequently because ruminal flora reduces nitrate to ammonia, with nitrite as an intermediate product.

   ii. Sheep are more efficient at converting nitrite to ammonia, so they are comparatively less susceptible to nitrite poisoning than cattle.

   iii. Non-ruminants such as horses and pigs have no mechanism for converting nitrate to nitrite in their digestive tract, so they are less susceptible to nitrite poisoning from excessive intake of nitrates (Figure 12.1) (Nitrate reduction and the associated nitrite production is reported to occur to some extent in caecum of horse, but not to the same extent as in ruminants). However, they are highly susceptible to poisoning from direct nitrite intake because they cannot convert nitrite to ammonia.

   iv. Pigs are highly susceptible to nitrite or nitrate but are affected only if they ingest it pre-formed.

b. *Age:* Young pigs and human infants are more susceptible to nitrite poisoning as they have GI microflora capable of reducing nitrate to nitrite. Adult monogastric species, including pigs and humans, are more resistant as this pathway is limited. Foetuses and neonates are more susceptible to nitrate/nitrite poisoning than the older young or adults.

c. *Weather conditions:* Weather conditions like draught, excessive rain, frost, low temperature, moisture, cloudy weather, etc. affect nitrate contents in plants to a great extent. In general, nitrate accumulates in plants when the soil nitrogen levels are high and readily absorbed by roots, but the plant due to adverse weather conditions cannot utilize it. Favourable conditions for excessive plant growth also enhance plant nitrate contents due to excessive uptake from soil.

   i. During periods of draught, the amount of nitrate in soil is greatly increased because of lack of leaching, reduced nitrate uptake by plants and decomposition of organic matter. When such a draught breaks by a rain, the plants resume their growth and increase nitrate uptake from soil. Consumption of such draught-stricken fodders, especially in the first week after rain, results in poisoning. Feeding of stunted fodder during a draught may also result in poisoning because plants may continue to absorb nitrate from soil to some extent even in such adverse conditions but cannot utilize it properly due to their retarded growth.

   ii. Frost and hail damage the leaf area of plants and reduce the photosynthetic activity causing accumulation of nitrate in stem or stalk. They also interfere with normal growth of plants, which continue to absorb nitrate from soil but cannot utilize it. Consumption of such frost/hail stricken plants may result in poisoning.

   iii. Most plants require an optimum temperature above 13°C for active growth and photosynthesis. In cool weather, plants continue to absorb nitrate from soil but it is not converted efficiently to amino acids and proteins due to decreased activity of enzyme nitrate reductase enzyme. This allows nitrate to accumulate in plants.

   iv. Cloudy weather or decreased light as seen early in the day before sunshine enhances nitrate levels in plants due to decreased activity of plant NO_3^- reductase enzymes. For these reasons, it is wise to cut hay or green chop relatively late on sunny days to minimise concentrations of nitrate.

   v. High nitrate concentrations are likely to develop when growth of plant is rapid during hot and humid weather. This is primarily due to excessive uptake of soil nitrate by the plants.

vi. Uptake of nitrate by plants is enhanced by rains due to adequate soil moisture and plant growth.

vii. Shading associated with crowding conditions can cause increased concentration of nitrate within plants.

d. *Plant parts:* Plant parts closest to the ground (stalks) contain the highest concentration of nitrate. Leaves contain less than stalks or stems, and the seed (grain) and flowers usually contain little or no nitrate. Most of the plant nitrate is in the bottom third of the stalk. Anything that stunts growth increases nitrate accumulation in the lower part of the plant.

e. *Stage of plant growth:* Young plants have higher nitrate concentrations than mature plants. However in favourable environmental and soil conditions, the mature plants can still have excessive nitrate concentrations.

f. *Storage:* Large, uncovered bales with xcess nitrate are potentially dangerous if stored outside; rain or snow can leach and subsequently concentrate most of the total nitrate present into the lower third of these bales. Green chop that has been heated after cutting or held overnight also contain high nitrate contents. Feeding of such hay to animals may be toxic.

g. *Water:* Water with high nitrate and significant coliform (bacteria) contamination has greater potential to affect health adversely than do either nitrate or bacteria alone due to the rapid conversion of nitrate to nitrite. Concentrations of nitrate are normally less in ponds with abundant plants or algae because algae bloom decreases nitrate.

h. *Soil:* Soils high in nitrogen readily supply nitrate to plants. Soils deficient in molybdenum, sulphur or phosphorus enhance nitrate intake by plants, where as soils deficiency of copper, cobalt and manganese tend to have opposing effects. Acidic soils, low soil temperature, and good soil aeration are conducive for nitrate accumulation.

i. Hungry ruminants are at a greater risk of nitrate poisoning than animals receiving regular and good fodder. This is because hungry animals consume more toxic feed and rumen microbes get little time to adapt to converting the nitrite to ammonia.

j. Large intake of nitrate over a short period is more toxic than same intake over a long period. This is because rumen microbes are more adapted to deal with the frequent intake of small amounts of nitrate-containing feed.

k. Toxicosis occurs more commonly in unaccustomed domestic animals which lack prior exposure to nitrates than animals which are used to such plants.

l. Ruminants receiving carbohydrate-rich fodders tolerate high nitrate and nitrite levels than those receiving low carbohydrate diets because energy from carbohydrates helps rumen microbes convert nitrite to ammonia.

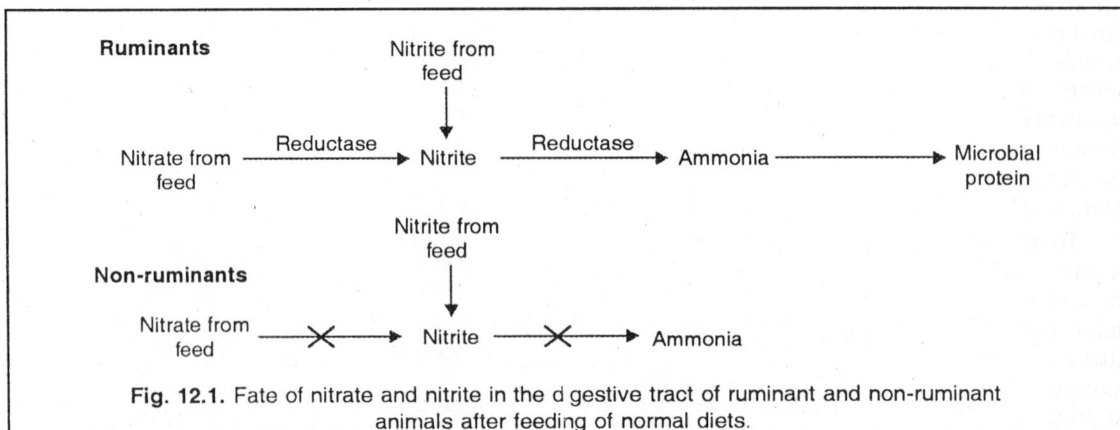

Fig. 12.1. Fate of nitrate and nitrite in the d gestive tract of ruminant and non-ruminant animals after feeding of normal diets.

m. Damaged and wilted plants contain high levels of nitrate. Herbicide damage to plants also lead to significant nitrate intake.

n. Animals in poor health and condition, especially cattle suffering from respiratory disease, are more susceptible to nitrate/nitrite poisoning.

o. Drugs like monensin facilitate the conversion of nitrate to nitrite in the rumen and may result in poisoning in animals on high nitrate fodder.

p. Pathological conditions and diseases like anaemia, methaemoglobinaemia, hypovitaminosis A and fasting aggravate the toxicity of nitrate and nitrite.

q. Pregnant animals are more susceptible to nitrate/nitrite poisoning than non-pregnant animals.

r. Restriction of water intake increases risk of toxicity; the greater the water intake, the faster is the elimination of NO_3^-/NO_2^- in urine.

Toxicity: The toxicity of the nitrate ion is approximately 10 times lower than that of the nitrite ion because nitrates are less reactive than nitrites. Nitrate is converted by rumen microbes to nitrite which is the main (not all) cause of poisoning in ruminants. Nitrate when ingested in large amounts may cause gastroenteritis, but mainly acts as source of nitrite which produces respiratory syndrome. As such, toxic doses of nitrate and nitrite are difficult to quantify precisely, varying according to the diet or with the food supply. In cattle, the acute oral median lethal dose of sodium nitrate is 650-750 mg/kg and that of sodium nitrite is 150-170 mg/kg body weight. The acute oral LD_{50} of potassium nitrate is 1000 mg/kg body weight. The acute oral lethal dose of sodium nitrite in some other species is: pigs = 70-75 mg/kg, sheep = 170 mg/kg, and rabbits = 80-90 mg/kg. It may be difficult to poison pigs with nitrate because of rapid passage of ingesta through intestinal tract and rapid conversion of nitrate to ammonia. Cattle and sheep can usually tolerate up to 0.5% nitrate on dry matter basis.

Toxicokinetics: Both nitrate and nitrite can be passively absorbed from the GI tract and reach the systemic circulation. However in ruminants, a major part of ingested nitrate is first reduced to nitrite in the GI tract and then to ammonia by the action of ruminal and intestinal microbes. Ammonia so produced is utilised as a source of nitrogen by the rumen microflora for protein synthesis. In case of excessive intake of nitrate, as observed in poisoning, the rate of reduction of nitrate to nitrite exceeds to that of nitrite to ammonia. This results in accumulation of nitrite in GI tract resulting in its quick absorption into the blood stream (before being reduced to ammonia). A suitable pH and sufficient bacteria producing nitrate reductases in the rumen and intestine help in quick reduction of nitrate to nitrite and its rapid absorption. Some nitrate is also absorbed as such and can probably undergo reduction to nitrite in liver and some other tissues. The rate of hepatic reduction of nitrate to nitrite is very slow and is not much important from toxicity point of view.

Once in blood stream, nitrite ion acts directly upon the vascular smooth muscle and easily enters the erythrocyte in exchange for chloride ion. Only small amounts of nitrate or nitrite are bound to plasma proteins. In the RBCs, nitrite converts haemoglobin to methaemoglobin (Met-Hb) and in the process gets itself converted to nitrate. Most nitrate thus produced is excreted by kidneys and some is recycled back into the gastrointestinal tract by salivary and GI tract secretion. Nitrite can also cross placental barrier and can convert foetal haemoglobin to methaemoglobin. In dogs and sheep, the biological half-life of blood nitrate is 44.7 and 4.2 hours and that of nitrite is 0.5 and 0.48 hours, respectively.

Mechanism of action :

Nitrite: Acute poisoning seen after nitrate or nitrite toxicity is due mainly to nitrite ions (administered as such or generated by reduction of nitrate). Nitrite has two important actions:

a. Interaction with haemoglobin: One molecule of nitrite interacts with two molecules of haemoglobin (Hb) and converts them to methaemoglobin (Met-Hb) by the process of oxidation i.e. oxidation of ferrous haemoglobin (Fe^{++}) to ferric haemoglobin (Fe^{+++}) or methaemoglobin. Methaemoglobin cannot carry oxygen. Under physiological conditions, some Met-Hb (1-2%) is always present which is converted back to ferrous haemoglobin by two reducing enzymes in blood viz. NAD-dependent diaphorase I and NADP-dependent diaphorase II. During nitrate/nitrite toxicity, the formation of methaemoglobin in blood

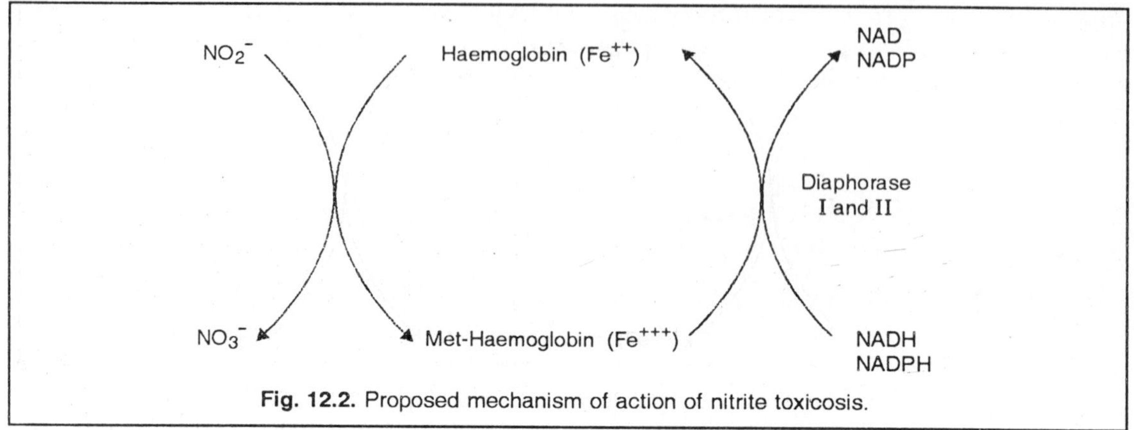

Fig. 12.2. Proposed mechanism of action of nitrite toxicosis.

exceeds the turnover rate of diaphorase I and II enzymes, which results in accumulation of abnormally high concentration of methaemoglobin. If 20-40% of the haemoglobin exists as methaemoglobin (depending on species and degree of physical activity of animal), clinical signs of anoxia develops. Death of animal occurs when 80-90% (in active animal 60%) of the haemoglobin exists as methaemoglobin.

b. The nitrite ions directly relax the smooth muscles, particularly the vascular smooth muscles. In this, increased concentration of nitrite ions lead to intracellular conversion to the reactive free radical nitric oxide (NO) which activates guanylate cyclase and increases production of cyclic GMP. Elevated cGMP ultimately leads to dephosphorylation of myosin light chains, resulting in vascular smooth muscle relaxation. The changes brought by vascular relaxation i.e. hypotension and decreased cardiac output may contribute to tissue oxygen starvation produced by methaemoglobin formation.

Nitrate: The primary action of large doses of nitrate is different from nitrite ions and resembles effect of excess common salt poisoning, producing signs of disturbed osmotic conditions in the body. In such cases, death may occur shortly after ingestion of very large doses of nitrate, even before the nitrite and methaemoglobin stages are reached. Water supplied in excess quantity decreases toxicity and hastens elimination of nitrate from the body. Nitrate is also irritant and caustic on the alimentary mucosa, kidneys and urinary tract.

Clinical signs :

Nitrite: Nitrite is much more toxic than nitrate and produces both acute and chronic toxicities.

Acute toxicity: Signs of acute nitrite poisoning usually appear suddenly with onset within 0.5-4 hours of ingestion and are related mainly to the gastrointestinal irritation and lack of oxygen in blood. Gastrointestinal irritation is manifested by salivation, diarrhoea and abdominal pain. After absorption, nitrite produces rapid respiration (predominant sign), rapid pulse (150+/min), weak heart beats, subnormal body temperature, muscular tremors, frequent urination, generalised weakness and ataxia. Brown cyanotic colour of membranes develops gradually. This results in dyspnoea with

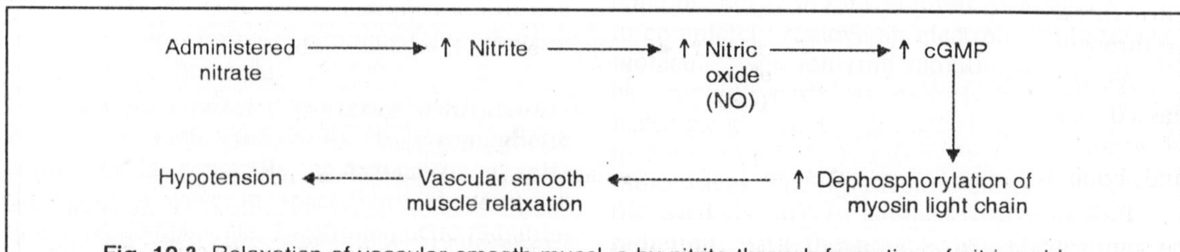

Fig. 12.3. Relaxation of vascular smooth muscles by nitrite through formation of nitric oxide.

rapid respiratory efforts. Exertion causes exacerbation of these signs. Finally there are violent respiratory efforts, open mouth breathing or gasping, collapse, coma and possible terminal clonic convulsions. Death in nitrate/nitrite poisoning occurs within a day or sometimes within hours. Severity of clinical signs show the degree of exposure i.e. cyanosis of visible mucous membranes occur when 5-15% of Hb is converted to Met-Hb, signs of anoxia appear when 20-50% of methaemoglobin is formed, and violent struggling is seen when more than 50-60% of the Hb is converted to Met-Hb. Direct nitrite poisoning has a shorter, but more acute course than nitrate poisoning.

In some peracute cases, animal may die without showing any signs or within 1 hour. Some monogastric animals because of excess nitrate exposure from non-plant sources may exhibit salivation, vomiting, diarrhoea (occasionally haemorrhagic), abdominal pain and gastric haemorrhage. Pregnant females that survive nitrate/ nitrite poisoning may abort due to lack of oxygen to the foetus. Abortion generally occurs approximately 5-10 days following exposure to nitrate.

Chronic toxicity: Chronic toxicity develops in some cases when the animal is eating nitrate containing forages for days to weeks. Signs of chronic poisoning in cattle may be those mentioned in acute toxicity (i.e. dyspnoea) or more commonly anorexia, loss of condition, weight loss or poor weight gain, decreased milk production, abortion, still birth or birth of weak and stunted calves, infertility; goitre (primarily in sheep due to interference with iodine metabolism) and increased susceptibility to infections. Death occurs if the offending feed is continued, but appetite returns with slow recovery when fresh feed is provided.

In swine, chronic nitrate toxicosis may cause thyroid dysfunction, avitaminosis-A, poor weight gain, arthritis, abortion, lymphocytosis and erythrocytosis.

Nitrate: Nitrate, if ingested in large quantities, has a direct caustic effect on the lining of gut. Signs of nitrate poisoning include diarrhoea, salivation and abdominal pain.

Post-mortem findings: In acute nitrate/nitrite poisoning, haemorrhagic gastroenteritis, congestion of internal organs (due to vasodilatory effect) and inflammation of kidneys and urinary bladder may occur. The blood becomes chocolate colour due to methaemoglobin formation. Tissues may also be stained brown and mucous membranes are cyanotic. However, brown colour is not apparent in every case of nitrate poisoning, especially if necropsy is conducted after long-time as there is conversion of methaemoglobin back to haemoglobin.

The characteristic lesions are absent, if the poisoning runs a peracute course. Lesions are also absent in chronic nitrate poisoning.

Diagnosis: Diagnosis of nitrate/nitrite poisoning is based on observed clinical signs, lesions, history of exposure to toxic plants or water, and chemical analysis. Outstanding signs of respiratory distress without evidence of lung lesions suggest a defect in oxygen carrying capacity of blood or a defect in ability of tissue cells to utilise oxygen. Excess nitrate exposure can be assessed by laboratory analysis for nitrate in both ante-mortem and post-mortem specimens. All specimens should be frozen in clean plastic or glass containers before submission (as both NO_2^- and NO_3^- alter rapidly) except when whole blood is collected for methaemoglobin analysis. Methaemoglobin analysis alone is not a reliable indicator of excess nitrate/nitrite exposure except in acute toxicosis because 50% of methaemoglobin present will be converted back to haemoglobin in 2 hours.

Evaluation of rumen contents for nitrate / nitrite concentration is not recommended. Plasma is the preferred ante-mortem specimen because some plasma-protein bound to nitrate could be lost in the clot if serum is collected. Additional post-mortem specimens from toxicosis or abortion include aqueous humour of eye, foetal pleural or thoracic fluid, foetal stomach contents and maternal uterine fluid. Urine, blood, suspected feed, water etc. also carry high nitrate concentration. Normal nitrate contents (mg/100 g wet weight) in some organs and body fluids of cattle are: blood 3.7, urine 1.5, liver 15.8, kidney 9.5 and heart 12.4. As nitrate is also a normal component of drinking water and plants, there should be multiple increases in nitrate concentration in the suspected sample.

In plants, 10,000 ppm (1%) concentration (dry weight) of nitrate may be toxic. Acute nitrate poisoning in ruminants may occur when nitrate concentration of feed is more than 5,000 ppm

Table 12.3: Safe and toxic concentration of nitrate in feed and water.

NO_3^- (ppm)		Recommendations for use in livestock
Forage	*Water*	
0– 6,500	0 – 400	Generally considered safe
6,500 – 20,000	400 – 1,300	Caution: Possible toxicity
>20,000	>1,300	Danger: Potential for toxicity high

(0.5%). Drinking water containing more than 1500 ppm of nitrate is associated with acute toxicosis in ruminants. Table 12.3 depicts safe and toxic concentrations of nitrate in livestock. The nitrate levels in the feed and water sources are additive.

Nitrate/nitrite toxicosis should be differentiated from compounds which also cause defect in oxygen-carrying capacity of the blood. Table 11.4 depicts the differential diagnosis of selected poisons that may be confused with nitrate/nitrite poisoning.

a. *Carbon monoxide*: Carbon dioxide also produces respiratory distress, but it converts haemoglobin into carboxy-haemoglobin which is bright red in colour but not brown.

b. *Haemolytic agents*: Haemolytic agents reduce oxygen carrying capacity of blood by rupturing the erythrocytes. The haemolysis can be detected by inspection of fresh plasma (not old serum which may be red due to other factors).

c. *Haemorrhage inducers*: Agents like warfarin also impair oxygen distribution to tissues but there are indications of massive haemorrhage and increased capillary permeability.

d. *Hypotensive agents*: Hypotensive agents mimic nitrate poisoning, but the history and absence of brown blood help to eliminate their possibility.

e. *Cyanide*: Cyanide also produces respiratory distress but colour of blood is bright red and not brown.

Table 11.4: Important features of selected toxicants that interfere with oxygen carrying capacity.

Toxicant	Mechanism of action	Blood colour	Treatment
Nitrate/Nitrite	Methaemoglobin formation	Brown	Methylene blue; ascorbic acid
Sodium chlorate	Methaemoglobin formation	Brown	Methylene blue; ascorbic acid
Paracetamol	Methaemoglobin formation	Brown	N-Acetylcysteine
Naphthalene	Methaemoglobin formation	Brown	Methylene blue; ascorbic acid
Silo gases (Nitrogen dioxide, nitric oxide)	Lung irritation; slight methaemoglobin formation	Slight brown	Methylene blue
Cyanide	Cytochrome oxidases inhibition	Cherry red	Sodium nitrite and sodium thiosulphate
Carbon monoxide	Carboxyhaemoglobin formation	Bright red	Oxygen + 5% Carbon dioxide
Methylene chloride	Carboxyhaemoglobin formation	Bright red	Oxygen + 5% Carbon dioxide
Carbon dioxide	Oxygen displacement	Dark	Oxygen

Treatment and management :

Specific therapy

a. *Methylene blue*: Methylene blue (Methylthioninium chloride) is a thiazine dye and an oxidizing agent that is used as an antidote for treating methaemoglobinaemia caused by nitrite/ nitrate or chlorate poisoning. It occurs as dark green, odourless crystals with bronze lustre, which when dissolved in water gives a dark blue solution. After intravenous administration, methylene blue is converted in blood and body tissues to a reducing agent leucomethylene blue by a $NADPH_2$-dependent system (Figure 12.4). The leucomethylene blue then reduces methaemoglobin (Fe^{+++}) back to haemoglobin (Fe^{++}). In the reaction, leucomethylene blue is oxidised back to methylene blue, which in turn can be reconverted to leucomethylene blue as long as there is sufficient $NADPH_2$. The $NADPH_2$ system may get saturated if there is too much methylene blue, with the result excess methylene blue may directly oxidise haemoglobin to methaemoglobin. It may also cause development of Heinz body anaemia or other red cell morphological changes, with decreased red cell life spans. So methylene blue should not be used in doses higher than recommended. Methylene blue is not approved for use in food-producing animals.

Dogs: 5 – 10 mg/kg, slow IV.

Cattle & sheep: 4 – 8 mg/kg, slow IV as 1% solution in normal saline (may be given up to 22 mg/kg, if severity of poisoning is high). Lower dosage may be repeated in 10 – 30 minutes, if the initial response is not satisfactory. Lower dosage can be used in all species, but only ruminants can safely tolerate higher ones. If additional exposure or absorption occurs during therapy, methylene blue should be repeated at 6-8 hours interval.

b. *Ascorbic acid:* Ascorbic acid is a reducing agent and can be used in the treatment of nitrite poisoning.

All species: 5-20 mg/kg body weight by I.V. route.

Supportive therapy and management

a. Rumen lavage with cold water and broad spectrum antibiotics may stop the continuing microbial conversion of nitrate to nitrite.

b. Blood transfusion and oxygen therapy may be instituted as these may speed recovery from toxicosis.

c. Saline purgatives may be used to empty the GI tract and mineral oils may help to soothe the GI lining.

d. If hypotension is severe, shock therapy can be instituted.

e. Plenty of water should be supplied to affected horses, pigs and ruminants in case of acute nitrate poisoning.

f. Chronic poisoning is treated by dietary supplements with vitamins A, D and E, additional iodised salt and trace minerals with plenty of water.

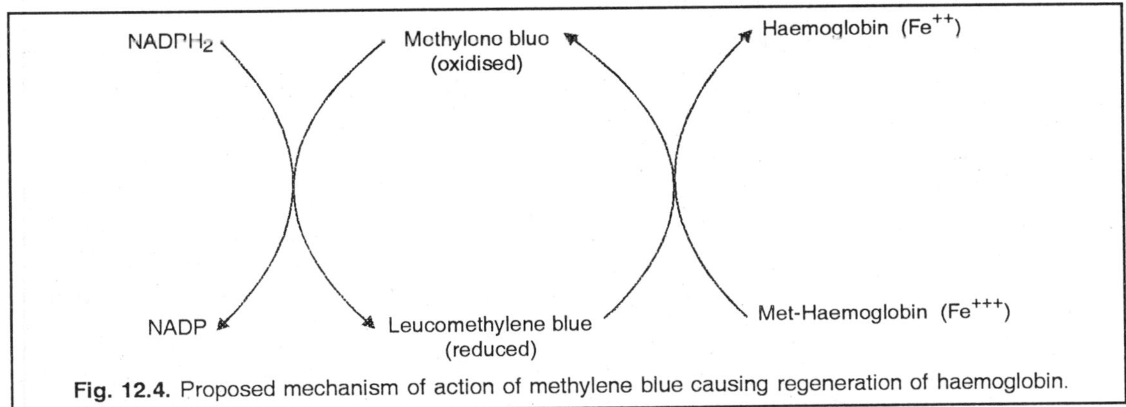

Fig. 12.4. Proposed mechanism of action of methylene blue causing regeneration of haemoglobin.

g. The source of nitrate or nitrite must be identified and eliminated.

h. Trace mineral supplements and a balanced diet may help to prevent nutritional/ metabolic disorders associated with long-term excess dietary nitrate consumption.

Contraindications: In shock condition, α-adrenoceptor agonists or antagonists should not be used to increase blood pressure and to produce vasodilation to increase blood supply, respectively, unless adequate haemoglobin is present to carry oxygen to the vital organs. Alpha- adrenoceptor agonists increase oxygen demand of tissues and α-adrenoceptor antagonists complicate hypotension.

Prevention: Prevention of nitrate poisoning is very essential and is best achieved by controlling type and quality of forages offered to livestock. As nitrate levels in plant fluctuates rapidly with weather and other conditions, it is better to observe following steps to reduce risk of poisoning.

a. Avoid excessive application of manure or nitrogen fertilizer to fodder plants.

b. When in doubt, analyse all feeds and forages for nitrate before grazing or feeding them to livestock. Test the draught stress forages of being high in nitrates before feeding.

c. Dilute high nitrate forages with other forages or feedstuffs which are low in nitrate.

d. Delay harvesting any stressed forages. A week of favourable weather is required for plants to reduce accumulated nitrate. Wait at least one week prior to harvest following a rain which ended a drought.

e. Cut the draught-stressed forages few inches above the ground level, as the lower stalk contains highest concentration of nitrate.

f. Do not feed the animal high-nitrate hay, straw or fodder that has been damp or wet for several days, or stockpiled after cutting as heating assists bacterial conversion of nitrate to nitrite.

g. Do not allow hungry cattle access to high nitrate forages or pastures. Feed cattle hays and forages low in nitrate before turning them onto suspect high nitrate pastures.

h. Graze cattle on high nitrate pastures during the day and remove them at night for first week of grazing. This reduces the amount of high nitrate forage consumed and helps cattle to acclimate to high nitrate levels.

i. Gradually introduce cattle to suspect forages over several days.

j. Consider harvesting and feeding high nitrate forages as silages. Nitrate levels are reduced by the fermentation process that occurs when feeds are ensiled.

k. If possible, cut forages late in the day on a warm sunny day.

l. Allow livestock access to fresh, nitrate-free water at all times.

m. Feed a grain supplement to increase the conversion of nitrate to protein. Supplement diet with vitamins A, D and E and iodized salt.

n. Do not feed monensin with diets high in nitrate.

Prognosis: Prognosis of nitrate/nitrite poisoning depends upon the time of institution of therapy. Early therapy may lead to recovery.

5. Chlorate

Chlorates are among the most widely used inorganic herbicides. The chlorate herbicide is considered phytotoxic to all green plant parts and mainly used on non-crop land for spot treatment and for total vegetation control on roadsides, fence ways, ditches, etc. Chlorate is a powerful oxidizer and should be kept away from organics or easily reducible materials. Though the use of chlorate compounds has declined recently due to availability of organic preparations, yet cases of acute or chronic poisoning are reported in all species of animals.

Properties: A chlorate is a compound that contains chlorine in oxidation state +5 (chlorate radical) and a metal or hydrogen. The most important chlorates are sodium chlorate ($NaClO_3$) and potassium chlorate ($KClO_3$). Sodium chlorate is a white hygroscopic substance, readily soluble in water and is primarily used as a non-selective herbicide. Potassium chlorate is a colourless crystalline substance that decomposes violently at about 400°C and is used in making explosives and matches and used occasionally as herbicide.

Chlorates are highly inflammable when mixed with a dry organic substance. They may persist in soil for 6 months to 5 years, depending on the rate applied, soil type, fertility, organic matter, moisture and weather conditions. Toxicity in soil is decreased considerably by high nitrate contents, alkaline conditions and high soil temperatures.

Sources of toxicity:

a. Chlorate salts (e.g. potassium and sodium chlorate) are occasionally used as herbicides and defoliants. Poisoning in animals may occur due to accidental ingestion of agrochemical products or consumption of freshly treated vegetation.

b. Because of its salty appearance and taste, chlorate may be accidentally mixed in animal feed in place of common salt by misidentification.

c. Careless disposal of chlorate is an important source of toxicity. Salt hungry animals may consume chlorate from improper disposal of dry salt.

d. Chlorate is used to make fireworks, matches and explosives. These are rare source of toxicity in animals.

Toxicity: Toxicity of chlorate depends on the type of compound and species involved. Sodium chlorate is not very toxic, but it is extremely palatable which can result in massive ingestion of the substance. Monogastrics and ruminants are of similar sensitivity. The lethal doses of sodium chlorate in different species are: dogs 0.2-2 g/kg, horses 0.5 g/kg, cattle 1 g/kg, sheep 2 g/kg, and poultry 5 g/kg. Sodium chlorate is considered non-toxic to fish. The possible 48-hour LC_{50} for various species of fish is 10,000 mg/l.

Toxicokinetics: The detailed toxicokinetics of chlorate in domestic animals is not known. Chlorate appears to be readily absorbed from the gut and is excreted largely unchanged.

Mechanism of action:

a. Chlorate is a strong oxidising agent which converts haemoglobin (Fe^{+2}) to methaemoglobin (Fe^{+3}) by the same mechanism as described for nitrite toxicity. However, as compared to the nitrite, the process of methaemoglobin formation by chlorate is slower and continues until chlorate is completely excreted as it is not inactivated in the reaction. The methaemoglobin formation continues even after death of the animal as long as chlorate is present in the blood.

b. In addition to methemoglobinaemia, chlorate also results in the formation of a small concentration of sulph-haemoglobin. The sulph-haemoglobin is a partially oxidised and denatured mixture of pigment due to non-specific oxidation. There is no mechanism in the erythrocytes for the reversal of sulph-haemoglobin.

c. Chlorate is an irritant of gastrointestinal tract and causes abdominal pain and diarrhoea.

Clinical signs :

Acute toxicity: In acute poisoning, onset of action is generally fast and occurs within 1 hour because chlorate, unlike nitrate, does not require reduction before it is active. Therefore the monogastrics are just as sensitive as ruminants. Except for the early onset, the general signs of chlorate poisoning are similar to that of nitrite toxicity and include signs of gastric and haematological disturbances. Important clinical manifestations are diarrhoea, salivation, violent abdominal pain, ataxia, prostration, convulsions, cyanosis and dyspnoea. Blood is chocolate brown in colour. Haemolysis, haematuria, haemoglobinuria or myoglobinuria and effusion of dark tarry blood from natural orifices, which clots readily, are quite characteristic of chlorate poisoning. In severe cases, death may occur even without any apparent sign of toxicity.

Subacute or chronic toxicity: In subacute or chronic chlorate toxicosis, the clinical manifestation may be similar to acute toxicity. In addition, there may be anorexia, loss of weight and body condition, haemolytic jaundice, oliguria or anuria, and coma. The long-term toxicity of sodium chlorate to birds results in reduced egg production and fertility. A prolonged chronic exposure to inhalation of sodium chlorate may cause mucous membrane irritation.

Post mortem findings: Important post mortem lesions of chlorate poisoning include generalised cyanosis, dark brown tissues and blood, blood-stained urine and exudation of blood from natural orifices. Musculature is dark or almost black and cut surfaces become some what lighter on exposure to air. Gastroenteritis and erosions in stomach (abomasum) and duodenum are observed due to the irritant action of chlorate on GI tract. In subacute or chronic cases, the necrotic lesions are identical to those observed in acute poisoning but with fatty degeneration of the liver and kidneys and splenomegaly.

Diagnosis: Diagnosis of chlorate poisoning is made from history, clinical signs and post mortem lesions, especially dark chocolate coloured blood and tissues. Chlorate determination in plasma, urine and aqueous humour may be useful in confirming the diagnosis. Estimation of met-Hb in blood during clinical signs period, on mortality and after death is very important. The concentration of methaemoglobin increases with passage of time as the process of met-Hb formation continues even after death.

Chlorate poisoning should be differentiated from other poisonings or diseases that cause respiratory distress (Table 12.3). These should include nitrate/nitrite poisoning (blood is brown, but there is no oozing out of blood from natural orifices), carbon monoxide poisoning (blood is bright red), cyanide poisoning (blood is bright red and bitter almond smell), hydrogen sulphide (blood is dark in colour), warfarin poisoning (haemorrhages, but colour of blood is normal), and haemolytic agents like copper, dimethyl sulphoxide, etc.

Treatment and management :

Specific treatment:

Objective of specific therapy in chlorate poisoning is similar to that of nitrate/nitrite poisoning i.e. to convert met-haemoglobin to haemoglobin.

a. Methylene blue: Methylene blue is the drug of choice in acute chlorate poisoning. It reduces the chlorate-induced methaemoglobin to haemoglobin by mechanism as discussed in nitrate/nitrite poisoning. However in chlorate toxicity, compared to nitrite poisoning, methylene blue needs to be administered more frequently and repeated until blood no longer turns dark red on standing. Methylene blue given in absence of methaemoglobin can cause Heinz body formation.

Dogs: 4 mg/kg by intravenous route (as 2-4% solution).

Cattle: 10 – 15 mg/kg by intravenous route (as 2-4% solution). The dose is repeated after every 8 hours during the first 24-48 hours post-ingestion.

b. Ascorbic acid: Vitamin C as a reducing agent is administered to small animals.

Dogs & cats: 20 mg/kg by intravenous route.

Supportive and symptomatic therapy

a. The excess chlorate should be removed from GI tract by gastric lavage and/or saline purgative.

b. Cardiopulmonary stimulants may be used in severe cases, as required by condition.

c. Gastrointestinal sedative may be advised in case of gastroenteritis.

d. Blood transfusion may help to reduce hypoxia.

Prevention :

a. Remove animals from the area treated with chlorate.

b. Properly dispose of all unused chlorate, away from domestic animals.

6. Sulphur

Sulphur is an essential element for life and normally present in many foods. It is found in two amino acids cysteine and methionine, which make polypeptides, proteins and enzymes. Sulphur is also an important component of coenzyme A, glutathione and inorganic sulphate and is involved in disulfide bonds between polypeptides. Sulphur is primarily used in agriculture in fertilizers and as a broad spectrum fungicide and insecticide. It has also been used for medicinal purposes in man and animals for many years and utilized in industries for manufacturing of a number of compounds. Sulphur poisoning in not common in domestic animals but may be observed in all species.

Properties: Sulphur (S) is a multivalent non-metal with atomic number 16. It exists as tasteless, odourless, yellow crystalline solid. In nature, it can be found as pure element or as sulphide and sulphate minerals. It burns with blue flame that emits sulphur dioxide, notable for its peculiar suffocating odour. Sulphur is insoluble in water but soluble in carbon disulfide and to lesser extent in other organic solvents such as benzene. Common oxidation states of sulphur include -2, +2, +4 and

+6. Sulphur forms stable compounds with all elements except the noble gases.

Sources of toxicity :

a. Sulphur is widely used in fertilizers and as a broad spectrum insecticide and fungicide. Accidental ingestion of agrochemical sulphur from storage sacks, sulphur mixed seeds or sprayed fields may cause toxicity in animals.

b. Sulphur is occasionally used topically for treatment of ringworm and other dermal infections in animals. Inadvertent use of higher doses may cause toxicosis in animals.

c. Some breeders use sulphur as a tonic for improving conditions of the fur of animals. Administration of high doses or use of micronized sulphur instead of flowers of sulphur causes poisoning

d. Sulphur is commercially used in industries for various purposes including preparation of batteries, detergents, gunpowder, fireworks, matches and phosphate fertilizers. It is also used as the light-generating medium in the rare lighting fixtures known as sulphur lamps. Sulphur from these sources is a rare cause of poisoning in animals.

e. Sulphur occurs naturally in volcanic emissions. Exposure to sulphur dust is harmful to animals.

Toxicity: Toxicity of sulphur depends on the type of sulphur and species involved. Sublimed or titrated sulphur is less toxic and does not present a particular toxicological problem. Micronized sulphur is more toxic and appears to be involved in most incidents of sulphur poisoning in animals. The oral lethal dose of sulphur in cattle is 100-1000 mg/kg and in sheep and horses is 1000-1500 mg/kg.

Toxicokinetics: Following oral administration, sulphur is absorbed either in form of sulphur containing amino acids (ruminants) or as sulphides, which are rapidly oxidised to sulphate. Absorbed sulphate enters the normal sulphate body-pool and is excreted via kidneys. Following topical application, little or no sulphur is absorbed into systemic circulation.

Mechanism of action: The exact mechanism of sulphur poisoning is not still clear.

a. After ingestion, sulphur has local effect on gut membranes which results in laxative effects. It also produces irritant action on GI mucosa that causes abdominal pain and colic.

b. Sulphur is an antagonist of copper, potassium and calcium. Some of its adverse effects may be attributable to its antagonism of essential metals in body. High sulphur in human beings is associated with some diseases like Crohn's disease, Lou Gehrig's disease, nerve degeneration, and inflammatory vascular/joint degeneration.

Clinical signs: Ingestion of sulphur in domestic animals produces primarily gastrointestinal effects with abdominal pain, diarrhoea (often haemorrhagic), anorexia and colic. In ruminants, tympany with or without rectal spasms, rumen hypomotility or atony, staggering gait and difficulty in getting up may also be observed. In some cattle, constipation instead of diarrhoea may be noticed. Neurological signs in ruminants and other species include dullness, lassitude, ataxia, abnormal behaviour, mydriasis, prostration, tremor and convulsions. Respiratory signs with difficult respiration are also observed. In horses, additional signs may include sweating, jaundice and petechiae or ecchymoses. Death in acute cases occurs mostly within several hours.

Inhalation of sulphur dust may be irritating to the eyes, nose, throat and lungs. Solid sulphur (especially when freshly produced) may release hydrogen sulphide gas, which can accumulate in confined, non-ventilated areas and may cause irritation, breathing failure, coma and death, without necessarily any warning odour being sensed. Residual effects after exposure can include shortness of breath, wheezing and delayed pulmonary oedema (may be fatal). Long term effects of sulphur exposure may include respiratory problems and inflammation of eyes. Frequent or prolonged contact may irritate the skin and cause a skin rash.

Post-mortem findings: Lesions of sulphur poisoning are not significant and poorly characterised. Congestion, haemorrhagic suffusions and petechiae along the digestive tract may be observed. Congestion of some internal organs such as lungs and urinary bladder may be noticed.

Diagnosis: Diagnosis of sulphur poisoning may be made by clinical signs and history of animals being overdosed with sulphur. At necropsy, a smell of hydrogen sulphide from the rumen may also indicate sulphur poisoning.

Treatment and management: Treatment of acute sulphur poisoning is only symptomatic and supportive.

a. Gastrointestinal sedative may be used in case of gastroenteritis.

b. Appropriate fluids may be administered to combat loss of fluid and electrolytes due to diarrhoea.

BIBLIOGRAPHY

Ballantyne B, Marrs T and Turner P (1995) General and Applied Toxicology. Macmillan, London.

Bartik M and Piskac A (1981) Veterinary Toxicology. Elsevier Scientific Publishing Company, Amsterdam.

Beasley V (1999) Veterinary Toxicology. International Veterinary Information Service, Ithaca NY (www.ivis,org).

Booth NH and McDonald LE (1982) John's Veterinary Pharmacology and Therapeutics. 5th edn. (Eds.). Kalyani Publishers, Ludhiana-New Delhi.

Burrows GE (1984) Methylene blue: Effects and disposition in sheep. *J. Vet. Pharmacol. Therapeut.* 7 : 225.

Chen L, Hogan GR and Azniak SL (1994) Tissue distribution of selenate, selenite, selenocysteine and selenomethionine in mice. *J. Environ. Sci. Hlth.* A29 : 2023.

Clarke ECG and Clarke ML (1967) Garner's Veterinary Toxicology. 3rd edn. Williams and Wilkins, Baltimore.

EXTOXNET (1995) Sodium chlorate. (http://extoxnet.orst.edu/pips/sodiumch.htm).

Frasher CM, Bergeron JA, Mays A and Aiello SE (1991) The Merck Veterinary Manual: A Handbook of Diagnosis, Therapy and Disease Prevention and Control for the Veterinarians. 7th edn. Merck and Company, Rahway.

Garg SK (2000) Veterinary Toxicology. CBS Publishers & Distributors, New Delhi.

Glasser G and Jones J (2007) Dental fluorosis: Smile please, but don't say cheese. National Pure Water Association, Ltd. (http://homepage.circom.net/~fluoridefree/lawandfluorosis.htm).

Helwig DM and Setchell BP (1960) Observations on the diagnosis of nitrate poisoning in sheep. *Aust. Vet. J.* 36 : 14.

Lorgue G, Lechenet J and Riviere A (1996) Clinical Veterinary Toxicology. Blackwell Science Ltd., United Kingdom.

Lu FC and Kacew S (2002) Lu's Basic Toxicology: Fundamentals, Target Organs and Risk Assessment. Taylor & Francis, New York.

Maas J (2001) Nitrate toxicity. UCD Vet Views, *California Cattleman.* (http://www.vetmed.ucdavis.edu/vetext/INF-BE_cca/INF-BE_cca01/INF-BE_cca0111.html).

National Academy of Sciences (1960) The fluorosis problem in livestock production: A report of the committee on animal nutrition agricultural board. Publication: 824. National Academy of Sciences - National Research Council, Washington DC.

Osweiler GD (1996) Toxicology. Williams and Wilkins, Philadelphia.

Polson CJ and Tattersall RN (1980) Clinical Toxicology. 2nd edn. Pitman Medical, London.

Prasad B, Mishra SK and Gupta PP (1984) Pathological changes in experimental nitrite poisoning in buffalo calves. *Ind. J. Anim. Sci.* 54 : 1081.

Radeleff RD (1970) Veterinary Toxicology. 2nd edn. Lea and Febiger, Philadelphia.

Rand WE and Schmidt HJ (1952) Water of high fluoride content. *Am. J. Vet. Res.* 13 : 50.

Randhawa SS, Randhawa CS, Brar RS, Dhillon KS, Dhillon SK and Singh B (1992) Biomedical profile of bovines fed on selenium rich fodders. Proceedings of International Symposium. Nutrient Management for Sustained Productivity. Vol. II. p 166, P.A.U., Ludhiana.

Robson S (2007) Nitrate and nitrite poisoning in livestock. *Primefact* 415. (http://www.dpi.nsw.gov.au/aboutus/resources/factsheets/primefacts/nitrate-nitrite-poisoning).

Rogers P (1999) Poisoning in cattle and sheep by urea, nitrates and nitrites: Sources, toxic doses, treatment and prevention. (http://homepage.eircom.net/~progers/ureanitr.htm).

Rogers P, Arora SP, Fleming GA, Crinion RAP and McLaughlin JG (1990) Selenium toxicity in farm animals: treatment and prevention. *Irish Vet. J.* 43 : 151.

Rosenfeld I and Beath OA (1964) Selenium. Academic Press, New York.

Rumbeiha KW and Oehme FW (1992) Methylene blue can be used to treat methaemoglobinaemia in cats without inducing Heinz body anaemia. *Vet. Hum. Toxicol.* 34 : 120.

Stoltenow C and Lardy G (1998) Nitrate poisoning of livestock. (http://www.animalrangeextension.montana.edu/Articles/Beef/Q&A2003/nitrate.htm).

Undersander D, Combs D, Shaver R and Thomas D (2007) Nitrate poisoning in cattle, sheep and goats. (http://www.uwex.edu/ces/forage/pubs/nitrate.htm).

White ME (2005) Cornell Consultant Toxicity Data. Alphabetical Search for the Cornell Consultant for Data on Intoxication, Poisoning or Toxicity in Animals. Cornell University College of Veterinary Medicine (Online service, http://homepage.eircom.net/~progers/consultox.htm).

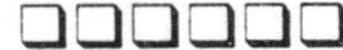

13 PESTICIDES

Insecticides
- Organochlorine insecticides
- Organophosphorus insecticides
- Carbamate insecticides
- Pyrethrins and Pyrethroid insecticides
- Formamidine insecticides
- Neonicotinoid insecticides
- Natural products
  - Rotenone
  - Nicotine

Herbicides
- Inorganic herbicides
  - Arsenicals
  - Chlorates
- Organic herbicides
  - Chlorophenoxy herbicides / Phenoxy acid derivatives
  - Dinitro herbicides /Dinitrophenols
  - Bipyridyl herbicides
  - Triazine herbicides
  - Substituted urea herbicides
  - Other herbicides

Fungicides
- Inorganic fungicides
  - Sulphur
  - Metals
- Organic fungicides
  - Organomercury fungicides
  - Chlorophenols / Pentachlorophenol
  - Dithiocarbamates
  - Organotin fungicides
  - Phathalimides
  - Benzimidazoles
  - Other fungicides

Fumigants
- Inorganic fumigants
  - Aluminium phosphide
  - Hydrogen cyanide
  - Carbon disulphide
  - Sulphur dioxide.
- Organic fumigants
  - Chloropicrin
  - Methyl bromide
  - Ethylene dibromide
  - 1,3-Dichloropropene
  - Dibromochloropropane (DBCP).

Rodenticides
- Inorganic rodenticides
  - Arsenic compounds
  - Elementary phosphorous
  - Thallium sulphate
  - Zinc phosphide
- Organic rodenticides
  - Anticoagulants
  - Fluoroacetic acid and its derivatives
  - Vitamin D compounds
  - Alphanaphthylthiourea (ANTU)
  - Bromethalin
  - Strychnine
  - Red squill
  - Pyriminil
  - Norbormide
  - Crimidine
  - Chloralose

Molluscicide
- Metaldehyde

Pesticides are a heterogeneous group of substances used for preventing, destroying or repelling the pests. They are among the most widely used groups of chemicals in modern world and have provided immense benefits to mankind by contributing significantly in enhancing food production and improving health and nutrition.

However, their massive and indiscriminate use in crop protection, food preservation, and insect pests' control has led to acute or chronic poisoning incidents in humans, domestic animals and wild life, and resulted in widespread ecological adverse effects. Pesticides fall into numerous chemical classes such as insecticides, herbicides and rodenticides, which have widely different biological activities and thus differing potential to produce adverse effects in animals.

Major sources of toxicity

There are number of possible ways in which humans and/or animals can be exposed to pesticides. These include accidental, malicious and occupational exposures.

a. *Accidental/Unintentional poisoning:* Accidental or unintentional exposure to pesticides is the most common source of poisoning in animals and can result in a number of ways:
    - *i.* Accidental ingestion of pesticides from storage containers or sacks.
    - *ii.* Consumption of freshly sprayed crops.
    - *iii.* Ingestion of contaminated concentrates i.e. when pesticide sprayed grain unfit for human consumption is fed to animals.
    - *iv.* Drinking of water from pesticide treated paddy fields or from ponds/streams contaminated with pesticides due to mosquito fogging, aerial spray, and effluent from pesticide factory or run-off from fields.
    - *v.* Consumption of dairy products (i.e. eggs, meat, milk, etc.) from intoxicated animals.
    - *vi.* Licking of freshly sprayed walls and pillars.
    - *vii.* Spillage of pesticides onto food during storage or transport.
    - *viii.* Secondary poisoning in predator animals (e.g. dogs eating poisoned rats, birds eating insects).
    - *ix.* Exposure of animals to products intended for other species (e.g. cats treated with dips for dogs).
    - *x.* Use of insecticides on stressed animals.
    - *xi.* Exposure to spray or spray drift due to poorly conducted aerial crop spraying.
    - *xii.* Watering and feeding of animals in bucket previously used for mixing pesticides.
    - *xiii.* Faulty storage i.e. keeping pesticides at the same place where animal feed is stored.
    - *xiv.* Use of pesticides in concentrations higher than that recommended for pest control.
    - *xv.* Absorption of ectoparasicitide from abraded skin, eyes or other mucous membranes of body.
    - *xvi.* Residues in agricultural products.
    - *xvii.* Birds get intoxicated from consumption of pesticide treated seeds in fields.
    - *xviii.* Dogs get intoxicated while playing in lawns treated with insecticides or herbicides.
    - *xix.* Inhalation from polluted environment.

b. *Malicious/Intentional poisoning:* Malicious and intentional poisoning is also an important source of pesticide poisoning in humans and animals. In recent years, this type of poisoning is on rise because most people have easy access to pesticides and they use these chemicals to kill animals.
    - *i.* Intentional mixing of pesticides in the feed or fodder of animals.
    - *ii.* Suicide/Homicide in humans.

c. *Occupational poisoning:* Occupational exposure is an important source of acute and chronic poisoning in humans.
    - *i.* Exposure of workers in the factory engaged in manufacturing, handling or storage of pesticides.
    - *ii.* Faulty operational procedures like use of leaking spray pumps or mixing of pesticides with naked hands.
    - *iii.* Spraying of fields by untrained and unskilled workers.

Classes of Pesticides

The classified lists of pesticides include more than 1500 compounds, which have been divided into several major classes, depending on their use in agriculture and related fields. Each major group of pesticides (e.g. insecticides) is further subdivided into chemical or other classes (e.g. organochlorines and organophosphates). Individual compounds can occur in more than one group or class, and at more than one place within a group or class. Although all classes are not important from toxicology point of view and have not been discussed in the present section, a list of major groups of pesticides is given below for knowledge:

A. Insecticides e.g. malathion, DDT and deltamethrin.
B. Herbicides e.g. 2,4-D, paraquat and atrazine.
C. Fungicides e.g. zineb, captan and dinocap.
D. Fumigants e.g. aluminium phosphide and ethylene dibromide.
E. Rodenticides e.g. zinc phosphide, warfarin and red squill.
F. Molluscicides e.g. metaldehyde, pentachlorophenol and copper sulphate.
G. Avicides e.g. 4-aminopyridine, chloralose and endrin.
H. Acaricides e.g. azobenzene, amitraz and clofentezine.
I. Nematicides e.g. acetoprole and benclothiaz.
J. Algicides e.g. bethoxazin, dichlone and hydrated lime.
K. Bird repellents e.g. guazatine, thiram and copper oxychloride.
L. Mammal repellents e.g. ziram, copper naphthenate and trimethacarb.

A. INSECTICIDES

Insecticides are a heterogeneous group of chemicals which are specifically used for preventing, destroying or repelling the insect pests. The use of insecticides in agriculture has grown tremendously since World War II and they have become an integral part of agriculture. Though insecticides have been designed to selectively kill insect pests, yet they are not very selective and result in poisonings in many non-target species including man and domestic animals. Their large scale use has also brought many problems like residues in food stuffs, ecological imbalance and environmental pollution.

Classes of Insecticides

The number of substances that fall into the major descriptive class of insecticides as such is enormous and include insecticides, attractants, repellents, growth regulators, chemosterilants etc. However, from toxicology point of view, following are the major groups of insecticides:

I. Organochlorine (Chlorinated hydrocarbon) insecticides e.g. DDT, BHC and methoxychlor.
II. Organophosphorus insecticides e.g. malathion, dichlorvos and monocrotophos
III. Carbamate insecticides e.g. carbaryl, methomyl and propoxur.
IV. Pyrethroid insecticides e.g. pyrethrum, allethrin, deltamethrin and fenvalerate.
V. Formamidine insecticides e.g. amitraz.
VI. Neonicotinoid insecticides e.g. imidacloprid.
VII. Natural products e.g. rotenone, nicotine, and avermectins.

I. ORGANOCHLORINE (CHLORINATED HYDROCARBON) INSECTICIDES

The organochlorine (OC) insecticides are chlorinated hydrocarbon compounds. They were the first major class of synthetic organic chemicals to become widely used as insecticides and are often called the first generation insecticides. They are mainly used as contact insecticides in agriculture and malaria control programmes and as ectoparasiticides in animals. Nowadays the use of OC insecticides has declined tremendously mainly due to their persistence in environment, animals and wildlife, and potential for chronic toxicity.

Chemistry: The organochlorine insecticides constitute a large group of insecticides with varying chemical structures and toxicological properties. However, all of these organic compounds contain chlorine atom in their structure (organochlorine) and appear to share the same mechanism with regard to neurotoxicity. Some of the important points related to the chemical structure of organochlorine insecticides are:

a. Presence of carbon, chlorine, hydrogen and sometimes oxygen atoms with a number of C-Cl bonds.
b. Presence of cyclic carbon chains (including benzene ring).
c. Lack of any particular intramolecular active site.

d. Apolarity and lipophilicity.

e. Chemical unreactivity and high stability in the environment (e.g. half-life of OC insecticides in soil varies from 1-12 years with DDT = 3-10 years and toxaphene = 10 years).

Classification: For toxicological purposes, the organochlorine insecticides may be broadly divided into three groups based on their chemical structures. In spite of similarity of chemical structure and toxicological effects, the individual insecticides within each group may differ in degree of toxicity and properties.

1. Diphenyl aliphatic compounds or DDT group, e.g. DDT, methoxychlor and dicofol.
2. Aryl hydrocarbons, e.g. BHC, mirex and kepone.
3. Cyclodiene (polycyclic chlorinated) insecticides, e.g. aldrin, dieldrin, endrin, chlordane, heptachlor, toxaphene and endosulfan.

Properties: Organochlorine insecticides are lipid soluble compounds with poor solubility in water, so these are mainly used as dusts, wettable powders, emulsions or suspensions. Volatility is characteristic of this group of insecticides. With few exceptions (e.g. endosulfan and perthane), OC insecticides are highly persistent in the environment because they resist chemical or microbial decomposition, especially when protected by soil. The high lipid soluble nature of these compounds, combined with their environmental persistence, favours bioaccumulation upward in food chain from environment to animal or human tissues.

Factors affecting toxicity :

a. Young animals are more sensitive than adults.

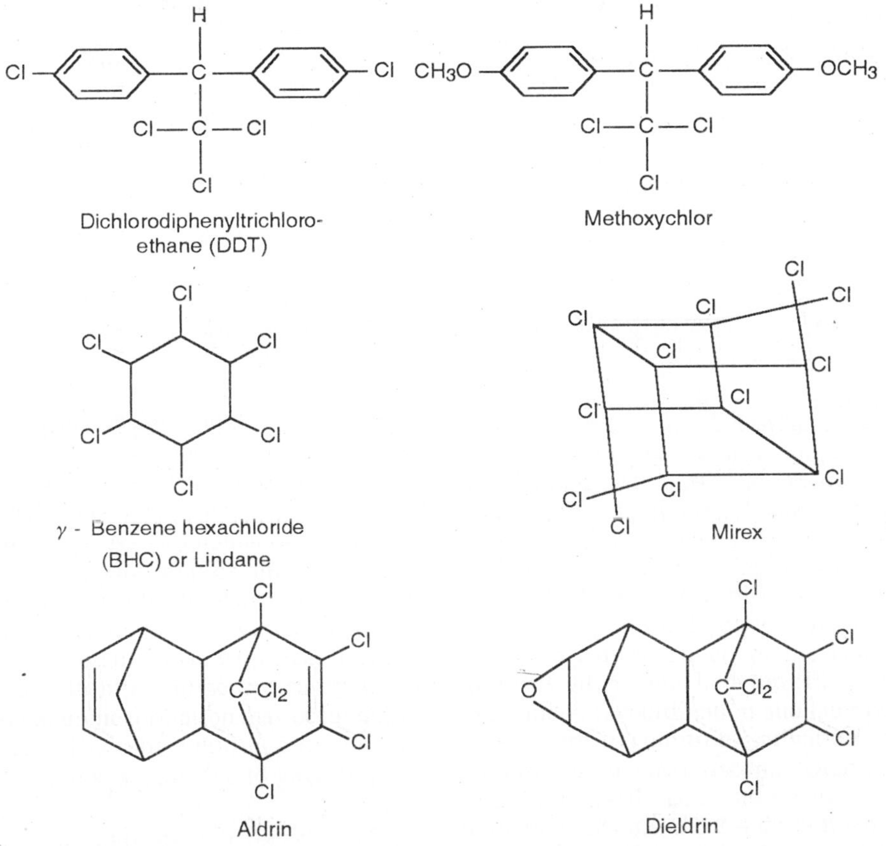

Dichlorodiphenyltrichloro-ethane (DDT)

Methoxychlor

γ - Benzene hexachloride (BHC) or Lindane

Mirex

Aldrin

Dieldrin

Fig. 13.1. Chemical structures of some important organochlorine (OC) insecticides.

b. Females are more sensitive than males.

c. Fatty and lactating animals are more sensitive than emaciated and non-lactating animals.

d. Stress or illness enhances toxicity.

e. The OC compounds are more toxic in oily vehicle than in suspensions and dry powders, (e.g. DDT is 10 times more toxic in oils than aqueous solution).

f. Agents of cyclodiene group are generally the most toxic, whereas chemicals of DDT group are least toxic (Table 13.1).

g. Cats are more susceptible than other domestic animals to OC insecticides. Fishes are more susceptible than mammals and birds (Fishes > mammals > birds).

h. The OC compounds are less toxic if absorbed slowly from skin or gut, especially when small doses have been ingested over a period of time.

Toxicity: The toxicity potential of chlorinated insecticides varies greatly with the type of compound, formulation and species of animal. Median lethal dose of diphenyl aliphatic compounds in most species tend to be relatively high, whereas that of cyclodiene agents tend to be less. The lethal doses of some of commonly employed organochlorine insecticides in different species of animals are given in Table 13.1.

Toxicokinetics: Organochlorine insecticides are lipid soluble, so these can be absorbed through the skin as well as by the respiratory and oral routes. However, the extent of absorption from dermal and oral routes varies greatly for different compounds and type of formulation. The intestinal absorption of these insecticides is also influenced by fibre and fat constituents of the diet as well as the total food intake. DDT is poorly absorbed from skin and GI tract, except in oily solution. In contrast dieldrin is effectively absorbed through the skin and gut even in solid form.

After entry into the blood stream, organochlorine insecticides may bind to serum lipoproteins and are stored in body fat (even at 1 ppm) and go on accumulating there Organochlorines are also found in other organs like liver, kidney, adrenals and brain. Although storage in fat can be partly explained by the lipophilicity of these insecticides, other factors such as chemical structure and competition between binding sites in tissues are also important. These compounds are mainly metabolised by liver microsomal cytochrome P-450 system. Cyclodiene insecticides are converted to epoxides, and diphenyl aliphatics are dechlorinated by mixed function oxidases. In many cases, metabolites are more toxic than the parent compound. Other routes of metabolism involve conjugation with glutathione or formation of glucuronides.

After ingestion much of the dose is excreted through faeces unchanged due to poor absorption. From body OC insecticides are mainly excreted through bile, urine and milk. The half-life of some OC insecticides may range from days to weeks. Residue elimination may be described by a two

Table 13.1: Oral lethal doses of selected organochlorine insecticides in different species of animals.

Insecticide	Lethal Dose-50 (mg/kg)							
	Rats	*Rabbits*	*Dogs*	*Cats*	*Sheep*	*Goats*	*Chickens*	*Quails*
DDT	100-5000	300	500-750	400	>1000	>1000	–	840
Dicofol	800	1870	>4000	–	–	–	–	–
Methoxychlor	6000	–	–	–	–	–	–	–
Lindane	80-125	–	30-200	35	100	100	70	–
Aldrin	40	50-80	65	10-15	40-50	180	–	7
Dieldrin	40-80	45	65	300-500	90	100	20	70
Endosulfan	40-110	–	200	2	–	–	–	150-200
Endrin	5	7	–	3-6	–	25	2-4	–
Toxaphene	40	–	15	60	200	200	–	85

– = Data not available

compartment model. The first phase is rapid and may account for 40-50% elimination during the first 3-4 days after exposure. The subsequent slow phase of elimination may require months due to slow mobilisation of insecticides from storage fat. Moreover, even after one-half of the dose of insecticide has been eliminated from the body, the remaining one-half can cause residues in meat, milk or egg for several months, possibly years. The lipid contents of milk and high blood flow to mammary tissue can lead to considerable concentration of OCs in milk, which may be harmful to consumers and young ones suckling the mother. Milk fat values may approximate body fat concentrates.

Mechanism of action: Organochlorine insecticides are non-specific stimulants to the CNS. They have no stereo selective receptors and therefore no known competitive antagonist. The molecular mechanism of acute toxicosis has not been clearly determined but interference with sodium channel kinetics in nerve membranes is considered the primarily action of many OC insecticides.

a. Diphenyl aliphatic OC insecticides by virtue of their high lipid solubility easily enter neural membranes and alter the electrophysiological and associated enzymatic properties of nerve membranes causing a change in kinetics of Na^+ and K^+ ion flow through membranes. This is produced mainly by slowing down the closure of Na^+ channel and by inhibiting the opening of K^+ channel. Accordingly, the time during which some of the sodium channels in the membrane open during depolarization is significantly enhanced and the sodium inflow is increased and the potassium outflow is decreased. This imbalance of ions results in decreased transmembrane resting potential (inside of membrane is more positive), enhanced initiation of action potentials and thus increased neuronal excitability. Sensory nerves are more readily affected by the DDT and analogues than are motor nerves, so there is increased tendency for seizures. Over depolarization of medullary neurons often results in respiratory failure. Both central and peripheral parts of the nervous system are affected by DDT and analogues, although the cerebellum and motor cortex have been considered to be of greatest importance.

b. The primary targets for cyclodienes in mammalian brain are γ-aminobutyric acid (GABA) receptors at GABA-ergic nerve terminals. Cyclodiene and some aryl hydrocarbon (e.g. lindane) insecticides bind to a site close to or in the Cl^- channel on $GABA_A$ receptors and inhibit the binding of inhibitory neurotransmitter gamma-aminobutyric acid (GABA) to the receptor. As a result of which there is inhibition of GABA-dependent opening of chloride channel and hence chloride influx into the neuron. This results in only partial repolarization of the neuron and a state of uncontrolled excitation. So cyclodienes cause intense stimulation of the nervous system.

c. Other actions of organochlorine insecticides include inhibition of some ion transporters like Na^+/K^+-ATPase, Ca^{2+}-ATPase, and Ca^{2+}-Mg^{2+}-ATPase. Disturbance in the activity of ion transporters in neuronal tissues causes imbalance in ion concentrations across the nerve membranes and hence alteration in neuronal excitability. Inhibition of calmodulin-Ca^{2+} binding is associated with altered release of neurotransmitters.

d. Organochlorine insecticides produce changes in the concentration of various biogenic amines in CNS, which are associated with manifestation of some adverse effects. It has been suggested that changes in the metabolism of serotonin and noradrenaline in CNS may be responsible for hyperthermia, and acetylcholine changes may be related to tremors and convulsions.

e. Small concentrations of OC insecticides depress mitochondrial respiration, possibly by hindering ion flux across the mitochondrial membrane. Large concentrations of insecticides cause lysis of mitochondrial membranes, uncoupling of oxidative phosphorylation and blockade of electron transport system. It is not clear, if these observations are relevant to brain mitochondria or to neurotoxicity of the insecticides.

f. Many of the organochlorine insecticides have endocrine disrupting properties perhaps by acting as either endogenous hormone mimetics or hormone blockers. DDT is an oestrogen agonist and DDE, its metabolic by-product, is a partial agonist and antagonist on oestrogen receptors. DDE can also act as an anti-androgen by binding to androgen receptors and may disrupt male reproductive development. The endocrine disrupting action is usually seen after a long time of insecticide use and affects primarily the reproductive performance.

g. Organochlorines, in particular diphenyl aliphatic compounds (e.g. DDT and its metabolites), are potent inducers of mixed function oxidases. Induction of microsomal enzymes alters metabolism of several endogenous substances (e.g. hormones) and produce specific adverse effects.

Clinical signs :

Acute toxicity: The clinical signs of acute toxicosis are nearly same in all species, but there are differences in onset, severity and duration of signs in individual animals depending upon the kind and quantity of insecticide involved. Onset of signs may take several minutes to several days, but in most cases first signs appear within 24 hours. Affected animal becomes timid, hypersensitive and apprehensive. Slowly twitching starts first from eyelids, face, and neck and extends to fore parts and then hind parts of body. Animal becomes restless, loses control over movements, staggers, moves in circle, strikes against obstacles or jumps over unseen objects. It often shows abnormal postures, such as resting the sternum on ground while remaining upright in the rear, or keeping the head down between forelegs. Some animals stand with their head pressed against a wall or fence. In advanced stages, intermittent clonic-tonic seizures are seen leading to convulsions (often elicitable by external stimuli) which occur repeatedly with some interval, but later on persistent convulsions, opisthotonos, paddling and clamping of jaws are common. Intense convulsions lead to high rise in body temperature (106° F- 108°F) and respiratory disorders. Affected animals may have intermittent periods of depression or appear almost normal between seizures. Autonomic manifestations such as emesis (in animals that can vomit), profuse frothy salivation, mydriasis, diarrhoea, urination, and bradycardia or tachycardia (depending on agent) may also occur.

Depression may be produced by some OC insecticides (cyclodienes) which may result from rapid depolarizing blockade of neurons of the reticular activating system.

Intoxicated birds may show sudden death, depression, disorientation, abnormal posture and apparent blindness.

Death may occur within minutes, hours or after several days which is due to respiratory failure.

Chronic toxicity: In chronic toxicosis, clinical signs may be similar to those of acute toxicosis, perhaps because of release of stored insecticide from storage in body fat. Severe stress such as starvation, freezing conditions or forced activity is known to cause release of adrenaline from adrenal medulla which initiates lipolysis. If body fat contains large amount of OC insecticide, sufficient amount of it may be released into the blood stream to cause clinical signs of intoxication or even death. In addition to acute nervous signs there may be interrupted oestrus cycle, decreased weight gain, decreased appetite, decreased milk or egg production or reproductive problems. Birds of prey, especially aquatic predators (e.g. bald eagle), exposed to organochlorines may show thinning of egg shells and decreased hatchability.

Post-mortem findings: Lesions of OC insecticide toxicosis are non-specific and unreliable for diagnosis. Animals may show signs of trauma, and carcass may be bruised, lacerated and dirty due to convulsions. Rigor may be prominent. Pale musculature may result after seizures or hyperthermia. Congestion and oedema may be present in several organs. Diffuse endocardial haemorrhage, excessive pericardial fluid and congestion of lungs may be seen. Petechiae on the heart, intestines and lungs and oedema of brain and spinal cord may also be observed. Dogs may have liver necrosis or adrenal gland haemorrhage.

In chronic poisoning, the carcass may be emaciated and devoid of fat and the liver and kidney may manifest degenerative changes.

Diagnosis: If there is a history of recent exposure to an OC insecticide and the clinical signs and lesions are classic as described above, then OC toxicosis may be suspected. For chemical analysis in acute toxicosis, liver, kidney, blood or milk may be taken as these may contain ppm concentrations of OC insecticides. Brain concentrations are better correlated with clinical signs than body fat. In addition, suspected sources, stomach contents, vomitus etc. should be analysed. Adipose tissue or milk fat are the preferred samples to assess residue contamination.

Organochlorine toxicosis should be differentiated from poisonings produced by some other toxicants having similar clinical findings.

a. *Sodium chloride (salt) poisoning:* Common salt can produce similar signs, but the history and absence of high body temperature exclude its poisoning.

b. *Strychnine poisoning:* Strychnine causes convulsions but they are tonic (not clonic) and are not preceded by behavioural aberrations or locomotor defects.

c. *Fluoroacetate poisoning:* Fluoroacetate also produces similar signs but convulsions are not elicitable by external stimuli and become weaker with time.

d. *Anticholinesterase poisoning:* In organophosphorus and carbamate insecticides poisoning, there are no behavioural changes and body temperature is not much elevated or even hypothermia may be seen. Intoxicated animal responds to treatment with atropine.

e. *Lead poisoning:* Lead does not cause abnormal posturing; convulsions are less common and there is usually no fever.

f. *Urea:* In urea poisoning, there is no abnormal posturing or jumping over unseen objects. Urea convulsions are severe and tonic in nature. Colic is an outstanding sign in urea toxicosis but not in OC insecticide poisoning. The odour of ammonia may be detected in the rumen of animals poisoned by urea.

Treatment and management: Organochlorine insecticides toxicosis has no specific treatment. The treatment of acute poisoning should mainly be directed towards checking the convulsions.

a. *CNS depressants:* Use of a sedative in organochlorine poisoning is often essential to control convulsions. Sedatives like benzodiazepines (e.g. diazepam in dogs and cats), xylazine, barbiturates (phenobarbitone or pentobarbitone in dogs, thiobarbitone in cats and pentobarbitone/phenobarbitone in farm animals) and chloral hydrate control most of the behavioural, nervous and locomotor signs. Sedation allows body temperature to subside slowly. Benzodiazepines are considered very useful in poisoning by cyclodiene group of insecticides because these drugs act by increasing the affinity of GABA for the $GABA_A$-receptor, the primary target of cyclodienes. Sedatives may be required for a period of 24-48 hours or, in some cases, for longer period. For prolonged CNS stimulation, the drug of choice is phenobarbitone that may also stimulate microsomal enzymes to shorten the half-life of organochlorine. However, barbiturates should be used with caution as they have narrow safety margins and may depress cardiac and respiratory functions.

Diazepam

Dogs & cats: 0.1 – 0.5 mg/kg, IV (repeated several times).

Cats: 0.3 –1 mg/kg, IM.

Phenobarbitone

Horses & cattle: 3-6 g, IV.

Sheep, goats & pigs: 1-2 g, IV.

Dogs & cats: 2 mg/kg, PO, 2 to 3 times daily.

Xylazine

Dogs & cats: 1 mg/kg, IV.

: 1 – 3 mg/kg, IM (preferred) or SC.

Cattle: 0.05 – 0.3 mg/kg, IM.

Horses: 0.6 – 1 mg/kg, IV.

: 2.2 – 3 mg/kg, IM.

Sheep & goats: 0.05 – 0.1 mg/kg, IV.

: 0.1 – 0.2 mg/kg, IM

Chloral hydrate

Horses & cattle: 40-60 g, orally.

: 30-40 g, I.V.

Sheep & goats: 4-8 g, orally.

: 2-4 g, I.V.

Note: If animal is already in a depressed state, CNS depressants should not be used. CNS stimulants are also contraindicated in depressed state as depression might have occurred due to excessive stimulation of CNS.

b. Calcium borogluconate (large animals, 200-400 ml, I.V.) may be given along with glucose in saline. This treatment prevents liver damage and neutralises effects of preconvulsive hyperkalaemia.

c. Activated charcoal is helpful for GI decontamination. Cholestyramine may be used alternatively to bind these highly lipophilic agents.

d. A saline purgative or gastric lavage may be used to remove the unabsorbed poison. Oily purgatives are contraindicated in OC poisoning as they hasten absorption of insecticides.

e. If exposure is by the dermal route, the animals must be scrubbed gently with soap and water and rinsed thoroughly.

f. Animals should be placed in a comfortable warm area to minimise trauma from seizures.

Prognosis: Prognosis in OC insecticide poisoning is guarded to good, depending on the dosage received and how quickly detoxification is accomplished. Signs of acute toxicosis abate in 1 or 2 days, but complete recovery may take weeks or months.

Public health and environmental concerns: The high lipid solubility and slow elimination of the organochlorine insecticides favour accumulation of residues in the edible tissues of food animals. Immediate sale or consumption of products (milk, butter) from animals that have recovered from toxicosis is not recommended.

The properties of lipophilicity, chemical persistence and induction of microsomal enzymes have led to accumulation of this group of insecticides in domestic animals, wildlife and birds. The persistence of OC insecticides in soil and sediments and contamination of ecosystem lead to their accumulation by organisms of the food chain and upward biomagnification of residues (concentrations in large fish and predators may go up to 100,000 times than in soil or water). Specific toxic effects can be observed which are clearly evident in animals at the top of food chain. Extensive contamination of ecosystem justifies their restricted use or even complete prohibition in some cases.

Some important agents :

a. Dichlorodiphenyltrichloroethane [DDT]: Prior to the placement of major restrictions on its use in many countries, DDT was the best known, least expensive and probably one of the most effective synthetic insecticides. As it is degraded very slowly in the environment and stored in the fat of animals, it is a prime substance for biomagnification. DDE is the principal metabolite of DDT and is the major storage form of the insecticide. This metabolite has low acute toxicity, but possesses chronic toxicity similar to DDT. It is the form that may persist in the world ecosystem for the longest time.

b. Methoxychlor: Methoxychlor is the only insecticide of DDT group which is still in use and is safest among the subgroup (DDT group). The substitution of CH_3O (methoxy) groups for chlorines renders the insecticide biodegradable and environmentally non-persistent. As such, it retains some of the advantages of DDT but without most of its disadvantages. It is stored in adipose tissue to about 0.2% of the extent of DDT, and half-life in rats is only about 2 weeks (DDT = 6 months).

c. Benzene hexachloride (BHC) and Lindane : Benzene hexachloride (BHC) is a mixture of eight isomers and the γ-isomer is often called lindane. Lindane is highly biodegradable and environmentally non-persistent. It is used clinically as ectoparasiticide in dogs (fleas, ticks, sarcoptic mange) and humans (scabies), but now its use is declining.

d. Mirex and Chlordecone : Mirex and chlordecone (Kepone) are extremely persistent OC insecticides and are concentrated several thousand-fold in the food chain. Mirex probably is oxidised to chlordecone.

e. Endosulfan : Endosulfan is one OC insecticide that is not stored in body fat. It is more biodegradable than others of this group (cyclodiene) and is widely used in agriculture.

f. Toxaphene: Toxaphene is not very biodegradable (i.e. slow biotransformation and degradation); it persists in environment and accumulates in biological systems (e.g. food chain of fish, poultry and cattle).

g. Other cyclodiene insecticides: Other important cyclodiene insecticides include aldrin, dieldrin, endrin and heptachlor. There are numerous problems with these cyclodiene insecticides like acute and chronic toxicoses, tumorigenicity, carcinogenicity, persistence in environment, biomagnification, etc. due to which great restrictions have been placed on them in recent years.

II. ORGANOPHOSPHORUS INSECTICIDES

Organophosphorus (OP) compounds are organic esters of phosphorus which have ability to inhibit cholinesterase enzyme. They are used as insecticides, acaricides, soil nematicides, fungicides, herbicides, defoliants, rodenticides, insecticide synergists, insect repellents, chemosterilants and warfare agents. As insecticides, organophosphates are one of the major groups in use at present time. Compared to organochlorines, OPs are much less environmentally persistent, much more biodegradable, less subject to biomagnification, and usually unstable in presence of sunlight. However, compared to organochlorines, they are much more acutely toxic to non-target species and several cases of poisoning frequently occur in man, domestic animals and wild life.

Chemistry: The term 'organophosphorus or organophosphate' is often used as a global synonym or generic name for the entire class of organic compounds containing phosphorus. Strictly speaking, however, organophosphorus compounds are esters of phosphoric, phosphonic, phosphorothioic or related acids. In the structure of organophosphorus insecticides, various atoms like O, S, C, N, halides or CN are attached to phosphorus. Based on these, different classes of OP insecticides have been identified. Most OP insecticides contain a P=S or thionate bond, whereas the remaining others contain a P=O bond. The OP compounds containing thionate (P=S) bond are useful insecticides, but they are inactive as such and require activation to oxon (P=O) form to inhibit acetylcholinesterase enzyme. This oxidative desulphuration can be carried out by chemical, biological or environmental agent. The organophosphorus insecticides containing P=S group are generally called indirect acting compounds and those containing P=O group are called direct acting compounds. Chemical names of organophosphorus pesticides generally contain all or part of the name of the chemical class i.e. "phosphate", "phos", "phoro", "phosphor" or some other derivative of the word phosphorus. This helps in the proper identification of pesticides of this class.

The general structure of OP insecticides is given by the formula given below, where R is an alkyl, aryl, alkoxy, alkylthio or amino group. The X is an acid radical, which may carry various substituents, particularly electron-withdrawing groups. It is called a 'leaving group' because it may leave by disruption of P-X bond when the OP molecule reacts with the hydroxide ion or serine enzymes like acetylcholinesterase (AChE), the primary target of OP insecticides.

$$(R_1)(R_2)P(=O(S))X$$

General formula

Classification

A. Classes Based on chemical structure

S.No.	Class	Structure	Examples
1.	Phosphates and pyrophosphates	$(-O)(-O)P(=O)O-$	Paraoxon, tetraethyl pyrophosphate (TEPP), schraden, dichlorvos
2.	Phosphorothioates	$(-O)(-O)P(=S)O-$	Parathion, fenthion, diazinon, ronnel
3.	Phosphonates	$(-O)(-O)P(=O)C\lessdot$	Trichlorfon
4.	Phosphoramidates	$(-O)(-O)P(=O)N<$	Phospholan, mephospholan
5.	Phosphorothiolates	$(-O)(-O)P(=O)S-$	Echothiophate, profenophos
6.	Phosphorohalides	$(-O)(X)P(=O)F$	Diisoprophyl fluorophosphate (DFP), sarin
7.	Phosphorocyanides	$(-O)(X)P(=O)CN$	Tabun

B. Classes Based on mode of action

1. *Direct acting OP insecticides:* These insecticides contain P=O group, so they directly inhibit cholinesterase enzyme and produce toxicity e.g. TEPP, trichlorfon and dichlorvos.
2. *Indirect acting OP insecticides:* These insecticides are basically phosphorothioates containing P=S groups. Sulphur is not electrophilic so such compounds are inactive as anticholinesterases. These agents require activation to oxon (conversion of P=S moiety to a P =O moiety) in the body, e.g. malathion, parathion and fenthion.

Properties: Organophosphorus insecticides are lipid soluble organic compounds. They are poorly soluble in water and must be used as dusts, wettable powders or emulsions. These compounds are soluble in organic solvents, fats and oils, so they can penetrate into waxy coatings of leaves or fruits or be absorbed directly through skin. The thionate (P=S) type insecticides are generally less polar, more stable, more penetrable to insect cuticle and less toxic to mammals in comparison with their oxon (P=O) analogues. Although OP insecticides exhibit a single mode of action i.e. AChE inhibition, the variety in structure reflects the broad range of their physical, chemical and biological properties. Although most OPs are not very persistent in environment and dissipate in 2-4 weeks, some OPs, such as chlorpyriphos, are sufficiently persistent to be used for control of termites.

Factors affecting toxicity: Toxicity of organophosphorus pesticides is influenced by number of physicochemical and other factors.

a. *Compound:* There is large variation in the toxicity potential of different compounds.

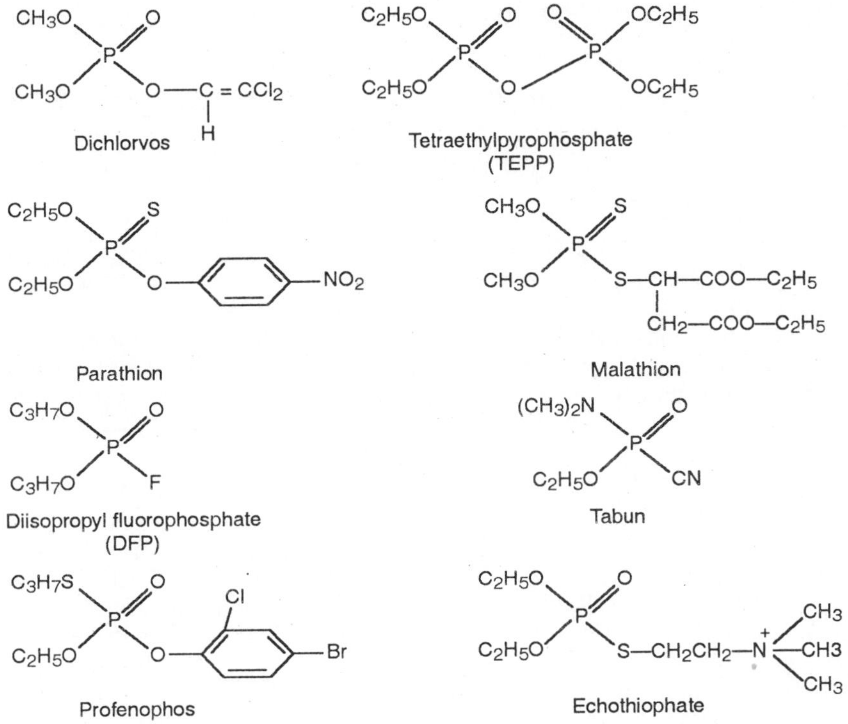

Dichlorvos

Tetraethylpyrophosphate (TEPP)

Parathion

Malathion

Diisopropyl fluorophosphate (DFP)

Tabun

Profenophos

Echothiophate

Fig. 13.2. Chemical structures of some important organophosphorus insecticides.

Some OP compounds are relatively low in toxicity (e.g. tetrachlorvinphos) and others are extremely poisonous (e.g. nerve agents).

b. *Storage:* Storage generally enhances toxicity of most OP compounds due to formation of toxic isomers. Therefore, technical grade organophosphates are often more toxic than the pure compounds. These changes are induced by contamination, heat induced isomerization and pH changes.

c. *Ambient temperature:* High ambient temperature increases toxicity of parathion in mice but low temperature increases toxicity of malathion in rats. Ambient temperature also influences volatility of certain fumigant compounds such as dichlorvos (more toxic at higher temperature).

d. *Species:* There is large species variation in the toxicity of OP insecticides. Some compounds are more toxic in one species while others in another species e.g. cattle is more sensitive than sheep to dimethoate, ronnel, crufamate and phosmet. Cats are highly sensitive to acute OP poisoning. Species differences are mainly due to difference in enzymatic activation or degradation of OP compounds. Suffolk sheep appear to be genetically predisposed to delayed neuropathy of OP compounds.

e. *Age:* Compounds that do not require enzymatic activation (direct acting OPs) are more toxic in young animals due to less development of metabolising enzymes. But agents that require enzymatic activation (indirect acting) are not so toxic in very young animals due to the same reason. Adult hens are highly sensitive to delayed neuropathy and are often used in organophosphate-induced delayed neuropathy (OPIDN) screening, whereas young chickens and probably the young of other species are resistant to OPIDN.

f. *Interaction:* Presence of other compounds can alter OP toxicity due to interactions. Combined effects of two OPs can either

Table 13.2: Oral lethal doses of selected organophosphorus insecticides in different species of animals.

Insecticide	Lethal Dose-50 (mg/kg)						
	Rats	*Dogs*	*Cattle*	*Buffaloes*	*Sheep*	*Goats*	*Chickens*
Malathion	1375-3300	–	500	55	150-200	>1000	150-400
Dichlorvos	50-80	100-300	–	–	–	–	15
Chlorpyriphos	135-160	–	–	50	–	–	–
Fenitrothion	570-740	–	220	435	–	–	280
Chlorfenvinphos	10-40	>12000	–	–	70	70	30
Monocrotophos	18-25	–	–	20	–	20	4
Trichlorfon	450-630	420	–	–	300	100	75
Acephate	600-1000	680	–	800	–	–	570
Ethion	200	–	–	20	–	–	–
Phorate	1.6-3.7	–	–	0.8	–	–	–
Triazophos	64-82	320	–	2.5	–	–	–

be additive/synergistic (malathion plus EPN, coumaphos or trichlorfon; methyl azinphos plus trichlorforn) or antagonistic (malathion plus parathion; EPN plus trichlorfon). Drugs that have neuromuscular blocking properties may enhance OP toxicity or vice versa.

g. *Formulation:* Vehicles that are organic solvents or oils increase OPs toxicity due to better absorption. Vehicles containing a sticking agent can cause pesticides to adhere to animals (dermally).

h. *Impurities:* Impurities in technical grade OP insecticides often increase toxicity. These impurities arise mainly as by-products of OP insecticide synthesis and are known to cause toxic action other than cholinesterase inhibition, several days after exposure to the insecticide (e.g. malathion).

i. *Other factors.* Toxicity of OP compounds decreases due to degradation by sunlight, water, microbes, alkali, or metal ions such as iron or copper.

Toxicity: Organophosphorus insecticides toxicity vary from extremely toxic to slightly toxic in different species of animals e.g. oral LD_{50} in rats varies from 1-5 mg/kg (dimefox) to about 4000 mg/kg (tetrachlorvinphos). In buffaloes, oral-lethal dose varies from 0.8 mg/kg (phorate) to 800 mg/kg (acephate). Most of the OPs have cumulative effect on repeated exposures. The toxic nerve agents (e.g. soman, sarin and tabun) are potent OP compounds, but they are primarily used as warfare agents and not insecticides.

Toxicokinetics: Organophosphorus insecticides are lipid soluble compounds, so they are absorbed from all body surfaces including the gastrointestinal tract, lungs and eyes. After absorption they are distributed rapidly throughout the body but, unlike organochlorine insecticides, do not accumulate in any particular tissue or fat depots. Some agents (e.g. phosphorothioates) require oxidative activation in the liver by microsomal enzymes, which makes OP insecticides more reactive or stronger inhibitor of AChE. Others (e.g. phosphates and phosphorothiolates) can act directly and inhibit cholinesterases immediately upon entry into the blood stream. Some OPs are transformed to quaternary compounds in body (e.g. phosphoramidates) and cannot enter the brain easily.

Organophosphorus compounds undergo a variety of metabolic reactions. In liver and to some extent in other tissues, a variety of enzymes (mainly esterases) may attack the OPs to form water-soluble metabolites which are rapidly excreted in urine. Hydrolysis of the ester linkage in OPs markedly decreases the toxicity. Most OPs are rapidly and nearly completely eliminated so that tissue or blood residues are minimal within few hours of exposure. Chlorinated organophosphates (e.g. chlorpyriphos) are more lipid soluble; therefore their residues persist longer than other OP insecticides.

Mechanism of action :

a. The organophosphorus insecticides owe their toxicity to their ability to inhibit acetylcholinesterase (AChE) enzyme, which is responsible for the hydrolytic degradation of acetylcholine (ACh), the neurotransmitter released at cholinergic synapses of nervous system. The mechanism of AChE inhibition by OP compounds closely resembles the catalytic hydrolysis of ACh but, unlike ACh, OP compounds interact with only the active esteratic site of the enzyme and the enzyme-OP complex formed is extremely stable that does not undergo significant spontaneous hydrolysis (Figure 13.3). Restoration of acetylcholinesterase activity often requires synthesis of new enzyme molecule that may take several weeks. In initial stages, some spontaneous hydrolysis may occur (mostly negligible) or complex can be dissociated with the use of chemical agents called cholinesterase enzyme reactivators like pyridine-2-aldoxime. However once covalent modification of enzyme occurs and the phosphorylated enzyme looses one of its alkyl group (called ageing), it is impossible for chemical reactivators to break the bond between the inhibitor and the enzyme. Ageing is very rapid for nerve gases like soman (ageing half-life 2 minutes), less for DFP (~4 hours) and more (up to 36 hours) for many other organophosphates. The ultimate result of AChE inhibition is accumulation of ACh which causes excessive synaptic neurotransmitter activity in the parasympathetic (cholinergic) nervous system and at neuromuscular (nicotinic) sites.

In addition to acetylcholinesterase enzyme (also called true cholinesterase), OP insecticides inhibit plasma cholinesterase (also called pseudocholinesterase or

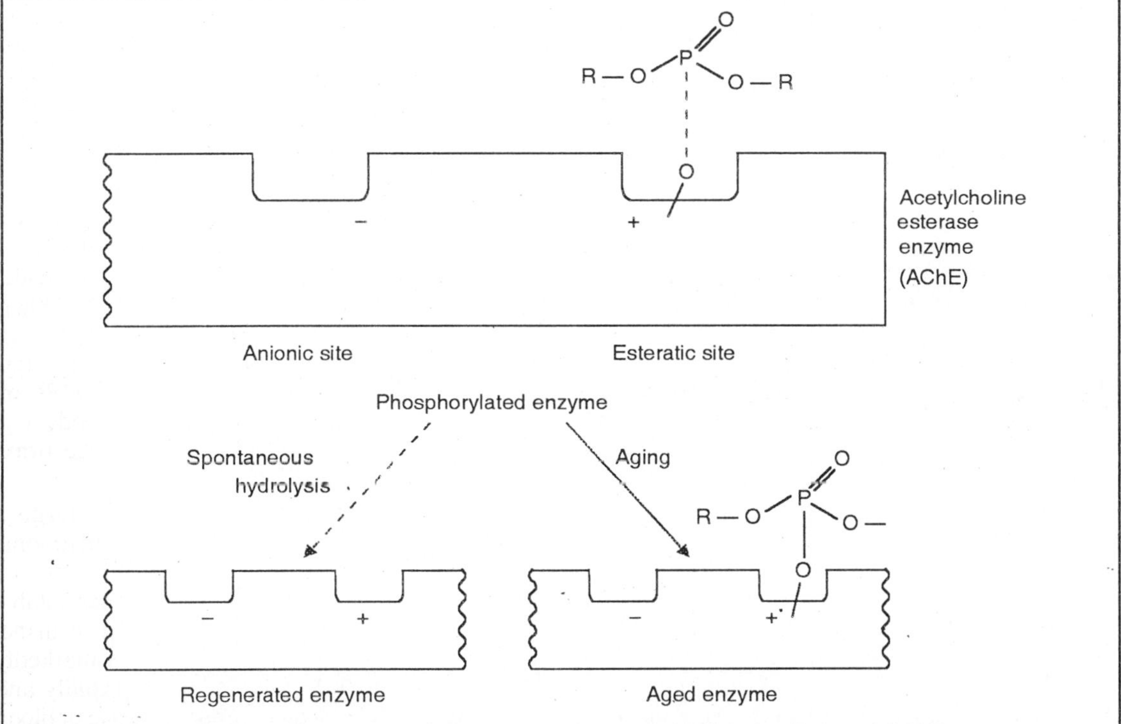

Fig. 13.3. Mechanism of action of organophosphorus insecticides. Phosphorylation of AChE enzyme occurs when organophosphate occupies esteratic site of the enzyme. Spontaneous hydrolysis resulting in regenerated enzyme may occur poorly. When aging occurs (loss of an esterified moiety 'R'), recovery of cholinesterase does not occur due to formation of irreversible stable bonds. This needs synthesis of new enzyme.

butyrylcholinesterase), a non-specific enzyme, and some other esterases with serine residue in their active sites (e.g. neurotoxic esterase). Inhibitions of these non-specific enzymes may interfere with metabolism of a wide variety of esters that occur in plasma, nervous tissue and some other systems in the body.

b. In delayed acute, subacute or chronic toxicity cases, some (not all) OP insecticides also inhibit an enzyme called neuropathy target esterase (NTE) or neurotoxic esterase. This esterase is present in peripheral nerves, lymphocytes, brain, placenta and some other sites. The NTE does not have an identified function in the body, but is thought to facilitate in axonal transport of nutrients. The inhibition of NTE results in demyelination leading to paralysis. This delayed toxic axonopathy is called organophosphorus-induced delayed neuropathy (OPIDN) or dying back axonopathy (so called because it starts at periphery and then goes upward into spinal cord and up into spinocerebellar, vestibulospinal and other tracts). Large diameter fibres appear to be more affected than small diameter fibres. The development of OPIDN does not correlate with inhibition of acetylcholinesterase and is produced only by selected OP insecticides (e.g. fenitrothion, monocrotophos, DFP, haloxon and trichlorfon). This syndrome can result from single or multiple exposures to OP insecticides. Some species are susceptible to OPIDN (e.g. humans, chickens, cats, pigs, cattle, horses, sheep, dogs, rats, and rabbits), whereas some other species are non-susceptible (e.g. mouse, rabbit and guinea-pig).

Clinical signs :

Acute toxicity: Acute toxicity of organophosphates varies widely with type of compound and species of animal. Depending upon the exposure, toxicity may be local or systemic.

Local exposure to vapour, aerosol or inhalation of OPs results in nasal discharge, tightness of chest, wheezing respiration due to bronchoconstriction and increased bronchial secretions. Exposure to eye results in lachrymation, constriction of pupil (miosis) and increased intraocular pressure with conjunctival hyperaemia. Percutaneous application of OP insecticides may result in muscular fasciculation.

In systemic toxicity, acute toxic signs may have quick (few minutes) or delayed onset (few hours) depending upon the type of compound and quantity taken. Initial toxic symptoms include apprehension, hyperexcitation, salivation, lachrymation, frequent urination, serous nasal discharge, broncho-constriction leading to dyspnoea and open mouth breathing, diarrhoea, miosis, excess bronchial secretions, etc. These manifestations are observed due to action of acetylcholine on muscarinic receptors. Signs of nicotinic cholinergic overstimulation appear soon after the onset of muscarinic signs and include muscle fasciculation, tremor, twitching, spasms, hypertonicity causing a stiff gait or rigid stance. Animal falls on ground and shows clonic or clonic-tonic convulsions. Central signs may include ataxia, stimulation followed by depression (due to excessive stimulation), convulsions, loss of reflexes and coma. Death of the animal may occur within few minutes to several hours. Death occurs mainly due to respiratory failure from bronchoconstriction, excessive respiratory secretions, paralysis of respiratory muscles and central depression of respiratory centre in medulla oblongata. Secondary cause of death is bradycardia.

Not all animals manifest all these signs, not all OPs produce the same sequence of signs and not all species react the same way to a given organophosphate.

Neurotoxicity: Single or cumulative doses of some OPs result in OPIDN, which may occur after several days of insecticide administration. The species most sensitive to delayed neurotoxicity are humans, chickens, cats, cattle, sheep, and pigs. Initially there are mild sensory disturbances, ataxia, weakness and muscle twitching which slowly develops into complete flaccid paralysis. The condition could progress to the point that the animal can not stand upright and is unable to eat or drink and dies. This condition is usually irreversible.

Post-mortem findings: Post-mortem lesions of acute OP poisoning are not specific. Lesions are not manifested in animals that die quickly. In animals that take several hours to die, pulmonary oedema and congestion, cyanosis, cerebral oedema, patches of necrosis in skeletal muscle and haemorrhages in heart, skeletal muscle and other organs may occur. The intestinal tract may be dilated and filled with fluid. If death is delayed for several hours or weeks, the carcass is dehydrated and emaciated.

Delayed neuropathy (OPIDN) is characterized as a central-peripheral distal axonopathy. The axon degeneration occurs largely in spinal cord tracts and peripheral nerves in hind limbs. The distal nerves of the peripheral nervous system are affected more severely than proximal fibres and large fibres are affected more than small diameter fibres. Lesions are symmetrical and involve both sensory and motor pathways.

Diagnosis: Diagnosis of acute OP insecticide intoxication is readily made from history, clinical signs and finally estimation of cholinesterase enzyme levels in blood and tissues (brain). Depression of ChE activity in blood (erythrocytes, whole blood or plasma) indicates anticholinesterase (OPI or carbamate) exposure. Clinical manifestations of poisoning are generally observed when 50-70% of cholinesterase activity is inhibited in the body. If blood AChE activity is less than 25% of normal, OP or other anticholinesterase agent exposure may be assumed. Brain cholinesterase is very important in assessing the probability of OP poisoning in dead animals. Desirable response (i.e. dry mouth, mydriasis, and normal/rapid heart rate) to test dose (pre-anaesthetic dose) of atropine remains a valuable diagnostic aid, but it should be supported with a blood AChE determination.

Treatment and management :

Specific therapy : Specific treatment of acute OP insecticide poisoning is available and is aimed to abolish the muscarinic effects due to accumulation of acetylcholine and to regenerate the inactivated AChE enzyme. No effective therapy is recognized for long-term OPIDN.

a. *Atropine sulphate:* Atropine is an antimuscarinic agent that counteracts the effect of excessive ACh at muscarinic receptors at all cholinergic sites. It is a specific and effective antidote to both organophosphorus and carbamate insecticides poisoning and counteracts all muscarinic signs (i.e. bronchoconstriction, salivation, bradycardia). However, it has no effect on nicotinic receptors and hence does not correct nicotinic signs. Atropine has relatively short half-life and requires to be repeated several times on the reappearance of clinical signs. Adequate atropinization exists when the respiratory distress and heart rate appears to become normal. Dilatation of pupil, cessation of salivation and dilation of pupil also indicate atropinization, but these effects are not of concern in survival and should not be taken as therapeutic end point for subsequent atropine administration. Over treatment with atropine should be avoided because it may result in atropine toxicosis i.e. behavioural changes, tachycardia, tachypnoea, excitation, delirium and even death. In horses atropine causes gut stasis, so it is carefully used only in life threatening pulmonary and cardiac effects.

   Dogs & cats: 0.2 – 2 mg/kg, ¼ IV and ¾ IM or SC, followed by same or half dose at 3 to 4 hour intervals by IM or SC until clinical signs subsides.

   Cattle, horses, sheep, goats & swine: 0.2 – 0.5 mg/kg, ¼ IV and ¾ IM or SC, followed by same or half dose at 4-6 hour intervals by IM or SC until clinical signs subside. In horses, atropine is added to IV fluids and administered carefully while auscultating the abdomen; administration is stopped prior to or on reduction of GI sounds.

   Birds: 0.1 – 0.2 mg, IM or SC, as needed.

b. *Cholinesterase reactivators / Oximes*: Several agents are capable of dephosphorylating inhibited acetylcholinesterase enzyme because of their nucleophilic properties and high affinity for phosphorus. The most effective cholinesterase reactivators have a strongly ionisable oxime group (=NOH) and include drugs like pyridine-2-aldoxime (2-PAM), diacetylmonoxime (DAM), monoisonitrosoacetone (MINA), and obidoxime. Early treatment with oximes is essential for positive results because once the phosphorylated enzyme becomes 'aged', it becomes refractory to dephosphorylation by oximes. Oximes should not be used after 24-36 hours of OP poisoning and are generally not recommended in the treatment of overdose of carbamate insecticides. However in case of dermal exposure, oximes may prove useful for several days because some of the topically applied OP compounds accumulate in skin layers or in subcutaneous fat before systemic absorption and hence the enzyme is largely protected from aging. Overdoses of 2-PAM can cause tachycardia and cardiac arrhythmias and DAM can cause excitation.

Pyridine-2-aldoxime (2-PAM)

Dogs & cats: 20 mg/kg, slow IV or IM to be followed by IM or SC, 2 to 3 times daily.

Cattle: 25 – 50 mg/kg, slow IV or infusion, followed by IM route at 8-12 hours intervals.

Horses: 10 - 40 mg/kg, slow IV or infusion.

Diacetylmonoxime (DAM)

Cattle: 30 mg/kg, slow IV, followed by 15 mg/kg, IM at 12 hour intervals for 2 to 3 times.

Supportive therapy

a. Emesis or gastric lavage is indicated if exposure has been less than 4 hours.

b. Activated charcoal is highly effective adsorbent for recent oral exposure of OP pesticides.

c. On dermal exposure, the animal should be washed with soap (or mild detergent) and water and rinsed thoroughly.

d. Oxygen therapy is advised, if cyanosis and dyspnoea are prominent. Assisted ventilation also helps to counteract respiratory acidosis.

e. Nutritional and fluid therapy is indicated, if there is prolonged anorexia.

f. Excessive seizures m[illegible] be controlled with diazepam or barbitur[illegible] sedatives.

Contraindications

Following drugs should not be used in OPs intoxication:

a. Neuromuscular blocking drugs e.g. d-tubocurarine or suxamethonium and gallium triethiodide. These drugs generally precipitate or worsen paralysis of respiratory muscles.

b. Anaesthetics e.g. inhalant anaesthetics, magnesium ions and local anaesthetics (procaine).

c. Atropine in cyanotic cats.

Public health and environmental concerns: Residues in food of animal origin are usually not a problem because OPs are rapidly metabolised and excreted. However, milk from poisoned animals should not be used until analysis indicates no evidence of residue. The excessive use of granular insecticides on lawns or crops may be harmful to wild birds. Pesticide spills and runoff can poison fishes and aquatic animals.

Some important agents :

a. *Malathion:* Malathion is one of the most common types of OP insecticide being used. Mammals have a great ability than insects to detoxify the insecticide by hydrolysis of carboxyl ester group by carboxylesterase enzyme, so it is considered relatively safe for mammals.

b. *Chlorpyriphos:* Chlorpyriphos is a non-systemic OP insecticide with contact, stomach and respiratory action to be used for control of many types of insect pests in agriculture. It is also used for control of household pests including termites.

c. *Coumaphos:* Coumaphos is occasionally used in veterinary medicine for control of nematodes and ectoparasites on cattle. Its toxic manifestations usually appear at twice the therapeutic dose, so is mainly used internally in feed.

d. *Parathion :* Parathion is one of the earliest OPs and is still widely used. It is very effective against large number of insects.

e. *Dichlorvos:* Dichlorvos is a phosphate which is less stable than other OPs and is frequently used on space sprays (e.g. mosquito fogging) and on crops near the harvest time where its quick breakdown poses minimum of residue problems. It is also used as flea collars for pets and as anthelmintic and ectoparasiticide.

f. *Diisopropyl fluorophosphate (DFP):* Diisopropyl fluorophosphate is best known and most extensively studied compound of the class. It is highly potent and lipid soluble compound, so easily penetrates into the CNS. Therapeutically it is sometimes used topically as an instillation into conjunctival sac for treatment of glaucoma.

g. *Tabun, sarin, soman :* Tabun, sarin and soman are nerve gases and are among the most potent synthetic toxic agents known. They are lethal to laboratory animals in submilligram doses.

h. *Echothiophate:* Echothiophate is a quaternary OP compound which interacts with both anionic and esteratic subsites in the active centre to produce a stable complex. It is highly potent and can be stored for several weeks in aqueous solution. It is employed clinically in the treatment of glaucoma.

III. CARBAMATE INSECTICIDES

The carbamate insecticides represent the third major group of synthetic organic insecticides developed after World War II. Carbamate insecticides are widely used in agricultural, veterinary and household practices by virtue of their broad-spectrum of activity, low mammalian toxicity and rapid environmental inactivation. Similar to organophosphorus insecticides, carbamates inhibit cholinesterase enzymes and produce clinical signs of over stimulation of the cholinergic system, but their toxic action as inhibitors of AChE is reversible. Poisoning from carbamate insecticides is common in animals and often indistinguishable from OP insecticides toxicosis.

Chemistry: Carbamates are cyclic or aliphatic derivatives of carbamic acid. These compounds may be viewed as mixed ester-amides. The carbamate functional group, also called urethane, is given below. The R_1 and R_2 attached to the carbamate nitrogen are usually hydrogen and/or methyl; other groups like ethyl, propyl or other short chain alkyls are also found, but they are generally more reactive toward AChE and hence more toxic to target and non-target species. The ester R_3 may be derived from alcohols, phenols, naphthols, oximes, or cyclic hydrocarbon rings. The carbamates are usually not sulphurated.

$$R_3-O-\overset{\overset{\displaystyle O}{\|}}{C}-N\begin{matrix}\diagup R_1\\ \diagdown R_2\end{matrix}$$

Basic Structure

Classification: Based on the chemical structures, carbamate insecticides are categorised into following groups:

1. Naphthyl carbamates e.g. carbaryl (sevin)
2. Phenyl carbamates e.g. propoxur
3. Heterocyclic methyl carbamates e.g. pyrolan and isolan
4. Heterocyclic dimethyl carbamates e.g. carbofuran and furadan.
5. Oximes e.g. aldicarb, methomyl and thiodicarb.

Properties: Carbamate insecticides are similar to organophosphorus insecticides in most of their properties, mode of action, range of toxicity, lack of environmental persistence and lack of safety for beneficial insects and non-target species. Similar to OP compounds, they do not have cumulative properties. However, carbamates differ from OP compounds in following aspects:

a. They are reversible inhibitors of cholinesterase (ChE) enzyme.

b. They inhibit cholinesterase at both anionic and esteratic sites.

c. They are selective inhibitors of cholinesterase enzyme and do not inhibit carboxylesterase enzyme.

d. Decarbamoylation (reactivation) of inhibited ChE enzyme is easier.

e. Cholinesterase enzyme reactivators like 2-PAM are ineffective in the carbamate intoxication.

Toxicity: Carbamate insecticides contain some compounds which are relatively low in toxicity and some which are extremely toxic. Carbaryl, one of the least toxic carbamate (oral LD_{50} in rats = 300-850 mg/kg and in dogs =250-800 mg/kg), may be applied topically in 1-4% aqueous solution as ectoparasiticide, while carbofuran (oral LD_{50} in rats = 5-11 mg/kg and in dogs =19 mg/kg) and aldicarb (oral LD_{50} in rats= 0.6-1 mg/kg and in dogs = 5-10 mg/kg) are more hazardous and should not be sprayed or sprinkled freely on or around animals. Factors that affect toxicity of carbamate pesticides are probably very similar to those affecting toxicity of organophosphates.

Toxicokinetics: Carbamate insecticides are well absorbed from skin, lungs and GI tract and are distributed throughout the body. They do not accumulate in any particular tissue. Blood esterases cause hydrolysis of ester linkage and inactivate a portion of circulating carbamates. Carbamates do not require activation by liver enzymes and

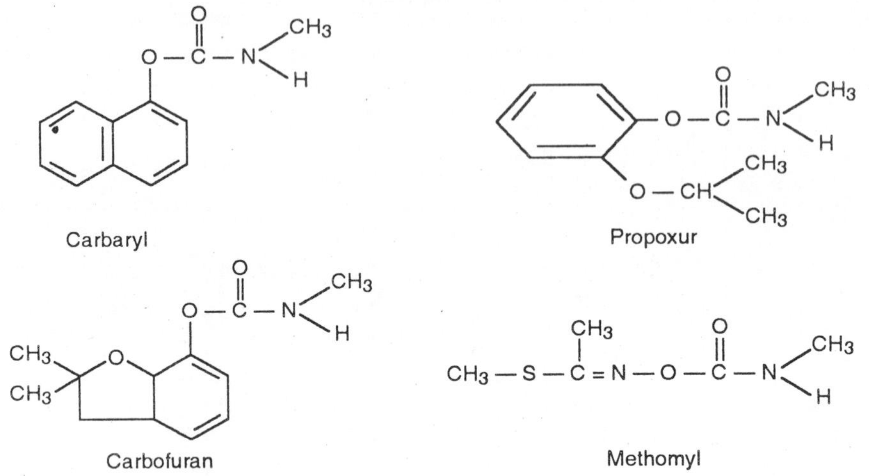

Carbaryl

Propoxur

Carbofuran

Methomyl

Fig. 13.4. Chemical structures of some important carbamate insecticides.

therefore may be more toxic for very young animals. Most of the carbamates are rapidly metabolized and excreted in urine mainly as sulphate of glucuronide conjugates within 24 hours. A small portion is also eliminated in faeces and milk. After carbaryl administration, 80% of dose appears in urine after 24 hours as sulphate or glucuronide conjugate; 0.5% - 15% is excreted in faeces and 0.1 - 1% in milk.

Mechanism of action: The mechanism of action of carbamates closely resembles to that of organophosphorus insecticides. Carbamates inhibit acetylcholinesterase enzyme, but these insecticides occupy both anionic and esteratic sites of AChE. The inhibition in case of carbamates results from a chemical reaction between the carbamoyl moiety of carbamate compound and the active site serine hydroxyl group of AChE to form carbamoylated enzyme rather than phosphorylated as with the organophosphates. Unlike the stable phosphorylated intermediate formed by reaction of AChE with OP compounds, the carbamoylated enzyme is relatively less stable and susceptible to hydrolysis, although rate of hydrolysis is not very fast as with acetylcholine. Therefore the decarbamoylation is easier in comparison to dephosphorylation (OPs). Because of relatively rapid reactivation of carbamoylated AChE, the carbamate insecticides are often called reversible anticholinesterase agents. Toxicosis develops when the amount of carbamate pesticide in the body is so large that the rate of carbamoylation of AChE exceeds the rate of hydrolysis of pesticide by the enzyme.

Clinical signs :

Acute toxicity: Clinical manifestations of acute carbamate intoxication occur primarily due to inactivation of sufficient amount of AChE and subsequent accumulation of ACh in neuromuscular junctions and neural synapses. The excess ACh results in over stimulation of muscarinic and nicotinic receptors of autonomic organs and skeletal muscles as well as cholinergic receptors of the CNS (as discussed in organophosphates). In general the clinical signs produced by carbamate insecticides are similar to those produce by OP insecticides, but the signs are likely to be less severe and/or much shorter in duration.

Chronic toxicity: The chronic carbamate toxicity produces signs of neuromuscular type, which are characterised by incoordination, ataxia, recumbency and prostration. Carbamates may also produce teratogenic effects but, unlike OPs, there are no signs of delayed neuropathy or demyelination of nerves.

Post-mortem findings: Lesions of carbamate poisoning are non-specific. The post–mortem findings are in general similar to that of organophosphates intoxication.

Diagnosis: Diagnosis of carbamate poisoning is made from history, clinical signs and response to atropine therapy. As clinical signs of carbamate intoxication resembles those of OPs, so it is difficult to differentiate the two poisonings from each other. It is also difficult to diagnose carbamate poisoning merely from AChE depression because inhibition of AChE resulting from carbamate poisoning is labile and the enzyme activity often spontaneously returns to normal. Also, carbamates are rapidly metabolised in the body, so they may not be detected in tissues, body secretions or blood. Testing blood or homogenized brain tissue for cholinesterase activity at several times before and during a period of laboratory incubation may provide some information on the type of poisoning. In case of OP toxicosis there is minimal or no change in the levels of inhibited cholinesterase enzyme (no reactivation), but in carbamate poisoning the enzyme level may recover to almost normal (or less than normal) due to substantial regeneration of activity.

Treatment and management :

Specific therapy

a. Antimuscarinic drug atropine sulphate is the specific agent in acute carbamate toxicosis. Atropine is administered in a similar manner and in same dosage schedule as that in case of OP insecticide toxicity. Atropinization should be maintained for 1-2 days and atropine is repeated on reappearance of toxic signs.

Supportive therapy : Supportive therapy may be given depending upon the condition of the animal as discussed in organophosphorus insecticides.

Contraindications : Cholinesterase enzyme reactivators like 2-PAM and DAM should not be used in carbamate poisoning. These drugs are not effective as they do not get binding site on the cholinesterase enzyme (both anionic and esteratic sites are occupied by carbamate insecticide). They may worsen the animal's condition as they themselves block the free cholinesterase enzyme to some extent.

Prognosis: The prognosis is generally good if treatment is instituted soon after onset of clinical signs. Animals may even survive without treatment if clinical signs are not severe because carbamates are metabolised very quickly.

Public health and environmental concerns: Public health and environmental concerns are similar to OP insecticides.

Some important agents :

a. Carbaryl: Carbaryl (Sevin) is a broad-spectrum insecticide of fairly low toxicity in mammals. It is a contact and stomach insecticide and is used for the control of chewing and sucking insects in a number of crops. It is also used as an ectoparasiticide in animals.

b. Carbofuran: Carbofuran is extensively used as a soil insecticide, where it has replaced cyclodienes for the control of seed-eating pests of grain crops. It is highly toxic to mammals as well as to insects.

c. Propoxur: Propoxur is a carbamate of moderate mammalian toxicity. It is used to control house-hold insects such as cockroaches, bedbugs and wasps. It is also used as a replacement of DDT for malaria control and is applied against a number of food storage, vegetable and ornamental pests.

d. Aldicarb: Aldicarb belongs to oxime carbamates which are the most recent members of this group of insecticides. Aldicarb is a plant systemic insecticide which is probably the most toxic insecticide to mammals (oral LD_{50} in rats <1 mg/kg). Its high toxicity to mammals has limited its usefulness.

e. Methomyl: It is a broad-spectrum oxime carbamate which is highly effective against many plant feeding insects and also has high ovicidal activity.

IV. PYRETHRIN AND PYRETHROID INSECTICIDES

Pyrethrins (also called pyrethrums) are natural insecticides produced from extracts of pyrethrum flowers (genus *Chrysanthemum*) and pyrethroids are their synthetic analogous. Pyrethrins possess significant insecticidal properties and still retain a useful role, but they have largely been surpassed by synthetic pyrethroids. Due to rapid degradation and non-persistence in environment, pyrethroids are among the most widely used group of insecticides nowadays. Intoxication of animals usually occurs due to their excessive use on animals as ectoparasiticide or due to accidental ingestion.

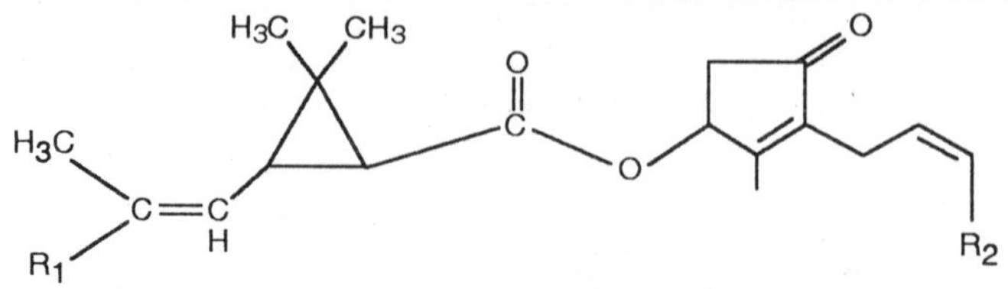

General Structure

Esters	R_1	R_2	Name
Pyrethrin I	$-CH_3$	$-CH=CH_2$	Pyrethrins I
Cinerin I	$-CH_3$	$-CH_2-CH_3$	
Jasmolin I	$-CH_3$	$-CH_3$	
Pyrethrin II	$-CO-O-CH_3$	$-CH=CH_2$	Pyrethrins II
Cinerin II	$-CO-O-CH_3$	$-CH_2-CH_3$	
Jasmolin II	$-CO-O-CH_3$	$-CH_3$	

Fig. 13.5. General structure of pyrethroids and naturally occuring pyrithrins.

Agricultural use rarely results in residues or toxicosis.

Chemistry: Most of the pyrethroids are ester of carboxylic acid. Natural pyrethrins have six insecticidally active components or esters viz. Pyrethrin I, Cinerin I, and Jasmolin I which are called pyrethrins I, and Pyrethrin II, Cinerin II, and Jasmolin II that together are called pyrethrins II. These are formed by substitution at R_1 and R_2 in the general structure. The active ingredient content of commercial pyrethrin products is expressed in terms of pyrethrin I and pyrethrin II.

Structure of synthetic pyrethroids range from very similar to natural pyrethrins (e.g. allethrin) to highly dissimilar compounds (e.g. flucythrinate). They comprise different numbers of asymmetric carbon atoms (chiral centres), which allow large number of stereoisomers to exist. Several synthetic pyrethroids contain halogen atoms.

Classification: Pyrethroids have been classified in a number of ways based on their chemical structure, physicochemical property, stereochemical configuration, history (generation), and biological activity. The most common classification used in toxicology is based on the clinical signs and structure and it comprises of 2 main groups – Type I and type II pyrethroids.

a. Type I or Non-cyano pyrethroids : These pyrethroids resemble natural pyrethrins in their structure and activity and are relatively less toxic to mammals e.g. pyrethrin, allethrin, bioallethrin, bioresmethrin, phenothrin and permethrin.

b. Type II or Cyano-pyrethroids: These pyrethroids contain an α-cyano group in their structure and are comparatively more active and more toxic to mammals than the natural pyrethrins or Type I agents e.g. deltamethrin, cypermethrin, fenvalerate, flucythrin, and flucythrinate.

Properties: Resembling the organochlorine insecticides, all pyrethroids are nonpolar compounds with very low water solubility. They have high potency, wide efficacy and relatively low mammalian toxicity. They are easily biodegradable and pose no serious residue problems. Pyrethroids are used in numerous formulations including aerosols, sprays, dusts, tags, dips, and shampoos. Some commercial formulations include additional insecticides and/or synergists to widen the spectrum of activity.

Factors affecting toxicity

a. Toxicity of pyrethroids varies with the type of species involved. They are highly toxic to arthropods, followed by fish, birds and least toxic to mammals. Fish are often extremely sensitive to pyrethroids.

b. In general, type I pyrethroids are less toxic than type II pyrethroids. Toxicity of a

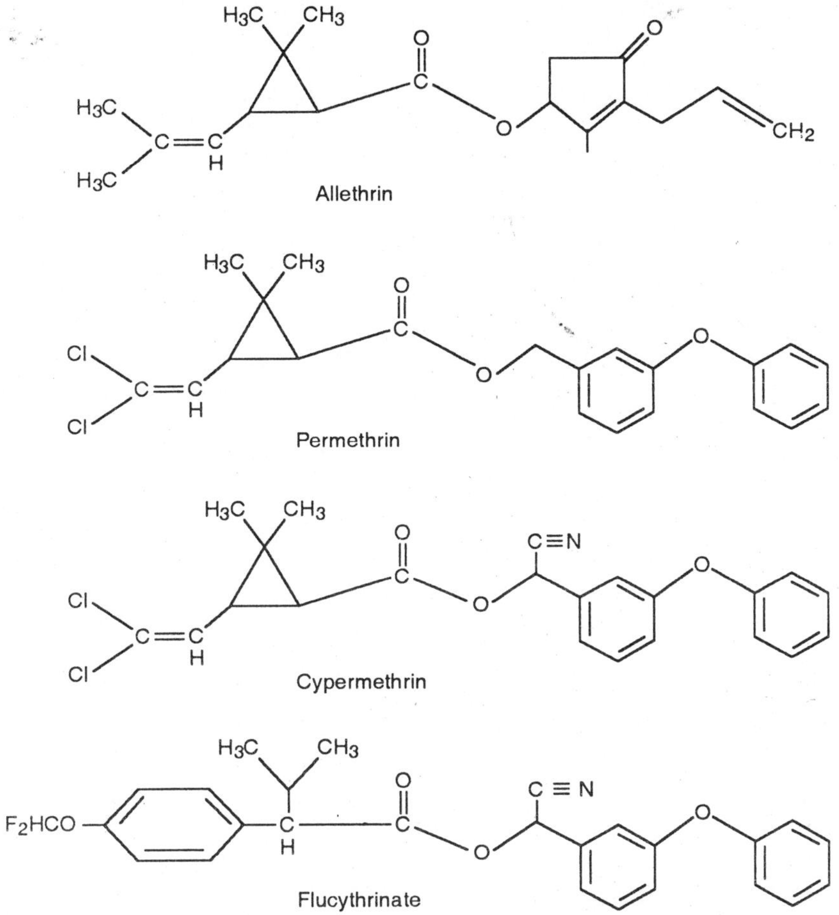

Allethrin

Permethrin

Cypermethrin

Flucythrinate

Fig. 13.6. Chemical structures of some important pyrethroid insecticides.

pyrethroid compound depends also on the number of halogens present in its structure i.e. more the number of halogens in a pyrethroid structure, more toxic it will be.

c. Toxicity of a pyrethroid insecticide is less by oral route than by parenteral route. Dermal toxicity is variable depending upon the compound.

d. Pyrethroids are usually less toxic by single exposure as compared to repeated doses.

e. Females are more susceptible to pyrethroid toxicity than males.

f. Toxicity of pyrethroids increases as the ambient temperature decreases and vice versa (–ve temperature coefficient).

Toxicity: The toxicity of synthetic pyrethroids varies with the specific compound and route of exposure. The natural and synthetic pyrethroids are relatively safe for mammals and other non-target species but are extremely toxic to arthropods. Pyrethroids show considerable selectivity for insects as compared to mammals with LD_{50} selectivity ratio (rat oral compared to insect topical application) of 4500 : 1. However, the introduction of some new pyrethroids, especially the α-cyano pyrethroids, has changed the selectivity, toxicity and/or type and site of action. Oral acute toxicity of pyrethroids varies from low toxicity (bioresmethrin, rat oral LD_{50} 8000 mg/kg) to high toxicity (fenproponate, rat oral LD_{50} 28 mg/kg). The oral lethal dose of cypermethrin in buffalo is 80 mg/kg. The potential for secondary toxicity is very limited because of the low acute toxicity and rapid detoxification of pyrethroids.

Toxicokinetics: After oral exposure, absorption of pyrethroids from gut is incomplete, with tendency of these lipophilic molecules to remain in the organic solvent or oil used in formulation. Pyrethroids also adsorb to other organic matters in the GI tract and are excreted largely unchanged in faeces. Rapid hydrolysis of ester linkage in digestive tract also allows low absorption and toxicity of some pyrethroids. Absorption from lungs after inhalation of dust or aerosol droplets may be good due to high lipid solubility of pyrethroids. Dermal exposure allows variable, but slow absorption due to incomplete penetration of skin and also due to local metabolic destruction of some pyrethroids in the skin. In case of severe contamination of skin, pyrethroids are continuously absorbed for several weeks, possibly due to a reservoir of insecticide bound to the epidermis.

After absorption, pyrethroids rapidly distribute through the body. Their high lipid solubility allows ready entry into the brain. Most pyrethroids are rapidly and extensively metabolised in the body, so their toxicity is relatively less. Rate of metabolism also determines their toxicity in a species as metabolites generally have low toxicity. During metabolism, plasma and liver esterases rapidly hydrolyse the ester linkage of the insecticide. Liver microsomal enzymes are also involved in rapid degradation of pyrethroids. Metabolites are usually conjugated with glycine, glucuronic acid or sulphates and are excreted in urine. There is little or no accumulation of pyrethroids in body tissues.

Mechanism of action: Pyrethroids, like other major classes of insecticides, interfere with the functions of nervous system and produce hyperexcitability. Many different mechanisms of action have been proposed for the pyrethroids, but their interaction with sodium channels in nervous system appears to be the primary action.

a. Like organochlorine insecticides, pyrethroids are non-specific stimulant to CNS and interact primarily with sodium channels. The sodium channels in the nervous system are highly sensitive to pyrethroids, especially to type II compounds which produce effects at very low concentrations. Pyrethrins and Type I pyrethroids interfere with axonal sodium gating to produce enhanced inward sodium flow and suppressed potassium outflow resulting in a delayed repolarization, decreased amplitude of action potential and repetitive discharges of nerve membranes. The Type II pyrethroids also interact with sodium channels and have the effect of slowing of inactivation of sodium channels. However, they can extend the time constant for sodium current inactivation by many milliseconds to seconds and are able to cause a persistent depolarization. The slower rate of inactivation of pyrethroid-modified sodium channels also generates a prolonged depolarizing 'tail' current that follows the normal action potential. The tail current can trigger a second action potential when depolarized even slightly; hence a single action potential can become converted into a train of abnormal discharges. These actions of Type II pyrethroids produce repetitive firing of sensory end organs and muscle fibres leading to a stable hyper-excitable state (Figure 13.7).

b. Type II pyrethroids are also believed to have an inhibitory effect on the voltage-dependent chloride channels in the brain, nerves, muscles and salivary gland. They interfere with the binding of GABA with its receptor sites and inhibit GABA-gated chloride channels in the nervous system. The pyrethroid induced decrease in chloride channel current in nervous system serves to increase excitability and therefore would synergise pyrethroid action on sodium channels. Pyrethroid action on voltage-gated chloride channels in muscle and salivary gland plays a major role in the generation of myotonia and salivation.

c. Pyrethrins and pyrethroids inhibit various adenosine triphosphatases including the Ca^{++}-ATPase and Ca^{++}/Mg^{++}-ATPase in nervous systems. These actions may affect the cation conductance at axonal membranes.

d. Pyrethroids are reported to produce several other biochemical changes in the nervous system. These include marked increase in cerebellar cyclic GMP and changes in the concentration of several neurotransmitters.

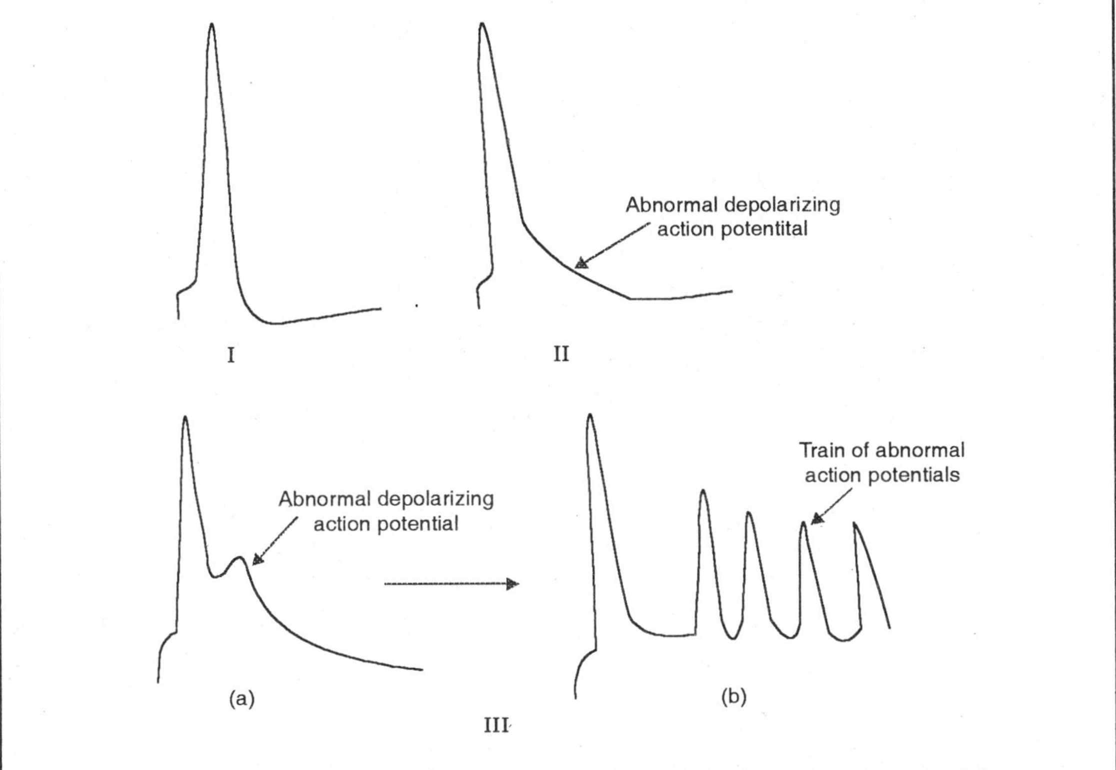

Fig. 13.7. Effect of Type I and Type II pyrethroids on skeletal muscle action potential.

I : Normal action potential in absence of pyrethroid insecticide.

II : Type II pyrethroid develops a short abnormal depolarizing action potential after the normal action potential spike.

III : Type II pyrethroid develops a long abnormal depolarizing action potential at the end of the normal action potential spike (a). When large enough, this abnormal depolarization causes a train of abnormal action potentials to follow the normal one (b).

These biochemical changes appear to be secondary to the increased motor activity produced by pyrethroid intoxication.

Clinical signs :

Acute toxicity: Clinical signs of acute pyrethroids intoxication may appear within minutes to few hours of oral exposure; however the onset may be significantly delayed after topical exposure due to slow dermal absorption. Pyrethroids are classified into Type I and Type II on the basis of clinical signs in rats. Type I pyrethroids in rats produce restlessness, incoordination, hyperactivity, sensitivity to external stimuli, fine tremors progressing to gross whole body tremors, hyperthermia, etc. Type II insecticides produce CS (choreoathetosis and salivation) syndrome in rats characterised by pawing and burrowing behaviour, salivation, coarse tremors progressing to sinuous writhing (choreoathetosis) and clonic seizures. They produce a pronounced convulsive phase with decline in body temperature.

In small and large animals, the clinical signs are usually similar for both types of pyrethroids. In dogs and cats, clinical signs may include hypersalivation, vomiting, diarrhoea, mild tremors, hyperexcitability, seizures or depression, dyspnoea and death. In cattle and buffaloes, Type II pyrethroids produce incoordination, staggering gait, salivation, mucoid nasal discharge, regurgitation of ruminal contents, and diarrhoea. More severely affected animals can have hyperthermia or hypothermia, dyspnoea, open mouth breathing, severe tremors, recumbency, seizures or CNS depression (due to excessive excitation), paralysis and coma. Death may occur within 24-72 hr due to respiratory failure.

Dermal toxicosis may produce allergic reactions i.e. dermatitis, burning and itching sensation in skin, and blister formation.

Chronic toxicity: In long-term oral exposure, most synthetic pyrethroids are considered non-hazardous to experimental or domestic animals. No carcinogenic, mutagenic or teratogenic effect has been observed. Some pyrethroids are known to induce microsomal enzymes and suppress immune systems. In birds deltamethrin has shown some embryotoxicity.

Post-mortem findings: Gross lesions of pyrethroid poisoning are not specific and are not usually associated with clinical toxicosis. Hepatic and renal degeneration may be observed.

Diagnosis: Diagnosis of pyrethroid insecticide intoxication is made from history and clinical signs. The presence of pyrethrins and pyrethroids or their metabolites in blood or tissues suggest exposure, however, a confirmatory diagnosis is difficult because confirmatory concentrations of most pyrethroids in tissues are not well established and also because the tissue levels are not well-correlated with the severity of signs or death. Generally brain and liver tissues are taken for analysis.

Differential diagnosis is made from organochlorine insecticides, OP and carbamate insecticides, strychnine, and nicotine poisonings. Diseases and conditions like pseudorabies and meningitis also produce clinical signs similar to pyrethroid intoxication.

Treatment and management: There is no specific treatment for pyrethroid poisoning at present. Only symptomatic and supportive therapy is recommended.

a. *Sedative:* Seizures can be controlled with sedatives such as diazepam, barbiturates or chloral hydrate. Clinical usefulness and dosage of CNS depressants are the same as discussed earlier for organochlorine poisoning.

b. *CNS muscle relaxants:* CNS muscle relaxants like methocarbamol have been found useful in pyrethroid insecticide poisoning. They decrease muscle hyperactivity by selective action in the cerebro-spinal axis. Methocarbamol also produces generalized CNS depressant effect, which is useful in hyper-excitation.

   Methocarbamol: 50-220 mg/kg, I.V., not exceeding 200 mg/min.

c. Atropine can be used sparingly to alleviate excessive salivation or gastrointestinal motility.

d. Emetics or gastric lavage can be used to empty the stomach, if exposure is recent (within 4 hours) and there is no seizure.

e. Cathartics like saline purgatives or sorbitol can be used.

f. Activated charcoal is used to reduce oral absorption of pyrethroids.

g. Animal should be bathed with soap or detergent and water, if exposure is dermal.

h. Increasing the ambient temperature may be a life saving measure as it decreases toxicity.

Contraindications

a. Oil and fats promote the intestinal absorption of insecticides so these should be avoided.

b. Phenothiazine tranquilizers are contraindicated in pyrethroid toxicosis.

Prognosis: Prognosis of pyrethroid poisoning is generally good unless exposure is massive or the animal is otherwise compromised.

Public health and environmental concerns: Human and animals exposure to pyrethroids generally occurs through careless use, as these products are considered quite safe. Residues in foods of animal origin are not likely because of rapid metabolism and excretion of pyrethrins and pyrethroids. Improper disposal can contaminate aquatic environment. Fish and some birds are very sensitive to pyrethroids.

Some important agents :

a. *Pyrethrins:* Pyrethrins are a group of closely related, naturally occurring compounds which are active insecticidal ingredients of pyrethrum. Synergists, such as piperonyl butoxide, sesamex, piperonyl cyclonene, etc. are added to increase their stability and effectiveness. By inhibiting MFOs, the synergists also potentiate mammalian toxicity.

b. *Allethrin:* Allethrin was the first commercially available pyrethroid, still in use today. It belongs to group I (non-cyano) of synthetic pyrethroids and structurally resembles natural pyrethrins. It is commonly used for repelling insects e.g. mosquitoes (available as anti-mosquito mats).

c. *Deltamethrin:* Deltamethrin is a broad spectrum synthetic pyrethroid having stomach and contact actions and is widely used in agriculture against large number of pests. It is extensively used as an ectoparasiticide in farm and companion animals against flies, fleas, ticks, mites, etc. It is available in the form of dip, spray, wash and pour-on formulations.

d. *Fenvalerate:* Fenvalerate belongs to group II compounds of pyrethroids having broad spectrum biocidal activities. In addition to crops, it is also used on non-crop lands (forests, parks, recreational areas) and to control ectoparasites in domestic animals.

e. *Cypermethrin:* Cypermethrin is a broad-spectrum highly potent biocide with wide use against large varieties of household and agricultural pests. It is widely used as ectoparasiticide in farm and companion animals against ticks, lice and biting flies and has application in slaughter houses and food storage rooms.

f. *Alphamethrin:* Alphamethrin is a highly potent, broad spectrum synthetic pyrethroid insecticide. In addition to its use on crops, it is capable of controlling nuisance organisms such as spiders, lizards, houseflies, cockroaches, etc.

V. FORMAMIDINE INSECTICIDES

The formamidines (amidines) are a novel group of compounds with insecticide-acaricide action. Formamidines are the first pest control chemicals that have shown to exert useful effects through actions on biogenic amine systems mainly on adrenergic and octopaminergic neurotransmission. Amitraz is the most widely used formamidine insecticide.

Amitraz

Amitraz is a formamidine pesticide that is widely used as insecticide and acaricide in agricultural and veterinary practices. It is active against all forms of worms i.e. eggs, larvae and adults. In veterinary medicine, it used as topical miticide in flea collars and for ectoparasite control in animals e.g. against ticks affecting cattle and sheep and against mange mites in variety of species. Animals are exposed to harmful effects when amitraz is used carelessly as a spray or dip or when dogs eat flea collars. It is usually not used as ectoparasiticide in horses due to increased incidence of toxicity.

Chemistry and properties: Chemically amitraz is N-methylbis (2, 4-xylyliminomethyl) amine. It is sparingly soluble in water but soluble in most organic solvents. Amitraz is formulated mainly as dips and flea collars for use as ectoparasiticide.

Toxicity: Toxicity of amitraz depends on the type of formulation and species involved. Incidence of toxicity is common in dogs and cats. Cats and puppies up to 3-4 months old seem to be especially sensitive to amitraz. Its acute oral LD_{50} is 100 mg/kg for dogs, >100 mg/kg for rabbits, 400-800 mg/kg for guinea pigs, 800 mg/kg for rats, and >1600 mg/kg for mice. Its use in horses is prohibited. Amitraz is slightly toxic to birds and moderately toxic to fish.

Toxicokinetics: Amitraz is poorly absorbed when applied topically to the skin. However after oral exposure, amitraz is rapidly and extensively absorbed from GI tract. Once in blood, amitraz is widely distributed in body and concentrated mainly in liver, skin, eyes, bile, kidneys, brain, lungs, spleen and gonads. It is metabolised to an inactive metabolite 4-amino-3-methylbenzoic acid which is excreted in urine and to lesser extent in bile.

Mechanism of action: Toxicity of amitraz in mammalian species is produced in part by stimulation of alpha$_2$-adrenoceptors and inhibition of monoamine oxidase (MAO) enzyme. Stimulation of alpha$_2$-adrenoceptors in CNS results in lethargy and CNS depressant effect and inhibition of MAO enzyme alters metabolism of neurotransmitter amines present in the

H_3C—C_6H_3(CH_3)—N=CH—N(CH_3)—CH=N—C_6H_3(CH_3)—CH_3

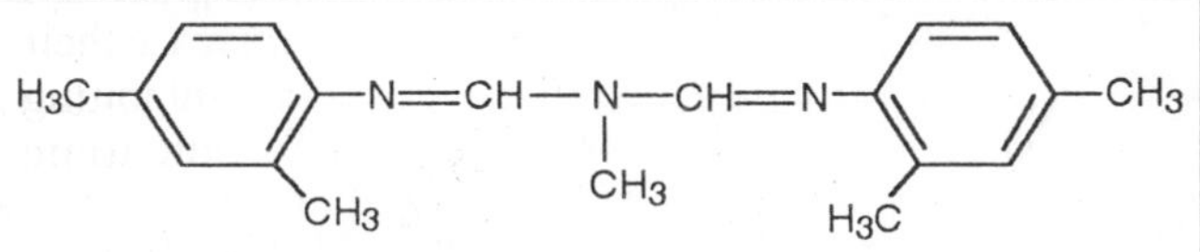

Fig. 13.8. Chemical structure of amitraz.

nervous system. It is also possesses other effects including prostaglandin E_2 (PGE_2) synthesis inhibition, but its role in amitraz poisoning is not clear. The central nervous system and cardiovascular system are the main target tissues of amitraz resulting in cardiovascular collapse and respiratory depression.

Clinical signs :

Acute toxicity: Acute toxicity of amitraz produces predominant CNS depression in domestic animals. Important signs in various species include sedation, incoordination, ataxia, disorientation, anorexia, vomiting, diarrhoea or constipation, decreased pulse rate, and hypothermia. In dogs and cats, additional signs may include abdominal distension, abnormal response to light, mydriasis, ataxia, muscular weakness, hypotension, and hyperglycaemia. Horses are more susceptible to amitraz poisoning with manifestations of anorexia, congestion of mucous membranes, ataxia, intestinal stasis and constipation, colic, dullness, generalized weakness, sweating, trembling and tremors. The intestinal stasis in horses often progresses to impaction colic; for this reason amitraz is not approved for use in equines. Amitraz toxicity can be significant if insecticide is ingested.

Topical application of amitraz in most species may produce only transient sedation. However in horses, even dermal application may produce different signs such as depression, ataxia, muscular incoordination, impaction, colic and swelling on face.

Chronic toxicity: Chronic toxicity of amitraz has not been well described in domestic animals. In an experimental study, anorexia, sedation, listlessness, intermittent diarrhoea, moderate to acute swelling of hock joints and jowl have been reported in cattle. Opacity of eyes in some animals is also associated with chronic amitraz exposure.

Post-mortem findings: The lesions of amitraz poisoning are non-specific. The size and weight of the liver may increase. Repeated exposures may produce hepatic periportal hyperplasia and thinning of adrenal zonae fasciculata and reticularis.

Diagnosis: Diagnosis of amitraz poisoning is made from history of exposure and clinical signs. Gas chromatography can detect and quantitate amitraz. For this purpose, samples may be taken from liver, kidneys, skin, brain, lungs, adipose tissue or spleen.

Treatment and management :

Specific therapy

a. *Alpha$_2$-adrenoceptor antagonists:* Acute toxicity of amitraz is treated by using a specific α_2-adrenoceptor antagonist such as yohimbine or atipamezole. These agents competitively block alpha$_2$-adrenoceptors in the CNS and periphery and reverse the adverse effects (i.e. sedation, GI hypomotility, bradycardia, and hypotension) of amitraz.

Atipamezole

All species: 50 μg/kg, IM.

Yohimbine

Dogs: 0.1 mg/kg, slow IV.

Cattle: 0.125 mg/kg, slow IV.

Supportive therapy

a. Emetics should be used to remove the recently ingested amitraz.

b. Activated charcoal and saline cathartics may be administered to remove the insecticide from gut.

c. Skin should be thoroughly washed with liquid detergents to remove excess amitraz in case of dermal exposure.

d. Intravenous fluids should be administered to hypotensive animals. However, fluids should not be used in case of marked bradycardia or hypertension.

Prognosis: Prognosis of amitraz toxicosis is good, provided the treatment is done timely. Mildly affected animals may recover spontaneously.

Public health concern: Residues of amitraz in foods of animal origin are unlikely because of its rapid metabolism. Labelled instructions should be followed to avoid potential residue problems.

VI. NEONICOTINOID INSECTICIDES

Neonecotinoids are a novel group of insecticides with action different from conventionally used synthetic insecticides. This group of pesticides are also referred to as 'chloronicotinyls' to emphasize the importance of chlorine atom for insecticidal potency. They possess broad spectrum of activity against insect pests, but are not very toxic to vertebrates. Neonicotinoids are widely used in crop protection and some like imidacloprid are used against animal ectoparasites.

Imidacloprid

Imidacloprid is the principal representative of neonicotinoid insecticides. It was introduced in market in 1992 for use in agriculture and is now used frequently in small animal medicine against ectoparasites on dogs and cats. It is commercially available as dustable powder, granules, suspension, emulsion, and tablet for agricultural use and as flea collar for use in small animals. It has low toxicity to mammals and incidence of poisoning in domestic animals is less reported.

Chemistry: The chemical name of imidacloprid is 1-[(6-chloro-3-pyridinyl) methyl]-N-nitro-2-imidazolidinimine.

Toxicity: Imidacloprid exhibits mild to moderate acute oral toxicity to mammals. Its oral LD_{50} value is approximately 450 mg/kg in rats and 150 mg/kg in mice. Dermal LD_{50} value for rats is >5000 mg/kg. The acute toxicity of imidacloprid varies widely among bird species. It is highly toxic to certain species including house sparrow, Japanese quails, canaries and pigeons. The oral acute LD_{50} in different bird species is: chickens and pigeons 150 mg/kg, Japanese quail 31 mg/kg, and bobwhite quail 152 mg/kg. Imidacloprid is mild to moderately toxic to adult fish with juvenile fish being considerably more susceptible.

Toxicokinetics: The toxicokinetic data on imidacloprid in domestic animals is limited. In rats, imidacloprid is rapidly and almost completely (>92%) absorbed from GI tract following oral administration. After absorption it is distributed to all organs within 1 hour with highest concentration in liver, kidneys and lungs. However, it is not distributed to body fat and brain due to poor penetration through blood-brain barrier. It is metabolised in liver to inactive metabolites and eliminated rapidly and almost completely in urine (70-80%) and remainder in faeces. There are no indications of bioaccumulation of imidacloprid in body.

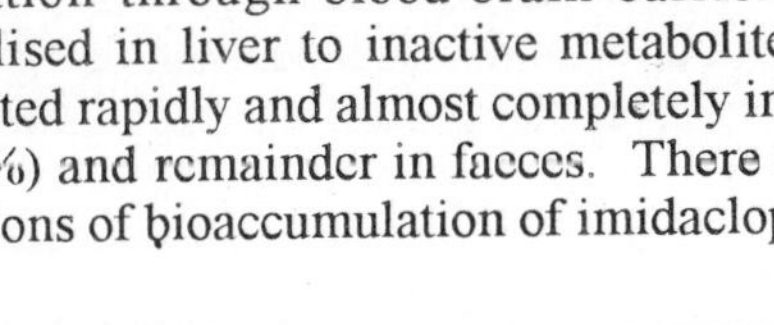

Fig. 13.9. Chemical structure of imidacloprid.

Mechanism of action: Imidacloprid acts and binds selectively to nicotinic cholinergic receptors on the post-synaptic membrane. This leads to disruption in the cholinergic neurotransmission causing nervous impairment and neuromuscular disturbance. The nicotinic receptors of mammals are less sensitive to imidacloprid than are insect receptors; therefore mammals are less susceptible to insecticide toxicity than insect pests.

Clinical signs: The clinical manifestations of acute toxicity of imidacloprid are related to nicotinic stimulation in nervous and neuromuscular systems. Clinical signs in animals include twitching of muscles, tremors, incoordination, and behavioural changes. Transient salivation may occur if animal licks the application site immediately after ectoparasiticide treatment. Eye/skin irritation and skin sensitization is generally not seen. In birds, imidacloprid causes transitory gastrointestinal distress (retching), ataxia, and abnormal behaviour such as lack of coordination, lack of responsiveness and an inability to fly.

The long-term imidacloprid toxicity produces reduction in body weight and food consumption and increased thyroid lesions in animals. It also has ability to cause eggshell thinning, reduced egg production and hatching problem in birds. Induction of hepatic microsomal enzymes has been reported following exposure to imidacloprid which may alter metabolism of several endogenous and exogenous substances. Imidacloprid is not mutagenic or carcinogenic.

Post mortem findings: Lesions of imidacloprid toxicosis are not specific. Slight hepatocellular hypertrophy and necrosis, and increase in liver weight may be found in some cases.

Diagnosis: Imidacloprid intoxication may be diagnosed from history and clinical signs.

Treatment and management: There is no specific treatment to imidacloprid poisoning. Intoxicated animals should be treated with symptomatic and supportive therapy. Emetics or activated charcoal and saline purgative may be administered to remove excess of insecticide from GI tract.

Prognosis: Prognosis of imidacloprid toxicosis is generally good. Mildly intoxicated animals may recover spontaneously.

Public health and environmental concerns: Residues of imidacloprid in foods of animal origin are unlikely due to its rapid metabolism.

Imidacloprid has low bioaccumulation in ecosystem. However, imidacloprid has raised ecological concerns because of its possible impact on bee populations, ability to cause eggshell thinning in birds, and reduced egg production and hatching success.

VII. NATURAL PRODUCTS

1. Rotenone

Rotenone is a natural contact insecticide derived from the roots of the *Derris* (tuba) and *Lonchocarpus* plants, particularly *Derris elliptica* and *D. chinensis*. Historically, rotenone was used to treat arrowheads for fishing. Rotenone is used in home gardens for insect control, for lice and tick control on pets, and for fish eradication (piscicide) as part of water body management. Excessive use of topical powders or dips and contamination of water (ponds, aquaria) used for fish rearing can cause toxicosis in animals.

Chemistry: The chemical name of rotenone is (2*R*,6a*S*,12a*S*)-1,2,6,6a,12,12a-hexahydro-2-isopropenyl-8, 9-dimethoxy-chromeno[3,4-*b*] furo(2,3-h)chromen-6-one. Rotenone is produced by extraction from the roots (also leaves) of several tropical and subtropical plant species belonging to the genus *Derris* or *Lonchocarpus*.

Properties: Rotenone (Synonyms: derrin, nicourine, and tubatoxin) is a highly lipophilic compound, which is practically insoluble in water but soluble in chloroform. Rotenone is stable on storage, but when exposed to light and air in the field it decomposes rapidly and loses activity within few days. Rotenone is available commercially in various formulations like dusts, emulsifiable concentrates, wettable powders, solutions and resins for use in gardens, and dips, sprays and powders for application on small animals, cattle and birds. Rotenone is often combined with other insecticides like pyrethrins or is synergized by piperonyl butoxide to broaden its spectrum of action and insecticidal activity.

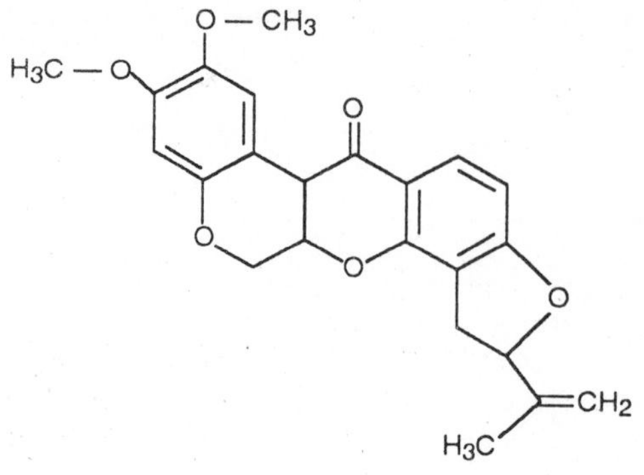

Fig. 13.10. Chemical structure of rotenone.

Factors affecting toxicity :

a. Species: Rotenone is highly toxic to fish and birds, but it may affect any species. Among domestic animals, cats are most commonly affected.

b. Formulation: Rotenone in emulsifiable concentrates is much more toxic than other formulations such as dusts.

c. Particle size: Rotenone in smaller particles is more toxic by oral and inhalation routes than when it is present in bigger particle size.

d. Route: In rats and dogs, dust formulation is more toxic by inhalation than by oral route.

e. Dietary factors: Fatty and oily food enhances absorption of rotenone from GI tract.

Toxicity: The toxicity of rotenone appears to vary considerably between species. The inherent toxicity of rotenone to vertebrates is very high (e.g. intraperitoneal LD_{50} in mice = 1.6 mg/kg), but other factors like route of exposure, concentration, formulation, and particle size of rotenone in the powder derived from various plant sources considerably affect the acute toxicity. The oral acute LD_{50} of rotenone in different species is: rats 130 mg/kg, guinea-pigs 100 mg/kg, dogs 300 mg/kg and rabbits 1600 mg/kg. Chickens are relatively resistant with lethal dose ranging from 1000-3000 mg/kg. The LC_{50} for fish is 12-75 μg/L. Rotenone may be intentionally added to water tanks to kill unwanted fish.

Toxicokinetics: The oral absorption of rotenone from GI tract is limited, but is increased by oily or fatty foods. Rotenone is metabolised in liver by hydroxylation to form equally toxic rotenoids. It also undergoes demethylation process to form non-toxic products. Rotenone is eliminated primarily in the faeces.

Mechanism of action :

a. Rotenone is a classical inhibitor of the respiratory chain of mitochondria. It forms a complex with reduced nicotinamide adenine dinucleotide (NADH) dehydrogenase (Complex I) and inhibits electron transfer between flavoprotein and ubiquinone (coenzyme Q). The inhibition of Complex I ultimately results in loss of oxidative phosphorylation, so that adenosine triphosphate (ATP) levels fall rapidly and cell death ensues.

b. Rotenone also inhibits mitosis, probably by binding to the mitotic spindle apparatus. This action of rotenone either occurs directly by binding of insecticide to tubulin or is mediated indirectly through decrease in ATP levels.

Clinical signs: Oral exposure of rotenone causes clinical signs of gastric irritation and vomiting. Dermal or very high oral exposure in animals may cause vomiting, lethargy, stupor, dyspnoea and respiratory depression, hypoglycaemia and death. In some cases excitation, muscular twitching, incoordination and tremors accompanied by seizures may also be seen. Inhalation of rotenone dust may produce additional signs of respiratory tract irritation. Death in acute poisoning occurs due to respiratory depression and asphyxia.

Chronic toxicosis may produce increased incidence of vomiting, diarrhoea, reduced body weight, reduced food consumption, growth retardation, anaemia, hypoglycaemia and hypoproteinemia. Chronic exposures to rotenone in rats produce features of Parkinson's disease due to highly selective nigrostratial dopaminergic degeneration.

Post-mortem findings: Lesions of rotenone poisoning are not specific. These include mild to moderate gastroenteritis and pulmonary congestion. In chronic exposure, microscopic lesions include passive congestion with midzonal necrosis in liver as well as fatty changes in liver and kidneys.

Diagnosis: Diagnosis of rotenone toxicosis is made from history, clinical signs and chemical analysis. Vomitus, blood, urine or faeces may be analysed for the insecticide.

Treatment and management: Specific antidotes are not available, so symptomatic and supportive therapy is indicated for rotenone intoxication.

a. Diazepam can be used to control seizures.

b. Menadione (Vitamin K_3) at a dose of 0.5 mg/kg, IM, has been found useful in rotenone poisoning.

c. Emetics, adsorbents and saline purgatives should be used to remove recently ingested poisons. Bathing with detergent is recommended in case of dermal exposure.

d. Cardiorespiratory stimulants may be recommended, as required by the condition.

Contraindication

a. Phenothiazine tranquilizers should be avoided.

b. Fatty or oily food should be avoided in case of oral exposure, because oil increases the absorption of rotenone.

Prognosis: Prognosis is excellent in most cases of rotenone poisoning.

Public health and environmental concerns: Residues of rotenone in foods of animal origin are unlikely. Rotenone is toxic to fish, thus its use near water may be hazardous to aquatic life.

2. Nicotine

Nicotine is a liquid alkaloid obtained from leaves of tobacco plant *Nicotiana tabacuum*. It is a potent poison and is occasionally used as a general purpose contact insecticide. Rarely, it is used therapeutically as an anthelmintic and immobilizing agent via projectile syringe. Nicotine has no therapeutic use, but it is of considerable interest in human toxicology because of its wide use in tobacco smoking and chewing. Nicotine is one of the most toxic substances known and has low margin of safety.

Chemistry: Nicotine is [3 - (1′-methyl-2′-pyrrolidyl) pyridine].

Properties: Pure nicotine is a colourless oily liquid. It is hygroscopic and freely miscible with water, ethanol, ethyl ether and most organic solvents. As a nitrogenous base, nicotine forms salts with acids that are usually solid and water soluble.

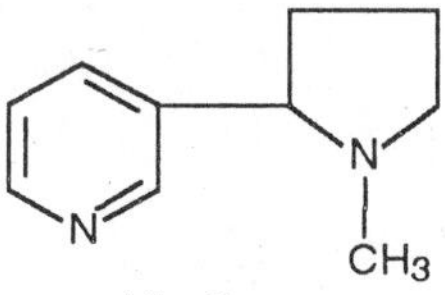

N
N
CH_3
Nicotine

Fig. 13.11. Chemical structure of nicotine.

Upon exposure to air, pure nicotine turns brown with a characteristic smell reminiscent of tobacco. Nicotine free base is commercialised as a concentrated 40% aqueous solution or a fumigant formulation of 0.5-4%. The insecticide called 'Black leaf 40' contains 40% nicotine sulphate.

Sources of toxicity :

a. Animals may ingest nicotine sulphate insecticide (Black leaf 40) from spills of the solution or sprayed foliage.

b. Use of nicotine sulphate dusts or sprays (0.05-4%) on animals to control insect pests may produce toxicosis.

c. Tobacco plants are unpalatable and animals generally avoid consumption. However in scarcity of fodder, animals may consume excessive amounts of tobacco leaves and get intoxicated.

d. Nicotine is occasionally used to capture and restrain dangerous, unmanageable or wild animals. For this purpose, a projectile-type syringe is loaded with nicotine solution and fired from a special CO_2-powdered rifle. Excessive amount of nicotine or improper handling of gun is harmful to the animal as well as to the operator.

e. Cigarettes contain up to 20 mg of nicotine each, cigarette butt contains about 5 mg nicotine each, and chewing tobacco contains 2.5-8 mg nicotine/gram dry material. Inadvertent ingestion of these nicotine products causes toxicity in birds and small animals. A pack of cigarette is lethal to a dog.

f. Tobacco smoke is occasionally used as a fumigant. Nicotine fumigation in animal houses or sheds may cause toxicosis in animals.

Toxicity: Nicotine is highly toxic to most mammals with low therapeutic ratio. The lethal dose in many species is 1-2 mg/kg. The oral LD_{50} in different species is: rats =50-60 mg/kg, mice = 24 mg/kg, dogs and cats = 20-100 mg/animal, horses = 100-300 mg/animal, and sheep 100-200 mg/animal. A total dose of 40 mg is lethal to an adult human.

Toxicokinetics: Nicotine base is readily absorbed from the skin, mucous membranes and lungs (when inhaled). Absorption of nicotine from acidic solution is less, so the commercial nicotine sulphate salt is safer on dermal contact. Accordingly nicotine is less absorbed from the acidic stomach, but readily absorbed from intestine. Alkalinization of stomach enhances absorption. As nicotine enters the body, it is distributed quickly through the bloodstream and can cross blood-brain barrier. Most of nicotine (up to 90%) is rapidly metabolised in the liver, kidneys and lungs to form various metabolites (e.g. cotinine and nornicotine). The metabolites and the remainder unaltered nicotine are excreted in urine. The half-life of nicotine in animals is in range of 2 to 3 hours, but the half-life of cotinine is 4-8 times longer.

Mechanism of action :

a. Nicotine exerts its toxic effect primarily by binding to nicotinic cholinergic (nACh) receptors located in skeletal muscle motor end-plates, autonomic ganglia, adrenal medulla and CNS. Toxicosis is produced by initial stimulation followed by depolarizing type blockade of all nACh receptors, including those present in autonomic ganglia (both sympathetic and parasympathetic). The activation of nACh receptors, occurring at lower dosage or initially with higher dosage, causes a rapid increase in cellular permeability of Na^+ and Ca^{++} leading to depolarization and excitation. Prolonged application of nicotine results in desensitization of the cholinergic receptor site and lasting blockade.

i. The initial activation of nicotinic receptors in autonomic ganglia facilitates release of neurotransmitter noradrenaline (sympathetic ganglia) or acetylcholine (parasympathetic ganglia), which in turn stimulates sympathetic and parasympathetic nervous systems, respectively. The subsequent blockade of autonomic ganglia suppresses both sympathetic and parasympathetic systems to produce complex actions in body.

ii. Similar to autonomic ganglia, nicotine possesses a biphasic action on neuromuscular junctions causing initial stimulation of skeletal muscles in small doses to be followed by persistent depression and paralysis in large doses.

iii. Stimulation of adrenal medulla results in enhanced secretion of catecholamines (e.g. adrenaline and noradrenaline) followed by their decreased release.

b. Nicotine is also known to stimulate a number of sensory receptors like mechanoreceptors that respond to stretch or pressure, chemoreceptors of carotid body, thermal receptors of skin, and pain receptors.

Clinical signs: The toxic manifestations depend largely on dose and rate of absorption, which in turn reflect the activity of nicotine on autonomic ganglia and skeletal muscle. At low dosage or in slow absorption nicotine stimulates autonomic ganglia, whereas at high doses or in faster absorption it initially stimulates then depresses the autonomic ganglia.

Clinical signs of nicotine poisoning appear rapidly within few minutes (15-45 minutes) and are characterised by excitement, rapid respiration, salivation, lachrymation, vomiting, diarrhoea, and convulsions of clonic-tonic type which may be very severe. The transient phase of stimulation is followed by depression, muscle weakness, incoordination, rapid pulse, shallow and slow respiration, collapse, coma, and flaccid paralysis. Death is from respiratory paralysis of diaphragm and chest muscles resulting from descending paralysis and depolarisation block of the neuromuscular junction.

Teratogenic effects have been observed in pregnant sows and ewes eating tobacco plants. Teratogenic effects include arthrogryposis (a form of limb deformity) in pigs and facial deformities and cleft palate in sheep.

Post-mortem findings: No characteristic lesions are produced by nicotine. Engorgement of subcutaneous tissues and blood vessels may be evident. There may be pale mucous membranes, dark blood, haemorrhages on heart and lungs, and congestion of brain. Stomach contents may give distinctive odour of nicotine.

Diagnosis: Diagnosis of nicotine poisoning can be made from history, clinical signs and chemical analysis. For chemical analysis, vomitus, stomach contents, liver, skin or urine can be taken. Urine content of the metabolite cotinine can be used to confirm absorption of nicotine.

Initial signs due to over stimulation of cholinergic receptors resemble organophosphorus insecticide poisoning.

Treatment and management: Treatment of acute nicotine poisoning is usually unsuccessful.

a. In very early stages of poisoning, a non-depolarizing type of ganglion blocker that can also cross blood brain barrier (e.g. mecamylamine) may be of some use. However in later stages, it may precipitate toxicity.

b. Removal of the toxicant by washing or gastric lavage with tannic acid or potassium permanganate may be successful in early stages.

c. If exposure is by dermal route, the animals must be bathed carefully with liquid dish detergent. Human exposure must be avoided by wearing thick rubber gloves.

d. Severe hypersecretion (especially salivation and diarrhoea) or bradycardia may be treated with intravenous atropine sulphate.

e. Parenteral fluid therapy may be given if hypotension occurs.

f. If the animal is already in depressed state and muscles are flaccid, no drug can help. Artificial respiration becomes the only means of keeping the poisoned animal alive but this too usually fails.

Contraindications

Antacids should not be administered in nicotine poisoning since alkaline medium facilitates absorption of nicotine from stomach.

Prognosis: Mildly affected animals recover rapidly and spontaneously. In acute nicotine poisoning, prognosis is poor.

B. HERBICIDES

Herbicides are phytotoxic chemicals used for destroying unwanted plants and weeds or inhibiting their growth. Most of these chemicals, particularly the most recently developed organic synthetic herbicides, are quite selective for specific plants and have low mammalian toxicity; other less selective compounds (e.g. arsenicals, chlorates, and paraquat) kill all green plants and are more toxic to animals. Very few problems occur when these chemicals are used properly. Most animal health problems result from exposure to excessive quantities of herbicides because of their improper use or careless disposal of containers. Residues of herbicides are less likely to occur in food than insecticides and fungicides as they are not/less used on food crops. However in recent days there is increasing concern about their effects on health because of run-off from agricultural applications and their entrance into drinking water supply.

Classification: There are large numbers of chemicals which are used for herbicidal action. Some important groups are given below:

I. Inorganic herbicides

1. Arsenicals e.g. sodium arsenite.
2. Chlorates e.g. sodium chlorate.

II. Organic herbicides

1. Chlorophenoxy herbicides e.g. 2, 4-D, 2,4,5-T, mecoprop, MCPA and MCPB.
2. Dinitro herbicides e.g. dinitroorthocresol (DNOC) and dinoseb.
3. Bipyridyl herbicides e.g. paraquat and diquat.
4. Triazine herbicides e.g. atrazine, simazine and propazine.
5. Substituted urea herbicides e.g. monuron, diuron and isouron.
6. Carbamates and thiocarbamates e.g. barban, propham, cycloate and butylate.
7. Uracils e.g. bromacil, isocil and terbacil.
8. Chlorobenzoic acid e.g. chloramben and dicamba.
9. Chloracetanilides e.g. alachlor, butachlor and metolachlor
10. Organophosphates e.g. glyphosate and glufosinate.

I. INORGANIC HERBICIDES

Herbicides of inorganic origin were formerly used on large scale in agriculture, but their use has gradually declined due to availability of better and selective organic preparations.

1. Arsenicals

Inorganic arsenicals (e.g. sodium arsenite and arsenic trioxide) are used as desiccants or defoliants on cotton and some other crops. Ruminants are attracted to and lick plants poisoned with arsenite. The highly soluble arsenicals can also concentrate in pools in toxic quantities after a rain has washed them from recently treated plants. Overall, the use of inorganic arsenicals as herbicides has been reduced greatly due to their harmful effect on animal health and the environmental persistence.

Signs and lesions caused by inorganic arsenical herbicides (also organic arsenical herbicides i.e. DSMA, MSMA, cacodylic acid) resemble inorganic arsenic poisonings (see Metals, Chapter 11). Dimercaprol by I.M. route is the recommended therapy.

2. Chlorates

Chlorates such as sodium chlorate ($NaClO_3$) are now seldom used as herbicide. Sodium chlorate treated plants and contaminated clothing are highly combustible and constitute fire hazards. Many cases of chlorate poisoning of livestock have occurred from ingestion of contaminated feed and treated plants. Ingestion of chlorates result in conversion of haemoglobin to met-haemoglobin. The detailed toxicology and treatment of sodium chlorate toxicosis in animals have been described earlier in Chapter 12.

II. ORGANIC HERBICIDES

1. Chlorophenoxy Herbicides /Phenoxy Acid Derivatives/Phenoxy Herbicides

The chlorophenoxy herbicides were the first commercially available organic herbicides in 1946. This group comprises the most important and most frequently used herbicides. These may be employed as growth regulators which stimulate plant growth in small doses and suppress it in large doses. The important members of the group are 2,4-D, 2,4,5-T, MCPA, MCPB, 2,4-DB, mecoprop (MCPP) dichlorprop (2,4-DP) and silvex (Table 13.3). The 2,4-dichlorophenoxyacetic acid (2,4-D) is the most widely used and best-studied herbicide and may be taken as the representative compound of this group.

Chemistry: This group of herbicides contains a chlorophenoxy ring that is esterified to simple acids (e.g. acetic, propionic and butyric acids). Their structures usually contain 1 to 3 chlorine atoms and sometimes a methyl group. Some early formulations (2,4, 5-T) contain dioxin contaminants that increases the toxicity of technical grade herbicides.

Properties: The chlorophenoxy compounds are primarily used as herbicide in agriculture, forestry and lawn care practices to eliminate broad leaf plants. In addition to their own toxic properties, phenoxy herbicides can potentiate the toxic effects of some plants. They may increase the nitrate content of some plants and can increase the palatability of certain toxic plants (e.g. sudan grass), thus increasing poisoning risks from these plants. The basic form of 2,4-D is the acid, but it is often formulated as an inorganic salt, amine or ester through various manufacturing processes and is used in many commercial products.

Toxicity: The toxicity of 2,4-D and other phenoxy herbicides primarily depends of the species and type of formulation. Dogs are the most sensitive animals, whereas pigs, sheep, cattle and poultry are less susceptible. The oral LD_{50} of 2,4-D in olive oil is 300-500 mg/kg for rats and 100 mg/kg for dogs. Toxicity of 2,4-D may be observed in calves at 200 mg/kg and swine at 100 mg/kg. The oral LD_{50} of 2,4,5-T (2,4,5-trichlorophenoxyacetic acid) in dogs and rats is 100 mg/kg and 500 mg/kg, respectively. Silvex is unusual for this group because as little as 2-6 mg/kg body weight may cause ill effects in dogs. The use of 2,4,5-T has been discontinued or curtailed because extremely toxic contaminants collectively called dioxins (See for detail Chapter 17) are found in it, mainly due to some manufacturing defects.

Toxicokinetics: Absorption of phenoxy herbicides occur rapidly from stomach and intestine. Their dermal absorption is slower and less complete. The herbicides are protein bound *in vivo* and are rapidly distributed to the liver, kidneys and brain, but they do not accumulate in animals. 2,4-D pass the placental barrier and is detected in the uterus, placenta foetus and intrauterine fluid of exposed animals. The phenoxy herbicides are not extensively metabolised but are actively excreted in the urine. Esters may be metabolised by hydrolysis and small amounts are conjugated with glycine or taurine. Excretion is markedly enhanced by ion-trapping using alkaline agents as most of

Table 13.3: Nomenclature of important chlorophenoxy herbicides.

Abbreviation/ Common name	Chemical name
2,4-D	2,4-Dichloro-phenoxyacetic acid
2,4,5-T	2,4,5-Trichloro-phenoxyacetic acid
2,4-DB	4-(2,4-Dichlorophenoxy) butyric acid
2,4-DP/Dichlorprop	2-(2,4-Dichlorophenoxy) propionic acid
MCPP/Mecoprop	2-(4-Chloro-2-methyl-phenoxy) propionic acid
MCPA	2-Methyl-4-chloropheno-xyacetic acid
MCPB	2-Methyl-4-chloropheno-xybutyric acid
Silvex	2-(2,4,5-trichlorophenoxy) propionic acid

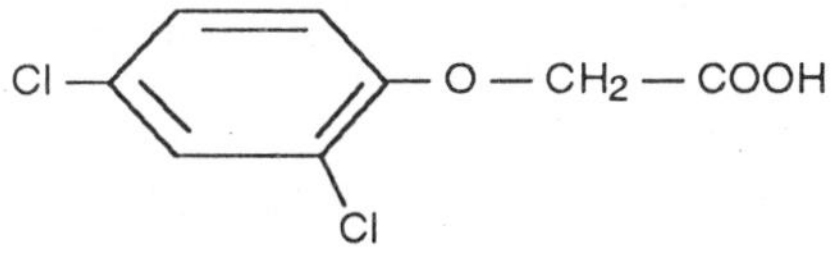

Cl — O — CH_2 — COOH, Cl

2,4–Dichlorophenoxyacetic acid (2,4–D)

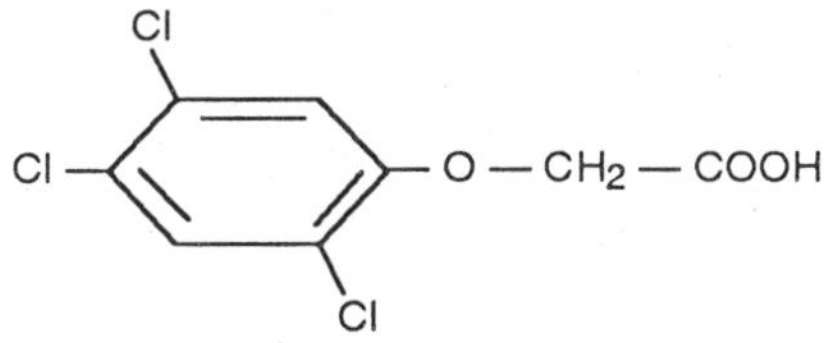

Cl, Cl — O — CH_2 — COOH, Cl

2,4,5–Trichlorophenoxyacetic acid (2,4,5–T)

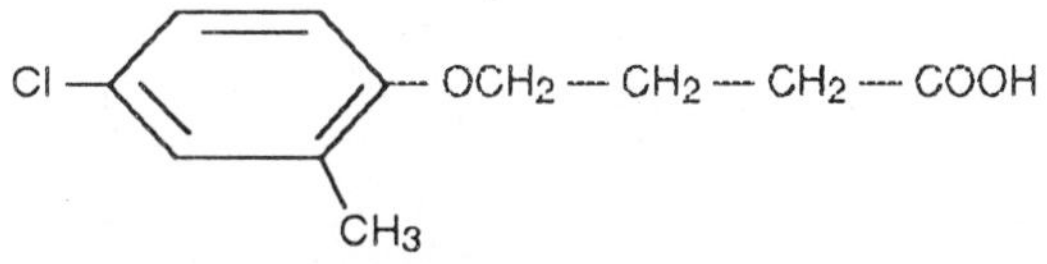

Cl — OCH_2 — CH_2 — CH_2 — COOH, CH_3

2–Methyl–4–chlorophenoxybutyric acid (MCPB)

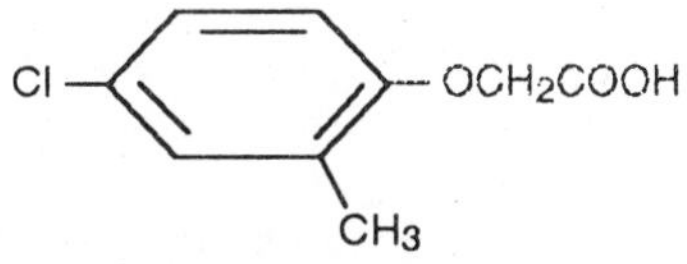

Cl — OCH_2COOH, CH_3

2–Methyl–4–chlorophenoxyacetic acid (MCPA)

Fig. 13.12. Chemical structures of some important chlorophenoxy herbicides.

these herbicides are organic acids. Half-life of 2,4-D is approximately 18 hours. The 2,4,5-T may undergo enterohepatic circulation and have longer half-life.

Mechanism of action: The exact mechanisms of toxicosis of phenoxyacetic acids are not known. These herbicides depress ribonuclease synthesis, uncouple oxidative phosphorylation and increase number of hepatic peroxisomes. The relationship of these biochemical changes to clinical effect is not clear. 2,4-D has a direct effect on muscle membranes causing increased irritability and rigidity followed by paralysis.

Clinical signs: Phenoxy herbicides produce clinical signs primarily related to GI tract and/or nervous system. Gastrointestinal signs include anorexia, rumen atony, diarrhoea, ulceration of oral mucosa, bloat and rumen stasis in cattle, and vomiting, diarrhoea (sometimes bloody), salivation, oral ulceration etc. in dogs and pigs. Neuromuscular signs include depression, muscular weakness in cattle, and ataxia, posterior weakness (particularly pelvic limbs) and periodic clonic spasms (at high doses) in dogs.

Sublethal doses, singly or repeatedly, produce tenseness, muscular weakness and weight loss.

Post-mortem findings: Lesions of phenoxy herbicides include gastritis, and swollen and fragile liver. Erosion and ulceration of lips, mouth, and buccal and oesophageal mucosae may be observed. Bright green, undigested feed may be present in the rumen due to rumen stasis. The kidneys are enlarged and show renal congestion and tubular degeneration. The mesenteric lymph nodes and vessels are hyperaemic and enlarged. Hydropericardium with epicardial haemorrhage may also be seen.

Diagnosis: Diagnosis of phenoxy herbicides is made from history, clinical signs, lesions and chemical analysis. Chemical analysis of forages, urine or renal tissue confirms exposure to these herbicides; however the exact concentration of phenoxy herbicides in tissues or urine that confirms toxicosis is not well-established.

Treatment and management: Specific antidotes for phenoxy herbicides are not available. Treatment is usually symptomatic and supportive.

a. Activated charcoal and a saline cathartic may be used for very recent exposure.

b. Ion trapping by administering fluids containing 1-2 mEq/kg bicarbonate may enhance removal of insecticide from the tissues and promote its excretion in the urine.

c. Diarrhoea and rumen atony should be treated and renal functions closely monitored.

d. Intravenous fluids should be administered to promote diuresis.

e. Drugs which aid the restoration of liver functions are recommended.

f. A bland diet and good nursing care should be provided.

Prognosis: Prognosis is good, if exposure is moderate and therapy is instituted immediately.

Public health concerns: Residues in foods of animal origin are infrequent because of the rapid excretion and short tissue half-life of phenoxy herbicides. Some reports have linked phenoxy herbicides use to increased incidence of non Hodgkin's Lymphoma in human beings.

2. Dinitro Herbicides/Dinitrophenols

The substituted dinitrophenols are non-specific biocides, mainly used as herbicides, insecticides, fungicides and acaricides. At one time, a considerable number of dinitrophenol derivatives were registered for use, but now as a result of their adverse effects, particularly their high toxicity and tendency to cause birth defects and chronic reproductive effects, only a few are available in market. These include 2,4-DNP, DNOC, dinocap, dinoterb and dinobuton . All compounds are highly toxic to all species of animals. The main sources of poisoning for domestic animals include human negligence in removing the preparation if it spills, in disposing off the containers, and allowing animals' access to the treated fields.

Chemistry: The dinitrophenol pesticides are all derivatives of 2,4-dinitrophenol. Pesticides having an additional alkyl substituent in the ring 'ortho' to hydroxy moiety generally increases lipophilicity and toxicity of the compound. The common and chemical names of important dinitrophenols are dinitrophenol (DNP; 2,4-dinitrophenol), dinitroorthocresol (DNOC; 2 - methyl - 4, 6-dinitrophenol), dinoseb (DNBP; 2-methylpropyl-4, 6 dinitrophenol) and dinoterb (2-dimethylpropyl-4,6-dinitrophenol). Dinocap, another dinitrophenol herbicide, is a complex mixture of 2,6-dinitro-4-octylphenyl and 2,4-dinitro-4-octylphenyl crotonates.

Properties: The dinitrophenol compounds are crystalline substances having pale yellow/yellow colour. 2,4-Dinitrophenol has a sweet, musty odour, which sublimes when carefully heated. It is sparingly soluble in water (its crystalline sodium salts are soluble in water), but soluble in alcohol, acetone, chloroform, carbon tetrachloride and other organic solvents. The 2,4-Dinitrophenol is used in the manufacture of dyes and wood preservatives and as a pesticide. As herbicides, they are used mainly on grass and broadleaf weeds.

Toxicity: The dinitrophenol compounds tend to have relatively high acute toxicity in all mammals. The LD_{50} of dinitrophenol in rats is 0.027-0.1 mg/kg. The oral acute LD_{50} of DNOC in different species is: rats = 20-50 mg/kg, rabbits = 45 mg/kg, dogs and pigs = 50 mg/kg and goats = 100 mg/kg. The acute LD_{50} of dinoseb in rats is 40-60 mg/kg. The LD_{50} of dinocap in dogs and pigs is 50 mg/kg and in goats is 100 mg/kg. In sheep, dosage of 25 mg/kg/day causes lethality in 5 days. Factors affecting toxicity of chlorophenols (see Fungicides) also affect dinitrophenols toxicosis.

Toxicokinetics: The dinitrophenols are readily absorbed from all routes including oral, dermal and inhalation. However, variations in lipophilicity and form of phenol employed (free acid, alkoxyamine salts, etherified, etc.) lead to differences in the absorption and hence the toxicity of different dinitrophenol compounds. These compounds have relatively slow clearance from body with half-life in humans in range of 5 to 7 days. The bright yellow colour of dinitrophenol compounds imparts yellow colour to urine and body tissues.

Mechanism of action

a. Dinitrophenol pesticides act as cellular metabolic poisons. They interfere with electron transport chain by causing the uncoupling of mitochondrial oxidative phosphorylation. This decreases the production of ATP. Cells counteract the lowered yields of ATP by oxidising the stored reserves such as carbohydrates and fat. Instead of formation of ATP, the cellular energy is lost as heat resulting in severe hyperthermia. This action of dinitrophenol is just like chlorophenols (See for detail Fungicides).

b. In ruminants, the ruminal microflora reduce the dinitro compounds to diamine metabolites that induce methaemoglobinuria.

Clinical signs

Acute toxicity: Acute toxicity clinical signs of dinitrophenols may appear within few minutes to several hours depending upon the amount of herbicide ingested. The toxic manifestations include dullness, listlessness, restlessness, loss of appetite, rapid respiration, occasional sweating, thirst, muscular weakness, hyperthermia, colic, mild jaundice, prostration, cyanosis, convulsions and coma. The urine and faeces have a chrome-yellow colour, which turns black on exposure to air. The illness generally runs a rapid course and death occurs within 24 to 48 hours. Death may arise from hyperthermia (when production of heat exceeds the capacity for heat dissipation) or respiratory or cardiovascular failure. Abortions have been observed in sows. Hepatotoxicity marked by jaundice is also a possible sequel. In ruminants, the clinical signs are the same as mentioned above, but animals are more susceptible for production of methaemoglobinaemia (blood chocolate brown in colour), intravascular haemolysis and hypoproteinaemia.

Exposure by inhalation can lead to pulmonary oedema in addition to systemic signs. Some of these compounds (e.g. dinocap) are irritant to skin, eye and mucous membranes. The bright yellow colour of these compounds leads to staining of site of exposure (skin and hair).

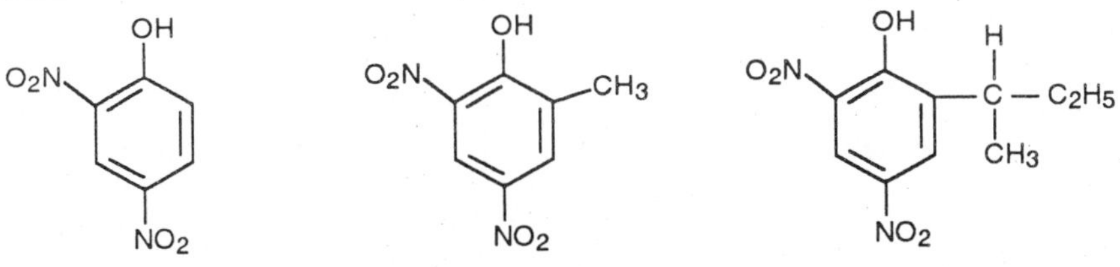

OH, O_2N, NO_2 — Dinitrophenol (DNP)

OH, O_2N, CH_3, NO_2 — Dinitroorthocresol (DNOC)

OH, O_2N, H, C, C_2H_5, CH_3, NO_2 — Dinoseb (DNBP)

Fig. 13.13. Chemical structure of some important dinitrophenol herbicides.

Chronic toxicity: Chronic exposure to dinitro orthocresol may produce fatigue, restlessness, excessive sweating (humans), unusual thirst and loss of weight (DNOC in controlled dose is also used to reduce body weight in obese persons). Chronic (long-term) oral exposure to 2,4-dinitrophenol in humans and animals may result in formation of cataracts and skin lesions and adverse effects on the bone marrow, central nervous system, and cardiovascular system.

Post-mortem findings: The gross post-mortem lesions of dinitrophenols are non-specific. Rigor mortis occurs quickly after death. The body tissues, urine and external surfaces (e.g. skin, hair, and paws) in contact with chemicals are yellow in appearance. Degenerative changes in parenchymatous organs may be observed. There may be generalized congestion, pulmonary and cerebral oedema and cyanosis, and blood is usually dark.

Diagnosis: A history of exposure, signs of rapid overheating and respiratory distress, and lesions like fast rigor mortis, dark blood and yellow tissues help in the diagnosis of dinitrophenol toxicosis. Laboratory analysis may confirm the diagnosis. Contents of stomach/rumen and urine are collected for laboratory analysis. The samples should be frozen immediately as these compounds degrade rapidly.

Dinitrophenol toxicosis should be differentiated from heat stroke and nitrate/nitrite (chocolate coloured blood, but absence of hyperthermia) and carbon monoxide (bright red blood and no pyrexia) poisonings.

Treatment and management: There is no specific antidote to dinitrophenols toxicosis. The treatment is only symptomatic and supportive (See also Chlorophenols in Fungicides).

a. Respiratory distress and anoxia should be treated with adequate oxygen supply (necessary in carnivores, where ever possible).

b. High fever should be reduced by cold water rinsing and ice-packs.

c. Fluid and electrolyte imbalance should be corrected. Dextrose saline may be infused in combination with diuretics.

d. In ruminants, methaemoglobinaemia is treated with methylene blue or ascorbic acid (See for detail Nitrate/Nitrite poisoning, Chapter 12).

e. The affected animal should be kept in shaded place.

f. Non-barbiturate sedative and tranquilizers may be used, if required.

g. Decontamination of skin and hair with soap and water may be done, if exposure is dermal.

Contraindications: Salicylate antipyretics should not be used to decrease fever in dinitrophenol pesticide poisoning because these agents can also act as uncouplers of oxidative phosphorylation and may exacerbate the poisoning. Other antipyretic drugs are also of little help since the dinitrophenol hyperthermia is a general tissue response rather then a disorder of central temperature regulation.

Public health and environmental concerns: 2-4-Dintrophenol is considered an important environmental contaminant. Dinocap is moderately toxic to birds, but its toxicity to fish and aquatic invertebrates is extremely high.

3. Bipyridyl Herbicides

The bipyridyl (dipyridyl, bipyridilium, dipyridilium) compounds are non-specific broad-spectrum desiccant contact herbicides. These are extensively used in agriculture for weed control and include paraquat and diquat. These compounds are highly toxic to animals, but they are used at low rates (150 ml/hectare) that do not pose serious threats. Poisoning in animals arise mainly due to direct ingestion of the herbicide or consumption of freshly treated crops. These herbicides are frequently used for malicious poisoning in dogs.

Chemistry: Paraquat and diquat compounds are derived from bipyridyls. Paraquat (1,1'-dimethyl 1-4, 4'-bipyridilium ion) is available as dichloride or dimethyl sulphate salt. Diquat (1, 1'-ethylene-2, 2' bipyridilium) is available as dibromide salt. Other members of this class include cyperquat, diethamquat, difenzoquat and morfamquat.

Properties: Bipyridyl herbicides are non volatile, water soluble herbicides which are degradable in sunlight within 3 weeks and rapidly and completely inactivated in soil by bacterial activity. They strongly bind to clay in soil. Paraquat and diquat are available commercially in the form of highly soluble concentrates for mixing in water. They are widely used as herbicides in no-till or minimum tillage programmes. They are also used

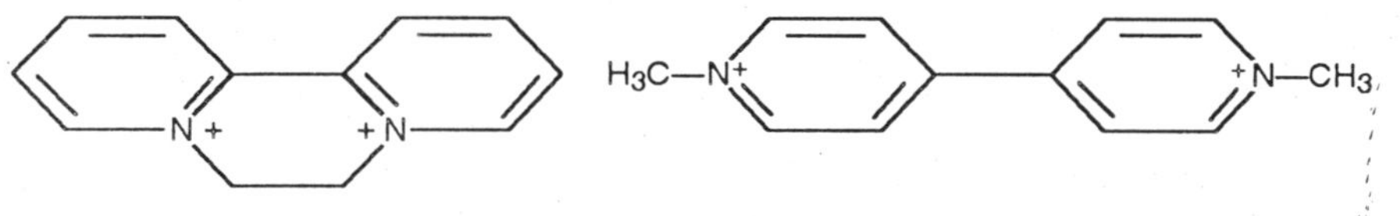

Fig. 13.14. Chemical structures of some important bipyridyl herbicides.

for general weed control on non-crop land, as defoliant on cotton and hops, and as desiccant to remove herbage prior to the harvest of soybeans, potatoes, and fruits. Paraquat and diquat become biologically inactive upon contact with soil.

Toxicity: The toxicity of bipyridyls depends on the concentration or dose of herbicide and the species involved. The local toxicity of paraquat depends mainly on its concentration in the formulation, whereas the systemic toxicity depends on the dose of herbicide. The oral LD_{50} of paraquat in different animals is: rats 110-200 mg/kg, dogs & pigs 25-50 mg/kg, cats 35-50 mg/kg, sheep 50-100 mg/kg, cattle 50-75 mg/kg and chickens 100-350 mg/kg. Dogs consuming 170 ppm dietary paraquat for 2 months develop anorexia, respiratory distress and pulmonary lesions leading to death. The oral LD_{50} of diquat in different species is: rats 200-400 mg/kg, dogs 100-250 mg/kg, cats, 35-50 mg/kg, cattle, 20-40 mg/kg and chickens 200-400 mg/kg. The dermal LD_{50} is similar to oral LD_{50}.

Toxicokinetics: Absorption of bipyridyl herbicides is limited from various routes. Diquat is poorly absorbed (<20%) from the GI tract. In cases of dermal exposure, less than 10% of paraquat and diquat are absorbed through skin. After absorption, paraquat mainly concentrates in lung tissues because of a specific energy dependent uptake system. Its concentration in lung tissues may be up to 10 times than that of other tissues. Bipyridyl herbicides are less metabolised in body and are excreted mostly unchanged mainly in the urine (paraquat) or faeces (diquat).

Mechanism of action: All bipyridyl compounds have similar mechanisms of toxicity. They are easily reduced to the radical ion, which generates superoxide radical that reacts with unsaturated membrane lipids.

Paraquat: Paraquat is a very reactive compound. It is actively taken up by the alveolar cells via a diamine or polyamine transport system where it readily accepts an electron from NADPH to become reduced paraquat. When the reduced paraquat is reoxidized by loss of electron it has previously accepted, a superoxide anion radical O_2^- is generated. The superoxide radical is unstable and spontaneously breaks down to the reactive singlet oxygen. The reactive singlet oxygen attacks the polyunsaturated lipids associated with cell membranes to form lipid hydroperoxides (Figure 13.15). These lipid hydroperoxides are normally converted to non toxic lipid alcohols by the selenium-containing glutathione dependent enzyme glutathione peroxidase. Selenium deficiency, depletion of glutathione or excess lipid hydroperoxides allows the lipid hydroperoxides to form lipid free radicals. Lipid hydroperoxides are also unstable in the presence of trace amounts of transition metal ions and decompose to lipid free radicals, which in turn can also cause further peroxidation of polyunsaturated lipid in a process that is slowed down by vitamin E. The action of paraquat in lungs is similar to that produced by carbon tetrachloride in liver. Small amounts of superoxide that are produced normally in tissues are also scavenged by superoxide dismutase, an enzyme that converts superoxide to H_2O_2. The H_2O_2 is detoxified by catalase or glutathione peroxidases. If the detoxification of H_2O_2 does not happen fast enough, the H_2O_2 may form highly reactive hydroxyl radical. Lung tissue is deficient in super oxide dismutase, so it is more susceptible to the excess superoxides generated by paraquat.

The excess of superoxide anion radical O_2^- and H_2O_2 cause damage to the cellular membrane in lungs, which reduces the functional integrity of lung cells, affects efficient gas transport and exchange, and results in respiratory impairment. The development of pulmonary lesions as a result of cellular lipid peroxidation can be divided into two distinct phases. The first phase, which occurs within one to three days after ingestion, is characterized by destruction of the alveolar epithelial cells. This leads to alveolitis and is characterized by pulmonary oedema and infiltration of air spaces of the lungs and the intestinal tissues with neutrophil polymorphs. The second phase involves the development of extensive fibrosis as a response to acute alveolitis occurring in the first phase. During this stage, the proliferation of fibroblasts and deposition on collagen will further reduce the effectiveness of gaseous exchange. The consequence is death resulting from severe anoxia.

Diquat: Diquat is also a very reactive compound and exerts its action in a manner somewhat similar to that produced by paraquat. It enters the cell in various organs including liver, lungs and kidneys and undergoes an alternate reduction followed by re-oxidation to form the super oxide anion O_2^-. A cascade of events is triggered leading to NADPH depletion and lipid peroxidation of membranes. The major difference being that diquat can more readily accept an electron than paraquat and it has most harmful effects on the GI tract. It causes severe loss of body water into the lumen of GI tract resulting in tissue dehydration and hypovolaemia. Diquat also produces some effects on the lungs, but does not cause pulmonary oedema or alter lung function. Signs of CNS excitement and renal impairment occur in severely affected animals.

Clinical signs :

Paraquat: Clinical signs in paraquat toxicity has delayed onset (several hours to 3 days) because of the time involved in toxification of the herbicide. Important clinical signs include gastroenteritis, vomiting and depression (early action) and finally (2-7 days) difficult respiration due to pulmonary oedema and alveolar fibrosis. Animals that survive first few days develop dehydration, pallor or cyanosis, tachycardia, tachypnoea, harsh respiratory sounds and emphysema. Pneumomediastinum occasionally occurs as a result of respiratory distress. Death of animal may occur within 8 days. In cattle, anorexia, depression and diarrhoea may occur and respiratory signs are somewhat less prevalent. Paraquat is capable of producing local toxicity on skin, cornea, larynx, and mucosa of upper GI tract by direct injury to tissues.

In subacute or chronic toxicosis, signs may develop after 7 days and gradually worsen for up to 3 weeks. In chronic phase, there is progressive pulmonary fibrosis and increased respiratory distress.

Diquat: Diquat toxicosis occurs within few hours resulting in anorexia, gastritis and severe loss of water into the lumen of GI tract. Signs of renal impairment and CNS excitement occur in severely affected animals and include lethargy, cerebral haemorrhage, coma and renal failure. Death usually is due to multiorgan failure. As with paraquat, local effects can occur and include damage to upper GI tract on ingestion and skin burns on dermal contact.

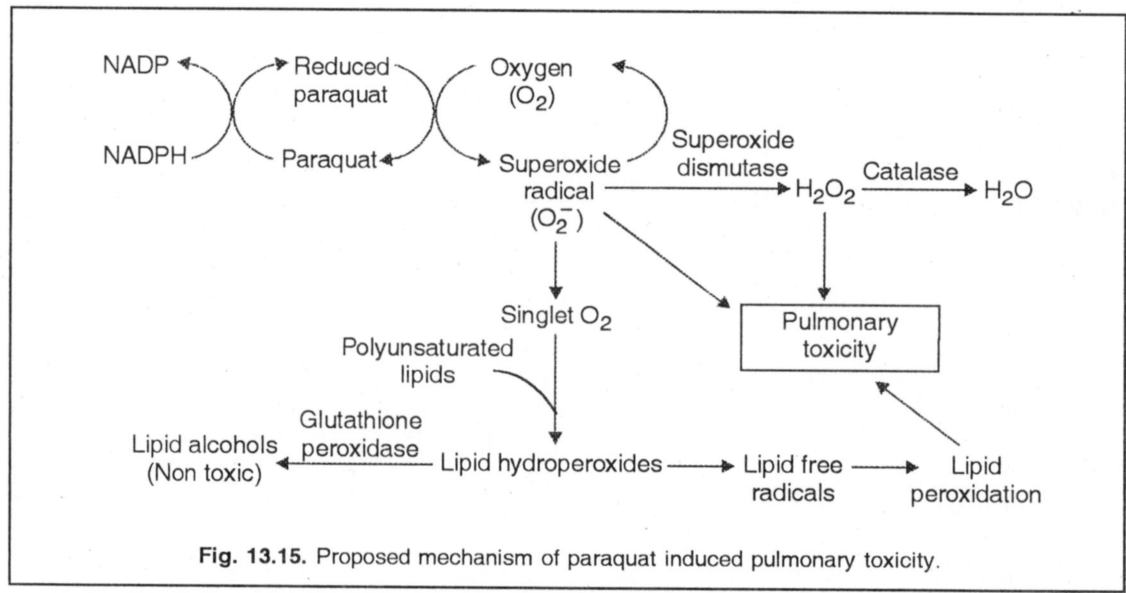

Fig. 13.15. Proposed mechanism of paraquat induced pulmonary toxicity.

Post-mortem findings: Gross lesions include pulmonary congestion, oedema and haemorrhage. Deep caustic burns and erosion and ulceration of buccal and pharyngeal tissue may be observed. Other findings include failure of lungs to collapse when chest is opened, areas of haemorrhages, fibrosis and atelectasis. In chronically affected animals, the lungs may be shrunken and fibrotic. Microscopic lesions of toxicosis include necrosis of alveolar type I epithelium followed by progressive alveolar and interstitial fibrosis and alveolar emphysema. Renal proximal tubular degeneration and moderate centrilobular hepatic degeneration may also be seen.

Diagnosis: Diagnosis of bipyridyl herbicide toxicosis is made from history, clinical signs and lesions. Chemical analysis in early stages is also helpful. Chemical analysis for paraquat may be performed on suspected sources, gut contents, tissues, blood or urine taken in the first 48 hours. Differential diagnosis of paraquat is made from following conditions:

a. *Common pneumonia:* This should be ruled out by clinical tests and radiography.

b. *ANTU poisoning:* Poisoning by ANTU is more acute and more rapidly fatal. It primarily causes lung oedema, whereas paraquat causes other lung lesions plus damage to other organs.

c. *Bovine pulmonary oedema:* A history of paraquat use or access is a valuable aid in diagnosis.

Treatment and management: There is no specific treatment for bipyridyl herbicides poisoning.

a. Removal of herbicide from the GI tract is very effective and should be carried out by gastric lavage and/or cathartics.

b. Due to slow absorption of bipyridyl herbicides, oral administration of adsorbents may be helpful. Bentonite is preferred (due to high adsorbent properties of clays for paraquat and diquat) but charcoal will suffice.

c. Vitamin E and selenium with supportive therapy may be helpful in early stages.

d. Excretion of herbicide may be accelerated by forced diuresis induced by mannitol infusion and frusemide administration. However, care must be taken not to aggravate the pulmonary oedema.

Contraindications

a. Oxygen therapy should not be given because it may generate more singlet oxygen in the lungs.

b. Fluid therapy may worsen pulmonary oedema in case of lung damage.

Prognosis: Prognosis of bipyridyl herbicide toxicosis is guarded to grave in spite of therapy. Early detoxification may be the most beneficial approach.

Public health and environmental concerns: Residues in foods of animal origin are not likely because of paraquat's low concentration in edible tissues and its relatively short half-life in the body.

4. Triazine Herbicides

Triazine compounds like atrazine, simazine, and propazine are widely used in agriculture and forestry as herbicide. Incidence of poisoning is not common because most members of this class have low oral acute toxicities ranging above 1000 mg/kg body weight. However, sensitivity of sheep and cattle to these compounds is appreciably high.

Chemistry: Most of the triazines are derivatives of the symmetrical 1,3,5-triazine-2,4-diamine, but other possibilities also exist. The compounds in this group include anilazine, atrazine, cyanazine, cyprazine, ipazine, propazine, proglinazine, simazine, terbuthylazine and trietazine. Atrazine is the most widely used compound in this group and is considered the prototype triazine herbicide. The chemical name of atrazine is 2-chloro-4-(ethylamino)-6-(isopropylamino)-1,3,5-triazine and that of simazine is 2-chloro-4,6-bis(ethylamino)1,3,5-triazine.

Toxicity: Generally triazines are not considered to be very toxic. The oral LD_{50} of atrazine for rats is 2000 mg/kg. Cattle and sheep exposed to atrazine at a dose of 250 mg/kg for 2 days are killed with acute toxic signs. Non-ruminants appear to be more sensitive to atrazine

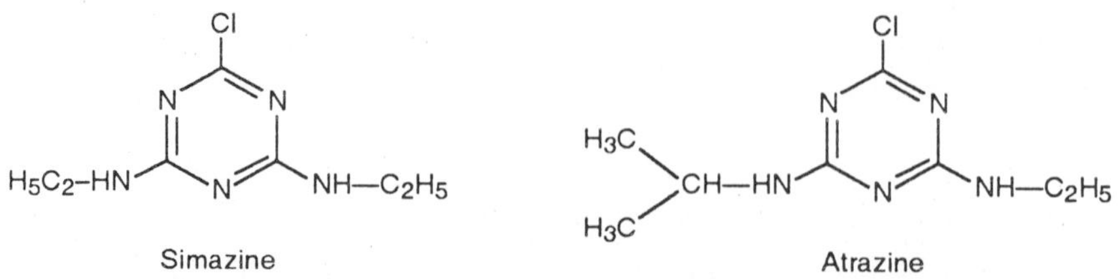

Fig. 13.16. Chemical structures of some important triazine herbicides.

than other types of animal. Simazine is non-toxic to a variety of animal species including mice, rats, rabbits, but is toxic to sheep and cattle which are killed by 3 daily doses of 250 mg/kg. Its oral LD_{50} for rats is 5000 mg/kg. Cyanazine is comparatively more toxic than atrazine and simazine with oral LD_{50} in rats about 150-350 mg/kg.

Mechanism of action: The mechanism by which triazines produce toxicity in animals is not well understood.

Clinical signs: Important clinical signs of triazine herbicides include anorexia, weakness, hypersalivation, dyspnoea with coughing, and muscle atonia occasionally accompanied by trembling, locomotor ataxia, weakness and paraplegia. Diarrhoea, hyperexcitability and loss of weight are possible. Atrazine is excreted in milk, so is of public health concern.

Post-mortem findings: Lesions of triazine toxicosis are non-specific and not pronounced. These may include gastrointestinal and pulmonary congestion and haemorrhages in heart, liver and kidneys.

Diagnosis: Diagnosis is based on history of exposure and clinical signs.

Treatment and management: There is no specific antidote to triazine herbicide poisoning. Therapy involves detoxification and symptomatic and supportive care only.

5. Substituted Urea Herbicides

Substituted ureas/Phenylureas are a group of herbicides used for general weed control in agricultural and non-agricultural practices. This group of herbicides include anisuron, diuron, fenuron, isoproturon, linuron monuron, parafluron, and tetrafluoron. Although over 20 different phenylureas have been marketed for use as herbicides, little information is available on the toxicity of most of these compounds. Isoproturon has been reported to be most widely used phenylurea herbicide in India.

Toxicity: Substituted phenylureas have relatively low toxicity in animals. Poisoning in animals is rare as a massive quantity of the herbicide needs to be ingested for toxicosis to occur, which is possible only if the compound is directly ingested. Ingestion of forage plants treated with herbicide usually does not result in poisoning. The oral LD_{50} of diuron and isoproturon in rats is approximately 3400 mg/kg and 1800-2400 mg/kg, respectively. Diuron produces toxicosis in cattle when it is given daily at a dose of 100 mg/kg for 10 days. Substituted ureas are non-toxic to fish.

Clinical signs: Phenylurea herbicide toxicosis produces clinical signs of anorexia, periods of depression, motor incoordination, prostration, and occasional respiratory difficulties. Haematuria and hypersalivation may occur.

Treatment and management: There is no specific treatment of substituted ureas toxicity. Symptomatic and supportive therapy generally provides recovery. Parenteral fluid administration or forced diuresis hastens early excretion of toxicant. The toxicosis has good prognosis.

6. Other Herbicides

Several other groups of herbicides are currently available for use in agriculture for chemical control of weeds and undesirable plants. These groups include carbamates and thiocarbamates, uracils, chlorobenzoic acids, chloroacetanilids and organophosphates. Most of the compounds belonging to these groups of herbicide have low mammalian toxicity. There is no specific antidote to their poisoning; treatment involves only symptomatic and supportive care. Important examples and clinical features of these herbicides are given in Table 13.4.

Table 13.4: Clinical features of other herbicides in domestic animals.

Class	Examples	Important clinical signs	Treatment
Carbamates and Thiocarbamates	*Carbamates:* Asulum, barban, chlorbufam, chlorpropham, fenasulam and phenmedipham. *Thiocarbamates:* Butylate, cycloate, di-allate, ethiolate, isopolinate, molinate, orbincarb, sulfallate and tri-allate.	Anorexia, salivation, diarrhoea, flatulence, ataxia, muscular incoordination and prostration.	Symptomatic and supportive.
Uracils	Bromacil, butafenacil, flupropacil, isocil, lenacil and terbacil,	Anorexia, depression, tympany, ataxia and convulsions.	Symptomatic and supportive.
Chlorobenzoic acids	Chloramben, dicamba, dinoben, TBA and tricamba.	Salivation, tympany, depression and possible convulsions.	Symptomatic and supportive.
Chloroacetanilides/ Acetanilides	Alachlor, acetochlor, butachlor, delachlor dimetachlor, metazachlor, metolachlor, and propachlor.	Dullness, depression, muscular weakness, weak pulse, hypothermia, and occasional paralysis.	Symptomatic and supportive.
Organophosphates	Glyphosate and glufosinate.	Nausea, vomiting, diarrhoea, dyspnoea, hypotension, tremors and metabolic acidosis.	Symptomatic and supportive.

TBA = 2,3,6-trichlorbenzoic acid.

C. FUNGICIDES

Fungicides are agents that are used to prevent or eradicate fungal infections from plants or seeds. In agriculture, they are used to protect tubers, fruits, and vegetables during storage or are applied directly to ornamental plants, trees, field crops, cereals and turf grasses. The main hazard to livestock from fungicides is likely to arise from their use as seed dressings for the protection of stored grains, potatoes, etc. Fungicides vary widely in chemical structure and, thus, in toxicity to livestock. In general, fungicides are of low to moderate mammalian toxicity, but they are believed to have greater potential than other pesticide groups to cause developmental defects and cancer.

Classification: Fungicides are classified in a number of ways on the basis of source, mode of action, mode of application and chemical structure. The most widely accepted classification is one based on the chemical structure and source.

I. Inorganic fungicides

1. Sulphur
2. Metals e.g. copper sulphate, bordeaux mixture (copper sulphate + calcium hydroxide), cadmium chloride and mercuric chloride.

II. Organic fungicides

1. Organomercury compounds e.g. phenylmercuric chloride, phenylmercuric acetate, ethylmercury acetate and methylmercury.
2. Chlorophenols, e.g. pentachlorophenol and trichlorophenol.
3. Dithiocarbamates e.g. ferbam, maneb, thiram and zineb.
4. Organotin compounds e.g. triphenyltin, tributyltin and triethyltin.
5. Phathalimides e.g. captan, folpet and captafol.
6. Benzimidazoles, e.g. benomyl, thiophanate methyl and fuberidazole.

7. Azoles e.g. cyproconazole, etridazole and penconazole.
8. Halogenated substituted monocyclic amines e.g. chlorothalonil, tecnazine and dichloran.
9. Morpholines e.g. dodemorph, fenpropiomorph and tridemorph.
10. Miscellaneous fungicides, e.g. cyclohexamide, pentachloronitrobenzene (PCNB), pyrazophos, terrazole and dinocap.

I. INORGANIC FUNGICIDES

1. Sulphur (Lime Sulphur or Flowers of Sulphur)

The use of sulphur as a pesticide is evident from the writings of ancient Greek. In the 19th and early 20th century, elemental sulphur and crude lime sulphur (calcium polysulphide and barium polysulphide) preparations were commonly used for control of fungus. Now the use of sulphur has declined due to availability of organic fungicides.

Lime-sulphur after ingestion may cause irritation, abdominal discomfort, colic, gastroenteritis, superpurgation and depression. However, death is rare. There are no specific lesions. There is no specific treatment to sulphur poisoning; removal of the residual material from GI tract and supportive therapy as required by condition is indicated. The detailed toxicology of sulphur has been described earlier in Chapter 12.

2. Metals

Inorganic metallic salts were among the first fungicides used in agriculture. They have both protective and preventive antifungal actions. However, metals are moderately to highly toxic and non-specific in action. Therefore, their use as fungicides has declined. The inorganic mercuric (-chloride and -oxide) and mercurous herbicides have been withdrawn from market in many countries because of their adverse effects and environmental concerns. Copper sulphate (also -carbonate, -chloride, and -hydroxide) and Bordeaux mixture (slurry of calcium hydroxide and copper sulphate) are still used occasionally on potatoes, apple, vine or hops to prevent growth of fungus. Copper products have low toxicity to mammals, but their excessive use may give rise to an unwanted build-up of copper in soil. Cadmium salts (-chloride and -sulphate) are also rarely used as fungicides.

II. ORGANIC FUNGICIDES

1. Organomercury Fungicides

The alkyl and aryl mercurials such as methylmercuric chloride, methylmercuric hydroxide, ethylmercuric chloride, phenylmercuric chloride, phenylmercuric acetate and methoxyethyl mercury -acetate and –chloride have been used extensively as seed fungicides for post-harvesting application to grain and other seed crops. However, large scale poisoning epidemics in some countries after consumption of treated seeds has led to their ban or restricted use. The organomercurial compounds possess moderate to high toxicity and have resulted in many deaths or permanent neurological disabilities in man and animals. Poisoning in farm animals due to mercury fungicides has declined in recent years but environmental problems are still widespread as methylmercury is readily formed from inorganic mercury (from industrial wastes) by aquatic microorganisms. The detailed toxicology of organomercurials has been discussed in Chapter 11.

2. Chlorophenols

Pentachlorophenol (PCP) : Pentachlorophenol or penta, commonly abbreviated as PCP, and its salts are used as fungicide, molluscicide, insecticide, herbicide, algicide and wood preservative. It is used to control termites and has been used extensively as wood preservative to protect timber against rot and marine borers. Animals may be poisoned either by licking wood

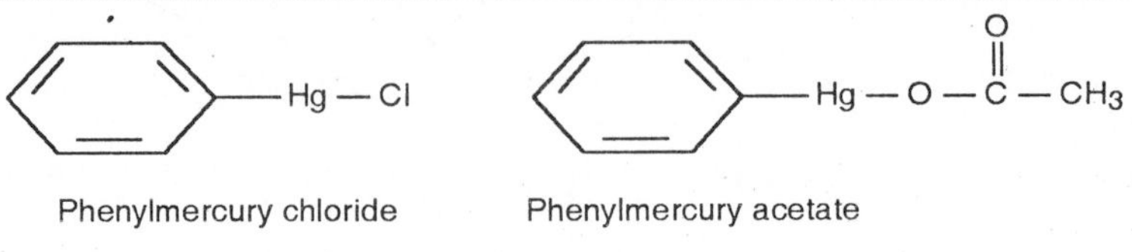

C_6H_5—Hg—Cl

Phenylmercury chloride

C_6H_5—Hg—O—C(=O)—CH_3

Phenylmercury acetate

Fig. 13.17. Chemical structures of some important organomercury fungicides.

that is treated with PCP or eating from treated feed bunkers. Animals may also inhale toxic amount of PCP from treated walls in sheds or barns. Some preparations of PCP may contain toxic contaminants such as carcinogenic dioxins. Pentachlorophenol has high potential for contamination of ecosystems. Now its indoor use has been restricted but is still sometimes used for outdoor wood treatment (timbers, poles).

Chemistry: Pentachlorophenol (PCP) is a chlorinated derivative of phenol. It is almost insoluble in water, freely soluble in alcohol or ether, and soluble in benzene. Sodium pentachlorophenate (NaPCP) is freely soluble in water. Pentachlorophenol is volatile and can give off toxic vapour especially at high ambient temperature which in sufficient concentration can kill animals confined in small quarters. Pentachlorophenol is synthesised by the successive chlorination of phenol. During the chlorination of phenol, a small amount of PCP forms a dimer by means of an oxygen bridge resulting in dioxin isomers containing five to eight chlorines. Technical grade PCP has historically contained dioxins (e.g. tetra-, hexa- and octo-chlorodibenzo-p-dioxin) and hexachlorobenzene as manufacturing by-products. The toxicity occurs due to either PCP or dioxin contents of penta.

Toxicity: Pentachlorophenol, in common with other chlorophenols, has a broad range of biocidal activity. The acute oral or dermal LD_{50} of PCP in domestic animals is in the range of 10-200 mg/kg. The acute oral LD_{50} in different species is: 70 mg/kg in dogs, 100 mg/kg in guinea pigs, 120 mg/kg in sheep and 140 mg/kg in calves. Adult ruminants may tolerate more ingested PCP than calves or non-ruminants. The LC_{50} of PCP in birds is 3400-5200 ppm. PCP is toxic to fish at 30-300 ppb and fish kills have resulted from spills into lakes and streams, primarily after a rain has flushed PCP from treated wood areas. Toxicity is enhanced by high temperature, physical activity, poor condition, oily or organic solvent as vehicle, prior exposure, hyperthyroidism, etc. Toxicity is diminished by cold temperature, antithyroid drugs, presence of body fat, etc. The acute toxicity of PCP appears to be greatest when the route of exposure is inhalation.

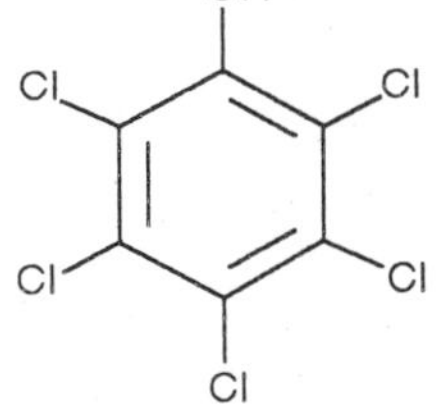

OH
Cl Cl
Cl Cl
Cl

Fig. 13.18. Chemical structure of pentachlorophenol.

Toxicokinetics: Chlorophenols are lipid soluble, so they are rapidly absorbed by all routes including GI tract, skin, and lungs. After ingestion, the peak plasma concentration of PCP is reached within few hours. Pentachlorophenol is highly protein bound in the blood and distributed throughout the body with highest concentrations detected in liver and kidneys. Some PCP is stored in body fat. Pentachlorophenol is metabolized mainly by conjugation with glucuronic acid and eliminated as the glucuronide conjugate. Other metabolites like tetrachlorophenol, tetrachlorocatechol and tetrachlorohydroquinone have also been reported. The metabolites as well as some unchanged PCP are rapidly excreted from the body in urine i.e. 50% is excreted within 24 hours in most species. Single doses of PCP have half-lives in blood of 15 hours in rats, 78 hours in monkeys, and 30 to 50 hours in humans.

Mechanism of action :

a. Chlorophenols such as pentachlorophenol are classic uncouplers (agents possessing ability to disconnect electron transport chain from production of ATP) of mitochondrial oxidative phosphorylation. Like other uncouplers, the chlorophenols are small amphipathic molecules which dissolve in phospholipid bilayers and enormously increase their ionic permeability. They shield the electric charge as the ion passes through the membrane, providing a polar environment for the ion and a hydrophobic face to the outside media. Their ability to act as proton ionophore leads to dissipation of the proton gradient across the inner mitochondrial membrane and inhibition of ATP generation.

In oxidative phosphorylation, the flow of electrons from NADH and $FADH_2$ to oxygen in mitochondria results in pumping of protons (H^+) by complexes I, III and IV from the mitochondrial matrix to the intermembrane space. This creates a proton gradient across the inner mitochondrial membrane, which is essentially required to drive the F_0F_1-ATPase/ATP synthase (Complex V) and produce ATP. In the process, when the protons move from intermembrane space back into the mitochondrial matrix through the ATP synthase, the osmotic energy of the gradient is converted into chemical energy in the form of ATP. Pentachlorophenol, being lipid soluble weak acid, act as proton ionophore (carriers of H^+ across biological membranes). It dissolves in the mitochondrial membrane and forms a pentachlorophenate ion (anionic form). The anionic form binds a proton on one side of membrane and carries it as a neutral molecule across the mitochondrial membrane. On the other side of membrane, the neutral molecule dissociates to reform the anionic form and releases the proton (Figure 13.19). This way PCP continues to carry/ or shuttle protons across the mitochondrial membranes, in particular from intermembrane space back into the matrix through the mitochondrial inner membrane. This proton shuttling leads to dissipation or destruction of proton gradient. As the protons are not passed during this shuttling process through the Complex V, the ATP synthase fails to function and there is no generation of ATP. Instead the proton energy is lost as heat, which is reflected in the form of fever. In absence of ATP, the cells meet the energy requirement by oxidizing more and more of stored carbohydrates and fats. Accordingly in PCP poisoning, the oxygen requirement increases, energy reserves are depleted and free energy generated is lost as body heat (fever). The Figure 13.19 depicts the possible mechanisms of action of pentachlorophenol and some other toxicants inhibiting the electron transport chain.

b. Other possible mechanisms of PCP include inhibition of glycolytic phosphorylation and respiratory enzymes, and damage to mitochondrial structure. Inhibition of the binding of T_4 to thyroid

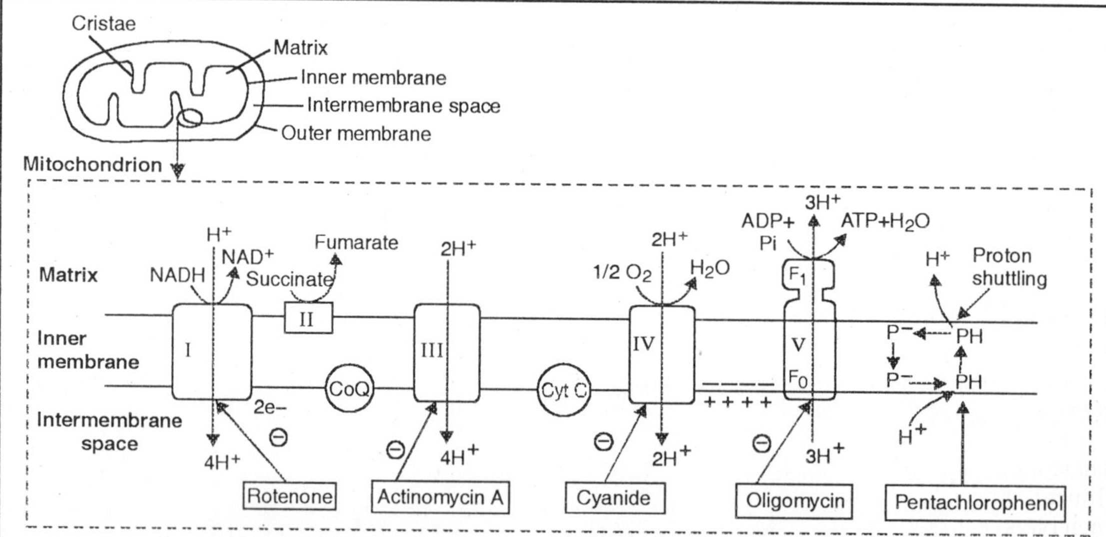

Fig. 13.19. Proposed mechanisms of action of pentachlorophenol and some other toxicants affecting the electron transport chain in mitochondria. Pentachlorophenol uncouples oxidative phosphorylation by shuttling protons and destroying proton gradient across inner mitochondrial membrane (See text for detail).
Abbreviation : P/P^- = Pentachlorophenol / pentachlorophenate ; H^+ = proton ; e^- = electron ; CoQ = coenzyme Q ; Cyt C = cytochrom C ; ADP = adenosine diphosphate ; ATP = adenosine triphosphate ; NADH = nicotinamide adenine dinucleotide (reduced form) ; NAD^+ = nicotinamide adenine dinucleotide (oxidized form) ; Pi = inorganic phosphate.
I : Complex I (NADH dehydrogenase). Rotenone blocks electron flow in complex I.
II : Complex II (Succinate dehydrogenase).
III : Complex III (Cytochrone C -coenzyme Q-oxidoreductase). Actinomycin A blocks electron flow in complex III.
IV : Complex IV (Cytochrome oxidase). Cyanide blocks cyt_{a3} in complex IV.
V : Complex V (ATP-synthase /F_0F_1 -ATPase). Oligomycin damages F_0 subunit of complex V.

hormone receptors has been associated with decreased T_4 levels in PCP-exposed animals.

Clinical signs :

Acute toxicity: In acute PCP exposure, the onset and duration of toxicosis may be so fast that no sign may be seen. Signs of acute poisoning include nervousness, weakness, muscle tremors, anorexia, lethargy followed by accelerated respiratory rate, hyperpyrexia (106-108° F), cyanosis, collapse, terminal convulsions and death. Less severely affected animals may not die but merely manifest hyperthermia and signs of oxygen deficiency. Signs of dermal exposure include erythema, dermatitis and acne. Hyperkeratosis also develops.

Chronic toxicity: In chronic PCP exposures, there may be abortion, stillbirth, foetal malformation, weight loss, decreased milk production, anaemia and increased leucocyte count in milk. Respiratory illness and fever may be absent. In poultry, there may be loss of weight, decreased egg production and increased mortality.

Post-mortem findings: Post-mortem lesions are non-specific in PCP poisoning. However, rigor mortis occurs quickly after death. Parenchymatous organs may manifest degenerative changes consistent with oxygen starvation and high body temperature. Agonal haemorrhages may be found on the heart and lungs. The blood would be dark because of ante-mortem deprivation of oxygen. Gastroenteritis may be present, if poison is ingested. In chronic cases, the carcass may be thin and devoid of fat. Fatty degeneration of liver and nephritis may be observed.

Diagnosis: History, signs of rapid overheating and respiratory distress, post-mortem findings and whole blood or urine analysis for pentachlorophenol may be helpful in the diagnosis. Clinical signs of PCP toxicosis generally occur when blood concentrations are from 40 to 80 ppm and acute lesions develop when concentrations in blood and tissues reach 100 ppm and 200 ppm, respectively.

Intoxication by chlorophenols has to be differentiated from other poisons causing respiratory insufficiency.

a. *Nitrate/Nitrite poisoning:* Colour of blood is brown and there is no fever.

b. *Carbon monoxide and cyanide poisoning:* Colour of blood is bright red and there is no fever.

c. *Insecticides poisoning:* Marked neuromuscular signs are present with variable autonomic manifestations.

Chronic pentachlorophenol toxicosis may be differentiated from other toxicoses like aflatoxins, nitrate, lead, pesticides, toxic plants, etc.

Treatment and management: No specific therapy is indicated for chlorophenol compounds toxicosis.

a. In the initial stages, use of emetics, gastric lavage or activated charcoal may be helpful.

b. Oxygen should be provided immediately to satisfy oxygen demand.

c. Body temperature should be lowered by cold water rinsing, ice-packs or ethanol spraying.

d. Acidosis may be corrected by administration of bicarbonate fluid.

e. Phenothiazine tranquilizers by I.M. route are indicated to decrease exertion and stress and to facilitate handling of animal for cooling. However, these should not be used to sedate or comatose the animal.

f. Dermal contamination should be removed by bathing the skin with liquid detergent.

g. Balanced electrolyte solutions without glucose should be administered to prevent dehydration.

h. Animal should be removed immediately from the exposure site.

Contraindications

Antipyretics like aspirin and paracetamol should not be used as they have minimal effect on the PCP-induced hyperpyrexia.

Prevention:

a. Remove all PCP treated wooden material from the immediate vicinity of animals.

b. Avoid contact of feed with penta-treated surfaces (e.g. wooden mangers).

c. Control temperature of interior surface of sheds to reduce volatilization of PCP from treated areas.

d. Increase ventilation, if PCP treated material is present in animal sheds.

Prognosis: If the animal survives the PCP poisoning for 24 hours, chances of complete recovery are fair. But in such cases, there are chances of secondary bacterial infections.

Public health and environmental concerns: Pentachlorophenol is slightly toxic to practically non-toxic to bird species, but it is highly to extremely toxic to fish. Biomagnification is not thought to be significant because of PCP's rapid break down in living organisms.

3. Dithiocarbamates

Dithiocarbamates are a broad chemical class of pesticides including fungicides. This group of fungicides have enjoyed wide spread use in agriculture and include metham, ferbam, thiram and ziram. They have low order of acute toxicity with oral LD_{50} values in rats ranging from several hundred milligrammes to several grammes per kg body weight. Although there are less chances of acute toxicosis from these agents, evidence of effects like endocrine disruption, teratogenesis and carcinogenesis from chronic exposure are available.

Chemistry and classification: Dithiocarbmates are the sulphur derivatives of carbamates. However, unlike carbamates, they are not or poor inhibitor of cholinesterase enzyme. Depending on the monoamine used in synthesis of fungicide, two groups of dithiocarbamates have been identified:

a. *Dialkyldithiocarbamates:* These are derived from secondary amines e.g. ziram, ferbam, thiram and NaDDC.
b. *Monoalkyldithiocarbamates:* These are derived from primary amines e.g. metham, zineb, nabam and maneb.

The fungicides in the metallodithiocarbamate group derive their names from the attached metal (See Fig. 13.20).

Toxicity: In general, dithiocarbamate fungicides are of low environmental persistence and low cumulative potential. They have low to moderate acute mammalian toxicity. The oral LD_{50} of various dithiocarbamate fungicides in rats is: metham 1800 mg/kg, ferbam >4000 mg/kg, thiram 780-865 mg/kg, ziram 1400 mg/kg, zineb 4400 mg/kg, and maneb >5000 mg/kg. Thiram is lethal to cats at a dose of 230 mg/kg. At level of 500 ppm in the diet, ziram inhibits egg laying in quails and partridges. In addition to fungicidal action, ziram and thiram are occasionally used as bird and mammal repellent (e.g. deer, stags and hare), probably because the birds and animals dislike their scent and keep away.

Toxicokinetics: Toxicokinetic data on dithiocarbamate fungicides are limited. Metham-sodium acts, in part, by decomposition to methyl isocyanate. Thiram produces carbon disulphide, which may contribute to the hepatotoxicity

Sr.No.	Name	Chemical name	Cation
i.	Ziram	Zinc dimethyldithiocarbamate	Zinc
ii.	Ferbam	Ferric dimethyldithiocarbamate	Iron
iii.	Na DDC	Sodium dimethyldithiocarbamate	Sodium
iv.	Thiram	Tetramethylthiuram disulphide (TMTD)	
iv	Metham	Sodium N-methyldithiocarbamate	Sodium
v.	Zineb	Zinc ethylenebisdithiocarbamate	Zinc
vi.	Nabam	Disodium ethylenebisdithiocarbamate	Sodium
vii.	Maneb	Manganese ethylenebisdithiocarbamate	Manganese

Fig. 13.20. Chemical names and structures of some important dithiocarbamate fungicides.

produced by it. Other dithiocarbamates also release carbon disulphide, which is responsible for some adverse effects.

Mechanism of action: Dithiocarbamates have multiple actions in the body, but their exact mechanism of action has not been elucidated.

a. The primary action of dithiocarbamate fungicides appears to be inhibition of –SH containing enzymes like α-ketoglutar-oxidase, pyruvate dehydrogenase and succinic dehydrogenase.

b. Dithiocarbamates have potential to cause metal chelation. They inhibit synthesis of some neurotransmitters, particularly noradrenaline, via chelation of copper-containing portion of enzyme dopamine-β-hydroxylase.

c. Dithiocarbamates have potential to cause endocrine disruption. They cause thyroid gland dysfunction with reduced plasma T_4 levels, perhaps due to decreased uptake of iodine or due to decrease TSH release. Interference with the release of gonadotrophin-releasing hormone from hypothalamus has been suggested to disrupt the hormonal control of ovulation in females. These actions may lead to long-term adverse effects.

d. Some dithiocarbamates (e.g. ziram and thiram) have ability to inhibit alcohol dehydrogenase enzyme. This may not be directly involved in toxicity, but leads to potentiation of toxicity of co-administered ethanol. Disulfiram, a commonly used alcohol deterrent, is a structural analogue of thiram.

Clinical signs: Toxic signs produced by various dithiocarbamate fungicides appear to be similar. A large dose of thiram and some other dithiocarbamates causes digestive disorders (nausea, vomiting, diarrhoea and abdominal pain), hypothermia, hypotension, ataxia, laboured breathing and clonic convulsions. Some of these compounds (e.g. ferbam and zineb) are reported to be carcinogenic in high doses. In addition, some compounds (e.g. maneb and zineb) break down to form ethylenethiourea (ETU) *in vivo*, in environment and during cooking of food. Ethylenethiourea is carcinogenic, mutagenic, teratogenic as well as antithyroid. Some of these agents (e.g. maneb, nabam and ziram) are irritant to eyes, skin and mucous membranes.

Long term exposure of dithiocarbamate fungicides may produce loss of body weight, retardation in growth and reproductive problems in animals. Reports of goitres in occupational workers handling thiram-treated seeds have been documented in literature.

Post mortem findings: Lesions of dithiocarbamate fungicide toxicosis are non-specific. Ingestion of these fungicides may cause focal necrosis of alimentary tract. Hepatic and renal pathology and increase in thyroid gland weight with histological evidence of hyperplasia may be observed in chronic toxicosis.

Treatment and management: No specific antidote is available for dithiocarbamates intoxication. Only supportive and symptomatic therapy is recommended.

4. Organotin Fungicides

Organotin compounds have been extensively used in agriculture as fungicides, acaricides and molluscicides. However, their use has declined in recent years mainly due to high toxicity potential, availability of better compounds and environmental concerns. Some agents like triphenyltin (acetate and oxide) possess good fungicidal activity, whereas others like tributyltin oxide are used in paints and wood preservatives (Table 13.5).

Chemistry and properties: Typical organotin compounds possessing fungicidal activities are di- and tri-alkyl and triphenyl tin. The triorganotin compounds are biologically very reactive and are mainly used as biocides. Important members

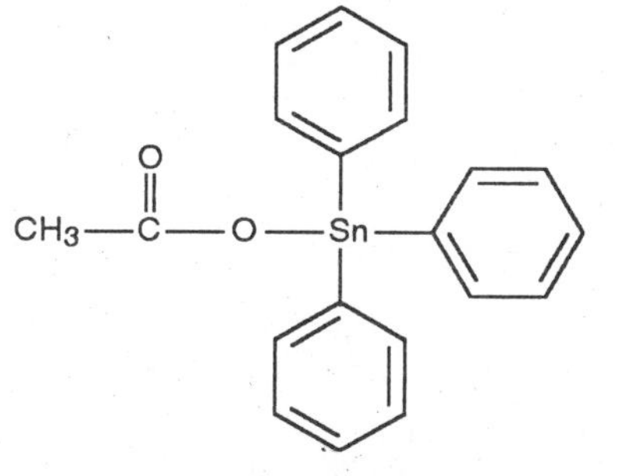

Fig. 13.21. Chemical structure of triphenyltin acetate.

possessing antifungal activity include tributyltin, trimethyltin, triethyltin and triphenyltin (Table 13.5). These compounds are lipid soluble and are used in wood preservatives and antifouling marine paints, and in paper mills.

Toxicity : Organotin compounds are highly to moderately toxic to animals. The toxicity of organotin compounds depends on the type of compound, type of salt used (e.g. acetate and oxide) and species involved. The oral LD_{50} of triphenyltin acetate for the laboratory rats is 136-238 mg/kg and triphenyltin oxide is 550 mg/kg body weight. Triphenyltin (fentin) is highly toxic to fish, but is moderately toxic to mammals. Organotin compounds are extremely toxic to invertebrates like snail.

Toxicokinetics: Organotin compounds are lipid soluble, so they are absorbed after ingestion or dermal exposure. After absorption, they are distributed to various organs including the CNS but highest concentration may be detected in liver. Metabolism of organotin occurs in liver and some other tissues. The mode of excretion of organotin compounds largely depends on the type of the compound. Ethyltin trichloride seems to be mainly excreted in urine, but diethyltin is eliminated in faeces, urine, and bile. Triethyltin is also excreted to some extent in milk. The biological half-life of different organotin compounds varies and many compounds are slow to disappear from the organs. Usually the biological half-life seems to be longer in the brain than in other organs.

Mechanism of action: Organotin compounds are neuro-, hepato-, reno- and immuno-toxic. They produce their action in different ways.

a. Organotins, particularly triethyltin, uncouples the oxidative phosphorylation.

b. They inhibit Na^+/K^+-ATPase and interfere with ion movement across cell membranes.

c. Some organotin compounds act by interfering with sulphydryl groups of mitochondrial enzymes.

d. Short-chain trialkyltins (e.g. trimethyltin and triethyltin) are neurotoxic. They decrease neurotransmitter concentration and appear to disrupt myelin production.

e. Trialkyltins inhibit T-cell lymphocyte proliferation and are immunotoxic. They decrease lymphopoiesis and increase susceptibility to infections.

Clinical signs: Clinical signs of poisoning occur very soon after triphenyltin acetate and after some time in triphenyltin oxide exposure. Similar to organomercurials, the clinical signs are primarily

Table 13.5 : Important agricultural and other uses of organotin compounds.

Organotin compound	Important uses
Triphenyltin acetate and triphenyltin hydroxide	Agricultural fungicide.
Tributyltin oxide	In paints and wood preservatives, for protection of jute, and production of paper.
Tributyltin benzoate	Disinfectant for use in hospitals and stables.
Dibutyltin dilaurate and tetraisobutyltin	As anthelmintic in poultry.
p-Bromophenoxy triethyltin	As nematocide.
Trivinyltin chloride	As herbicide.
Tributyltin chloride and triphenyltin chloride and acetate	As rodent repellent.
Triphenyl- and tributyltin compounds	As molluscicide.
Trialkyl- and triaryltin chlorides in combination with DDT or pyrethrins	As ovicide.
Triphenyl- and tributyltin compounds	As antifoulants in ship paints and underwater coatings.
Tricyclohexyltin hydroxide	As miticide.
Triphenyltin compounds	As insect chemosterilant.

related to nervous system. The important toxic manifestations are depression, irritability, weakness, nausea, vomiting, disorientation, aggressive behaviour and paresis or paralysis. In humans, they cause increased intracranial pressure, headache, vertigo, photophobia, blurred vision, amnesia, tremors, convulsions, and other neurobehavioural disturbances. Local exposure produces irritation to skin, eye and mucosae.

Post-mortem findings: Post mortem findings are non-specific. Nervous system lesions consistent with organotin poisoning may be noted on histopathological studies.

Diagnosis: Diagnosis depends on history of exposure to organotin compounds, clinical signs and laboratory analysis. Source material includes stomach contents and tissues like brain and kidney.

Treatment and management: There is no specific treatment to organotin poisoning. Detoxification limiting the absorption of poison and supportive therapy is required.

Public health and environmental concerns: Organotin compounds are associated with undesirable accumulation in invertebrates and fish and are regarded as one of the most serious environmental pollutant pesticide groups. Tributyltin (also triphenyltin) is associated with endocrine disruption in snail and oyster.

4. Phthalimides

Phthalimides (Chloroalkylthiodicarboximides) are a group of broad-spectrum protectant fungicides. They have been in use for more than 50 years and include captan, folpet and captafol. These fungicides possess low mammalian toxicity and there are only a few reports of acute toxicity in animals.

Chemistry: The phthalimide fungicides are sometimes referred to as R-SCCl compounds or chloroalkylthio fungicides due the presence of side chains that contain chlorine, carbon and sulphur (Figure 13.21). The phthalimide ring provides certain physical properties to the compound, but the toxicological action of fungicides is determined mainly by the side chain. They have some structural similarity with thalidomide and have teratogenic activities. They are less soluble in water and have low volatility.

Toxicity: Phthalimide fungicides generally have low toxicity to mammals (oral LD_{50} in rats: captan 9000-12,500 mg/kg, folpet >10,000 mg/kg, and captafol 5000-6200 mg/kg). However in ruminants, captan may produce acute toxicity (oral toxic dose 250-500 mg/kg). Low protein diet makes rats more sensitive to captan (oral LD_{50} 480 mg/kg) than those receiving normal protein diet (oral LD_{50} 9000-12,500 mg/kg).

Toxicokinetics : The toxicokinetic data on phthalimide fungicides in domestic animals are limited. After ingestion, some amount of fungicide is degraded by non-enzymatic as well as enzymatic chemical reactions in gut. After absorption, these compounds undergo rapid metabolism and are eliminated (24-48 hours) from the body.

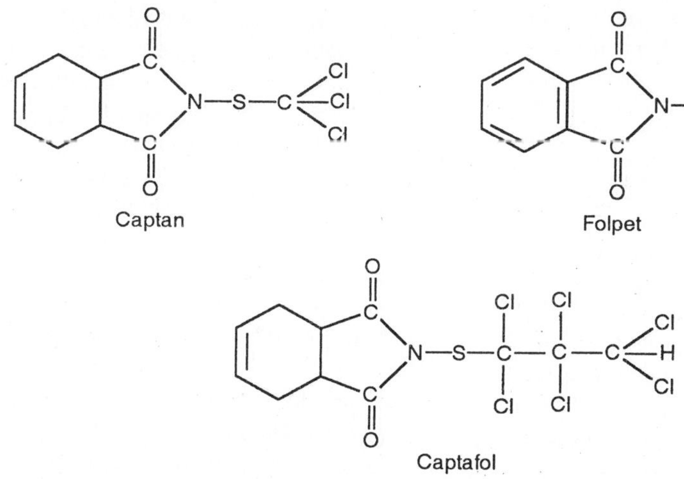

Captan

Folpet

Captafol

Fig. 13.22. Chemical structures of some important phthalimide fungicides.

Mechanism of action :

a. The phthalimide fungicides have affinity for sulphydryl (thiol, -SH) groups. However, their rapid degradation and the resultant limitation in exposure prevent many of these reactions from resulting *in vivo* toxicological actions.

b. Captan and folpet react with DNA and induce point mutations and clastogenic changes *in vitro*, but the mechanism by which such effects are induced has not been elucidated.

Clinical signs: The phthalimide fungicides have low acute toxicity. Important clinical signs with massive oral doses include laboured respiration, anorexia, depression, hydrothorax, ascites and gastroenteritis. Adverse skin reactions to these fungicides due to delayed contact hypersensitivity are possible. Phthalimide fungicides irritate mucous membranes and there is potential for damage when they contact eye. Chronic toxicosis may produce reduced feed intake, reduced weight gain, carcinogenicity, mutagenicity and teratogenicity.

Post mortem findings: There is no specific lesion to phthalimide fungicide toxicosis. Occasionally hydrothorax, gastroenteritis and petechiae on gall bladder are visible.

Treatment: There is no specific antidote to phthalimide fungicides toxicosis. Therapy involves symptomatic and supportive care only.

6. Benzimidazoles

Benzimidazoles are nitrogen heterocyclic compounds with systemic curative and protective fungicidal actions. These include benomyl, thiabendazole, thiophanate, fuberidazole, and imazalil. Some of these agents are also used as antifungal agents in veterinary medicine. Inhibition of microtubule polymerization by binding to α-tubulin is the primary action of benzimidazoles. Many of these fungicides also inhibit mitochondrial fumarate reductase, reduce glucose transport and uncouple oxidative phosphorylation, but these actions occur at significantly higher concentrations in mammals than that observed in fungi. The oral LD_{50} of different benzimidazole fungicides in rats is: benomyl >5000 mg/kg, thiabendazole 3000 mg/kg, thiophanate methyl 7500 mg/kg, fuberidazole 330 mg/kg, and imazalil 345 mg/kg. Benzimidazoles are unlikely to cause acute toxicosis in animals in the concentrations they are used, but may cause skin sensitization on contact. Some benzimidazoles (e.g. benomyl) have been associated with fetotoxicity and teratogenicity in the absence of obvious maternal toxicity, indicating possible adverse effects.

7. Other Fungicides

Several other groups of fungicides are currently used to eradicate or prevent the undesirable growth of fungi in many agricultural, horticultural and industrial situations. These fungicide groups include azoles (e.g. cyproconazole, diniconazole, etridazole, hexaconazole, penconazole, and tebuconazole), halogenated substituted monocyclic aromatics (e.g. chlorothalonil, chloroneb, dicloran, hexachlorobenzene, quintozene and tecnazine,), morpholines (benzamorph, dodemorph, imethomorph and tridemorph), organophosphates (e.g. ediphenphos, pyrazophos and tolclophos methyl), dinitrophenols (e.g. binapacryl, dinocap and dinosulphon), antibiotics (e.g. cycloheximide and validomycin) and several miscellaneous agents. All these fungicides are lowly to moderately toxic to humans and animals. The therapy of toxicosis in most cases involves only the symptomatic and supportive care.

D. FUMIGANTS

Fumigants are non-specific acute toxicants that are effective by inhalation. They are effective as pesticide only in gaseous forms and are generally used to control insects, rodents and soil nematodes. These are more useful in the control of pests in grain, food and feed-stuff stores. Fumigants as rodenticide are not as economical as poisonous baits, but they can be used when baits are ineffective, impractical or hazardous to use. Fumigants are effective only when used in closed situations such as storage containers, warehouses, ships, burrows, etc. With these types of application, fumigants are very specific for target species.

A large number of fumigants were available few years back, but some of these (e.g. carbon disulphide, carbon tetrachloride and ethylene dibromide) have been withdrawn from market owing to their excessive toxicity. However, fumigant related poisonings from these agents are still reported in literature and are included in the present section. Fumigants are available as liquids that readily vaporize, solids that release a gas by chemical reaction (e.g. HCN release from $Ca(CN)_2$ plus water), or gases contained in cylinders or ampoules (e.g. methyl bromide). Fumigants can be toxic to non-target species after inhalation, accidental ingestion or dermal exposure. Great care is required in their use and in many countries only professionals are permitted to apply them.

Advantages of fumigants

a. Fumigants can be eliminated from the treated area simply by ventilation.

b. As fumigants exert their action in gaseous form, they easily penetrate to areas otherwise inaccessible for pesticidal action (e.g. burrows).

c. Fumigants are useful for very big installations or structures (e.g. aeroplanes and ships) that can be sealed or enclosed effectively.

d. Chances of secondary poisoning with fumigants are negligible.

Classification

Fumigants can be broadly divided into 2 groups: inorganic and organic fumigants.

I. Inorganic fumigants

1. Aluminium phosphide/Phosphine gas
2. Hydrogen cyanide
3. Carbon disulphide
4. Sulphur dioxide.

II. Organic fumigants

1. Chloropicrin
2. Methyl bromide
3. Ethylene dibromide
4. 1,3-Dichloropropene
5. Dibromochloropropane (DBCP).

I. INORGANIC FUMIGANTS

1. Aluminium Phosphide/Phosphine Gas

Aluminium phosphide (or Magnesium phosphide) is one of the most commonly used fumigants for stored cereals and grains. It is also used as rodenticide to kill moles, rabbits and small rodents. Phosphine (PH_3) gas released gradually from aluminium phosphide in the presence of atmospheric moisture is mainly responsible for pesticidal action. Though aluminium phosphide is highly toxic, yet it is said to be safer for use as grain fumigant under practical condition because it is required in lesser amount than other fumigants. In India, aluminium phosphide tablets (Trade name Celphos) are widely used for suicidal purposes in humans and for malicious poisoning in animals due to their easy availability in homes and rapid onset of action. Accidental poisoning may occur following fumigation. On inhalation, it produces severe pulmonary oedema. Its toxicity is similar to zinc phosphide (See for detail Rodenticides).

2. Hydrogen Cyanide

Hydrogen cyanide (HCN) gas is used to fumigate ships, buildings, closed chambers and soil. It is also used for rabbit control in some countries and is applied as sodium cyanide powder. Cyanide is one of the most rapidly acting poisons; victims may die within minutes of exposure. Cyanide has very high affinity for iron in the ferric form. When absorbed, it reacts with the trivalent iron of cytochrome oxidase (Complex IV) in mitochondria, thus inhibiting cellular respiration. The mechanism of action, course of poisoning and line of treatment are the same as discussed in cyanogenetic plants (see Poisonous plants, Chapter 14).

3. Carbon Disulphide

Carbon disulphide (CS_2) has been used as a grain fumigant mainly in combination with carbon tetrachloride. It is also used as soil fumigant, general insecticide and industrial solvent. Now its use has greatly declined due to high toxicity. The use of CS_2 as a fumigant is the primary source exposure to man and domestic animals.

Properties: Carbon disulphide is a colourless, non-viscous explosive liquid having a sweetish aromatic odour. However, the industrial grade CS_2 may have a yellowish colour and a rotten cabbage or radish odour. When heated, CS_2 decomposes to form sulphur dioxide and carbon monoxide. Carbon disulphide is not miscible with water, but freely dissolves in alcohol, ether and chloroform.

Toxicity: Carbon disulphide is highly reactive and may cause serious toxicosis in domestic animals and man. In human beings, 5 ml of CS_2 when taken internally causes serious symptoms and about 10 ml is fatal. A concentration of about 600 ppm produces serious symptoms if inhaled for one hour, while double this amount is dangerous in thirty minutes.

Toxicokinetics: Carbon disulphide is well absorbed from all routes including oral, dermal and inhalation. After absorption, it binds with RBCs for which it has special affinity. Initially it tends to accumulate in liver followed by distribution to other body organs including the brain. It binds to various body tissues and about 20-40% is excreted unchanged in breath and urine.

Mechanism of action: Carbon disulphide is a highly reactive compound. Carbon disulphide is structurally analogous to CO_2, but is more reactive towards nucleophiles and bases and more easily reduced. It reacts with various amino acids, catecholamines, vitamins and steroid hormones and produces multiple actions in body. Its primary effect is neurotoxicity.

a. *Neurotoxicity:* Carbon disulphide affects nervous system in a number of ways. It reacts with nucleophiles such as amines and afford formation of dithiocarbamates ($2R_2NH + CS_2 \longrightarrow [R_2NH_2^+][R_2NCS_2^-]$), which are potent neurotoxicants. It inhibits synthesis as well as metabolism of several biogenic amines in both central and peripheral nervous systems and causes neuropathy.

   i. Carbon disulphide reacts with amino acid tryptophan and forms tryptophan dithiocarbamate, which inhibits certain enzymes (e.g. dopamine-β-hydroxylase) and impairs the synthesis of biogenic amines such as noradrenaline. This impairs neurotransmission in adrenergic neurons.

   ii. The reaction products of CS_2 with adrenaline and noradrenaline block monoamine oxidase enzyme. Inhibition of MAO affects metabolism of biogenic amines.

   iii. The dithiocarbamates formed from CS_2 chelate metals such as copper and zinc. These metals are essential part of some enzymes required for proper neuronal functions. Chelation of these metals also produces biochemical lesions of copper and zinc deficiency.

   iv. Carbon disulphide produces thiamine deficiency, mainly through its hepatotoxic action, which leads to a generalized neuropathy.

   v. Carbon disulphide disrupts activity of peripheral and central nervous systems by virtue of demyelination, vacuolization and cellular death.

   vi. There are evidences that CS_2 causes distal axonopathy by covalent cross-linking of neurofilaments through a series of reactions.

   vii. Carbon disulphide produces destruction of microcirculation in CNS, which contribute to neurotoxicity.

b. *Hepatotoxicity:* Carbon disulphide causes hepatotoxicity mainly via conversion to active metabolite sulphur. Sulphur reacts with microsomal enzymes as a result of which cytochrome P-450 activity is lost. Carbon disulphide also inhibits proteins synthesis through formation of amino dithiocarbamates. Carbon disulphide associated liver disease may result in deficiency and derangement of vitamin B_1 (thiamine) metabolism.

c. *Cardiovascular toxicity:* Carbon disulphide is believed to cause interference with elastase-inhibiting factors in the plasma. Together with a functional copper deficiency (metal chelation), this action disrupts the elastic elements in the walls of blood vessels. This leads to generalized destruction of microcirculation, particularly the microcirculation of the brain.

d. *Endocrine disruption:* Carbon disulphide interferes with the production of testosterone and adrenal steroids. Formation of tyrosine dithiocarbamate may interfere with thyroid hormone production and/or receptor site activity.

e. *Inhibition of vitamins and enzymes:* Carbon disulphide reacts with vitamin B_6 (Pyridoxamine) to form pyridoxine dithiocarbamic acid that causes blockade of a number of pyridoxine-dependent enzymes, especially transaminases and amino oxidases.

f. *Irritation and corrosion:* Carbon disulphide is an irritant and caustic. On contact, it causes severe burns on the skin and degenerative changes in the nearby peripheral nerves. Eye exposure may cause degeneration in the retina and optic nerve.

Clinical signs :

Acute toxicity: Acute poisoning may occur after inhalation of carbon disulphide vapour or swallowing the liquid. After ingestion, it produces intense burning pain in throat, nausea, vomiting, colic (horses), drowsiness, unconsciousness, dilated pupils, cyanosed mucous membranes, dyspnoea, laboured breathing and muscular weakness. Ataxia, abnormal reflexes and fine tremors occur followed by pulmonary oedema, convulsions, possible blindness, collapse, coma and death from respiratory paralysis. Death may occur in few hours or may be delayed for several days. Urine, faeces and breath usually smell of CS_2. Inhalation of CS_2 produces coughing and dyspnoea followed by systemic signs. Local exposure produces blisters on the skin.

Chronic poisoning: Chronic poisoning is usually seen in occupational workers who get constant exposure of carbon disulphide fumes in ill-ventilated rooms. Main signs include muscular weakness, ataxia and paralysis of extensor muscles. Amblyopia with optic atrophy occurs in some cases. Reproductive problems with sterility, chronic metritis, abortions, etc. have been reported in human occupational workers. The adverse effects on reproductive performance are generally permanent. Death may occur from inanition and hepatic insufficiency.

Post-mortem findings: There is no specific lesion in CS_2 poisoning. On opening the body cavities, there is smell of carbon disulphide. The blood is dark and fluid. Congestion and haemorrhages in the stomach and lungs may be seen and the lungs are oedematous. In chronic poisoning, there may be degenerative changes in the cerebral cortex, heart and liver.

Diagnosis: Diagnosis of carbon disulphide poisoning is made from history, circumstantial evidences, clinical signs and necropsy findings. Confirmational diagnosis can be made for laboratory analysis of suspected tissue samples.

Treatment and management: Carbon disulphide has no specific antidote. Symptomatic and supportive therapy is recommended.

a. The animal should immediately be removed into the fresh air and given oxygen.

b. Activated charcoal and a saline cathartic should be given, if the toxicant has been ingested recently.

c. Exposed eyes should be washed with water for at least 15 minutes; skin should be washed with liquid detergent if exposure is dermal.

d. Convulsions are controlled with an appropriate CNS depressant e.g. barbiturates or diazepam.

e. Free carbon disulphide in the blood may be inactivated by intravenous administration of urea (0.5-1.5 g/kg).

f. Vitamin B_6 should be administered in large doses to compensate its CS_2-induced inactivation in body.

Contraindication

Adrenergic agonists such as amphetamine should not be administered in CS_2 poisoning due to inhibition of monoamine oxidase.

4. Sulphur Dioxide

Sulphur dioxide (SO_2) is a heavy, colourless, non-inflammable gas possessing a pungent, suffocating smell of burning sulphur. It dissolves freely in water. Sulphur dioxide is a powerful antiseptic and disinfectant and sometimes used as fumigating agent. It is now mostly used in industry as a refrigerant and a bleaching agent. It is very destructive to vegetable life and intensely poisonous to mammalian and insect life. Its detailed toxicology and line of treatment have been discussed in the air pollutants (see Environmental Pollutants, Chapter 17).

II. ORGANIC FUMIGANTS

1. Chloropicrin

Chloropicrin (CCl_3NO_2) has been used as an insecticide since 1917 and as a soil fumigant since 1920. Its primary use today is for pre-plant soil fumigation to control soil borne fungi, diseases and nematodes. It is also used to treat wood poles and timbers for internal decay by fungi and insects, and as a warning/clearing agent for sulphuryl fluoride (structural fumigant) and methyl bromide (soil and structural fumigant). Chloropicrin is highly toxic to mammals (class I toxicant) and was used in World War I as a chemical weapon.

Properties: Chloropicrin is a colourless or faintly yellow, oily liquid with a strong, sharp, highly irritating odour. It smells like chlorine and is about 4 times more toxic than chlorine. It is a strong irritant and sensory irritation gives early warning of its presence. It is, therefore, sometimes added in small amounts to other relatively odourless fumigants to act as a warning agent. Chloropicrin liquid decomposes in the environment. Photochemical reactions with chloropicrin produce phosgene; other decomposition products include nitrogen oxides and chlorine compounds.

Toxicity: Undiluted chloropicrin is highly toxic by ingestion or direct contact with the skin or eyes. Inhalation exposure to 0.15-0.37 ppm for 3-30 seconds results in eye irritation and lachrymation; 4 ppm for a few seconds may cause some degree of incapacitation and an exposure of few seconds to 15 ppm can cause injury to respiratory tract. Exposure to concentrations above 15 ppm can result in lachrymation and vomiting and if allowed to continue for a minute or longer can cause pulmonary oedema and possibly death. Animal studies established that the 4-hour inhalation LC_{50} for chloropicrin vapour in rats is 11.9 ppm and the respiratory irritation potential threshold in mice is 7.98 ppm. Chloropicrin is toxic to fish.

Mechanism of action: Chloropicrin is a strong irritant and a lachrymator. Although the exact mechanism of chloropicrin action has not been defined in animals, most adverse effects are attributed to strong irritation of tissues. Respiratory tissues are the primary target for chloropicrin inhalation toxicity.

Clinical signs: Undiluted chloropicrin is severely and immediately irritating to the upper respiratory tract, eyes and skin upon direct contact. Accordingly, clinical signs of chloropicrin poisoning depend on the route of exposure. When inhaled, it causes lachrymation, coughing, dyspnoea, feeling of pain, vomiting, etc. These symptoms are followed by marked restlessness, rapid and laboured breathing, cyanosis and death. Death may occur from acute pulmonary oedema within 24-28 hours or later from bronchopneumonia. If ingested, chloropicrin can cause burns to the mouth, throat, and oesophagus. Other signs are similar to those of overexposure through inhalation. Ingestion of large quantities of chloropicrin liquid can be fatal.

Dermal exposure to chloropicrin can lead to chemical burns or dermatitis manifested by red, cracked and irritated skin. The extent of skin injury depends on the concentration and duration of exposure. Contact with the eyes can cause pain, redness and tearing. Prolonged eye exposure to chloropicrin can cause blindness. Entrance through damaged skin causes similar signs as those seen in overexposure through inhalation.

Diagnosis: Diagnosis of chloropicrin toxicosis should be made from history and clinical signs.

Treatment and management: Chloropicrin has no specific antidote. The treatment consists of supportive therapy only.

a. On inhalation, the intoxicated animal should immediately be removed to fresh air or provided with assisted ventilation to support pulmonary function.
b. On ingestion, the intoxicated animal should be given milk, egg white or lot of water.
c. On dermal exposure, the skin should be washed with running water. Eyes should be thoroughly rinsed gently with water for at least 15 minutes.

Contraindication

Emetics should not be used in chloropicrin poisoning.

2. Methyl Bromide

Methyl bromide (CH_3Br) is a broad-spectrum pesticide primarily used for soil fumigation, seed fumigation, commodity fumigation, structural fumigation and quarantine treatment. It is also used in some fire extinguishers and as an intermediate in the manufacture of other chemicals. It is the most important organic fumigant which is responsible for large number of occupational deaths in human beings. Accidental poisoning incidents also occur in man and animals due to entry into buildings, green houses or fields being fumigated with methyl bromide. Individuals or animals living in close proximity to fumigated fields or buildings are also occasionally exposed to its harmful effects. Methyl bromide use and application should be strictly controlled and allowed only by professional, certified applicators.

Properties: Methyl bromide (Bromomethane) is a colourless, odourless non-flammable gas, which is heavier than air at room temperature. It is manufactured commercially but also is produced naturally by marine algae and other plants and as a by-product of the combustion of plant materials (i.e. forest fires). It is easily compressed into liquid form and is contained in cylinders and ampoules. Methyl bromide is 3 times heavier than air and can accumulate in poorly ventilated or low-lying areas. Under adverse conditions, it can remain in air for days after application as a fumigant. A gas at room temperature, methyl bromide readily penetrates skin, cloth, and other protective materials such as rubber and leather. Due to its high toxicity and odourless nature, chloropicrin (a powerful irritant and stimulator of lachrymation) is added to methyl bromide as a warning of exposure.

Toxicity: Methyl bromide is highly toxic to human beings and animals. Exposure to methyl bromide mainly occurs by the inhalation route; the dermal and oral route being of minor relevance. If administration of methyl bromide takes place at a concentration of 1 mg/litre, it may kill a rat within 22 hours; and 2 mg/litre may kill a rat within 6 hours. The oral LD_{50} value in rats for liquid methyl bromide is 100 mg/kg. Children and young animals exposed to the same levels of methyl bromide as adults may receive larger doses because they have greater lung surface area : body weight ratios and increased minute volumes : weight ratios. In addition, they may be exposed to higher levels than adults in the same location because of their short stature and higher levels of methyl bromide found nearer to the ground.

Toxicokinetics: Methyl bromide is rapidly absorbed from all routes including oral, lungs and skin. However, ingestion of methyl bromide is unlikely because it is a gas at room temperature. After inhalation, it produces irritation of the upper respiratory tract before being absorbed. Peak concentrations in plasma, liver, adipose tissues and brain generally reaches within one hour of pesticide exposure. Methyl bromide is highly lipid soluble, so is widely distributed in different tissues including brain. Methyl bromide is metabolized mainly (about 50%) to carbon dioxide, which is primarily excreted in expired air. Some excretion of methyl bromide and its metabolites (CO_2, bromide, methanol, etc.) also occur in urine and faeces.

Mechanism of action: Methyl bromide has high affinity for sulphydryl (-SH) groups. So it methylates the sulphydryl groups of enzymes and proteins, causing cellular disruption and reduced glutathione levels. Cellular disruption, primarily in CNS, results in progressive dysfunction. Methanol, a metabolite of methyl bromide, may also contribute to the neurological and visual effects, but this is likely to be significant only at high levels of exposure.

Clinical signs :

Acute toxicity: Clinical signs have been described in human beings and dogs and depend on both the concentration and the duration of exposure to methyl bromide. Important clinical manifestations include nausea, vomiting, visual disturbances, ataxia, tremor, nystagmus, marked depression, inability to stand, paralysis of limbs, clonic and tonic convulsions and death. Pulmonary effects include acute pulmonary oedema. Death mainly results from respiratory or cardiovascular failure. Several non-fatal cases result in persistent neurological and psychiatric complaints in humans ranging from muscular soreness, headache, decreased libido, mental depression, phobias and paranoia.

On dermal exposure methyl bromide produces erythema, blisters, severe vesicular dermatitis and burns of second degree. Eye exposure to liquid methyl bromide or to high concentrations of vapour may cause corneal irritation and burns.

Chronic toxicity: Repeated exposures to methyl bromide in occupational workers have been associated with peripheral neuropathies, especially sensory neuropathy, impaired gait, behavioural changes, and mild liver and kidney dysfunction. Visual impairment secondary to atrophy of the optic nerve has also been reported in human beings. Methyl bromide is not considered a reproductive or developmental toxicant.

Post-mortem findings: The post-mortem findings of methyl bromide toxicosis are related mainly to nervous system and excretory organs. There is congestion and petechial haemorrhages of brain and lungs, and congestion and tubular necrosis of kidneys. Scattered minute haemorrhages in the brain, heart, lungs and spleen may also be seen.

Diagnosis: Diagnosis of methyl bromide poisoning can be made from history of exposure and clinical signs.

Treatment and management: Methyl bromide has no specific antidote.

a. Supportive and symptomatic therapy is advocated which include oxygen, if necessary.

b. Antacids and sodium bicarbonate therapy is given for acidosis.

c. Convulsions can be controlled by barbiturates.

d. Washing of the affected skin may be done.

Public health and environmental concerns: Methyl bromide is one of the ozone-depleting substances and its use has been curtailed. In coming years, the use of methyl bromide is likely to be phased out completely.

3. Ethylene Dibromide

Ethylene dibromide (Br-CH_2-CH_2Br; dibromethane; ethylene bromide; EDB) is used as a soil and post-harvest fumigant for crops and as a quarantine fumigant for citrus and tropical fruits and vegetables. It exists as a colourless liquid with a mild, sweet odour. It is a highly toxic compound with number of adverse effects reported in occupational workers. Inhalation is the most hazardous route of exposure to EDB, however it may also be toxic by skin contact or ingestion. The oral LD_{50} of EDB is 110 mg/kg for rats, 250 mg/kg for mice, and 55 mg/kg for rabbits.

In human beings, acute exposure to EDB produces moderate depression of central nervous system and pulmonary congestion after exposure by inhalation, and acute gastrointestinal distress (vomiting, diarrhoea) and pulmonary oedema after ingestion. Lung injury can also lead to secondary effects such as pneumonia and respiratory tract infections. Subacute or chronic exposure to ethylene dibromide may cause decreased weight gain, loss of appetite and impaired spermatogenesis in bulls and decreased egg production in laying hens due to impaired follicle growth. Ethylene dibromide is reportedly a severe skin and eye irritant and can cause skin blistering with contact. Histopathological changes in liver and kidneys have been observed following acute and repeated exposure to EDB. Ethylene dibromide is considered a carcinogen in rats and mice, due to which it use as fumigants has been restricted now.

4. 1,3-Dichloropropene

1,3-Dichloropropene (α-Chloroallyl chloride) is a soil fumigant nematocide used in agriculture for more than 50 years. It exists as white to amber coloured liquid with sweet-penetrating odour. Commercial preparations generally contain varying amounts of a mixture of *cis*- and *trans*-isomers. 1,3-Dichloropropene is irritating to the mucous membranes and skin and is moderately to acutely toxic to animals. Its oral lethal dose in rodents is approximately 100 mg/kg.

Toxicity of 1,3-dichloropropene in animals and man occurs mainly through inhalation and skin. Toxic effects observed in humans exposed to high levels of vapours or having extended dermal contact with the liquid appears to reflect the irritant nature of the pesticide. Acute (short-term) inhalation exposure of humans causes mucous membrane irritation, chest pain, and breathing difficulties. Dermal exposure to 1,3-dichloropropene causes redness, oedema, erythema and necrosis and possibly contact dermatitis. Irritation of eyes and upper respiratory mucosae accompanied with lachrymation may appear after exposure to its vapour. 1,3-Dichloropropene is rapidly and extensively metabolized upon absorption by animals and humans, so serious systemic effects are rarely observed.

5. Dibromochloropropane

Dibromo-chloropropane (DBCP) is 1, 2-dibromo-3-chloropropane ($ClCH_2CHBrCH_2Br$). It is a fumigant nematocide, but is rarely used now due to its adverse effects on reproduction. It has moderate to high toxicity in mammals with oral LD_{50} of 170 mg/kg in rats. Like ethylene dibromide, in human beings it produces moderate depression of CNS and pulmonary congestion after inhalation and gastrointestinal distress and pulmonary oedema after ingestion. Dermal exposure results in irritation and redness. Dibromochloropropane causes sterility and/or abnormally low sperm counts in workmen engaged in its manufacture. Studies in laboratory animals have suggested that repeated inhalation exposure to as little as 5 ppm of DBCP has an adverse effect on testes and on reproductive performance of male rats.

E. RODENTICIDES

Rodenticides are chemical preparations used to destroy rodents, particularly mice and field rats. They are required to control the over-population of rodents and to prevent losses caused by them. Rodenticides should be selectively toxic to rodents and non-toxic to man and farm animals. But unfortunately, there is no such rodenticide which fully meets this requirement. Rodenticides are second only to insecticides in the prevalence of pesticidal exposure and poisoning of farm and domestic animals. Farm animals, pets and wild life often gain access to these poisons via the baits or the carcass of intoxicated animal or by malicious intent. Following factors increase the likelihood of rodenticide toxicosis in domestic animals:

a. Rodenticides are readily available in market.

b. Animals have easy access to rodenticides as these chemicals are often used in places where pets and livestock have easy approach.

c. Susceptible biochemical pathways are similar among all mammals.

d. There is often a narrow margin between the safe dose and the lethal dose of most rodenticides.

e. Rodenticidal baits are often formulated to be attractive and palatable to rodents. They also attract other animals.

Classification: Rodenticides constitute a large number of chemicals. Some chemicals are more commonly used (newer organic compounds) while others have little place in this group (inorganic and older organic compounds). Rodenticides are broadly divided into two groups: inorganic and organic rodenticides. Each group further contains a number of compounds.

I. Inorganic rodenticides

1. Arsenic compounds e.g. arsenic trioxide and sodium hydrogen arsenite.
2. Elementary phosphorous
3. Thallium sulphate
4. Zinc phosphide

II. Organic rodenticides

1. Anticoagulants e.g. warfarin, diphacinone, difenacoum and brodifacoum.
2. Fluoroacetic acid and its derivatives e.g. sodium fluoroacetate and fluoroacetamide.
3. Vitamin D compounds e.g. ergocalciferol and cholecalciferol.
4. Alphanaphthylthiourea (ANTU)
5. Bromethalin
6. Strychnine
7. Red squill
8. Pyriminil
9. Norbormide
10. Crimidine
11. Chloralose

I. INORGANIC RODENTICIDES

1. Arsenic Compounds

Arsenic compounds such as arsenic trioxide and sodium hydrogen arsenite were once used commonly as rodenticides; however, they have largely been replaced by substances less toxic to humans and domestic animals. As discussed earlier, arsenic has high affinity for sulphydryl groups, so it interferes with functions of a variety of proteins and enzymes. The detailed toxicology and line of treatment of arsenic have been discussed in Chapter 11.

2. Elementary Phosphorous

Phosphorus in its white or yellow form is highly reactive and hazardous to all domestic animals, so it is less used as rodenticide. Whenever used, it is concealed in butter or some other type of oil-based bait due to its strong oxidising action. Careless baiting practices often cause toxicosis. Its detailed toxicity and line of treatment have been discussed in the Non-metals (Chapter 12).

3. Thallium Sulphate

Thallium is chemically similar to lead and is occasionally used as rodenticide. Its use has been banned in many countries because thallium is a general cellular poison that affects all species. Dogs and cats are poisoned mostly by eating baits intended for rodents. Its detailed toxicology and line of treatment have been discussed in Metals (Chapter 11).

4. Zinc Phosphide

Zinc phosphide (Zn_3P_2) and occasionally aluminium and calcium phosphides are used as rodenticide for the control of rats, mice and ground squirrels. Zinc phosphide is one of the most widely used rodenticides in developing countries because it is cheap and very effective. Zinc phosphide is often recommended as the rodenticide of choice because it is fairly specific for rodents and there is no true secondary poisoning, except possibly in dogs and cats. Zinc phosphide is highly toxic to all mammals.

Properties: Trivalent phosphorus binds to a metal salt (Zn, Ca or Al) to form the corresponding metal phosphide. Zinc phosphide (Zn_3P_2) is generally available as a grey-black powder with garlic like odour. It is practically insoluble in water (decomposes slowly) and ethanol. Zinc phosphide (also other metal phosphides) is stable when dry, but slowly decomposes in moist air or bait and loses its potency within 2 weeks. Under acidic conditions, it decomposes rapidly to liberate phosphine (PH_3), a flammbable gas, which has odour similar to acetylene or decaying fish. This reaction is violent with concentrated acids (e.g. stomach acid) and other oxidising agents.

Zinc phosphide contains 14-18% of phosphorous and 80-70% of zinc and insoluble sediments. Rodenticide-grade zinc phosphide usually comes as a black powder containing 75% of zinc phosphide and 25% of antimony potassium tartrate, an emetic to cause vomiting if the material is accidentally ingested by humans or domestic animals. It is applied in baits at concentrations of 1-5%; 2% is most widely used. The baits have to contain sufficient amount of zinc phosphide in sufficiently attractive food (e.g. bread, buns, soaked wheat, fruits, or sugar) in order to kill the rodents in a single serving; a sublethal dose may cause aversion towards zinc-phosphide baits encountered by surviving rodents in the future.

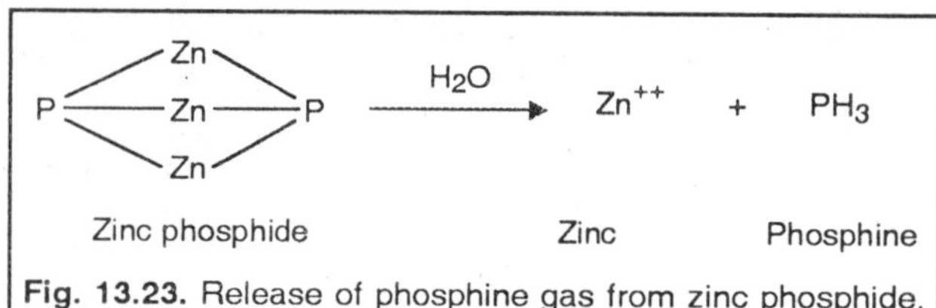

Fig. 13.23. Release of phosphine gas from zinc phosphide.

Toxicity: The acute toxicity of metal phosphides depends primarily on the speed at which phosphine is released from phosphide. Full stomach increases post-prandial acid production which enhances hydrolysis of phosphide to phosphine. Thus, metal phosphides are more toxic if taken with meals or baits than in the empty stomach. Lethal dose of zinc phosphide in most domestic animals is in range of 20-50 mg/kg. The oral LD_{50} of zinc phosphide on a full stomach in different species is: rats 45 mg/kg, poultry 20-30 mg/kg, and dogs 40 mg/kg. In empty stomach, a dog can take up to 300 mg/kg and survive.

Toxicokinetics: Toxicokinetic data on zinc phosphide in domestic animals are limited. On ingestion, zinc phosphide is rapidly hydrolysed in stomach acid to release phosphine gas. Once released, phosphine is rapidly absorbed from the GI tract and distributed throughout the body. Phosphine is labile and little is known of its metabolism and excretion. Some intact zinc phosphide and most of metabolised zinc (about 80%) are also absorbed from GI tract. Hypophosphite may be excreted in the urine as a metabolite of zinc phosphide.

Mechanism of action: Acute zinc phosphide toxicosis is primarily neither due to zinc nor phosphorus, but is due to the phosphine gas. Some adverse effects are due also to intact zinc phosphide. The exact mechanism of action of phosphine in body is not clear.

a. Phosphine gas is said to act as a 'general protoplasmic poison'. It causes direct damage to membranes of blood vessels and erythrocytes leading to cardiovascular collapse. Phosphine also causes depression of CNS, irritation of lungs and damage to liver and kidneys.

b. Phosphine inhibits cytochrome C oxidase, which causes tissue hypoxia.

c. Phosphine is a nucleophile and acts as a strong reducing agent. Its strong reducing properties are capable of causing several chemical and biological oxidant effects.

d. Oxidation of phosphine can lead to formation of reactive phosphorylating species. It releases free radicals capable of producing damage to membranes.

e. Zinc phosphide (also phosphine) is directly irritant to the gut and produces gastroenteritis. The irritant action of intact phosphide in body may cause hepatic and renal damage.

Clinical signs :

Acute toxicity: Clinical signs of phosphide poisoning are usually acute in nature, occurring within 0.5-4 hours of ingestion. These include vomiting (which is often life saving in non rodent species, if occurs early), often bloody vomiting, depression, tremors and abdominal pain. Acidosis is prominent in zinc phosphide poisoning, and there is usually hypocalcaemia. Other signs in different species include ataxia, weakness, prostration, dyspnoea, gasping, struggling, convulsions or hyperesthesia, increase in body temperature and coma. In dogs, aimless running (mad dog running), howling, barking, yelping, snapping of teeth, tremors, salivation, etc. may be present. Colic is seen in horses whereas bloat occurs in cattle. Large doses of zinc phosphide cause death within 3-5 hours, although some animals may live longer up to 48 hours. Death occurs as a result of heart failure and, more commonly, pulmonary oedema. In surviving animals, signs of renal and hepatic damage may be observed 5-14 days later.

Zinc phosphide is non-irritating to the skin and eyes.

Chronic toxicity: Subacute and chronic toxicities are not observed with metal phosphides.

Post-mortem findings: The stomach contents may have a characteristic acetylene or 'dead fish' odour. There is gastroenteritis which may be haemorrhagic. Less frequent lesions include venous congestion, capillary breakdown, visceral congestion and pulmonary oedema. Other non-specific and inconsistent lesions include myocardial degeneration, a pale yellow fatty liver and degeneration of liver and kidneys.

Microscopic examination may reveal congestion of the liver and kidney. Renal tubular necrosis and hepatic cloudy swelling and fatty degeneration can be seen in many instances.

Diagnosis: Diagnosis is based on the history of exposure to zinc phosphide, suggestive clinical signs and detection of zinc phosphide in stomach contents, liver and kidneys. Detection of phosphine gas is difficult because it readily dissipates; however, its presence in stomach contents may be detected by its acetylene odour. Rapid freezing of stomach contents and body tissues like liver and kidneys may sometimes even help detection of phosphine gas. In some cases, enhanced levels of zinc in body tissues may suggest zinc phosphide poisoning, but these assays are more difficult to interpret. Haematological and biochemical lesions are inconsistent.

Treatment and management: Specific antidote to zinc phosphide poisoning is not available. Supportive therapy must be instituted immediately to get a positive result.

a. Oral detoxification should be performed with gastric lavage (5% sodium bicarbonate) and activated charcoal.

b. Oral administration of sodium carbonate (cattle, 2-4 L of 5%) should be done to neutralise stomach acidity. In small animals, oral aluminium plus magnesium hydroxide gel may be preferred.

c. Oxygen or artificial respiration may be instituted to overcome pulmonary irritation and oedema.

d. Demulcents and protectants may be given to treat gastroenteritis.

e. Metabolic acidosis should be corrected by slow intravenous sodium bicarbonate administration.

f. Appropriate fluid therapy and corticosteroids may be needed to overcome shock.

g. Convulsions may be treated with diazepam or, if it fails, barbiturates.

h. B-vitamins and dextrose may be used for possible hepatic injury along with appropriate dietary therapy.

Prognosis: Prognosis depends on the dosage of zinc phosphide received and the degree of supportive therapy. The prognosis is considered grave, once the clinical signs become apparent.

Public health and environmental concerns: Zinc phosphide is highly toxic to wild mammals and birds when ingested directly. Secondary toxicity to mammalian predators (animals eating other animals those had been exposed to the compound) from zinc phosphide is rather low, primarily because the compound does not significantly accumulate in the muscles of target species.

II. ORGANIC RODENTICIDES

1. Anticoagulants

The anticoagulants are the most commonly used organic rodenticides and include warfarin and related anti-vitamin K compounds. These were initially discovered in the first half of 20th century during search for the cause of 'Sweet Clover Disease' in cattle in North America. These are readily available in a number of formulations and are used extensively by public and professionals. The anticoagulant rodenticides are potentially dangerous to all mammals and birds and are a frequent cause of poisoning in pets. Animals may be poisoned directly from baits or indirectly by consumption of poisoned rats.

Chemistry and classification: The anticoagulant rodenticides are derivatives of the 4-hydroxycoumarin or indan-1,3-dione. Accordingly, anticoagulant rodenticides have been divided into two groups: hydroxycoumarins and indanediones.

a. Hydroxycoumarins e.g. warfarin, coumafuryl, coumachlor, coumatetralyl, brodifacoum, bromadiolone and difenacoum.

b. Indanediones e.g. pindone, chlorophacinone and diphacinone.

Anticoagulant rodenticides can also be classified as first generation and second generation rodenticides depending on their origin and ability to kill warfarin-resistant rats.

a. *First generation anticoagulant rodenticides:* These rodenticides were developed before 1970. Their potency as vitamin K antagonist is low, so multiple doses are required to produce toxicosis. They have short half-life due to their rapid excretion. Some of these anticoagulants are also used therapeutically for treatment and prevention of recurrence of thrombotic conditions like venous thrombosis and aortic or pulmonary thromboembolism. Examples of first generation anticoagulant rodenticides include warfarin, dicoumarol, pindon and coumatetralyl.

b. *Second generation anticoagulant rodenticides:* These rodenticides were developed after 1970 and are capable of killing warfarin-resistant rats. They have high potency as vitamin K antagonists and retain all the advantages of first generation anticoagulants. However, they are effective usually after single feeding and have long action in the body due to their retention in body tissues (therefore, sometimes called long acting anticoagulants). The second generation rodenticides are more toxic to rodents (including warfarin resistant rats) and non-target species and are largely implicated in rodenticide toxicosis. The most common second-generation compounds that are encountered in veterinary practice are brodifacoum and bromadiolone (hydroxycoumarins), as well as diphacinone and chlorophacinone (indandiones).

Properties: Anticoagulant rodenticides are mostly odourless and tasteless compounds, so they do not produce bait shyness. Due to their relatively slow action, bait is carried to nesting places where other rodents may also eat. The concentration of warfarin and some other first-generation anticoagulants in baits ranges from 0.02% to 1.0 %, but 0.5% is the most common percentage. Second generation anticoagulants are marketed in 0.005% to 2% concentrations. The low concentration of most anticoagulant rodenticides in baits often requires multiple doses feeding over several days to produce death in rodents. The second generation compounds are more effective, so a lethal dose is ingested by rodents during a single episode of feeding on poisoned baits. The anticoagulant rodenticides are available in one or more of the following forms: bait packs, powders, concentrates, pellets, tablets and capsules.

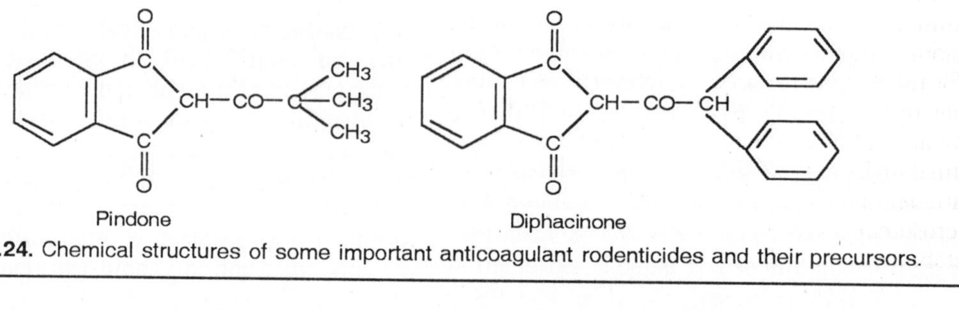

4–Hydroxy coumarin

Indan–1, 3–dione

Warfarin

Pindone

Diphacinone

Fig. 13.24. Chemical structures of some important anticoagulant rodenticides and their precursors.

Factors affecting toxicity :

a. Ruminants are less susceptible to anticoagulant rodenticides than simple stomach animals. Dogs and cats are most frequently involved, with occasional poisoning in other domestic animals.

b. Anticoagulants are more toxic when repeatedly ingested over several days than when an equal amount is consumed in a single feeding.

c. Drugs that reduce vitamin K synthesis by microflora in the intestinal tract (e.g. sulphonamides and broad spectrum antibiotics) are believed to exacerbate anticoagulants toxicity.

d. Drugs which displace anticoagulants from plasma protein binding sites (e.g. aspirin and phenylbutazone) may increase their toxicity by making available more of free anticoagulants.

e. Anticoagulants are more toxic in animals with deficient clotting factors production due to liver failure or gastrointestinal malabsorption syndrome.

Toxicity: The anticoagulant rodenticides are potential hazards to mammals, birds and possibly other species. Single dose of warfarin ranging from 20 to 50 mg/kg body weight is fatal for dogs. Repeated dose of 1 mg/kg/day for 1 week is lethal for dogs and cats. Dose of 3 mg/kg of diphacinone and 0.25-3.5 mg/kg of brodifacoum are median lethal dose (LD_{50}) in dogs. In ruminants, single oral LD_{50} of brodifacoum is higher (25-33 mg/kg). Pigs are usually more susceptible to warfarin in single (LD_{50} 30 mg/kg) and multiple (LD_{50} 0.05 mg/kg/day for 7 days) oral doses than other species. Poultry is more resistant and cases of poisoning from current baiting practices are rare.

Toxicokinetics: Anticoagulant rodenticides are absorbed slowly but fairly well (> 90%) from GI tract and peak plasma concentration may reach within 12 hours. Their distribution in plasma is prolonged by strong binding to plasma proteins (90-95% for warfarin). High concentrations may be found in liver, spleen and kidney. These compounds may accumulate with time, as in the case of an animal ingesting small amounts over several days. Anticoagulant rodenticides are metabolised by microsomal mixed function oxidases to inactive metabolites which are excreted in the urine. They are eliminated at various rates depending on the type of compound and the amount ingested. The half-life of various compounds is: warfarin 15 hours, diphacinone 5 days and bromadiolone 6 days. Brodifacoum may be detected up to 24 days in serum.

Mechanism of action: Warfarin and other anticoagulant rodenticides produce their action by two mechanisms: inhibition of vitamin K-dependent blood clotting factors (primary action) and capillary damage.

a. Inhibition of synthesis of blood clotting factors: The warfarin and other anticoagulant compounds are chemically related to vitamin K, so they apparently behave as competitive antagonists of vitamin K and interfere with the hepatic synthesis of vitamin K-dependent clotting factors II, VII, IX, and X. Normally these factors after their synthesis in liver undergo vitamin K dependent activation, whereby a number of their glutamic acid residues are carboxylated. In this carboxylation reaction, the vitamin K (reduced form) is converted to vitamin K epoxide (oxidised form). Vitamin K epoxide is then converted back to vitamin K by vitamin K epoxide reductase (Figure 13.25). All anticoagulant rodenticides block vitamin K epoxide reductase enzyme and interfere with regeneration of the active form of vitamin K, thereby inhibiting synthesis of prothrombin (Factor II) and Factors VII, IX, and X. When synthesis of clotting factors is reduced by more than 50%, a bleeding disorder occurs and animal dies of tissue hypoxia from massive internal bleeding. These compounds are slow acting with a latent period of several hours because of the persistence of clotting factors synthesised before drug administration.

b. Damage to capillaries: There are reports that warfarin-containing rodenticides cause direct damage to capillaries. This occurs perhaps via the benzalacetone moiety of warfarin. Damage to capillaries contributes to the primary action of bleeding disorder and leads to bleeding upon the very slightest trauma.

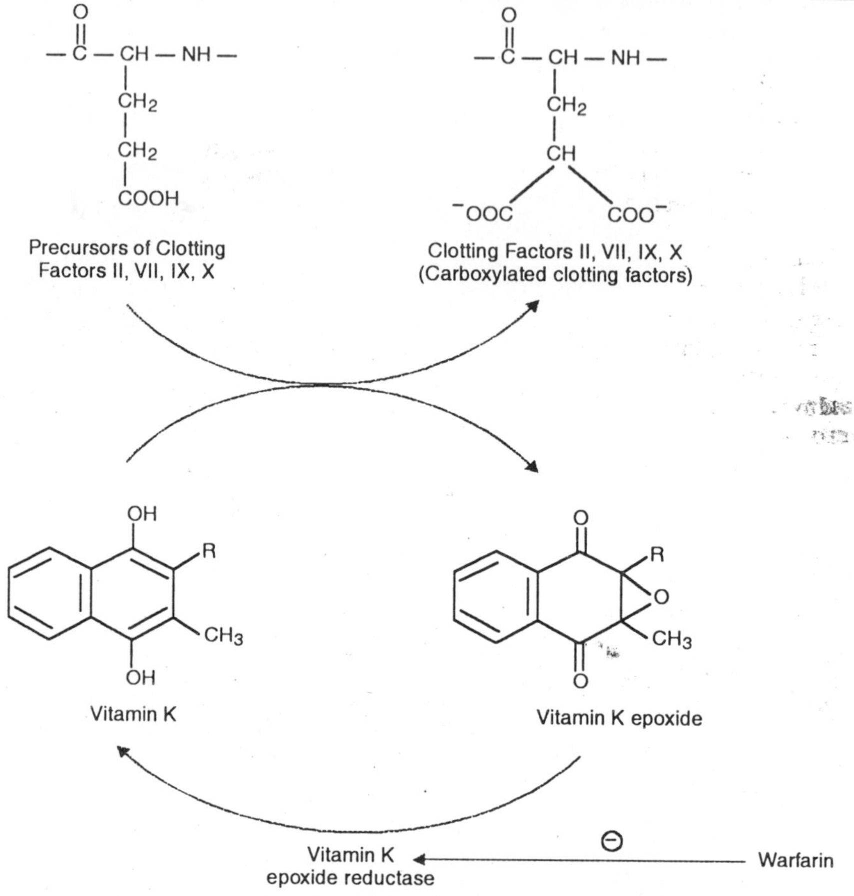

Fig. 13.25. Mechanism of action of warfarin (see text for detail).

Clinical signs: Clinical signs have late onset of action (1-3 days) after ingestion of anticoagulant rodenticide because the toxicosis occurs only after the clotting factors present in body are utilised. Initial clinical signs are rather non-specific and include lethargy, weakness and pallor. Important clinical signs relate to massive haemorrhage and include blood discharge from body orifices, visible haematomas under skin and around joints, purpurea, pale mucous membranes, dyspnoea, hypoxia, weakness and signs of shock. Capillary haemorrhages may occur in absence of trauma. Haemorrhages may be internal or external. Depending upon the site of haemorrhage, clinical signs may vary.

a. Sudden internal haemorrhage can lead to acute anaemia, shock and cyanosis. Animal may be found dead with no premonitory signs.

b. Haemorrhages in brain, spinal cord or subdural space are reflected as ataxia or staggering, paresis, depression, convulsions, etc.

c. Periarticular or intraarticular haemorrhages can cause lameness, joint swelling and pain.

d. Placental haemorrhages may cause abortion.

e. Pulmonary haemorrhages may cause coughing, epistaxis and dyspnoea.

f. Genitourinary tract haemorrhages may cause haematuria.

g. Gastrointestinal haemorrhages may cause tarry coloured faeces and haemorrhagic gastroenteritis.

h. In a case of castration or another surgical treatment, poisoned animal may suffer from long-lasting intense bleeding.

i. Extensive external haematomata may occur at pressure points or traumatized areas.

Death in case of anticoagulant rodenticides poisoning is similar to that from old age or general weakness and may occur unobserved. This is most common when haemorrhage occurs in brain, abdominal cavity, pericardial sac, mediastinum or thorax.

Post-mortem findings: Necropsy reveals haemorrhages on the mucous membranes, subcutaneous bleeding and internal haemorrhages in the body cavities. Most haemorrhages are ecchymoses or suffusions rather than petechiae. The blood does not clot. Centrilobular hepatic necrosis may result from anaemia and hypoxia. The heart is often flaccid and haemorrhagic.

Diagnosis: Diagnosis of anticoagulant rodenticide intoxication is made from history, clinical signs and lesions. Formation of large haematomas, persistent bleeding at venipuncture sites, and/or persistent bleeding during surgery strongly suggests anticoagulant rodenticide toxicosis. In laboratory, increased activated coagulation time (2 to 10 times) and activated partial prothrombin time (2 to 6 times) give indication. Radiography may reveal massive haemorrhages in abdomen and thorax. Chemical analysis may reveal anticoagulants or their metabolites in the blood, urine, or hepatic tissues. Warfarin and congeners are not natural constituents of the body; therefore, any concentration in plasma, liver, kidney or spleen is diagnostically significant.

Differential diagnosis of anticoagulant rodenticide poisoning should be made from inherited bleeding disorders (e.g. haemophilia A and B, Von Willebrand's diseases and clotting factors deficiency), medicinal warfarin overdose, heparin use, and vitamin K deficiency due to malnutrition and malabsorption.

Treatment and management :

Specific therapy

a. Phytomenadione (Vitamin K_1): Phytomenadione (Phytonadione, phylloquinone, or phyllomenaquinone) or vitamin K_1 is a specific antidote to anticoagulant poisoning. It is present in plants and mainly concentrated in the chloroplasts of plant leaves. Phytomenadione is available in several formulations for oral and parenteral administration and is the most commonly used vitamin K preparation in both human and veterinary medicines. Vitamin K_2 is not commercially available and vitamins K_3 and K_4 cannot be used in poisoning because they are provitamins that are converted slowly to their active forms. One week of vitamin K_1 therapy is required for first generation toxicants whereas 4-6 weeks therapy is required for second generation toxicants. Oral vitamin K_1 therapy should be given along with a small amount of food to hasten its absorption.

Dogs & cats: 2.5 – 5 mg/kg/day, IM or SC (several sites, with smallest possible injury) in divided doses for 1 to 3 days followed by oral administration. For severe cases, initial treatment may be given by slow IV injection. Rapid IV injection of vitamin K_1 may result in anaphylactic shock.

: 0.25 – 2.5 mg/kg/day, PO, in 2 to 3 divided doses.

Horses, cattle, sheep, goats, and pigs: 0.5 – 1 mg/kg/day, IM or SC (several sites) in divided doses.

Supportive therapy

a. Blood transfusion may be given to counter loss of blood at the dose rate of 20 ml/kg body weight or fresh or frozen plasma is given at the dose rate of 9 ml/kg body weight.

b. Emetics or activated charcoal should be administered for recently ingested poison.

c. The affected animal may be sedated to minimize the injury or trauma.

d. Oxygen therapy may be instituted, if required.

e. Thoracocentesis should be performed to prevent death from pulmonary or cardiac compression.

Contraindications

Corticosteroids, sulphonamides, antihistamines, adrenaline and aspirin should not be used during poisoning or recovery period.

Prognosis: Prognosis is good if haemorrhages are not massive and a full therapeutic and convalescent regiment is maintained.

Public health concerns: Residues in foods of animal origin are not likely because anticoagulants usually have short half-life, low lipid solubility and are also inactive.

Some important compounds :

a. *Warfarin:* Warfarin (3-[α-acetonylbenzyl]-4-hydroxycoumarin) was the first marketed anticoagulant and therefore became the best known and most widely used. Most warfarin-based baits contain 0.25 to 1.0 per cent warfarin and are available as white or tan pelleted or seed grain-based products. It has relatively limited sales today, due to the availability of more potent anticoagulants.

b. *Pindone:* Pindone (2-pivaloylindan-1,3-dione) is also one of the early anticoagulants which is still available for use in rodent control. It is slightly less effective than warfarin and is commercially available in baits containing 0.005-0.05% active ingredient for control of rats and mice.

c. *Diphacinone:* Diphacinone (2-[diphenylacetyl]indan-1,3-dione) is significantly more toxic than the anticoagulant compounds developed earlier, so it is formulated at lower concentrations. It is toxic to Norway rats, but is less toxic against house mice. It is used in many formulations.

d. *Brodifacoum:* Brodifacoum (3-[3-(4'-bromobiphenyl-4-yl)-1,2,3,4-tetrahydro-1-naphthyl]-4-hydroxycoumarin) is the most potent second generation anticoagulant rodenticide. It is available in 0.005% pellet formulations and wax blocks. Because of its acute toxicity, a lethal dose can be obtained in single feeding, although death is delayed for 4 or 5 days.

e. *Bromadiolone:* Bromadiolone (3-[3-(4'-bromobiphenyl-4-yl)-3-hydroxy-1-phenylpropyl]-4-hydroxycoumarin) is not quite as toxic to rodents as brodifacoum but can result in the same level of control. It is available in 0.005% pellet formulations and wax blocks. It is sufficiently potent to kill warfarin resistant rats.

2. Fluoroacetic Acid and its Derivatives

Sodium fluoroacetate (Compound 1080), sodium fluorocetamide (Compound 1081) and sodium fluoroethanol are potent rodenticides used for destruction of rats, mice, and other rodent pests. In some countries they are used for the control of foxes, wild dogs and wild pigs. Fluoroacetate also occurs naturally in at least 40 toxic plants in South Africa (*Dichapetalum cymosum* or gifblaar plant), Australia (*Acacia georginae* or Gidgee and *Gastrolobium grandiflorium* or poison peas) and Brazil. Sodium fluoroacetate is not a specific rodenticide as it is also highly toxic to other species. Accordingly its use has been restricted now.

Chemistry and properties: Sodium fluoroacetate (sodium monofluoroacetate), fluoroacetamide and fluoroethanol are fluorinated derivatives of acetic acid, usually present as the sodium salt. Highly toxic compounds either have two carbon atoms or are metabolized to this form. These rodenticides are odourless, tasteless and water soluble. Rodents do not develop bait shyness to these compounds due to characteristic lag period after ingestion. Sodium fluoroacetate is used in baits in concentration of 0.08-0.5%. Sodium fluoroacetamide is less potent than sodium fluoroacetate, so is used in higher concentration of 1 or 2 per cent.

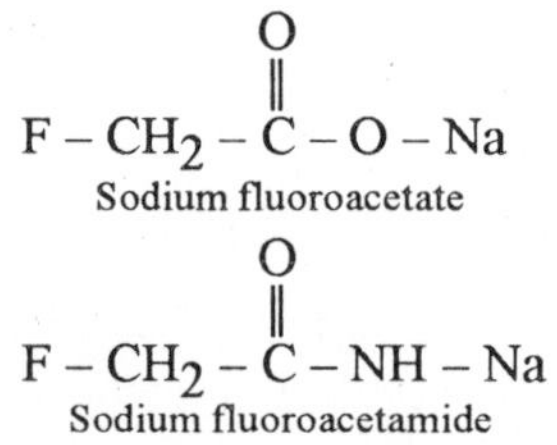

$$F - CH_2 - \overset{\overset{\displaystyle O}{\|}}{C} - O - Na$$

Sodium fluoroacetate

$$F - CH_2 - \overset{\overset{\displaystyle O}{\|}}{C} - NH - Na$$

Sodium fluoroacetamide

Fig. 13.26. Chemical structures of sodium fluoroacetate and sodium floroacetamide.

Toxicity: Fluoroacetic acid and its derivatives are highly toxic to all animals. Sodium fluoroacetate is extremely toxic to rats and other mammalian species with oral LD_{50} ranging between 0.1 to 8 mg/kg body weight and in most of the domestic species below 1 mg/kg body weight (dogs 0.06-0.2 mg/kg, cats 0.3-0.5 mg/kg, cattle 0.15-0.6 mg/kg, sheep 0.25-0.5 mg/kg, goats 0.3-0.7 mg/kg, pigs 0.3-0.4 mg/kg and horses 0.5-1.75 mg/kg). Due to very high toxicity in mammals, preparations containing fluoroacetate have a warning black colour (nigrosine) to prevent confusion from other substances. Sodium fluoroacetamide has moderate to high acute toxicity depending on the species with oral LD_{50} in different species: rats 15 mg/kg, mice 30 mg/kg and chickens 4.5 mg/kg. Sodium fluoroacetate does not bioaccumulate in organisms, but relay (secondary) toxicosis is possible, especially when carnivorous predators consume poisoned rats.

Toxicokinetics: Fluoroacetate is readily absorbed from gut, lungs or open wounds but not through the intact skin. The compound is carried throughout the body in blood stream and does not accumulate in a given type of tissue. However, its concentration in brain is more than in other tissues. A portion of fluoroacetamide *in vivo* is slowly converted to fluoroacetate. Therefore, fluoroacetamide is comparatively less potent and slower acting than the fluoroacetate. Fluoroethanol is relatively inactive and its toxicity depends on its oxidation to fluoroacetate by tissue alcohol dehydrogenase.

Mechanism of action: Sodium fluoroacetate, fluoroacetamide and fluoroethanol have the same mechanism of action. They cause toxicity by blocking Krebs cycle leading to lower energy production.

Fluoroacetate administered directly or formed *in vivo* from fluoroacetamide or fluoroethanol, acts as an antimetabolite. It enters into cells and condenses with oxaloacetate to form the active metabolite fluorocitrate (often called lethal synthesis). Fluorocitrate has structural similarity with citrate, so it competes with citrate for the active site of the enzyme aconitase in Krebs cycle. Inhibition of enzyme aconitase slows or blocks the Krebs cycle leading to lower energy production, reduced oxygen consumption, and reduced cellular concentration of ATP. Furthermore, since the citrate synthetase continues to work, citrate accumulates in the tissues. Citrate is a potent chilator of calcium. It is thought that toxicity of fluoroacetate is primarily due to blockade of energy metabolism and not due to accumulation of citrate in body. However, increased tissue and plasma citrate is probably responsible for some of the signs seen during acute poisoning. The heart and brain are affected first and most severely by cellular energy deficit. It takes some time for above processes to occur, so onset of poisoning has a latent period of 30 min to 2 hours; but once occur there is rapid increase in the toxicity.

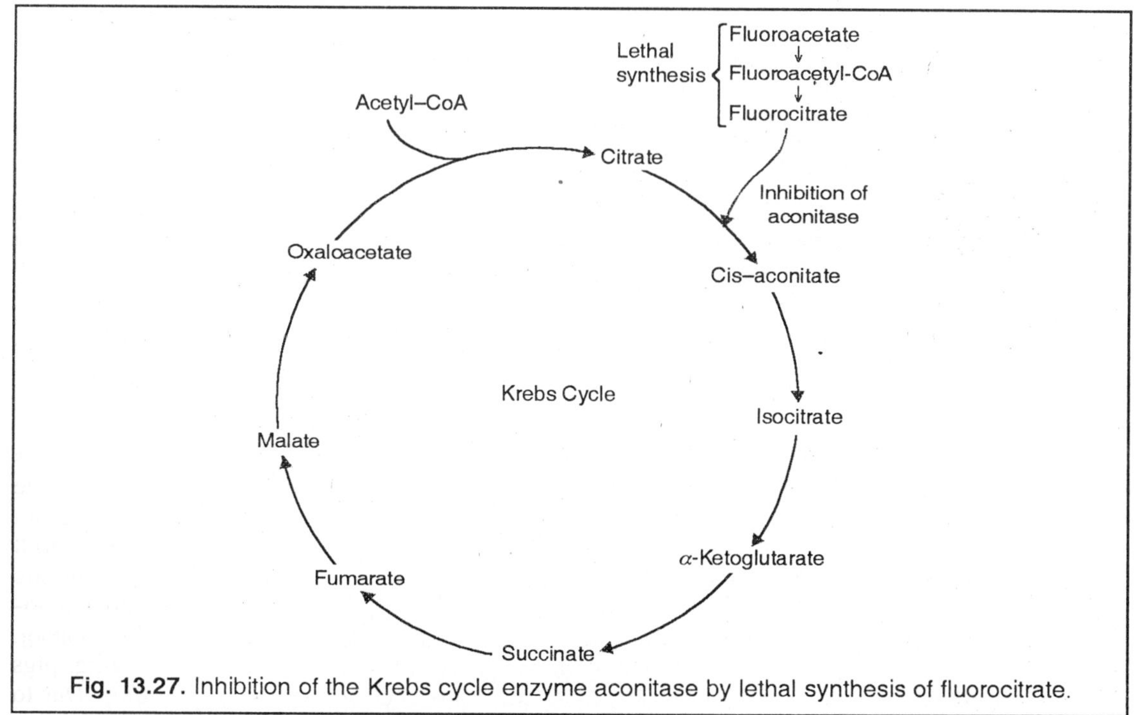

Fig. 13.27. Inhibition of the Krebs cycle enzyme aconitase by lethal synthesis of fluorocitrate.

Clinical signs: Clinical signs of fluoroacetate have an acute onset (0.5-2 hr after ingestion). Neurotoxic signs are most prominent in dogs and less in other species. Initial signs in dogs include restlessness, anxiety, hyperirritability and vomiting (often late to be life saving). Advanced signs include repetitive urination and defecation, tenesmus, dyspnoea, frothing and hyperthermia. The dogs periodically experience wild running, barking, etc. These are followed by intermittent tonic-clonic seizures with paddling movements. Breathing ceases before heart stops. Death generally occurs during seizures or from respiratory paralysis within 2-12 hours after ingestion.

In ruminants and horses, cardiac signs are predominant and include arrhythmia, rapid weak pulse, ventricular fibrillation, staggering, trembling, sweating (horses), grinding of teeth and terminal seizures. Cardiac arrest accompanied by sudden death is the prominent feature of fluoroacetate toxicosis in horses and ruminants. The overall course is rapid and affected animals die within hours after signs appear. Sheep, goats, cats and pigs exhibit a mixture of neurotoxic and cardiotoxic signs.

Post-mortem findings: Necropsy reveals no characteristic lesions. Rigor mortis is rapid. There are petechial haemorrhages in the intestine and on the epi-and endo-cardium. Heart usually stops in diastole. Congestion in liver and kidneys may be observed. Microscopically, the brain may manifest oedema and perivascular infiltration with lymphocytes.

Diagnosis: Diagnosis of sodium fluoroacetate poisoning should be based on detailed history, knowledge of clinical signs and lesions. Kidney tissue may be tested for excess citrate. Baits, stomach contents, vomitus, liver and kidney should be analysed for fluoroacetate presence.

In dogs, fluoroacetate poisoning may mimic any severe encephalitic disease, hypomagnesaemia, hypocalcaemia and poisoning by strychnine, zinc phosphide, lead, methylxanthines, cardiotoxic glycosides, organochlorine insecticides or bacterial food toxins.

Treatment and management: There is no specific antidote to fluoroacetate poisoning. Response to therapy is often poor.

a. Gastric lavage and adsorbents (activated charcoal) are recommended to remove the toxicant from GI tract.

b. Glyceryl monoacetate (monoacetin) has been used as a competitive antagonist of fluoroacetate at dose rate of 0.5 mg/kg/hour in 5 parts of normal saline by I.M. route until a total dosage of 2-4 mg/kg body weight is reached.

c. Ethanol (50%) and acetic acid (5%) at a dose rate of 8 ml/kg of each by oral route is given to add acetate to reduce the conversion of fluoroacetate to fluorocitrate.

d. Barbiturates (pentobarbitone or phenobarbitone) can be used for controlling seizures.

e. Calcium borogluconate (0.2-0.5 ml/kg of 5% solution, slow IV) has been recommended to control tetany.

f. Antiarrhythmics may be used, if required, in appropriate species.

Contraindications

Emetics are contraindicated, if clinical signs are present.

Prognosis: Prognosis of fluoroacetate poisoning is grave, if clinical signs are severe.

Public health and environmental concerns: Sodium fluoroacetate is highly toxic to birds, domestic animals and wildlife. It is readily broken down by naturally occurring bacteria and fungi, so it does not cause a build-up of toxic residues in soil, water or plants. However, its inadvertent use may pose high risk of secondary poisoning to carnivorous and omnivorous species from eating poisoned carcasses.

3. Vitamin D Compounds

Vitamin D rodenticides include ergocalciferol (vitamin D_2) and cholecalciferol (vitamin D_3). These were introduced in early 1980s as single- and multiple-feeding agents for control of commensal rats and mice. Baits are available as 'place packs' (packs designed to be placed into areas frequented by rodents) and packages to be mixed with seeds or grains. Incidence of acute vitamin D toxicosis in companion animals has been reported and is on rise with marketing of vitamin D rodenticides.

Properties: Ergocalciferol (Calciferol) and cholecalciferol are used commercially for rodent control either alone or in combination with some anticoagulants (e.g. warfarin and difenacoum). The technical procedures to prepare vitamin D compounds are based on irradiation of ergosterol to prepare ergocalciferol and of 7-dehydrocholesterol to form cholecalciferol. Both vitamin D compounds are insoluble in water and soluble in most organic solvents. Rodenticide baits are available in a number of formulations including granules, flakes, tablets and cakes in which the active compound is mostly present at concentrations of 0.075% cholecalciferol and 0.1% ergocalciferol when used alone. Vitamin D rodenticides are toxic to warfarin-resistant rats and often kill rodents within 1 week of ingestion.

Toxicity: The oral LD_{50} of ergocalciferol and cholecalciferol for dogs is 56 mg/kg and 85mg/kg, respectively; however, lethal intoxication can occur at dosages as low as 10-20 mg/kg. These compounds show cumulative effect on repeated use, so that much lower doses given over a period of several days can lead to toxicity. For example, when ergocalciferol is administered daily for 5 consecutive days to laboratory rats, the LD_{50} falls to 7 mg/kg/day. Younger animals appear at higher risk to the development of vitamin D toxicosis may be due to indiscriminate feeding habit, smaller body size or increased sensitivity to vitamin D compounds and their metabolites. No breed predilection has been observed for dogs and cats, although smaller breeds are reported to suffer most. Animals with pre-existing kidney disease may also be predisposed to vitamin D toxicosis.

Toxicokinetics: Absorption of vitamin D is rapid and complete in the small intestine, especially if the animal's diet is rich in lipids. Bile is essential for adequate absorption of vitamin D. After absorption, vitamin D circulates in blood in association with vitamin D binding protein, a specific α-globulin. The vitamin D requires activation to become biologically active. The ergocalciferol (D_2) is first converted to 25 hydroxyergocalciferol (25-OH D_2) in the liver and then to 1,25-hydroxyergocalciferol (1,25-$(OH)_2$ D_2) in the kidney. The 1,25-$(OH)_2$ D_2 is the active form of vitamin D_2. Similar to ergocalciferol, cholecalciferol is first metabolized in liver to 25-hydroxycholecalciferol (25-hydroxy vitamin D_3; 25-OH D_3) or calcifediol and then to 1,25-dihydroxycholecalciferol (1,25-dihydroxy vitamin D_3; 1,25-$(OH)_2$ D_3) or calcitriol in the kidneys. Calcitriol is the most potent cholecalciferol metabolite in terms of enhancing bone resorption and intestinal transport. Vitamin D_3 metabolites are excreted primarily via bile and in faeces, with about one-third excreted in urine.

Mechanism of action: Physiologically, vitamins D and its metabolites maintain normal calcium levels in blood by increasing intestinal absorption of calcium, stimulating bone resorption of calcium (mobilization of calcium from bones) and decreasing renal excretion of calcium (by enhancing calcium reabsorption from renal tubules). In high doses (as rodenticide), ergocalciferol and cholecalciferol accelerate these mechanisms many times leading to marked hypercalcaemia as a result of which calcium salts are deposited in soft tissues such as kidneys, blood vessels, heart and lungs. Thus, soft tissues tend to become calcified while the bone tends to be rarefied. Calcification of heart muscles leads to conduction dysfunctions and abnormal ECG. Deposition of calcium in blood vessels, particularly in small renal arteries and large vessels like aorta, results in vasoconstriction, hypertension and decreased blood supply to vital organs. Effects on kidneys include degeneration and necrosis of renal tubules (as a result of direct calcium deposition and renal ischemia from vasoconstriction) and interference with the ability of renal tubules to reabsorb water and salt. Death is thought to result from hypercalcaemia, calcification of tissues, and renal and heart failure. The whole mechanism is slow and takes many hours for effective calcium level to build-up. Therefore, the development of hypercalcaemia and occurrence of lethal lesions may take 4 or 5 days.

Clinical signs: Clinical signs associated with ergocalciferol and cholecalciferol develop within 18-36 hours of ingestion and can lead to lethargy, depression, polyuria and polydipsia. As serum calcium concentrations rise, clinical signs become more severe and renal failure may develop. Gastrointestinal smooth muscle excitability decreases, which is manifested by anorexia, vomiting and constipation. Haematemesis and haemorrhagic diarrhoea may develop as a result of dystrophic calcification of GI tract. Hypercalcaemia of blood vessels may lead to vasoconstriction and hypertension. As hypercalcaemia progresses, the heart sounds are slowed and become prominent and there is renal insufficiency. Acutely poisoned animal dies within 2-5 days of onset of clinical signs.

Post-mortem findings: Gross lesions of vitamin D toxicosis include petechial haemorrhages in tissues, pale streaks in kidney tissue and raised plaques in intima of large vessels. In microscopic lesions, renal tubules may be degenerative or necrotic and mineralization is seen in various tissues such as kidneys, coronary arteries, gastric mucosa, bronchioles, pancreas and urinary bladder. Myocardial degeneration, necrosis and mineralization may occur.

Diagnosis: Diagnosis of vitamin D rodenticide poisoning is based on history of ingestion, clinical signs and hypercalcaemia. Kidney calcium concentration may be in range of 1,000 ppm as compared to approximately 100 ppm for controls. Hyperphosphataemia, enhanced blood urea nitrogen (BUN) and elevated serum creatinine are also commonly noted.

Differential diagnosis should be made from other causes of hypercalcaemia such as hyperparathyroidism and juvenile hypercalcaemia.

Treatment and management: Treatment of vitamin D toxicosis is aimed primarily at lowering the elevated serum calcium levels.

a. *Corticosteroids:* Corticosteroids (e.g. cortisone and prednisone) are useful in the treatment of cholecalciferol poisoning. They decrease enhanced serum calcium levels by inhibiting release of osteoclast-activating factors, reducing intestinal absorption of calcium and promoting urinary excretion of calcium. Corticosteroids are often used in combination with calcitonin and diuretics for a period of about 1-2 weeks, followed by removal of therapy and retesting the calcium levels after 24 hours. Continuous monitoring of serum calcium and BUN levels may be needed throughout the therapy.

   Cortisone

   Dogs & cats: 1-2 mg/kg, PO or IM, once daily.

   Prednisone

   Dogs: 2-3 mg/kg, PO, 1 to 2 times daily.

b. *Salmon calcitonin:* Salmon calcitonin, a synthetic preparation of calcitonin, is considered useful in the treatment of vitamin D-based rodenticide poisoning. It reduces hypercalcaemia by reducing bone resorption and also to some extent by inhibiting tubular reabsorption of calcium. It is often used as adjunctive therapy with corticosteroids.

   Dogs & cats: 4 – 6 IU/kg, SC, 2 to 3 times daily.

   : 4 IU/kg, IV (loading dose for severe toxicity) followed by 4 – 8 IU/kg, SC, 1 to 2 times daily.

c. *Pamidronate:* Pamidronate is a bisphosphonate that inhibits bone resorption. It has been found useful in the treatment of cholecalciferol-induced hypercalcaemia in dogs and is considered useful only if administered before the soft tissue mineralization occurs. The advantage of pamidronate disodium compared with salmon calcitonin is that it has long-lasting effect and hence does not require repeated dosing. Pamidronate also does not require intensive fluid therapy and adjunct corticosteroid therapy often used in conjunction with calcitonin therapy.

   Dogs: 1.3 – 2 mg/kg, slow IV in 0.9% sodium chloride solution over a period 2 to 4 hour. It may be repeated once at 96 hours.

d. Fluid therapy with normal saline and frusemide (5 mg/kg, I.V. followed by 3 mg/kg thrice daily) should be initiated. Saline diuresis promotes calcium excretion. Thiazide diuretics should not be used because they decrease urinary excretion of calcium and hence contribute to poisoning.

e. Emesis or gastric lavage should be recommended, if patient has recently consumed a vitamin D-based rodenticide.

f. Administration of activated charcoal (2-8 g/kg in water slurry) and osmotic cathartic may be considered to remove unabsorbed toxicant from GI tract.

Prognosis: Prognosis of vitamin D-based rodenticide toxicosis is guarded, if the clinical signs are severe or advanced.

4. Alphanaphthylthiourea (ANTU)

Alphanaphthylthiourea, commonly abbreviated as ANTU, is a less commonly used thiourea rodenticide. It was introduced as rodenticide in 1945, but presently has been withdrawn from use in several countries because of the carcinogenicity of α-naphthylamines present as impurities. Although dogs, cats and pigs are susceptible, most domestic animals are resistant to ANTU.

Properties: ANTU is a thiourea derivative. Pure ANTU forms colourless crystals and the technical grade is a grey crystalline powder. It is insoluble in water and does not have detectable offensive taste or odour. The compound is extremely stable and does not deteriorate on prolonged storage. Baits are usually prepared by including 2% ANTU in cereals, meats or bread mashes. Baits containing ANTU are readily accepted by rodents, but there is rapid appearance of both tolerance and bait refusal. Although tolerance is lost within one month, the bait refusal may last longer.

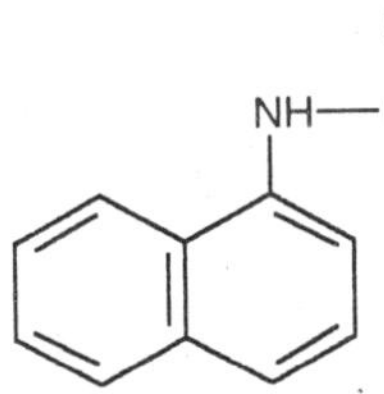

S
NH—C—NH_2

Fig. 13.28. Chemical structure of alphanaphthylthiourea (ANTU).

Toxicity: ANTU is a selective poison for rats with LD_{50} of 3-5 mg/kg body weight. The Norway rat is particularly susceptible, the young being slightly more resistant than the adults. Susceptibility of other species to ANTU is variable with oral LD_{50}: dogs 40 mg/kg, cats 75-100 mg/kg, and poultry 2500-5000 mg/kg body weight. In empty stomach dogs, it induces vomiting which many times save the animal.

Toxicokinetics: Alphanaphthylthiourea is rapidly absorbed from the gut and can cause illness in dogs in less than 1 hour. Death can occur within 6-48 hours; however, survival for 12 hours may indicate possible recovery. It is rapidly metabolised and quickly eliminated from the body. Tolerance develops after ingestion of sublethal doses of ANTU.

Mechanism of action: Alphanaphthylthiourea has selective action on lung capillaries caused by widening of pores between endothelial cells and formation of blebs on endothelial cell membranes. This leads to massive pulmonary oedema and leakage of fluid into air passages. The effusion is agitated to froth by the intense respiratory efforts of animal. Thus, the animal literally drowns in its own fluid and death occurs due to marked hydrothorax and pulmonary oedema. The exact mechanism by which ANTU damages lung capillaries endothelial cells and pneumocytes is not clear. Reaction of ANTU with sulphydryl groups in the tissue macromolecules may be a necessary part of mechanism of toxic action as use of sulphydryl group blocking drugs inhibits this action of ANTU.

Clinical signs: The initial clinical signs of ANTU include vomiting, occurring a few minutes to a few hours following ingestion. This is followed by irregular breathing (short, jerky inspiration) and cough. Then intoxicated animal becomes inactive with respiratory distress, laboured breathing and cyanosis. Auscultation of chest reveals bubbly respiratory sounds. Animal continues to vomit as the disease progresses and the vomitus may consist entirely of blood. In later stages, white foam is discharged from nostrils and oral cavity. The pulse is usually accelerated and heart beats are difficult to determine, owing to hydropericardium. The affected animal initially remains standing, then sits on its haunches to relieve thoracic pressure and finally assumes a position of sternal recumbency as it becomes weak. Body temperature may remain normal or may decrease. As asphyxiation proceeds, coma ensues and terminal clonic convulsions may occur. Pulmonary oedema and circulatory failure usually kill the animal within 12 hours. If the animal survives for 12 hours after ANTU exposure, the chances of survival are more.

Post-mortem findings: The most apparent signs of ANTU poisoning are observed in lungs. The thoracic cavity is partly filled with a colourless or pale reddish liquid. Severe oedema of the lungs is a consistent finding and the lungs are enlarged and of pasty consistency. A foamy liquid appear on the cut surface of the lung, either spontaneously or when lung is pressed. Hydrothorax and blood tinged fluid and froth may be present in bronchi or trachea. There is hyperaemia of tracheal, bronchial and GI tract mucosa, liver and kidneys. ANTU is moderately irritating to the stomach and intestine, so catarrhal inflammation is usually present in these organs. Cyanosis and dark-coloured arterial blood are also observed.

Diagnosis: ANTU poisoning is diagnosed from history, clinical signs and post-mortem lesions. Pulmonary oedema with pleural effusions and absence of marked signs and lesions of disease in other organs is characteristic of ANTU poisoning.

Treatment and management: There is no specific antidote to ANTU poisoning. Supportive and detoxification therapy may be used.

a. Emetic and gastric lavage may be tried to remove the toxicant in the early stages. Activated charcoal may be helpful if added in lavage fluid and left in the lumen thereafter.

b. Animal may be sedated or anaesthetised with barbiturates to reduce struggling, dyspnoea and production of foam.

c. The animal may be placed on an inclined surface so that fluid escapes from the bronchi. The chest may be periodically compressed to facilitate drainage.

d. Silicone aerosols might be of some value in preventing fatal foaming in bronchioles.

e. Agents providing sulphydryl groups like N-amyl mercaptan, N-acetyl cysteine or sodium thiosulphate (10%) are beneficial.

f. Competitive ANTU antagonists like ethylenethiourea or 1-ethyl-1-phenyl thiourea provide some protection against the toxicity, but their clinical utility is small.

g. An osmotic diuretic (e.g. mannitol) and atropine (0.02-0.25 mg/kg) may help to releive the pulmonary oedema.

Prognosis: Prognosis of ANTU poisoning is grave when severe respiratory signs develop or when the animal is in comatose condition. If the animal survives for 12 hours, then it implies a good prognosis.

5. Bromethalin

It is a diphenylamine rodenticide, developed in 1980s as an alternative to warfarin against warfarin-resistant rats and mice. However, it is less frequently used than anticoagulant rodenticides or cholecalciferol due to high toxicity. Secondary bromethalin poisoning can occur in dogs or cats that eat killed rodents.

Chemistry: Bromethalin is N-methyl-2, 4-dinitrc-N-(2, 4, 6-tribromophenyl)-6- (trifluoro methyl) benzeneamine. It exists as a pale yellow crystalline solid, which is insoluble in water but soluble is acetone and chloroform. Bromethalin is used in baits in concentration of 0.005% or 0.01% and is usually pelleted or dyed green. It is marketed as a single feeding rodenticide for use mainly against anticoagulant resistant rodents. It does not induce bait shyness.

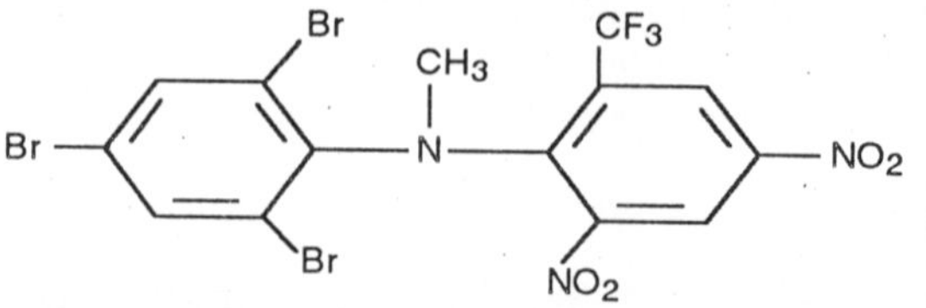

Fig. 13.29. Chemical structure of bromethalin.

Toxicity: Bromethalin is highly toxic to rodents and other mammalian species. Cats are more than 3 times as sensitive as dogs. The acute oral LD_{50} in different species varies from 1.5 to 5 mg/kg body weight (rats 2.0-4.0 mg/kg, mice 2-3 mg/kg, cats 1.8 mg/kg, dogs 4.7 mg/kg and pigs 0.25 mg/kg). In guinea pigs the LD_{50} is more than 1000 mg/kg.

Toxicokinetics: Bromethalin is rapidly absorbed after ingestion with peak plasma concentration reaching in 4 hours. However, its absorption from skin is poor. After absorption, bromethalin circulates through blood to most tissues. Metabolism is mainly through mixed function oxidases to desmethyl bromethalin which is also equally toxic or even more toxic than the parent compound. Excretion is mainly through the bile. The half-life of bromethalin in rats is 5-6 days.

Mechanism of action: Bromethalin and its active metabolite desmethyl bromethalin are uncoupler of oxidative phosphorylation in the mitochondria of central nervous system. Uncoupling of oxidative phosphorylation results in less production of ATP, which in turn leads to less energy for sodium-potassium adenosine triphosphatase ($Na^+ - K^+ -$ ATPase) activity. Inhibition of sodium pump in CNS subsequently results in cerebral oedema due to inability to maintain essential osmotic gradient. Fluid build-up is manifested by fluid filled vacuoles between myelin sheaths, cell swelling and degeneration. Accumulation of fluid and cerebral oedema may result in increased CSF pressure and increased pressure on nerve axons resulting in decreased nerve impulse conduction, paralysis and death. Bromethalin may also induce cerebral lipid peroxidation. Although cells of many organs are affected, damage to the CNS is predominant and mainly responsible for clinical signs exhibited by intoxicated animals.

Clinical signs: Bromethalin is somewhat slow acting, progressive neurotoxin. It displays two neurological syndromes: one at lower dosage and other at higher dosage. In the lower sub-lethal dosage (<2.5 mg/kg), toxic effects may appear 24-86 hours after ingestion. The syndrome in dogs is characterised by tremors, depression, hind limb weakness, ataxia, vomiting and lateral recumbency. These effects are reversible, if further exposure of toxicant is inhibited. Clinical signs following ingestion of lethal or higher dosage (> 5.0 mg/kg) in dogs appear within 4-24 hours and include hyperexitability, muscle tremors, grand mal seizures, hind limb hyper-reflexia, CNS depression and death. Body temperature usually rises. Death may occur from respiratory paralysis. In cats, bromethalin develops a similar syndrome of progressive depression, ataxia, abdominal swelling, focal motor seizures, vocalization, and respiratory depression.

Post-mortem findings: The gross lesions seen on post-mortem examination are limited to those caused by cerebral oedema (brain swelling), which include narrowing of sulci and flattening of gyri. Mild pulmonary congestion may be seen in some cases. The predominant histological change is seen in the brain. Spongy degeneration occurs in the optic nerve and in the white matter of brain and spinal cord. Electron microscopy may reveal vacuoles, oedema and splitting of myelin sheath.

Diagnosis: Diagnosis of bromethalin poisoning is made from history, clinical signs, lesions and chemical analysis. EEG changes may show marked voltage depression and abnormal high-voltage short-wave activity. Bromethalin can be identified in kidney, liver, fat, and brain tissues. Bromethalin toxicosis should be considered when cerebral oedema or posterior paralysis is present; however, facilities for the analysis of bromethalin in tissues are currently available only in selected diagnostic centres.

Bromethalin toxicosis should be differentiated from other diseases and poisonings that present convulsive syndromes such as cerebral trauma, spinal cord injury, larval migration, neoplasia, canine distemper and toxicity from lead, strychnine and organophosphate compounds.

Treatment and management: Specific antidote to bromethalin is not available. Treatment should be aimed at blocking the absorption of toxicant from gut and reducing the cerebral oedema.

a. Repeated oral administration of activated charcoal/sorbitol mixture decreases absorption of bromethalin and is considered useful in early stages of poisoning.

b. Use of mannitol (250 mg/kg, I.V. every 6 hour) as an osmotic diuretic and corticosteroids have been suggested, but these have shown variable responses.

c. Fluid balance should be maintained with oral fluids.

d. Seizures and hyperexcitability can be controlled with diazepam or phenobarbitone sodium.

Prognosis: Prognosis is guarded, if signs are severe or advanced.

6. Strychnine

Strychnine is an alkaloid extract obtained from the dried ripe seeds of Indian tree *Strychnos nux vomica*. Strychnine was isolated in pure form in 1818 and since then it is used for control of rodents, birds and stray dogs. Currently, strychnine is a restricted-use pesticide and is not freely available. Nevertheless, both malicious and accidental poisonings still occur with its illegal use.

Properties: Strychnine forms colourless crystals which are odourless, very bitter in taste and almost insoluble in water and readily soluble in ethanol and other organic solvents. Its salts (HCl or sulphate) are more soluble in water. It is relatively stable agent and persists in food or environment when used as bait. The baits are usually red- or green-coloured grains that contain 0.5% to 1%

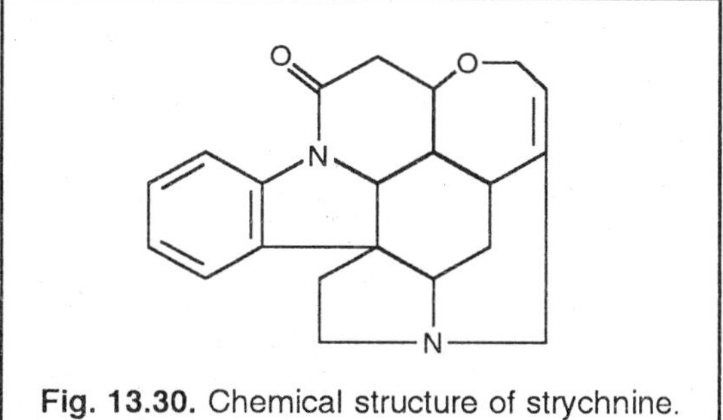

Fig. 13.30. Chemical structure of strychnine.

strychnine sulphate. Due to its bitter taste, strychnine readily produces bait shyness. Strychnine possesses some therapeutic values and has also been used in lower concentrations as a tonic and stimulant in veterinary and human medicine.

Toxicity: Strychnine is extremely toxic to all animals; however incidence of poisoning occurs mainly in birds and small animals, particularly dogs. The oral lethal dose of strychnine in various animal species is: dogs and cattle 0.5 mg/kg, horses and pigs 0.5-1.0 mg/kg, cats 2.0 mg/kg, rats 3.0 mg/kg and poultry 5.0 mg/kg. The female rats are more susceptible to strychnine than male rats perhaps due to not very efficient hepatic metabolism in females.

Toxicokinetics: Strychnine is rapidly absorbed from the gastrointestinal tract and nasal mucosa, but not through the skin. Once in blood, it is widely distributed in body with significant amounts found in the liver and kidneys. Some portion of strychnine reaches CNS, but it does not accumulate in nervous tissues. It is readily metabolized in liver by microsomal mixed function oxidases to several non-toxic polar metabolites including strychnine-N-oxide. Both parent compound (5-20%) and metabolites are excreted rapidly in the urine. The half-life of strychnine is approximately 10 hours. Acidic urine hastens excretion of strychnine by causing ionization and ion trapping.

Mechanism of action: Strychnine is a strong convulsant. It competitively antagonises the action of inhibitory neurotransmitter glycine in the central nervous system. Glycine normally interacts with glycine receptors at post-synaptic neuronal sites in the spinal cord and medulla and opens Cl^- channels, which hyperpolarizes neurons and thus decreases likelihood of depolarization. Inhibition of glycine receptors by strychnine results in loss of inhibitory effects leading to unchecked reflex stimulation and hence uncontrolled excitation of the spinal cord. Stimulation of extensor muscles, which predominates, results in extensor rigidity and tonic seizures. The major site of strychnine action is the recurrent inhibitory interneuron (Renshaw cells) of the reflex arc in spinal cord and medulla.

Clinical signs: Initial signs of strychnine poisoning usually appear within 0.5 to 2 hours after ingestion and include restlessness, anxiety, muscular twitching and neck stiffness. Later convulsions occur with intervening periods of relaxation which becomes progressively shorter. During periods of relaxation any external stimulus *i.e.* noise, touch or light induces reflexive spasms of increasing severity. Breathing becomes laboured and irregular. Advanced signs include spontaneous and nearly continuous tetanic seizures with marked rigidity sometimes known as a 'saw horse stance' (opisthotonos condition). Generally, there is no salivation, masticatory activity, paddling or running movement. Vomiting is rare and poisoned animals are in full consciousness until near death. Death mainly occurs from suffocation due to spasms of the respiratory muscles or paralysis of the respiratory centre.

Birds affected by strychnine poisoning exhibit ataxia, wing drop, tremors, muscle tenseness, feathers fluffed or held tightly against the body and convulsions.

Post-mortem findings: Post-mortem findings of strychnine poisoning are non-specific and reflect only the presence of violent convulsions and anoxia. Subcutaneous or intramuscular haemorrhages may result from trauma, animal may have food or bait in stomach and cyanosis results from asphyxia. The onset of rigor mortis is rapid.

Diagnosis: Diagnosis of strychnine poisoning is made from history, clinical signs and lesions. Chemical analysis of strychnine may confirm poisoning. Strychnine can be detected in the cadaver for several months after death. Urine from a live animal and stomach contents and urine from a dead animal are the samples of choice for laboratory analysis of strychnine.

The clinical signs of strychnine poisoning closely resemble many diseases and intoxications and should be carefully differentiated. These include rabies, tetanus, distemper, Aujesky's disease, epilepsy, hypoglycaemia, organophosphate poisoning, metaldehyde poisoning, phosphide poisoning and ethylene glycol poisoning.

Treatment and management: There is no specific antidote to strychnine. Therapy includes symptomatic and supportive care with primary goal to prevent asphyxia. Airway and seizure control may need to be instituted prior to decontamination procedures.

a. *Sedatives:* Sedation of the poisoned animal to prevent seizures while toxicant is metabolized and excreted is the primary therapy of strychnine poisoning. Sedation with a barbiturate (e.g. pentobarbitone sodium) to effect by intravenous route is the preferred drug in strychnine poisoning. Chloral hydrate may be useful in large animals. Although diazepam is normally the drug of choice for animals having seizure, its efficacy for strychnine-induced seizures may be variable.

Pentobarbitone

Dogs & cats: 5 – 15 mg/kg, IV to effect. Dose may be repeated in 4 – 8 hours.

b. Muscle relaxants which decrease central respiratory depression may be used for relaxation of tense muscles. These may include glyceryl guaiacolate (110 mg/kg) or methocarbamol (55-220 mg/kg, IV, followed by 90 mg/kg, if required).

c. Gastric lavage with potassium permanganate or tannins may be used in anaesthetised animal with endotracheal tube in place.

d. Fluid diuresis (5% mannitol in 0.9% normal saline) should be initiated to stimulate urine flow and excretion of strychnine.

e. Acidification of urine with ammonium chloride (100 mg/kg, PO, twice daily) may be useful for ion-trapping and urinary excretion of strychnine. Ammonium chloride is contraindicated, if animal is already acidotic.

f. Severely affected animal should be intubated and artificial respiration provided.

g. Animal should be maintained in a warm, quite environment away from external stimuli.

Contraindications

a. Ketamine and morphine are contraindicated in strychnine-intoxicated animals due to their motor stimulatory effect and respiratory depression effect, respectively.

b. Emesis is contraindicated due to potential for development of seizures.

Prognosis: Prognosis is good, if animal is treated promptly and supportive care is maintained for 24-48 hours. Strychnine is rapidly excreted from the body; so prognosis is bright if animal survives first 24-36 hours.

Public health and environmental concerns: Strychnine is generally less toxic to avian species than to mammals, but the way it is commonly applied poses danger to non-target birds. Poisoning to non-target animals and wildlife has led to its restricted use in several countries.

7. Red Squill

Red squill is one of the oldest rodenticides with selective action on rats and mice. It is obtained from the bulbs of the Mediterranean Sea onion *Urginea (Scilla) maritima*, a plant with large bulbs. Though considered good, it has limited use today.

Properties: Red squill contains a mixture of glycosides of which scilliroside is most toxic. Scilliroside is a potent emetic and bitter tasting bufadienolide glycoside that is found in all parts of the plant, but its concentration in the bulbs is high. The scilliroside content of the bulbs depends on the plant variety and the time of harvest, but is typically below 0.5% of dry weight. Dried red squill powder loses its scilliroside content upon storage and when exposed to atmosphere. Red squill is bitter in taste, so rodents quickly learn to avoid the baits. The squill is mixed in meat, fish and cereals or other type of baits mostly at a concentration of 10%.

Toxicity: Red squill is highly toxic to rats and nontoxic to other warm-blooded animals when used in recommended dosages. The specific toxicity to rats is due to their inability to vomit while the product induces vomiting in other animal species. Furthermore, it is unpalatable to domestic animals

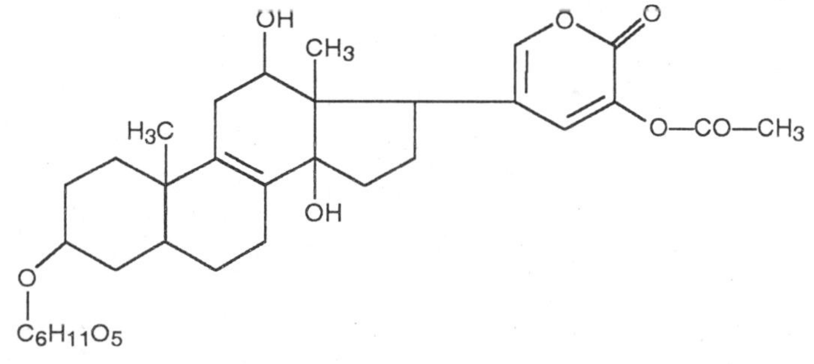

Fig. 13.31. Chemical structure of scilliroside, an important active constituent of red squill.

but not to rodents. Red squill is about twice as toxic to female rats (LD_{50} 200-250 mg/kg) as it is to male rats (LD_{50} 490 mg/kg). In dogs, oral LD_{50} of red squill is 145 mg/kg and in ruminants it is 250 mg/kg. The same implies to pure scilliroside which has oral LD_{50} of 0.7 mg/kg in male rats and 0.43 mg/kg in female rats. The lethal dose of scilliroside for pigs, cats and dogs ranges from 5-16 mg/kg body weight.

Mechanism of action: Scilliroside is a cardioactive glycoside which in higher dose produces digitalis-like action and cardiac arrest. It also acts on central nervous system, but the mechanism of neurotoxicity is not clear because scilliroside is unlikely to cross blood brain barrier to cause convulsions and paralysis. It is suggested that the scilliroside is metabolized by the gut microflora to its aglycone scillirosidin, which is equally toxic and produces some of the toxic effects of red squill.

Clinical signs: Clinical signs produced by ingestion of red squill or scilliroside include vomiting, abdominal pain, diarrhoea, ataxia, cardiac irregularities, and hyperesthesia followed by paralysis, depression or convulsions. Bradycardia and cardiac arrhythmias may end in cardiac arrest. The initial signs of poisoning occur within 12 hours and death usually follows within 3 days.

Post-mortem findings: Necropsy lesions of red squill poisoning include enlargement and congestion of abdominal and thoracic organs, gastritis and enteritis (due to strong irritant action). Kidneys, liver, lungs and myocardium show signs of congestion and swelling. Histopathological studies may reveal degenerative changes.

Treatment and management: No specific antidote is available for red squill poisoning. Treatment consists of supportive therapy and evacuation of the GI tract.

a. Gastric lavage and saline cathartic may be used to remove the toxicant from digestive tract.

b. Atropine sulphate given subcutaneously at 6-8 hours intervals may prevent cardiac arrest.

c. Phenytoin (35 mg/kg, PO, thrice daily) is given to dogs to suppress arrhythmias.

8. Pyriminil

Pyriminil (N-3-pyridylmethyl-N'-p-nitrophenylurea; Vacor; PNU) is a substituted urea rodenticide. It was introduced in 1975 for control of rats and mice and was considered effective against rodents resistant to warfarin. The compound has largely been withdrawn from market due to its adverse effects in humans, especially destruction of pancreatic beta cells and development of insulin-deficient, ketosis-prone diabetes mellitus.

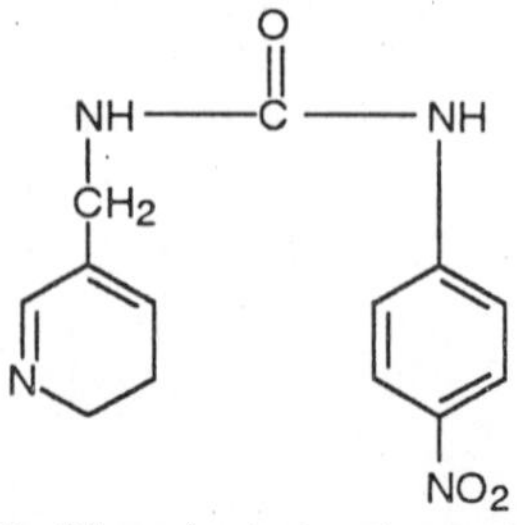

Fig. 13.32. Chemical structure of pyriminil.

Toxicity: Toxicity of pyriminil depends on the dose, species and individual susceptibility. It is highly toxic to rats (oral LD_{50} 4.5 mg/kg) and humans (lethal dose 5 mg/kg), and moderately toxic to cats (oral LD_{50} 62 mg/kg) and dogs (LD_{50} 500 mg/kg). It is sold for indoor use only as prepared bait containing 2% active ingredient and as 10% tracking powder.

Toxicokinetics: Pyriminil is rapidly absorbed after ingestion with peak plasma concentration achieving in 1-6 hours. In dogs, it is extensively metabolised and excreted in urine. Rats and humans are more sensitive to pyriminil toxicity than dogs perhaps due to less efficient metabolism of the rodenticide.

Mechanism of action: The exact mechanism of action of pyriminil is not clear. It is suggested that pyriminil selectively inhibits the NADH: ubiquinone reductase (Complex I) activity in mammalian mitochondria. It produces peripheral neuropathy, encephalopathy and diabetes mellitus. Inhibition of complex I activity also correlates well with the inhibition of insulin release from pancreatic islets, an action responsible for development of hyperglycaemia and diabetes mellitus.

Clinical signs: Clinical signs of pyriminil toxicosis begin within 4-48 hours and include weakness, nausea, vomiting, abdominal pain, hypotension, arrhythmias, tremors, ataxia and diabetic-type keto-acidosis (diabetes mellitus). In horses, weakness, anorexia, mydriasis, sweating, ataxia, muscle tremors and temporary glycosuria have been described. In horses and cats, pyriminil gives fishy odour to urine.

Post-mortem findings : Lesions of pyriminil poisoning are non-specific. These may include erosions, ulcers or perforations in the GI tract.

Diagnosis: Diagnosis of pyriminil poisoning should be based on history of exposure, clinical signs and clinical pathological changes. Clinical pathological findings may include glycosuria, hyperglycaemia and ketosis. Analysis of urine and tissues for pyriminil and its metabolites may be done, but is a possible only in well equipped laboratory.

Treatment: There is no specific antidote to pyriminil. Therapy of poisoning is only symptomatic and supportive.

a. Emetics, gastric lavage, activated charcoal or saline cathartic may be used to remove the recently ingested poison.

b. Nicotinamide administration has been found effective in rats, but may produce variable results in humans and animals.

c. Blood glucose should be closely monitored for development of diabetes mellitus.

9. Norbormide

Norbormide was developed as a safe rodenticide in 1964. It is a selective rodenticide, lethal to rats (oral LD_{50} 5.3 mg/kg) but not to other rodent species (oral LD_{50} in mice 2250 mg/kg). It is essentially non-toxic to cats, dogs, chickens, ducks, primates, sheep or swine. In dogs and cats, LD_{50} of norbormide is more than 1000 mg/kg body weight. It acts directly on the smooth muscles of peripheral vessels causing them to constrict irreversibly resulting in widespread ischaemia leading to death. It is selectively toxic to rats because it is assumed that norbormide receptors in smooth muscles of peripheral vessels exist uniquely in the rats. Rats show ataxia, restlessness, dyspnoea and weakness before the death. Treatment is not applicable in domestic animals as it is toxic to rats only. This compound as such has limited use as rodenticide.

10. Crimidine

Crimidine (2-Chloro-4-dimethyl amino-6-methyl pyrimidine) is an old rodenticide having limited use nowadays due to its non-selectivity. Poisoning in animals occur mainly due to ingestion of cereal-based baits containing up to 0.1% of the active ingredient. Oral LD_{50} of crimidine in various species is: rats 1.2-1.5 mg/kg, rabbits 5 mg/kg, dogs 0.5-1.0 mg/kg and poultry 5 mg/kg body weight. In body it acts as an antagonist of vitamin B_6-(pyridoxine). Clinical signs in animals appear 1 to 3 hours after crimidine ingestion and include staggering gait, bellowing, barking or howling, followed by hypersalivation, prostration, open mouth breathing, acute convulsive seizures and hyperthermia. Death occurs mainly due to asphyxia. Animal may recover quickly when treated with pyridoxine hydrochloride (20 mg/kg, I.V. or 25 mg/kg, S.C.). Diazepam or barbiturates can be used to control convulsive seizures.

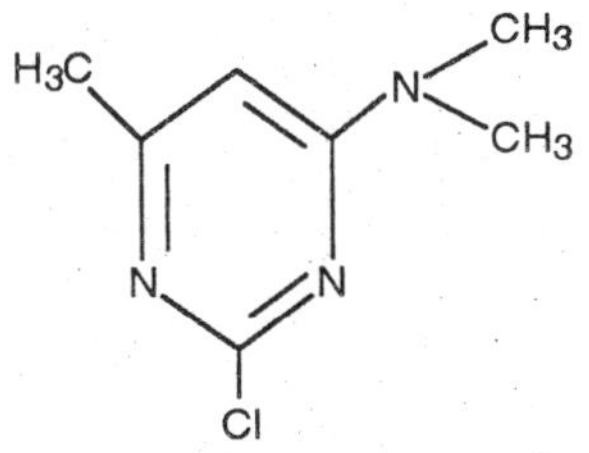

Fig. 13.33. Chemical structure of crimidine.

11. Chloralose

Chloralose (Alpha-chloralose) is a fast acting narcotic agent used occasionally as rodenticide and avicide. It is most active against small rodents such as mice, which have high surface area-to-volume ratio. Its narcotic properties are employed to immobilize birds and render them easier to capture or kill by other means. As a rodenticide it is used in baits at concentrations of 2-8%. The oral LD_{50} value of chloralose in different species is: rats and mice 300-400 mg/kg, cats 100 mg/kg, and dogs 600-1000 mg/kg. Chloralose possesses the unique characteristic of altering the mental component of central nervous system activity while increasing reflex activity. It acts by slowing down several metabolic processes in body causing hypothermia and virtually death. Important clinical signs of poisoning include incoordination, vertigo, disorientation, hypnosis, hypothermia and increased reactivity to sound and touch, but no response to pain. If stimulated, the intoxicated animals may respond reflexively and with full force. Death may occur due to respiratory failure. Treatment of poisoning include administration of analeptics such as methylamphetamine (0.5-4 mg/kg, orally or intramuscularly) or ephedrine (2.5 mg/kg, subcutaneously) and supportive therapy to correct hypothermia and respiratory problems.

F. MOLLUSCICIDES

Molluscicides are pesticides used to control molluscs such as slugs, snails and motts. These compounds are used mostly in temperate coastal and low land areas and in gardens. The group includes metaldehyde, pentachlorophenol, aluminium sulphate and copper sulphate. The use of copper sulphate in agriculture does not raise serious toxicological problems in domestic animals. Pentachlorophenol is highly toxic to both humans and animals and has been discussed along with fungicides.

1. Metaldehyde

Metaldehyde is a common molluscicide used world wide for the control of slugs and snails. Metaldehyde is toxic to all animals, but small animals and birds are frequently poisoned due to accidental ingestion of baits or eating of dead slugs. The World Health Organisation (WHO) classifies metaldehyde as a class II 'moderately hazardous' pesticide.

Chemistry and properties: Metaldehyde is an acetaldehyde polymer. It exists as a white or colourless crystalline solid with a mild characteristic odour and a powdery appearance. It is flammable and burns with a non-smoking flame. Metaldehyde is applied as molluscicide bait for controlling slugs and snails in a very wide range of agricultural and horticultural crops and in gardens. Molluscicide baits usually contain 3.5% metaldehyde. Some formulations contain a cat and dog repellent in order to avoid poisoning of these domestic animals.

Toxicity: Metaldehyde is highly toxic by inhalation, moderately toxic by ingestion and slightly toxic by dermal absorption. All species are susceptible to metaldehyde, but poisoning cases are commonly encountered in dogs, cats, sheep and birds. Toxic doses of metaldehyde for most species is in range of 100-500 mg/kg. Oral LD_{50} of metaldehyde in different species is: rats 220 mg/kg, mice and cats 200 mg/kg, dogs 100-500 mg/kg, sheep 300 mg/kg, pigs and cattle 400-500 mg/kg, and horses 300-400 mg/kg. In ducks the lethal dose is 500 mg/kg and in chickens 2000 mg/kg. Metaldehyde is toxic to game and wild birds and animals.

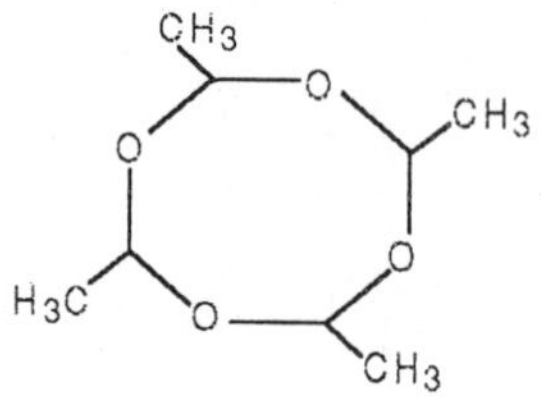

Fig. 13.34. Chemical structure of metaldehyde.

Toxicokinetics: Metaldehyde is readily absorbed from the gastrointestinal tract after ingestion. Metaldehyde is slowly decomposed in body to an active metabolite acetaldehyde, a chemical that acts like a narcotic. Gastric acid also promotes conversion of metaldehyde to acetaldehyde. Metaldehyde and its metabolites can cross the blood-brain barrier, as evidenced by their effect on the level of consciousness of animals. The metaldehyde and acetaldehyde metabolite is then excreted in urine.

Mechanism of action: The exact mechanism of action of metaldehyde is unknown.

a. Metaldehyde is a gastric irritant. Ingestion of metaldehyde causes irritation to the stomach and intestine and can cause kidney and liver damage.

b. Metaldehyde causes electrolyte and acid-base imbalance with development of acidosis perhaps from release of acetaldehyde and other effects such as convulsions and exhaustion. Metabolic acidosis is often associated with CNS depression and tachypnoea.

c. Metaldehyde decreases GABA levels in central nervous system. Decreased activity of GABA has been associated with enhanced excitation and decreased survival rate.

d. Metaldehyde decreases concentrations of serotonin and noradrenaline in brain. Brain concentrations of biogenic amines are often inversely related to the prevalence of seizures in animals.

e. Metaldehyde produces hyperthermia secondary to intense convulsions. As the body temperature increases, all organ systems begin to experience cellular necrosis within few minutes.

Clinical signs: The clinical signs of metaldehyde poisoning may appear within few minutes or up to three hours after ingestion. In dogs, the initial signs are anxiety, restlessness, mydriasis, hypersalivation (occasionally frothy), ataxia and incoordination. The initial signs are followed by tachypnoea, panting, tremor, tachycardia, opisthotonos clonic convulsions, cyanosis, nystagmus and severe hyperthermia. Liver failure may develop after 2 to 3 days of metaldehyde exposure. Death may occur from respiratory failure within few hours after onset of clinical signs. In cats, clinical signs are similar to that in dogs but nystagmus is more prominent. In sheep and goat, nervous signs predominate with significant ataxia, tremor and convulsions. Horses exhibit colic, hyperesthesia, diarrhoea, sweating, tremors, nystagmus and severe clonic seizures. In birds, clinical signs of metaldehyde poisoning include ataxia, opisthotonos, polypnoea and tremors.

Local exposure to metaldehyde causes skin and eye irritation. Inhalation of vapours of metaldehyde may cause severe irritation of the mucus membrane lining of mouth, throat, sinuses and lungs. Long-term repeated skin exposure to metaldehyde can result in dermatitis and prolonged eye exposure can cause conjunctivitis.

Post-mortem findings: Lesions of metaldehyde poisoning are non-specific. Gross lesions may include congestion of liver, kidneys, brain and lungs. Occasionally, haemorrhagic gastroenteritis, swollen red liver and epicardial haemorrhages may be observed. In birds, petechiation in gizzard and bloody fluid in air sacs may be seen. The stomach contents usually give smell of acetaldehyde. Microscopic lesions in different species may include hepatic and renal degeneration.

Diagnosis: Diagnosis of metaldehyde poisoning should be based on history, clinical signs, post-mortem lesions and laboratory analysis. Acetaldehyde odour in GI tract or from breath may help in diagnosis. Acidosis often results from metabolism of metaldehyde to acetaldehyde. Acetaldehyde may be evident in stomach contents or lavage fluid. Residues of metaldehyde are difficult to detect in tissues and may not be reliable for diagnosis.

Metaldehyde toxicosis should be differentiated from other poisonings such as strychnine, sodium fluoroacetate, zinc phosphide, organochlorine and organophosphorus insecticides, methylxanthines, lead, tremorgenic mycotoxins and amphetamine.

Treatment and management: Treatment of metaldehyde poisoning is non-specific and supportive.

a. Seizures should be controlled with appropriate sedatives such as diazepam (2-5 mg/kg, IV, to effect). In horses, xylazine with acepromazine has been recommended. Use of barbiturates should be discouraged in metaldehyde poisoning because they inhibit an enzyme involved in metabolism of acetaldehyde. Barbiturates should be used only if other sedatives fail to induce required sedation.

b. Muscle relaxants (e.g. methocarbamol) may be given to control severe tremors.

c. Attempts should be made to remove the recently ingested poison from GI tract by using an appropriate emetic, adsorbent, lavage or cathartic.

d. Appropriate fluid therapy should be administered to control dehydration, acidosis and electrolyte imbalance.

e. Artificial respiration may be instituted in severe cases.

f. Animal should be moved to a calm and quiet place.

Prognosis: Prognosis depends on the dose of molluscicide and time of institution of therapy. If treatment is started soon after poisoning, chances of survival are bright.

BIBLIOGRAPHY

Ashton FM and Crafts AS (1981) Mode of Action of Herbicides. 2nd edn. Wiley-Interscience, New York.

Ashworth B (1973) The frequency of animal poisoning by warfarin. *Vet. Rec.* 93 : 50.

Bahes D (1999) DNP (2,4-Dinitrophenol). (http://www.uk-muscle.co.uk/211319-post6.html).

Ballantyne B (2004) Toxicology of fungicides. In: Pesticide Toxicology and International Regulation. Mars T and Ballantyne B (Eds.) p. 193. John Wiley & Sons, Ltd., West Sussex.

Bartik M and Piskac A (1981) Veterinary Toxicology. Elsevier Scientific Publishing Company, Amsterdam.

Beasley V (1999) Veterinary Toxicology. International Veterinary Information Service, Ithaca NY (www.ivis.org).

Booth NH and Mcdonald LE (1982) John's Veterinary Pharmacology and Therapeutics. 5th edn. Kalyani Publishjers, Ludhiana-NewDelhi.

Boyd RE and Spyker DA (1983) Strychnine poisoning: Recovery from profound lactic acidosis, hyperthermia and rhabdomyolysis. *Am. J. Med.* 74 : 507.

Braund KG (2003) Neurotoxic disorders. In: Clinical Neurology in Small Animals – Localization, Diagnosis and Treatment. Braund KG (Ed.) International Veterinary Information Service, Ithaca, NY. (www.ivis.org).

Briggs SA (1992) Basic Guide to Pesticides: Their Characteristics and Hazards. Hemisphere Publishing Corp., Washington.

Buchel KH (1983) Chemistry of Pesticides. Wiley. New York.

Buffin D (2003) Imidacloprid. Pesticides News No. 62 : 22. (http://www.pan-uk.org/pestnews/Actives/imidaclo.htm).

Casida J E, Gammon D W, Glickman A H and Lawrence L J (1983) Mechanism of selective action of pyrethroid insecticides. *Ann. Rev. Pharmacol. Toxicol.* 23 : 413.

Cavalli RD and Fletcher K (1977) An effective treatment for paraquat poisoning. In: Biochemical Mechanism of Paraquat Toxicity. Autor, AP (Ed.). Academic Press, New York.

Clarke ECG and Clarke ML (1967) Garner's Veterinary Toxicology. 3rd edn. Williams and Wilkins, Baltimore.

Corbett JR, Wright K and Baille AC (1983) The Biochemical Mode of Action of Pesticides. Academic Press, London.

Dawson C (2007) Rodenticide poisoning: Rodent bait toxicity in dogs and cats. (http://petcare.suite101.com/article.cfm/rodenticide_poisoning).

De Bleeker JL, De Reuck JL and Willems JL (1992) Neurological aspects of organophosphate poisoning. *Clin. Neurol. Neurosurg.* 94 : 93.

Dettbarn WD (1984) Pesticide induced muscle necrosis: Mechanisms and prevention. *Fundam. Appl. Toxicol.* 4 : 518.

Diwan JC (2007) Oxidative phosphorylation: Chemiosmotic coupling. Molecular Biochemistry I. (http://www.rpi.edu/dept/bcbp/molbiochem/MBWeb/mb1/part2/oxphos.htm)

Dorman DC (1990) Anticoagulant, cholecalciferol, and bromethalin- based rodenticides. *Vet. Clin. North Am: Small Anim Pract.* 20 : 339.

Dougherty SA, Center SA and Dzanis DA (1990) Salmon calcitonin as adjunct treatment for vitamin D toxicosis in a dog. *J. Am. Vet. Med. Assoc.* 196 : 1269.

Duke SO (1990) Natural pesticides from plants. In: Advances in New Crops. Janick J and Simon JE (Eds.) p 511., Tmber Press, Portland.

Ecobichon DJ (1996) Toxic effects of pesticides. In: Casarett & Doull's Toxicology: The Basic Science of Poisons. 5th edn. Klaassen CD (Ed.) p 643. Mcgraw Hill Companies Inc., New York.

Eldefrawi A T (1983) Acetylcholinesterases and anticholinesterases. In: Comprehensive Insect Physiology, Biochemistry and Pharmacology. Vol. 12. Insect Control. pp 115-130. Kerkut G A and Gilbert L I (ed.). Pergamon Press, New York.

Eto M (1974) Organophosphorus Pesticides, Organic and Biological Chemistry. CRC Press, Boca Raton.

EXTOXNET (2006) Ethylene dibromide (EDB), dibromoethane. (http://extoxnet.orst.edu/pips/edb.htm).

Fest C and Schmidt KJ (1982) The Chemistry of Organophosphorus Pesticides. Springler Verlag, Berlin.

Fikes JD (1990) Organophosphorus and carbamate insecticides. In: The Veterinary Clinics of North America: Toxicology of Selected Pesticides, Drugs and Chemicals. Beasley VR (Ed.) 20 : 353.

Fitzwater WD and Prakash I (1989) Toxic chemicals. In: Handbook of Vertebrate Pest Control. Indian Council of Agricultural Research, New Delhi.

Garg SK (2000) Veterinary Toxicology. CBS Publishers & Distributors, New Delhi.

Guale FG, Stair EL and Johnson BW (1994) Laboratory diagnosis of zinc phosphide poisoning. *Vet. Hum. Toxicol.* 517.

Gupta PK and Salunkhe DK (1985). Modern Toxicology. Vol. III. Immuno and Clinical Toxicology Metropolitan Publishing Company, New Delhi.

Harrell TW, Latimer KS, Bain PJ and Krimer PM (2003) Anticoagulant rodenticide toxicosis in the dog and cat. Department of Pathology (Latimer, Bain, Krimer), College of Veterinary Medicine, The University of Georgia, Athens. (http://www.vet.uga.edu/vpp/ clerk/Harrell/ index.php).

Harris CR (1972) Factors influencing the effectiveness of soil insecticides. *Ann. Rev. Entomol.* 17 : 177.

Hatch RC and Funnel HS (1968) Strychnine levels in tissues and stomach contents of poisoned dogs, an 11 years survey. *Can Vet. J.* 9 : 161.

Hayes WJ (1975) Toxicology of Pesticides. The Williams and Wilkins Company, Baltimore.

Hollingshaus JG, Armstrong D and Toia RF (1981) Delayed toxicity and delayed neurotoxicity of phosphorothiolate and phosphonothionate esters. *J. Toxicol. Environ. Hlth.* 8 : 619.

Hollingworth RM (2001) Inhibitors and uncouplers of mitochondrial oxidative phosphorylation. In: Handbook of Pesticide Toxicology. 2nd edn. Vol. II: Agents. Krieger RI (Ed.). p 1169. Academic Press, San Diego.

Hovda LR and Hooser SB (2002) Toxicology of newer pesticides for use in dogs and cats. *Vet. Clin. North Am: Small Anim Pract.* 32 : 455.

IPCS INCHEM (1980) Tin and organotin compounds: A preliminary review. International Programme on Chemical safety - Environmental Health Criteria 15. (http://www.inchem.org/documents/ ehc/ehc/ehc015.htm).

IPCS INCHEM (2007) Strychnine. (http:// www.inchem.org/documents/pims/chemical/ pim507.htm).

Jewess PJ (2003) Acetylcholinesterase. In: Encyclopedia of Agrochemicals. Vol 1. Plimmer JR, Gammon DW and Ragsdale NN (Eds.). p 8. John Wiley &Sons, Inc., New Jersey.

Karczmar AG (1970) Anticholinesterase agents. Vol I. International Encyclopedia of Pharmacology and Therapeutics. Sect. 13. Pergamon Press Ltd., Oxford.

Kaur B, Brar R S and Sandhu H S (2002). Histopathological alterations in subacuter oral toxicity of amitraz in crossbred cow calves. *Ind. J. Vet. Path.* 26: 41.

Kaur B, Sandhu H S and Kaur R (2006) Toxic effects of subacute oral exposure of imidacloprid on biochemical parameters in crossbred cow calves. *Tox. Int.* 13: 43.

Kaur R, Rampal S and Sandhu H S (2005) Clinical and haematological studies on experimentally induced selenosis in crossbred cow calves. *Pak. Vet. J.* 25: 127.

Klaassen CD (2001) Non-metallic environmental toxicants: Air pollutants, solvents and vapours, and pesticides. In: Goodman & Gilman's The Pharmacological Basis of Therapeutics. 10th edn. Hardman JG, Limbird LE and Gilman AG (Eds.) p 1877. The McGraw-Hill Companies Inc., New York.

Krieger RI (2001) Handbook of Pesticide Toxicology. 2nd edn. Vol. I and II. Academic Press, San Diego.

Kumari V, Kaur B. and Sandhu H S (2002). Experimental cypermethrin toxicity in buffalo calves. *Ind. J. Anim. Sci.* 72: 658.

Lehninger AL (1978) Biochemistry. 2nd edn. Kalyani Publishers, Ludhiana-NewDelhi.

Lisella FS, Long KR and Scott HG (1971) Toxicology of rodenticides and their relation to human health. *J. Environ. Hlth.* 33 : 231.

Livezey KL, Dorman DC, Hooser SB and Buck WB (1991) Hypercalcaemia induced by vitamin D_3 toxicosis in two dogs. *Canine Pract.* 16 : 126.

Lorgue G, Lechenet J and Riviere A (1996) Clinical Veterinary Toxicology. Blackwell Science Ltd., United Kingdom.

Lotti M (2001) Clinical toxicology of anticholinesterase agents in humans. In: Handbook of Pesticide Toxicology. 2nd edn. Vol. II: Agents. Krieger RI (Ed.). p 1043. Academic Press, San Diego.

Lu FC and Kacew S (2002) Lu's Basic Toxicology: Fundamentals, Target Organs and Risk Assessment. Taylor & Francis, New York.

Majid MIA (2007) Know your pesticide: Paraquat. (http://www.prn2.usm.my/mainsite/ bulletin/ sun/1997/sun13.html).

Manning AM (2005) Rodenticide poisoning in dogs. (http://www.petplace.com/dogs/rodenticide-poisoning-in-dogs/page6.aspx).

Marrs TC (1993) Organophosphate poisoning. *Pharmacol. Ther.* 58 : 51.

Marrs T (1995) Toxicology of pesticides. In: General and Applied Toxicology. Ballantyne B, Marrs T and Turner P (Eds.) p 1199. Macmillan Press Ltd., London.

Marrs T and Ballantyne B (2004) Pesticide Toxicology and International Regulation. John Wiley & Sons, Ltd., West Sussex.

Matsmura F (1975) Toxicology of Insecticides. Plenum Press, New York.

Matsmura F (1984) Differential Toxicities of Insecticides and Halogenated Aromatics. International Encyclopedia of Pharmacology and Toxicology. Series 113. Pergamon Press Ltd., Oxford.

Means C (2001) Small animal toxicoses – rodenticides. (http://www.vspn.org/Library/misc/VSPN_M01287.htm).

Merola V (2002) Anticoagulant rodenticides: Deadly for pests, dangerous for pets. *Vet. Med.* 716. (http://www.aspca.org/site/DocServer/dbrief.oct2002.pdf?docID=304.).

Miyamote J and Kearney PC (1983) Pesticide Chemistry: Human Welfare and the Environment. Vol 1-4. Pergamon Press, Oxford.

Mosha RD (1993) The toxicology of organophosphorus insecticides: a review. *Vet. Bull.* 63: 1039.

Mount ME (1988) Diagnosis and therapy of anticoagulant rodenticide intoxications. *Vet. Clin. North Am: Small Anim Pract.* 18 : 115.

Murphy (2002) Rodenticides. *Vet. Clin. North Am: Small Anim Pract.* 32 : 469.

Nafe LA (1988) Selected neurotoxins. *Vet. Clin. North Am: Small Anim Pract.* 18 : 593.

O'Brien RD (1967) Insecticides: Action and Metabolism. Academic Press, New York.

Oehme FW and Mannala S (2001) Pesticide use in veterinary medicine. In: Handbook of Pesticide Toxicology. 2nd edn. Vol. I:: Principles. Krieger RI (Ed.). p 263. Academic Press, San Diego.

Ogg CL and Schulz CD (2006) Managing pesticide poisoning risk and understanding the signs and symptoms. University of Nebraska – Lincoln Extension Publications. (www.ianr.unl.edu/pubs/Pesticides/ec2505.htm).

Osweiler GD (1996) Toxicology. Williams and Wilkins, Philadelphia.

Pauluhn J (2003) Inhalation toxicity. In: Encyclopedia of Agrochemicals. Vol 1. Plimmer JR, Gammon DW and Ragsdale NN (Eds.). p 893. John Wiley &Sons, Inc., New Jersey.

Pelfrene AF (2001) Rodenticides. In: Handbook of Pesticide Toxicology. 2nd edn. Vol. II: Agents. Krieger RI (Ed.). p 1793. Academic Press, San Diego.

Pimentel D (1991) CRC Handbook of Pest Management in Agriculture. Vol. II. 2nd edn. CRC Press, Boca Raton.

Piccirillo VJ (2001) Methyl bromide. In: Handbook of Pesticide Toxicology. 2nd edn. Vol. II: Agents. Krieger RI (Ed.). p 1837. Academic Press, San Diego.

Plimmer JR (1982) Pesticide Residues and Exposure. ACS Symposium Series 182. American Chemical Society, Washington.

Plimmer JR (2003) Insecticidal carbamates. In: Encyclopedia of Agrochemicals. Vol 1. Plimmer JR, Gammon DW and Ragsdale NN (Eds.). p 924. John Wiley &Sons, Inc., New Jersey.

Plimmer JR, Gammon DW and Ragsdale NN (2003) Encyclopedia of Agrochemicals. Vol 1. John Wiley &Sons, Inc., New Jersey.

Radeleff RD (1970) Veterinary Toxicology. 2nd edn. Lea and Febiger, Philadelphia.

Ray DE (2001) Pyrethroid insecticides: Mechanisms of toxicity. In: Handbook of Pesticide Toxicology. 2nd edn. Vol. II: Agents. Krieger RI (Ed.). p 1289. Academic Press, San Diego.

Rebhun WC (1995) Miscellaneous toxicities and deficiencies. In: Disease of Cattle. p 503. Williams & Wilkins, Baltimore.

Rodostits O M, Gay C C, Blood D C and Hinchcliff K W (2000) Veterinary Medicine: A Textbook of the Diseases of Cattle, Sheep, Pigs, Goats and Horses. 9th edn. W. B. Saunders, London.

Rugman FP and Cosstick R (1990) Aplastic anaemia associated with organochloride pesticide: Case reports and review of evidence. *J. Clin. Path.* 43 : 98.

Sandhu HS and Bal MS (1998) Biochemical alterations following long-term oral administration of triazophos in buffalo calves. *Ind. Vet. J.* 75 : 507.

Sandhu HS and Malik JK (1988) Subacute toxicity of monocrotophos and its influence on circulating enzymes in *Bubalus bubalis*. *Pharmacol. Toxicol.* 62 : 290.

Sasser SM (1998) Rodenticides. In: Emergency Toxicology. 2nd edn. Viccellio P (ed.) p 425. Lippincott-Raven Publishers, Philadelhia.

Singh R and Sandhu H S (1999). Acute toxicity of acephate and its effects on biochemical parameters in buffalo claves. *Ind. J. Anim. Sci.* 69: 935.

Smith AG (2004) Toxicology of organochlorine insecticides. In: Pesticide Toxicology and International Regulation. Mars T and Ballantyne B (Eds.) p. 27. John Wiley & Sons, Ltd., West Sussex.

Smith BP (2001) Large Animal Internal Medicine. 3rd edn. Mosby, St. Louis.

Sonadgrass WR (2001) Diagnosis and treatment of poisoning due to pesticides. In: Handbook of Pesticide Toxicology. 2nd edn. Vol. I: Principles. Krieger RI (Ed.). p 589. Academic Press, San Diego.

Stenersen J (2004) Chemical Pesticides: Mode of Action and Toxicology. CRC Press, Boca Ratton.

Stephenson JPB (1967) Zinc phosphide poisoning. *Arch. Environ. Hlth.* 15 : 83.

Sultana M (1986) Toxicological and biochemical studies on O, O-diethyl-S-2-ethyl thiomethyl phosphorodithiolate "Phorate" in *Bubalus bubalis*. M.V.Sc. Thesis, Punjab Agricultural University, Ludhiana.

Talcott P A and Dorman D C (1997) Pesticide exposures in companion animals. *Vet. Med.* 78: 101.

Thomson WT (1992) Agricultural Chemicals. Book II: Herbicides. Thomson Publications, Fresno, CA.

Tomlin C (1984) The Pesticide Manual. 10th edn. pp 259. The Bath Press, Bath, U.K.

Ujvdry I (2001) Pest control agents from natural products. In: Handbook of Pesticide Toxicology. 2nd edn. Vol. I: Principles. Krieger RI (Ed.). p 109. Academic Press, San Diego.

Valentine WM (1990) Pyrethrin and pyrethroid insecticides. *Vet. Clin. North Am: Small Anim Pract.* 20 : 375.

Wedin GP and Benson BE (2004) Treatment of pesticide poisoning. In: Pesticide Toxicology and International Regulation. Mars T and Ballantyne B (Eds.) p. 473. John Wiley & Sons, Ltd., Weat Sussex.

Whisson D (1996) Rodenticides for control of Norway rats, roof rats and house mice. Poultry Fact Sheet No. 23, Cooperative Extension, University of California. (http://animalscience.ucdavis.edu/Avian/pfs23.htm).

White ME (2005) Cornell Consultant Toxicity Data. Alphabetical Search for the Cornell Consultant for Data on Intoxication, Poisoning or Toxicity in Animals. Cornell University College of Veterinary Medicine (Online service, http://homepage.eircom.net/~progers/consultox.htm).

Williams J (2005) CBRNE - Lung-Damaging Agents, Chloropicrin. eMedicine.(www.emedicine.com/emerg/topic907.htm).

World Health Organization (1990) Public Health Impact of Pesticides used in Agriculture. WHO, Geneva.

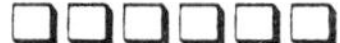

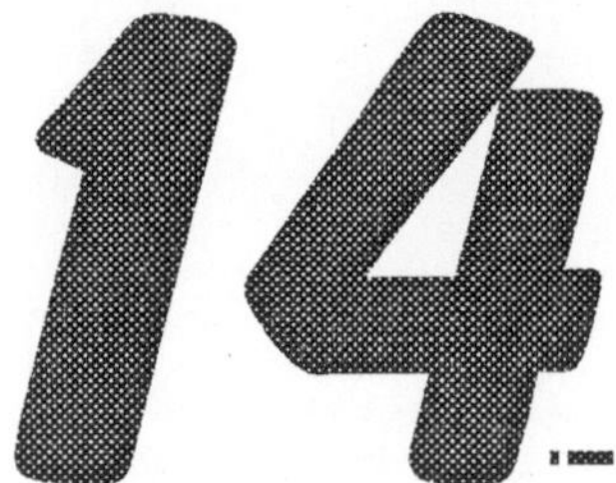

14 FUNGAL AND BACTERIAL TOXINS

Mycotoxins
- Hepatotoxic mycotoxins
  - Aflatoxins
  - Rubratoxins
  - Sporidesmin
  - Other hepatotoxic mycotoxins
- Nephrotoxic mycotoxins
  - Ochratoxin
  - Citrinin.
- Oestrogenic mycotoxins
  - Zearalenone (F-2 toxin)
- Cytotoxic mycotoxins
  - Trichothecenes
- Neurotoxic mycotoxins
  - Tremorgens
- Miscellaneous mycotoxins
  - Ergot
  - Fescue

Bacterial toxins
- Botulinum toxin
- Tetanus toxin

MYCOTOXINS

Mycotoxins are secondary fungal metabolites (i.e. metabolites not essential to the normal growth and reproduction of fungus) that cause illness or death in other species. Fungi make up a large part of the plant kingdom and are ubiquitous in occurrence. Out of large number of fungi, some genera and species are capable of producing toxins under specified conditions, particularly when temperature, moisture and aeration are favourable. These mould metabolites when produced in food stuffs and feeds and are consumed by animals exert toxic effects. The effects of poisoning by mycotoxins are referred to as mycotoxicoses. Mycotoxins have received considerable attention especially over the last three decades and mycotoxicology is currently a subject of international importance.

Characteristics of mycotoxins

a. Mycotoxins are not transmissible from one animal to another, so are not infectious.

b. Mycotoxin outbreaks are usually seasonal because a particular climatic sequence may favour fungal growth and toxin production.

c. Mycotoxins have specific association with a particular feed.

d. Treatment with drugs or antibiotics has little effect on the mycotoxins and the course of disease.

e. Several mycotoxins are immunosuppressive, which may allow viruses, bacteria, or parasites to cause a secondary disease that may be more obvious than the primary.

f. Presence of large number of fungi in feedstuff does not necessarily indicate excessive toxin production.

g. Mould infested feed along with nutritionally poor and inadequate diet makes animals more susceptible to mycotoxin-induced deleterious effects.

h. Environmental stress, insect damage and plant disease encourage colonization, growth and toxin production by fungi.

Although more than 250 mycotoxins have been detected chemically, the biological and veterinary-medical impact of many mycotoxins has not yet been defined. Some important mycotoxins having adverse biological effects have been discussed in the present chapter.

Classification

Mycotoxins may be classified according to the main organ system they affect. Important groups include:

I. Hepatotoxic mycotoxins e.g. aflatoxins, rubratoxins, sporidesmin and sterigmatocystin.

II. Nephrotoxic mycotoxins e.g. ochratoxin and citrinin.

III. Oestrogenic mycotoxins e.g. zearalenone (F-2 toxin).

IV. Cytotoxic mycotoxins e.g. trichothecenes (T-2 toxin, diacetylnivalenol and deoxynivalenol).

V. Neurotoxic mycotoxins e.g. tremorgens (penitrem, paspalitrem and roquefortine)

VI. Miscellaneous mycotoxins e.g. ergot and fescue.

I. HEPATOTOXIC MYCOTOXINS

1. Aflatoxins

Aflatoxins are toxic metabolites produced mainly by the toxigenic fungi *Aspergillus flavus* and the closely related species *A. parasiticus*. These moulds are present worldwide and invade and grow on all sorts of stored feed ingredients and organic matters and produce mycotoxins under favourable conditions. Aflatoxins were first discovered in England in 1960 when more than 10,000 turkeys and ducks died within a few months. The disease contracted by these animals was called Turkey X disease and its cause was traced to *Aspergillus flavus* contamination of peanut meal. Aflatoxicosis is not only a serious health hazard to animals but also a public health concern because food animals can retain residues of aflatoxins or their metabolites in the tissues.

Chemistry: The aflatoxins are a family of closely related polycyclic furan compounds. They contain a coumarin nucleus flanked by an apparently highly reactive bifuran system on one side and either a pentenone (B series) or a six membered lactone (G series) on the other. There are 18 compounds in the aflatoxin family; some of these occur naturally in feedstuffs and others are metabolites formed in animal body after ingestion of the contaminated feed. There are four important aflatoxins: B_1 and B_2 that fluoresce blue under long-wave ultraviolet light and G_1 and G_2 that fluoresce green. This grouping has been done according to their chromatographic and fluorescence characteristics. Aflatoxin B_1 is the most abundant and most toxic. These aflatoxins may occur together and their concentration may vary depending on the fungal strain and the substrate e.g. *A. flavus* growing on corn produces primarily B_1 and B_2, whereas *A. parasiticus* on corn produces all four major aflatoxins B_1 and B_2, G_1 and G_2; neither of these moulds produce B_1 toxin to an appreciable degree on soybeans.

Properties: Aflatoxins are lipid soluble, heat resistant and not soluble in water. They are, therefore, extractable from feedstuffs by a number of organic solvents. They are generally unstable when exposed to UV radiation. These moulds are not inherently toxigenic but can grow rapidly and become so in grains or feeds stored under aerobic

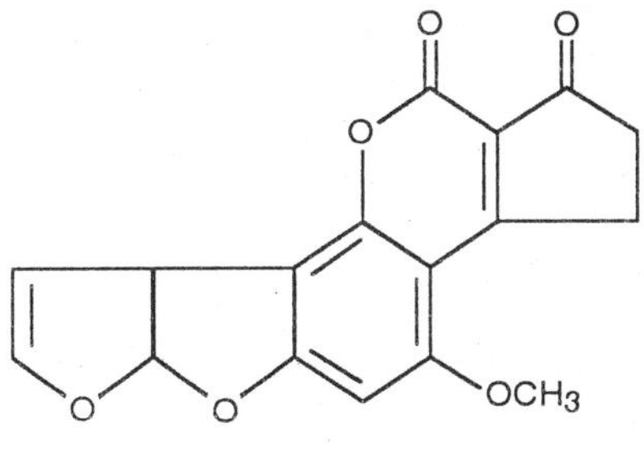

Aflatoxin B_1

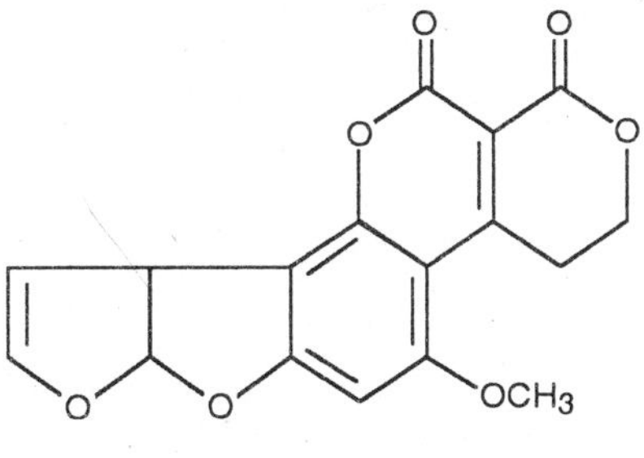

Aflatoxin G_1

Fig.14.1. Chemical structures of some important aflatoxins

conditions when moisture content of the feedstuff exceeds 15% and temperature is 25°C-32° C. Many feedstuffs like peanuts (groundnuts), soybean, and cottonseed meal and cake can support the growth of aflatoxin-producing moulds. Other products that can be associated with aflatoxicosis are shelled corn, cornmeal, silage, wheat, barley, oats, rice, and other grains or cereal products. Aflatoxins are produced by fungi when they have reached their maximum growth and may remain in food or feed product for years, even long after the mould has died. Contamination can occur in the field, during harvest, or in storage and processing.

Factors affecting toxicity:

a. *Species:* Dogs, rats, guinea-pigs, rabbits and ducklings are highly susceptible to aflatoxins, whereas sheep, adult cattle and goats are relatively resistant to toxicity.

b. *Duration:* Adult cattle, sheep and goats are relatively resistant to acute form of the disease, but show susceptibility to toxic diets fed over long periods.

c. *Dosage:* High doses of aflatoxins produce severe hepatocellular necrosis, whereas prolonged low dosages produce reduced growth rate and liver enlargement.

d. *Age:* Young animals of most species are more susceptible to aflatoxins than mature animals.

e. *Nutrition:* Nutritional deficiencies, especially deficiency of protein, selenium and vitamin C, increase susceptibilities to aflatoxins.

f. *Sex:* In general, males are more susceptible than females except during pregnancy.

Toxicity: Aflatoxins are acutely toxic, carcinogenic, mutagenic, teratogenic and immunosuppressive to most mammalian species. They are one of the most potent toxic substances that occur naturally and no animal species is resistant to the acute toxic effects of aflatoxins. Aflatoxin B_1 is the most toxic and is approximately twice as active as G_1 and M_1 (a metabolite of B_1 found in animals urine, milk or tissues). Aflatoxins B_2 and G_2 are approximately four and eight fold less active than B_1, respectively. A wide variation in LD_{50} values has been obtained in animal species tested with single doses of aflatoxins. For most species, the LD_{50} value ranges from 0.5 to 10 mg/kg body weight. The acute oral LD_{50} of aflatoxin B_1 in different species is : Horses, sheep, goats, swine 2.0 mg/kg, cattle 0.5 -2 mg/kg, dogs 0.5 - 1.0 mg/kg, cats 0.5 mg/kg, chickens 2.0 mg/kg, ducks 0.3 - 0.6 mg/kg, rabbits 0.3 - 0.5 mg/kg, mice 9.0 mg/kg and hamster 10 mg/kg. Dietary levels of aflatoxin (in ppb) generally tolerated are: young poultry ≤50, adult poultry ≤100, weaner pigs ≤50, finishing pigs ≤200, calves ≤100, and cattle ≤300. However, dairy cattle should not be exposed to more than 20 ppb because of danger of residues of the carcinogenic M_1 metabolites appearing in milk in concentrations greater than the allowable 0.5 ppb. Species susceptibility to aflatoxin mainly depends on its liver detoxification system, genetic make up, age and other nutritional factors.

Toxicokinetics: Aflatoxins are ingested in feedstuffs and may be partly transformed to water soluble conjugates by rumen flora, which may again be deconjugated in acidic stomach to release the original toxins. Aflatoxins are rapidly absorbed from the GI tract and are bound to serum albumin. The liver removes most of the toxins from blood stream and a variety of metabolites are produced by cytochrome P450 group of enzymes, depending on the genetic predisposition of the species. The metabolites may be water-soluble conjugates or lipid soluble forms. Aflatoxin B_1 is converted to at least seven metabolites including aflatoxicol, aflatoxin Q_1, aflatoxin P_1 and aflatoxin M_1. Along with the above metabolites, another metabolite called aflatoxin 8,9 epoxide is also formed, which is highly reactive. Of different aflatoxin metabolites, aflatoxin M_1 is toxic, carcinogenic and is excreted in milk. The primary metabolites are further detoxified by conjugation with glutathione, glucuronic acid, amino acids, sulphate and bile salts. The aflatoxins and their metabolites are excreted in urine and bile and may undergo entero-hepatic cycle. Complete elimination may require several days, although the toxins are not stored in any particular tissue.

Mechanism of action: Aflatoxins or their active metabolites (e.g. aflatoxin B_1 epoxide) binds covalently to cellular macromolecules such as DNA, RNA and proteins and cause dysfunction or destruction of hepatocytes and other metabolically active cells. The hepatocellular damage leads to impaired liver function, bile duct proliferation, bile stasis and liver fibrosis.

a. Aflatoxins modify DNA template and depress messenger RNA synthesis, thus interfering with transcription and subsequent inhibition of protein synthesis.

In particular, aflatoxin B_1 epoxide covalently binds to N-7 guanine residue of nuclear DNA resulting in pairing of adducted guanine with adenine rather than cytosine. The nucleotide mispairing leads to formation of an incorrect codon and insertion of an incorrect amino acid into the protein. Impaired protein synthesis interferes with formation of structural proteins and enzymes necessary for various biochemical processes. This action of aflatoxins affects the metabolic or biochemical pathways in one or more of the following ways:

i. Defective enzyme synthesis affects the energy metabolism and fat metabolism. Lack of formation of lipid acceptor protein in the liver leads to hepatic steatosis (accumulation of fat). There is also failure of transport mechanism of fat from liver (rather than its increased synthesis) resulting in excessive accumulation of lipids.

ii. Loss of enzymes results in reduced formation of structural proteins. Loss of tissue strength in blood vessels may lead to increased capillary permeability and bleeding.

iii. Defective enzyme and protein synthesis results in decreased prothrombin and other clotting factors synthesis in liver and decrease in vitamin K activities. This action in combination with weak capillaries results in haemorrhagic phenomenon.

iv. Defective enzymes may cause improper antibody formation and immunosuppression. Immunosuppression is also due to the reactivity of aflatoxins with T-cells and decrease in phagocytic activity in macrophages. The immunosuppressive effects lead to poor cell mediated and humoral immunity with more chances of secondary infections.

v. In correlation with the decrease in liver function and defective enzyme synthesis, there is development of jaundice and decrease in essential serum proteins synthesized by the liver.

b. Aflatoxins may directly affect the endocrine system (pituitary, thyroid, adrenal) thereby, resulting in hormonal imbalances.

c. Aflatoxin B_1 has been found to cause chromosomal aberration and DNA breakage to produce mutagenic effects. The mutagenic and carcinogenic properties of aflatoxins depend largely upon their metabolic activation to a DNA alkylating agent, the aflatoxin epoxide.

Clinical signs: Aflatoxicosis may occur in three forms: acute, subacute or chronic.

Acute toxicity: Acute toxicosis occurs sporadically as a farm disaster when high to moderate amount of toxin is consumed. In many cases death occur suddenly or after a short clinical course. Important clinical signs include weakness, anorexia, vomiting, depression, dyspnoea, coughing, nasal discharge, anaemia, epistaxis, petechiae on mucous membranes, bloody faeces, icterus, possible convulsions and death. In cattle, there may be general debility, ascites, diarrhoea and hepatic insufficiency. Clinical signs in birds may include anorexia, ruffled feathers, ataxia, circling, opisthotonos, convulsions, ecchymoses, oedema and rapid death.

Subacute toxicity: In subacute toxicity, animals may develop jaundice, hypoprothrombinemia, hematomas, haemorrhagic enteritis (warfarin like condition) and death. In cattle, there may be blindness, moving in circles, ear twitching, teeth grinding, photosensitive dermatitis, ataxia, etc. Subacute outbreaks are more common than acute toxicosis.

Chronic toxicity: Chronic aflatoxicosis is the most commonly occurring syndrome in domestic animals, birds and human beings due to continuous intake of low levels of aflatoxins in feed/food for weeks or months. Chronic toxicosis is manifested by gradual decrease in feed efficiency, productivity and weight gain. Rough hair coat, anaemia, enlarged abdomen, mild jaundice, depression and anorexia are also seen. Abortion may also occur. In ruminants, there may be reduced rumen motility. In poultry, aflatoxins interfere with absorption of lipids and transportation of yolk, so the egg production and egg size are reduced. Frequently, there is high incidence of concurrent infectious diseases (secondary infection), often respiratory, that respond poorly to usual chemotherapy.

Aflatoxicosis increases susceptibility of turkeys to coccidiosis, pasteurellosis and salmonellosis and of chicken to coccidiosis and Marek's disease. Signs may differ among different species but overall impression with aflatoxicosis is one of liver damage and blood coagulation defects. The chronic syndrome is characterised by high incidence of hepatic tumours.

Post-mortem findings: In acute cases, there are widespread haemorrhages and icterus. Gastroenteritis, ascites, hepatic necrosis and enlarged liver may also be seen. Microscopically, liver shows marked fatty accumulation and massive centrilobular necrosis and haemorrhages. In subacute cases, the hepatic changes are not so pronounced, but there is some liver enlargement and increased firmness. Microscopically, the liver shows proliferation and fibrosis of bile ductules and increase in size of the hepatocytes and their nuclei. Gastro-intestinal mucosa may show glandular atrophy and associated inflammation. Chronic toxicity may produce diffuse liver fibrosis, hydrothorax, ascites and oedema of the wall of the gall bladder. Hepatic neoplasms may also be seen.

Diagnosis: History, clinical signs, necropsy findings and microscopic examination of liver help in the diagnosis of aflatoxicosis. Aflatoxin M_1 can be detected in milk or urine for several days, if intakes of the toxins are high. Liver and kidney also retain measurable toxins or metabolites for few days. If bleeding disorders are found on clinical examination, determination of coagulation times may be useful. Serum liver enzymes including aspartate aminotransferase, alanine aminotransferase, alkaline phosphatase, ornithine carbamyl transferase, and isocitric dehydrogenase are elevated. Prothrombin activity may be reduced. Serum bile acids are elevated in early aflatoxicosis. Hyperbilirubinemia develops in chronic toxicosis. Laboratory tests of the feed can detect small amounts of aflatoxins.

Other conditions that may mimic aflatoxicosis include warfarin poisoning (primary coagulation defects), coal tar poisoning (variegated mottling of liver), copper poisoning (haemoglobinuria, haemolysis), infectious hepatitis, and other hepatotoxins such as carbon tetrachloride, pyrrolizidine alkaloids, etc.

Treatment and management: Aflatoxicosis has no specific treatment. With acute or subacute poisoning, dietary adjustments and supportive measures may not work.

a. Contaminated feed must be withdrawn immediately.

b. Hydrated sodium calcium aluminosilicate as feed additive (5 kg/tonne) can adsorb aflatoxins and hence reduce their absorption from the GI tract.

c. Vitamin E and selenium may be used to decrease the effects of aflatoxins; however they produce variable results.

d. Treatment of grains with anhydrous ammonia for 10-14 days to reduce its aflatoxin content may be recommended, but it is not approved by FDA. Several chemicals (e.g. hydrogen peroxide, chlorine and ozone) have been used to destroy aflatoxins but their efficacy has not been established.

e. Feeding of chronically poisoned animals with easily digestible, low-fat diet containing adequate protein is recommended.

f. Animals with secondary infectious diseases should be isolated and treated accordingly.

Prognosis: The prognosis depends on the extent and severity of liver dysfunction. In general, in acute and subacute aflatoxicosis prognosis is grave. Chronic toxicosis requires good managemental and nursing care.

Public health concerns: Because aflatoxins have proven to be carcinogenic in laboratory animals, milk should be routinely monitored for aflatoxins. Although estimates vary, aflatoxins in milk appear at approximately 1% of their dietary concentration.

2. Rubratoxins

Rubratoxins are acute toxins produced by the fungi *Penicillium rubrum* and *P. purpurogenum*. Rubratoxicosis was first recognized in 1950s as "Haemorrhagic Syndrome" in poultry after consumption of mouldy feed. Rubratoxins often grow in feedstuffs along with *Aspergillus* spp; therefore, rubratoxins and aflatoxins may coexist in the grain or feed product and the conditions favouring aflatoxins production in stored feeds can also favour rubratoxins.

Chemistry: The rubratoxins occur in two forms - rubratoxins A and B that have an unusual polycyclic structure containing stable anhydride functions. Their empirical formulas are

$C_{26}H_{32}O_{11}$ (A toxin) and $C_{26}H_{30}O_{11}$ (B toxin). Toxicity is due to the presence of an α, β-unsaturated lactone ring in their structure. Rubratoxin A is the minor metabolite while B is the major metabolite and most toxic rubratoxin. Rubratoxin B is hepatotoxic, mutagenic and teratogenic.

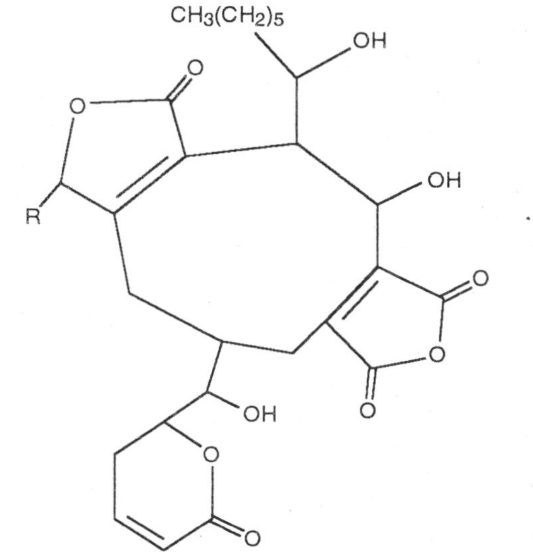

Rubratoxin A : R = –OH

Rubratoxin B : R = =O

Fig.14.2. Chemical structures of rubratoxins.

Properties: The rubratoxins are poorly soluble in water, insoluble in oils, and soluble in alcohol and esters. The toxins are stable at room temperature, but heating at 85-100°C for two hours may destroy rubratoxins in feeds.

Toxicity: Many domestic animals including dogs, cats, goats and horses are susceptible to rubratoxins, whereas some laboratory animals are relatively resistant to these mycotoxins. On equal weight basis, the rubratoxins are much less toxic than the aflatoxins. Rubratoxins occur usually along with aflatoxins in mouldy feeds and both these mycotoxins probably enhance each others toxic actions i.e. have synergistic effect. The acute oral LD_{50} of rubratoxin-B in rats is 400-450 mg/kg (when vehicle is dimethyl sulphoxide). Chronic toxicity of rubratoxins is not much important.

Toxicokinetics: After absorption into systemic circulation, rubratoxins are metabolised in the liver, producing number of metabolites. In rats, glucuronide and sulphate conjugates are excreted in bile and may undergo entero-hepatic cycle after deconjugation in liver. Much of the parent toxin is also excreted unchanged in the urine and faeces.

Mechanism of action: Mechanism of action of rubratoxins in some aspects is similar to that of aflatoxins. Rubratoxin B or its toxic metabolites due to the presence of lactone moiety can bind to cell macromolecules like DNA, RNA and others. It is postulated that binding of rubratoxin B might alter DNA, RNA polymerase or protein functions. There is also depression of oxidation of citrate, malate and pyruvate, possibly because rubratoxin or its metabolites block the electron transport chain. Rubratoxin B also inhibits adenosine triphosphatases (ATPases). The lethality of rubratoxin B is related to these basic effects on ATPases and the electron transport system.

Clinical Signs: Clinical signs of rubratoxicosis are related to severe liver damage and include anorexia, dehydration, depression, diarrhoea, jaundice and weight loss. Swine may manifest head pressing, colic and ventral erythema. Acute poisoning in horses is characterised by anorexia, depression, profuse bloody diarrhoea, foul smelling faeces, incoordination, recumbency and terminal convulsions. Death occurs after 12 hours or more.

Post-mortem findings: The lesions of rubratoxicosis include haemorrhages in various organs with severe haemorrhagic necrotising hepatitis. There may be jaundice, haemorrhagic enteritis and mild renal damage. In horses, there may be brain haemorrhages.

Diagnosis: Diagnosis on the basis of history, clinical signs and lesions may be difficult. Laboratory tests are required to identify causative fungi. Presence of rubratoxin in urine and feed may help diagnosis. Rubratoxins can be detected by chromatographic procedures.

Rubratoxicosis may be differentiated from other mycotoxicoses, particularly aflatoxicosis.

Treatment and management: There is no specific treatment for rubratoxicosis. Contaminated feed should be withheld and animals may be given symptomatic treatment and nursing care. Rubratoxicosis is usually complicated by aflatoxins and may be treated accordingly.

3. Sporidesmins

Sporidesmins are mycotoxins produced by soil fungus *Pithomyces chartanum* (*Sporidesmium bakeri*) that infest dead plant material. The fungus grows and sporulates on perennial ryegrass and other pastures during autumn following periods of draught. The ruminants grazing on short pasture consume the dead plant litters and get intoxicated. Sporidesmin poisoning is common in cattle and sheep in parts of New Zealand, Australia and South Africa, where the disease is commonly called ruminants' facial eczema.

Properties and toxicity: Sporidesmins are a group (Sporidesmins A to H) of epipolythiadioxopiperazine mycotoxins. Incidence of poisoning varies widely depending on climatic conditions. Outbreaks of poisoning typically occur when weather conditions suitable for rapid fungus growth and spore production are combined with abundant dead, recently killed plant material, which favours fungal growth. The fungus requires warm, humid weather and light rain (or irrigation) for growth, which is most likely in autumn. The fungus multiplies on most pasture plants (best on perennial ryegrass) by producing millions of spores which are coated with the toxin sporidesmin. At this stage, animals grazing short pasture are at greatest risk. Sheep are most susceptible followed by cattle; goats are less susceptible and rats are relatively resistant to the hepatotoxic effects of sporidesmin.

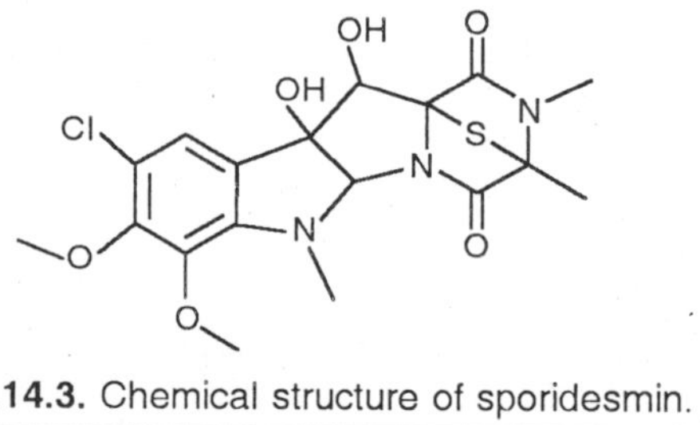

Fig.14.3. Chemical structure of sporidesmin.

Toxicokinetics: Sporidesmin is readily absorbed from intestine after ingestion. After absorption, the toxin reaches liver and causes hepatic damage.

Mechanism of action: Sporidesmin is a potent hepatotoxin. It causes extensive damage to liver and biliary epithelium leading to acute biliary obstruction and a resulting severe hepatic insufficiency. As a result of this liver dysfunction, chlorophyll absorbed from the gut is not completely metabolized and excreted. Instead, the partial breakdown products of chlorophyll, including phylloerythrin, enter the bloodstream. When the phylloerythrin (a fluorescent pigment and potent photodynamic compound) reaches the surface capillaries, it sensitizes skin to sunlight. This leads to photosensitization and blistering of the skin. The blistering of skin is common in lightly pigmented areas such as on the face of sheep or udder of cows. Hence the common name for this condition-facial eczema.

Clinical signs: The clinical signs of sporidesmin poisoning may appear 10-20 days following ingestion of the toxin. Important clinical findings in sheep and cattle are dullness, anorexia, jaundice, facial eczema and photosensitive dermatitis. The photosensitization usually affects exposed areas of the skin such as face, ears, teats and vulva, and areas of skin lacking dark pigmentation. The skin over these areas becomes reddened and then becomes crusty and dark. It eventually peels off leaving large raw areas, which are susceptible to infections. The photosensitization is often accompanied by watery swelling of the underlying tissues. Jaundice with yellowing of mucous membranes is often seen. Other associated signs are hyperirritability, lachrymation, nasal discharge and haemolysis with haemoglobinuria. Many animals die during acute stage and in the survivors conditions become poor. Some animals show no clinical signs, but have significant changes in serum enzyme systems indicative of hepatic damage.

Post-mortem findings: Important lesions of sporidesmin poisoning include swollen mottled liver, thickened bile duct walls and necrotic lesions on face and other lightly pigmented areas. In chronic cases, liver is tough and gets fibrosed. Microscopically, there is perilobular fibrosis, obliteration of bile duct and atrophy of hepatocytes. Spongy vacuolation of brain may be observed in some cases.

Diagnosis: Diagnosis of sporidesmin toxicosis should be based on history of exposure to contaminated pasture, clinical signs and necropsy lesions. Detection of sporidesmin in the feed and urine of affected animal may help diagnosis.

Treatment: There is no specific antidote to sporidesmin toxicosis. Therapy involves supportive care only.

a. Animals should be immediately shifted to shaded area, out of direct sunlight.

b. Supportive treatment for hepatitis and photosensitization should be started.

c. Antibacterials and antihistamines should be used to control secondary infections.

d. Zinc sulphate (6 g/100 l) in drinking water for 3-4 weeks may hasten recovery of affected wounds.

4. Other Hepatotoxic Mycotoxins

Some other hetapatotoxic mycotoxins causing poisoning in animals include sterigmatocystin, luteoskyrin and cyclochlorotine. Sterigmatocystin is structurally related to the family of aflatoxins and produced by fungi *Aspergillus versicolor* and *Bipolaris* spp. that infest groundnuts, barley and wheat. The sterigmatocystin is known to cause lung and liver tumours in laboratory animals and has been implicated as the cause of disease in calves that have consumed feed heavily invaded by the mould. Luteoskyrin and cyclochlorotine are produced by *Penicillium islandicum* and affect mainly chicken and rats. Luteoskyrin and cyclochlorotine cause great loss due to heavy mortality in chickens.

II. NEPHROTOXIC MYCOTOXINS

1. Ochratoxins

Ochratoxins are toxins produced by *Aspergillus ochraceus* and *Penicillium viridicatum* and some other species of *Aspergillus* and *Penicillium* that infest stored grains, corn, peanuts, cottonseed and decaying vegetation. In Denmark and Sweden these toxins cause significant losses in swine and poultry. Ochratoxins are potent nephrotoxins and produce renal damage in animals and birds, a syndrome commonly called mould nephrosis or mycotoxic nephropathy. The ochratoxin residues may also be carried over in pigs and poultry meats and affect persons eating contaminated meats.

Chemistry: Ochratoxins are group of at least 9 isocoumarin compounds synthesised from phenylalanine. Ochratoxin A is the most common of all the ochratoxins and has the greatest toxicological significance. Ochratoxin A consists of a polyketide-derived dihydroiso-coumarin moiety linked through the 12-carboxy group to phenylalanine. Ochratoxin B differs in structure only by the absence of chlorine atom. It can occur naturally but is much less toxic. Other related molecules include ochratoxin C, ochratoxin α and ochratoxin β.

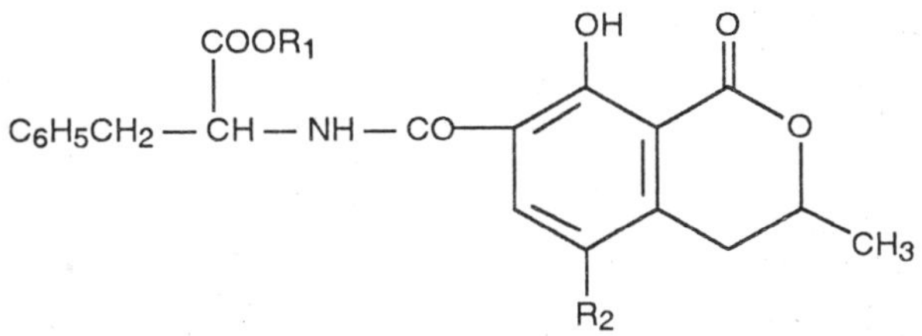

COOR1; $C_6H_5CH_2$ — CH — NH — CO—; OH; O; O; CH_3; R2

Ochratoxin A : $R_1 = -H$, $R_2 = -Cl$

Ochratoxin B : $R_1 = -H$, $R_2 = -H$

Ochratoxin C : $R_1 = -C_2H_5$, $R_2 = -Cl$

Fig.14.4. Chemical structures of some important ochratoxins.

Properties: The moulds belonging to the fungal genera *Aspergillus* and *Penicillium* infest corn, barley, wheat, rice, oats, rye, green coffee beans, pea nuts, etc. and extend ochratoxins under suitable conditions. Toxin production can continue during long term storage of grains especially when moisture content is >16% and relative humidity is > 85%. The optimal temperature range for toxin production is 12°C - 25°C; however reports of toxin production during low temperatures are also there. Ochratoxin A is a colourless crystalline compound, exhibiting blue fluorescence under UV light. It can be stored in ethanol for at least a year under refrigeration and protected from light. Ochratoxin A is a moderately stable molecule that survives most food processing to some extent.

Toxicity: Ochratoxins produce toxicity in many domestic species including pigs, poultry, horses, cattle and sheep. Pigs are most often involved, although birds are most susceptible. Cattle are less susceptible and are affected only at high concentrations. In acute toxicity studies, LD_{50} values vary greatly in different species, the dog being more susceptible. The acute oral toxic range of ochratoxins for swine and poultry is 1-5 ppm. Concentrations greater than 0.3 ppm for 2-6 weeks can produce tubular nephrosis and fibrosis in swine and poultry. For swine chronically exposed to ochratoxin A in feed, a no-effect concentration is less than 0.2 ppm. In broiler chickens, a no-effect concentration in acute studies is 0.5-1 ppm.

Toxicokinetics: Ochratoxins are absorbed from GI tract after ingestion and distributed mainly to liver and kidneys. Ochratoxin A accumulates in body tissues and fats of pigs and poultry. In the liver, ochratoxins are converted to active metabolites by microsomal MFOs. Metabolites of ochratoxin A include ochratoxin-Q and phenylalanine. Ochratoxin A disappears from the muscles and fat of affected pigs after two weeks and from liver and kidneys after 3-4 weeks. The half-life of ochratoxin A in swine is 3-5 days, but minute quantities can be detected in kidneys for about 30 days even after removal of the contaminated feed. Ochratoxins have been found to cross the placental barrier in sheep and produce residues in foetal lamb blood.

Mechanism of action: Ochratoxins have main action on renal proximal tubule where they cause decrease metabolite clearance and urine concentration ability, and inhibit anion transport and release of renal brush border enzymes (e.g. leusine aminopeptidase). At cellular levels, they have multiple actions like binding to proteins (e.g. albumin), interference with synthesis of transfer RNA and messenger RNA, interference with protein synthesis, disruption of carbohydrate metabolism, and increase in generation of free radicals via cytochrome P-450 reductase metabolism. Kidneys of affected pigs become enlarged and greyish in colour.

Clinical signs:

Acute toxicity: Acute clinical signs of ochratoxicosis include anorexia, vomiting, diarrhoea, dehydration and depression. In poultry, listlessness, crowding together, diarrhoea, ataxia, prostration and death may be observed. Acute toxicity is relatively rare.

Chronic or subacute toxicity: Subacute or chronic toxicity is more common and includes weight loss, reduced feed efficiency, polyuria, polydipsia, dehydration and severe anaemia followed by death. Immunosuppression, teratogenicity, carcinogenicity and haemorrhages are occasionally reported in cases of natural or experimental ochratoxicosis. Ochratoxin may also cause poor sperm quality in boars and foetal death, foetal resorption and abortion in sows.

Post-mortem findings: Renal lesions predominate and include pale, enlarged kidneys with a rough irregular surface. The cut surface of renal cortex reveals pale cortical streaking and multiple small cystic areas typical of fibroplasia. Enteritis, gastric ulcers and oedema may also be observed. Microscopic lesions include renal tubular swelling, degeneration of proximal tubules, atrophy of tubular epithelium, interstitial fibrosis in renal cortex and hyalinisation of some glomeruli. High concentrations of ochratoxin A may also cause hepatic necrosis and lymphoid depletion.

Diagnosis: Diagnosis of ochratoxicosis should be based on history of feeding mouldy feeds, clinical signs, lesions and laboratory analysis. Chemical analysis of grains and feeds using thin layer chromatography or high performance liquid chromatography reveals ochratoxin A. Ochratoxin A can also be detected in renal, hepatic and adipose tissues. Blood analysis indicates elevated BUN and serum creatinine levels.

Ochratoxicosis should be differentiated from poisoning by other mycotoxins and nephrotoxic agents.

Treatment and management: Ochratoxins have no specific therapy.

a. Activated charcoal may be used to reduce absorption of ochratoxin from GI tract, but usually is not practical in cases of chronic exposure.

b. Supportive therapy as required by the condition may be instituted.

c. Offending feed should be immediately removed.

d. Intake of protein in diet/ feed should be restricted.

Prevention:

a. Do not use animal feed if level of ochratoxin is more than 10 ppb.

b. Harvest and properly dry the animal feed before storage.

Public health concern: Ochratoxin residues have been detected as a carryover in pigs and poultry meats, which may produce harmful effect in human consumers.

2. Citrinin

Citrinin is a mycotoxin produced by various species of fungi *Penicillium* and *Aspergillus* including *P. citrinum, P. viridicatum, P. verrucosum, A. ochraceus* and *A. terreus*, which contaminate barley, oats, rye, wheat and corn. Citrinin mostly occurs as a co-contaminant with ochratoxins and produces mycotic nephropathy in livestock. Pigs are highly sensitive to citrinin. It causes kidney damage and mild liver damage in the form of fatty infiltration. Other effects include vasodilation, constriction of bronchi and increased muscular tone. Citrinin also affects domestic birds with clinical signs of watery diarrhoea, increased food consumption and reduced weight gain due to kidney degeneration in chickens Histopathological findings in different species include low-grade, long standing interstitial nephritis. There is no specific treatment of citrinin toxicosis.

III. OESTROGENIC MYCOTOXINS

1. Zearalenone

Zearalenone (also called F_2 toxin or RAL) is a potent non-steroidal oestrogenic mycotoxin that is produced as one of several toxic metabolites by the mould *Fusarium roseum (F. graminearum).* Zearalenone contaminated grains and fodders can produce hyperoestrogenism with reproductive disorders when animals consume them. Swine are most commonly affected but cases occur in other species as well.

Chemistry: Zearalenone is 6-(10-hydroxy-6-oxo-trans-1-undecanyl)-β-resorcyclic acid lactone. Therefore, it is a substituted resorcyclic acid lactone that is structurally similar to the anabolic agent zearalenol. Zearalenone has no structural similarity with oestrogen, but it produces the uterotropic and metabolic effects similar to that of excessive steroidal or synthetic oestrogens.

Properties: Zearalenone is a white crystalline compound, which exhibits blue-green fluorescence when excited by long wavelength UV light (360 nm) and a more intense green fluorescence when excited with short wavelength UV light (260 nm). The fungal species of *Fusarium* infest maize, wheat, sorghum, milo and oats and proliferate in warm weather. They elaborate zearalenone during a subsequent cold spell, particularly in stored grains (especially corn) that has high moisture content (23% or more). Fungal infections of corn and wheat are commonly known as "pink ear rot" and "scab" respectively. The toxin is heat-stable, and it is not destroyed by long storage, roasting, or by addition of propionic acid or mould retardants.

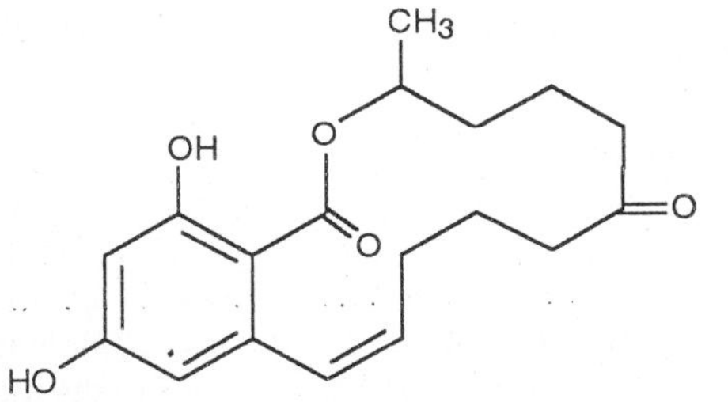

Fig.14.5. Chemical structure of zearalenone.

Toxicity: Zearalenone is probably one of the most widespread and economically important mycotoxins that affect swine, cattle, sheep, poultry and other species. Swine are the most susceptible domestic species to the reproductive effects of zearalenone and the condition in pigs is commonly called porcine vulvovaginitis or hyperestrogenic syndrome. Toxic effects of zearalenone are usually related to the concentration of mycotoxin in the diet of domestic animals. In prepubertal gilts, dietary zearalenone concentrations of 1-3 ppm may produce hyperoesterogenism, vulvovaginitis and vaginal and rectal prolapse. In cattle, dietary concentrations >10 ppm may cause reproductive dysfunctions like infertility, reduced conception rate and repeat breeding. Infertility in cattle has been of very low clinical incidence. Very high doses of the toxin are required to produce disease in poultry.

Toxicokinetics: Zearalenone is readily absorbed from the GI tract. It is metabolized to alpha and beta zearalenols, which conjugate with sulphates or glucuronides and are excreted mainly in bile, faeces and urine. Limited amount of zearalenone is excreted in milk. Alpha-zearalenol is the major metabolite in pigs and is 3-10 times more potent than the parent compound while the major metabolite in cattle is beta-zearalenol. The difference in the type of active metabolite is primarily responsible for more sensitivity of swine to zearalenone than the cattle.

Mechanism of action: The mechanism of action of zearalenone is similar to that of the oestrogens. Zearalenone and its active metabolites (α- and β-zearalenols) bind to cytosolic receptors for oestradiol-17β. The alpha-isomers of zearalenone metabolites have greater affinity of oestrogen receptors than the beta-isomers and thus the alpha-zearalenol is more potent than the beta-zearalenol or the parent compound. After binding, zearalenone (or zearalenol)-receptor complex migrates to the nucleus and binds to oestradiol sites on DNA, initiating specific RNA and protein synthesis. Physiologically, zearalenone functions as a weak oestrogen with potency two to four times less than that of oestradiol. It causes increased water and lowered lipid contents in muscles and increased permeability of uterus to glucose, RNA and protein precursors. It inhibits secretion and release of follicle-stimulating hormone (FSH), which inhibits preovulatory ovarian follicle maturation.

Clinical Signs: Clinical signs vary according to the animal's species, age and reproductive status. Usually the condition cannot be distinguished from excessive oestrogen administration. In pigs, zearalenone acts directly on the female reproductive tract and induces porcine "vulvovaginitis syndrome." It affects primarily weaned and prepubertal gilts in which it causes hyperaemia and enlargement of the vulva. There is hypertrophy of the mammary glands and uterus with occasional vaginal and rectal prolapse. Clinical signs appear 2-7 days after exposure and subside 4-10 days post-exposure. Mature sows may experience nymphomania (constant oestrus) or anoestrus and pseudopregnancy. In multiparous sows, effects of zearalenone include diminished fertility, anoestrus, reduced litter size, neonatal mortality, small foetal size, foetal malformation and probably foetal resorption.

Dairy heifers may show a range of clinical signs in relation to severity. These include weight loss, vaginal discharge, nymphomania, uterine hypertrophy; in pregnant heifers, abortion may occur 1-3 months after conception. Young males may become infertile with atrophy of testes and castrated males may develop enlargement of prepuce and nipples. In poultry, reduced fertility and lowered spermatogenesis have been noted following ingestion of high levels of zearalenone contaminated feeds. There are no reports on the adverse effects of zearalenone in man.

Post-mortem findings: Lesions of zearalenone are present only in the reproductive system. Prepubertal gilts exhibit swelling and oedema of vulva and mammary enlargement. The uterus is enlarged and oedematous with cellular proliferation and hypertrophy. Microscopic lesions of uterine and vaginal metaplasia and follicular atresia are characteristic. Mature sows with anoestrus exhibit retained and functional corpora lutea, uterine oedema, mammary alveolar development and ductular squamous metaplasia.

Diagnosis: Diagnosis of zearalenone toxicosis is based on the reproductive performance in the herd or flock, together with clinical signs and history of diet-related occurrence. Chemical analysis of grains or feeds is the most useful means of confirming significant exposure. The toxin can be identified by chromatographic analysis, and confirming the presence of specific fungus may not be necessary. The feed should not contain more than 10 ppb of zearalenone.

Zearalenone toxicosis may be differentiated from other oestrogenic toxicants.

Treatment and management: There is no specific treatment for zearalenone toxicosis. Unless stocks are severely or chronically affected, recovery of reproductive functions and regression of signs generally occur 1-4 weeks after the intake of zearalenone stops.

a. Supportive therapy for treating vaginal and rectal prolapse and physical damage to external genitalia must be initiated.

b. Administration of one 10 mg dose of prostaglandin F2α or two 5-mg doses on successive days usually resolves retained corpus lutea and corrects anoestrus in sows.

c. Activated charcoal binds zearalenone in the GI tract and helps to prevent its enterohepatic cycling.

d. Dehydrated alfalfa feed (15% in ration or feed) is protective as fibre reduces absorption of mycotoxin from the GI tract.

e. Offending feed should be withdrawn immediately.

IV. CYTOTOXIC MYCOTOXINS

1. Trichothecenes

The trichothecenes are a very large family of chemically related toxins produced by various species of *Fusarium, Myrothecium, Trichothecium, Trichoderma, Cephalosporium, Verticimonosporium,* and *Stachybotrys.* There are over 140 known metabolites in the trichothecene class, but most commonly found and studied are T-2 toxin, deoxynivalenol (vomitoxin, DON) and diacetoxyscirpenol (DAS). These toxins may occur in combination and cause more or less characteristic kinds of illness referred to under the blanket names of T-2 toxicosis or fusariotoxicosis. The toxic effects of the T-2 was first documented in 1940s when it was associated with an outbreak of alimentary toxic aleukia (ATA) in human beings. Trichothecenes affect all species including human beings and are amongst the most toxic mycotoxins. During the 1970s and 1980s, the trichothecene mycotoxins gained some notoriety as putative biological warfare agents when they were implicated in "yellow rain" attacks in Southeast Asia.

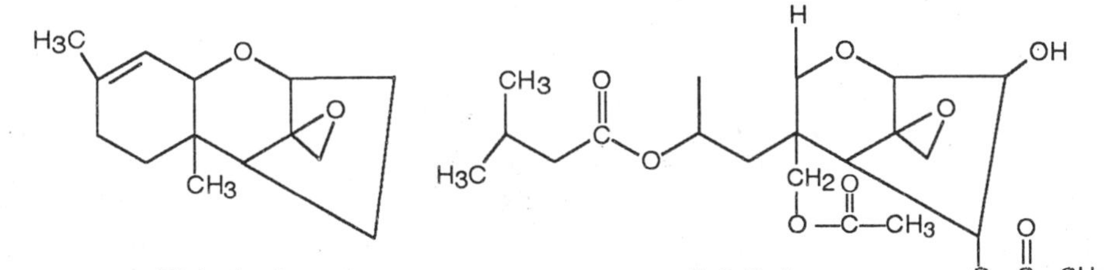

Trichothecin nucleus T–2 Toxin

Fig.14.6. Chemical structures of trichothecin nucleus and T-2 toxin.

Chemistry: Trichothecenes belong to a class of sesquiterpene lactones known as 12, 13-epoxy-trichothecenes. Toxicological properties depend in part on the presence of a 12, 13 epoxy group, as loss of the epoxide markedly reduces toxicity. On the basis of their molecular structure, trichothecenes are divided into two groups: the macrocyclic (e.g. satratoxin, verrucarin and roridin) and the non-microcyclic (e.g. T-2, diacetoxyscirpenol and deoxynivalenol) trichothecenes. Best known and of greatest concern are non-microcyclic trichothecenes and out of all trichothecenes T-2 is most cytotoxic.

Properties: The T-2, diacetoxyscirpenol and deoxynivalenol toxins are mainly produced by field fungi *Fusarium sporotrichioides* (T-2 toxin and DAS) and *F. roseum* (DON) that grow on corn, milo, wheat, rye, barley and other cereal crops. Mould growth and toxin production are favoured by alternating cool and warm temperatures ranging from 5°C to 15°C. Trichothecenes are poorly soluble in water, but are soluble in organic solvents and fats. These toxins resist chemical and environmental decomposition and persist in field indefinitely. Extraction of trichothecene mycotoxins from fungal cultures with organic solvents yields a yellow-brown liquid, which, if allowed to evaporate, forms a greasy, yellow crystalline product. In contrast, highly purified toxins form white, crystalline products that have characteristic melting points.

Toxicity: The trichothecene mycotoxins are toxic to mammals, birds, fish, many invertebrates, plants, and eukaryotic cells in general. The acute toxicity of trichothecene mycotoxins varies somewhat with the particular toxin and animal species studied. Mice are more resistant than rats, guinea pigs, swine and chickens. Cats appear to be more sensitive to T-2 toxin than other domestic species. The acute oral LD_{50} of T-2 toxin in various species is: rats 3.8 mg/kg, day-old broiler chicks 5-5.25 mg/kg and swine 4.0 mg/kg. For DAS, the acute oral LD_{50} is 1-2 mg/kg for guinea pigs, 7.3 mg/kg for rats and 3.8 mg/kg for day-old broiler chicks. For DON, the acute oral LD_{50} is 46 mg/kg in mice. Toxicity of a particular batch of mouldy grain or feed depends on factors such as temperature, humidity, moisture content, duration of exposure and degree of aerobiasis. Dietary levels of T-2 toxin capable of causing poor growth, decrease production or pathological effects are: cattle 2 ppm for several months, swine 1-8 ppm for 8 weeks, chicks 0.4 ppm for 7-9 weeks or 1 ppm for 3 weeks, and laying hens >16 ppm for 28 days. Some species (swine, cattle) refuse to eat feeds containing large amount of T-2 toxin, so it (toxin) is called as refusal factors in mould grain. DON produces vomiting due to its irritant nature, so is called vomitoxin.

Toxicokinetics: Trichothecene mycotoxins are lipophilic agents, so they are easily absorbed through skin, gut and pulmonary mucosa. Once trichothecene mycotoxins enter the systemic circulation, regardless of the route of exposure they affect rapidly proliferating tissues. However, they do not accumulate preferentially in any tissue. In liver, microsomal enzymes rapidly metabolise trichothecenes. Some of the metabolites are toxic. Compared with some of the other mycotoxins such as aflatoxin, the trichothecenes do not appear to require metabolic activation to exert their biological activity. Excretion of trichothecenes and their metabolites is mainly by faeces (from bile) and urine; to some extent they may be present in poultry eggs and cattle milk.

Mechanism of action: Trichothecenes are highly toxic at subcellular, cellular and organic system levels. They swiftly penetrate cell lipid bilayers and gain access to DNA, RNA and cellular organelles. Inhibition of protein synthesis appears to be the principal mechanism of action, but recent studies have indicated that effects of these toxins are much more diverse.

a. Trichothecenes are potent inhibitors of protein synthesis in mammalian cells. The T-2 toxin interacts with 60S subunit of ribosomes and inhibits protein synthesis possibly by degrading polyribosomes and blocking initiation, elongation and termination of protein synthesis. Lack of essential proteins and enzymes impairs various cellular activities such as mitochondrial electron transport mechanism ultimately resulting in cell death.

b. In doses higher than those required to inhibit protein-synthesis, trichothecenes inhibit DNA and RNA nucleic acid synthesis.

c. Low dosages of trichothecenes inhibit membrane transfer of glucose, calcium and some amino acids. These effects are independent of the inhibition of protein synthesis.

d. The trichothecene mycotoxins are directly cytotoxic to a variety of cells. The direct cytotoxicity is often referred to as a radiomimetic effect.

e. Trichothecenes induce some alterations in membrane structure, which consequently stimulates lipid peroxidation. Toxin-stimulated alterations in mitochondrial membranes contribute to the effects on cellular energetics and cellular cytotoxicity.

f. Trichothecenes affect immunity and hence increase susceptibility to certain infectious diseases. The main immunosuppressive effect of trichothecenes is at the level of T suppressor cell; however, they may also affect function of helper T cells, B cells, or macrophages or interaction between all of these cells.

g. Toxins cause haemorrhages by producing depression of clotting factors, thrombocytopenia, and inhibition of platelet function or possibly combination of these.

h. Trichothecenes are irritant to the skin and mucous membranes and produce gastroenteritis.

Clinical signs: The clinical signs of trichothecene intoxication can vary depending on whether the exposure is acute or chronic.

Acute toxicity: Acute oral or dermal exposures to trichothecene mycotoxins produce combination of clinical signs in domestic animals including vomiting, colic, poor appetite or anorexia (feed refusal), lethargy, weakness, mucous or bloody diarrhoea (due to gastro-enteritis), dehydration, hypothermia, unthriftiness, abortion, haematuria, epistaxis (defective coagulation), hypotension and shock. Paresis, tremors, seizures and paralysis occur in almost all species. Death could occur within minutes, hours, or days, and is mainly attributed to hypotension and shock. Following direct contact with contaminated feed, cutaneous areas could become red, tender, swollen, painful, pruritic or necrotic.

In horses, condition is characterized by retarded reflexes, bradycardia, disturbed respiration, cyclic movement, convulsions and death in 10-15% of the affected animals. In poultry, neurological effects (ataxia, abnormal posture) have been observed along with poor feathering, abnormal wing positioning, etc. Due to immunosuppression, secondary bacterial, viral or parasitic infections may mask the primary injury in all species.

Chronic toxicity: Chronic exposure to subacute doses of trichothecene mycotoxins is responsible for ATA (Alimentary Toxic Aleukia) toxicosis in humans and mycotoxicosis in domestic animals. The ATA toxicosis is characterised initially by weakness, salivation, abdominal pain, leucopenia, granulopenia and progressive lymphocytosis followed by appearance of bright red or dark cherry-red petechial rashes on the skin that may slowly spread and become numerous. In most severe cases, intensive ulceration and gangrenous processes develop in the larynx, leading to aphonia and death by strangulation. In most ATA cases, recovery is seen but the convalescence is prolonged and can last for several weeks. In animals, chronic trichothecene poisoning is not well characterised but may be seen in form of infertility or poor litters, poor weight gain, poor hatchability, decrease egg production and egg shell thickness. During this period, exposed animals are susceptible to various secondary infections.

Post-mortem findings: In animals, there may be oral, oesophageal, abomasal and ruminal erosions along with haemorrhagic enteritis and necrosis. Mucosal membranes and visceral organs may have petechial or ecchymotic haemorrhages. Liver may show necrosis. The lymphatic organs are smaller than normal. In chickens, there may be focal yellow-white caseous plaques at beak margins, on hard palate, or along edge of tongue. The spleen may be decreased in size, a finding seen only with T-2 mycotoxins in chickens and not with any other mycotoxin.

Diagnosis: Because clinical signs are non-specific or masked by secondary infections and diseases, the diagnosis of trichothecene poisoning in animals is difficult. Trichothecenes are rapidly metabolised and excreted, so diagnostic confirmation by chemical analysis is also difficult. Analysis of toxins in feed or grains can be done by TLC, HPLC and ELISA techniques. Extracts of mouldy corn produce a characteristic reaction when applied to the skin of laboratory animals if T-2 toxin is present.

Treatment and management: There is no specific treatment for T-2 toxicosis. Animals are treated symptomatically for GI signs, skin and oral lesions, toxemia and shock. Stress and exposure to animals with potential infectious diseases should be avoided to prevent potentially immuno-suppressed animals from becoming infected.

Prognosis: The prognosis of trichothecene toxicosis is grave in severely ill animals.

Public health concern: Residues in edible animal tissues are not a practical problem because trichothecenes are rapidly metabolised and excreted.

V. NEUROTOXIC MYCOTOXINS

1. Tremorgens

Tremorgens are a group of mycotoxins produced by fungi belonging to genera *Penicillium, Aspergillus and Claviceps*, which primarily affect the central nervous system. A large number of tremorgenic mycotoxins have been identified including paspalitrems, lotitrems, aflatrem, verruculogen, fumitremorgens, roquefortine and penitrems. Penitrem A is the most toxic tremorgen. The fungi that produce tremorgenic mycotoxins have been isolated from grains, cheese, silage and various forages, so they pose a health threat to both animals and humans who consume these commodities.

Properties and toxicity: Most of the tremorgens implicated in natural tremorgenic mycotoxicoses contain an indole moiety, presumably derived from tryptophan. Penitrems A, B and C, verruculogen and roquefortine are produced by *Penicillium* spp. and fumitremorgens A and B are produced by *Aspergillus* spp. Members of genus *Penicillium* are commonly found in feedstuff in temperate climate. The tremorgens affect all species, but the incidence of mycotoxicosis is more common in cattle and dogs. In cattle, paspalitrems, lotitrems, aflatrem and verruculogen have been implicated in a neurological disease commonly known as "staggers syndrome". In small animals, penitrem A and roquefortine are the two important tremorgenic mycotoxins associated with natural disease outbreak. The oral LD_{50} of penitrem A in mice is 10 mg/kg and the intraperitoneal LD_{50} is 1.1 mg/kg. Oral exposure to penitrem A from mouldy bread at a dose of 0.175 mg/kg is sufficient to produce severe muscle tremors in dogs.

Toxicokinetics: Tremorgenic indole alkaloids are lipophilic compounds, so they are readily absorbed from GI tract after ingestion. Once in blood, they are distributed to different body organs and can cross blood-brain barrier to enter the CNS. Penitrem A in dogs is excreted unchanged, although some tremorgens undergo some hepatic transformation. Enterohepatic recirculation and continued reabsorption may contribute to the prolonged recovery seen in animals exposed to these mycotoxins. Excretion of penitrem A and roquefortine are primarily through the bile.

Mechanism of action: The exact mechanism of action of tremorgens is not clear. Some studies suggested that they exert multiple effects on receptors and neurotransmitter release mechanisms

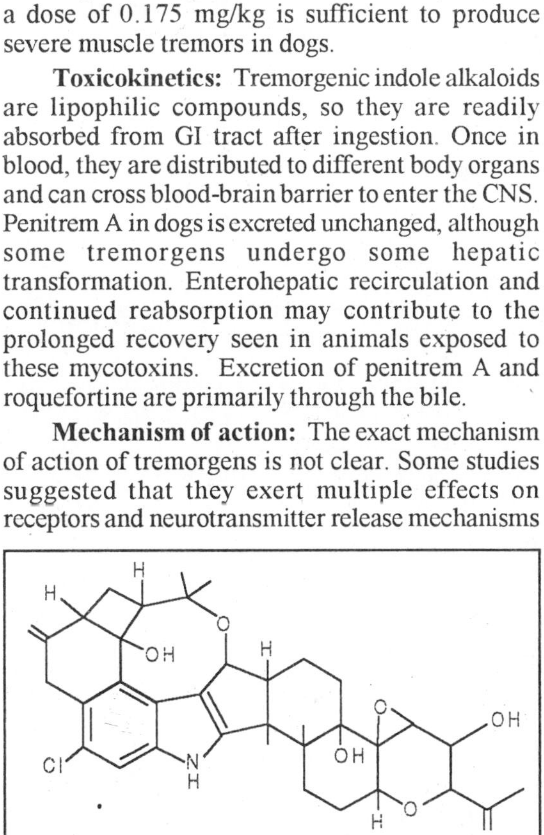

Fig.14.7. Chemical structure of tremortin A.

at central and peripheral levels. Penitrem A may affect presynaptic acetylcholine release, antagonise production of glycine, or act as a surrogate of GABA. Increased levels of excitatory neurotransmitter glutamate and decreased levels of inhibitory transmitter GABA in the brain have been noticed following treatment with some tremorgenic mycotoxins. Acute exposures to toxins may also result in degeneration of neuronal fibre processes.

Clinical signs: Clinical signs of penitrem A in dogs usually occur within 30 minutes after exposure, but may be delayed for a few hours. Early signs of poisoning in dogs include irritability, weakness, vomiting, muscle tremors, rigidity, hyperactivity and panting. Eventually the tremors may become more severe and there is appearance of opisthotonos, seizures, nystagmus, paddling movements, hyperpyrexia, dehydration and exhaustion. Death may occur during seizures, or animal may recover gradually over 1-2 days. Tremorgens in cattle produce a condition universally known as staggers syndrome. Staggers syndromes have different aetiologies and have been named differently like rye grass staggers, paspalum (Dallis grass) staggers, corn staggers and Bermuda grass staggers, but the clinical presentation in all is almost similar. The staggers syndrome is characterised by ataxia, muscle tremors, gait incoordination, rigid stance, falling on ground, recumbency and convulsions. Nystagmus and profuse salivation may occur sometimes.

Post-mortem findings: Tremorgenic mycotoxins do not produce specific gross and histopathological changes. Trauma from seizures may be observed.

Diagnosis: Diagnosis of tremorgenic mycotoxin poisoning should be based on history and clinical signs. Increased muscle activity and seizures may result in elevated levels of plasma creatinine phosphokinase, lactic dehydrogenase and aspartate aminotransferase. Detection of mycotoxin in vomitus, stomach contents or bile may help in diagnosis.

Tremorgenic mycotoxicosis should be differentiated from other poisonings producing tremors and seizures such as strychnine, metaldehyde, bromethalin, and organophosphorus and organochlorine insecticides.

Treatment and management: There is no specific antidote to tremorgenic mycotoxins. Treatment should be directed towards controlling seizures, metabolic acidosis and hyperthermia.

a. Emesis is recommended in recent poisoning in patients that have no risk for developing aspiration pneumonia.

b. Gastric lavage in small animals may be recommended when massive ingestion has occurred.

c. If acid-base imbalance has occurred, administration of sodium bicarbonate may be considered.

d. Seizures may be controlled with sedatives such as diazepam. If diazepam fails to give the desired result, seizures may be controlled with intravenous pentobarbitone or phenobarbitone.

e. Central muscle relaxants like methocarbamol or guaiphenesin may be used to relax muscles.

f. Fluids and corticosteroids may be recommended for shock.

g. Elevated body temperature may be decreased by using ice packs or cold water baths.

Prognosis: Prognosis in tremorgenic mycotoxicosis is good if decontamination occurs early. Most poisoned animals recover without sequelae within 24 to 48 hours with aggressive treatment.

VI. MISCELLANEOUS MYCOTOXINS

1. Ergot

Ergot is the longest known mycotoxin that affects animals and humans health. The disease ergotism had been well documented since the middle ages, but its aetiology was not well known. Ergot poisoning is caused by one or several alkaloids that are formed during the growth of *Claviceps purpurea,* and perhaps other *Claviceps* species in a variety of cereal grains and grass seeds. In livestock, ergot poisoning occurs mainly due to ingestion of fungus infested grasses while in humans poisoning is due to contamination of wheat flour with rye.

Chemistry: Ergot alkaloids are derivatives of lysergic acid. More than 40 derivatives are known, but important ergot alkaloids are ergotamine, ergometrine, ergocryptine, ergocornine, ergocristine and ergosine. The collective extract of ergot is called ergotoxin, which contains a number of biologically potent chemicals. Chemically, ergot alkaloids fall into two major categories, whether

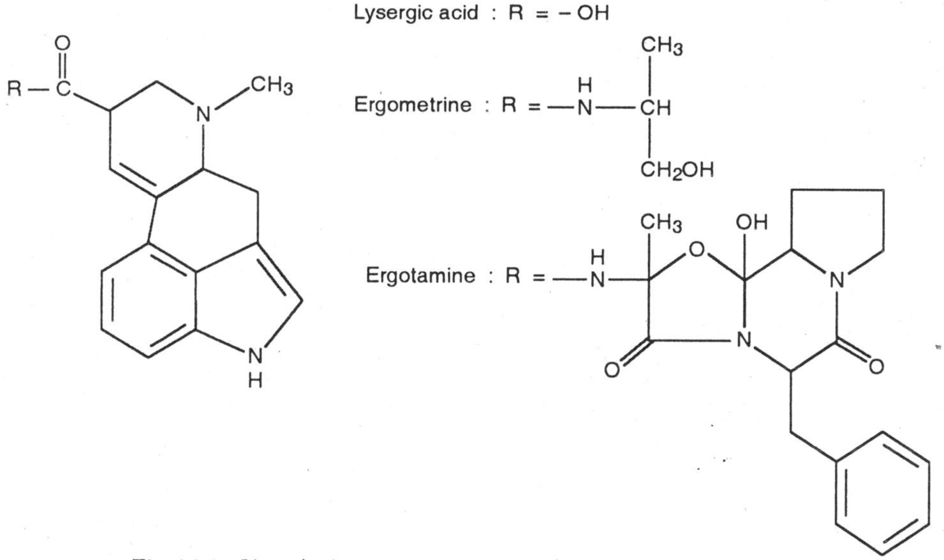

Fig.14.8. Chemical structures of some important ergot toxins.

they possess an amine or an amino acid side-chain. Compounds with an amine side-chain include ergometrine and those with an amino acid side-chain include ergotamine. Of various alkaloids, ergotamine and ergometrine are pharmacologically and toxicologically more important.

Properties: Ergot is the product of fungus *Claviceps purpurea* that grows upon rye and less commonly other cereals such as maize, wheat, barley, oats, wild grasses and fescue grass. Normally the fungal spores are carried by insects or wind to the ovaries of young rye, where they germinate into hyphal filaments under conditions of adequate warmth and moisture. The hyphal filament penetrates deep into ovary (seed) of the rye and forms a dense tissue, which gradually consumes the entire substance of the grain and hardens to form a lightly curved, black to purple body called sclerotium. The sclerotium contains varying quantities of ergot alkaloids and some other constituents. Ergot toxins, being alkaloids, have the same chemical and physical properties as alkaloids in general.

Factors affecting toxicity :

a. Ergotism depends on the amount of ergot ingested and duration of exposure. Although ergot is widespread in its distribution, it is seldom consumed in sufficient amount to cause poisoning.

b. Ergot poisoning mostly occurs in warm and wet season, which is conducive to the growth of the fungus.

c. Ergot poisoning occurs more commonly in cattle.

d. Ergot poisoning occurs mainly in stall fed animals feeding on heavily contaminated feed.

Toxicity: Ergotism occurs in chronic (gangrenous) and acute (nervous or convulsive) forms. Nervous ergotism occurs mostly in carnivores, horses and sheep but rarely in cattle. The amount of ergot sclerotia required to cause nervous signs varies with climate, location, species, and rate of ingestion of toxic feeds. Total alkaloid content and relative amounts of different alkaloids and other mould metabolites in ergot sclerotia also influence toxicity. Data are lacking on the LD_{50} of ergot sclerotia in various species. Autoclaving, exposure to high temperature (> 150°C) or application of 1% chlorine solution markedly reduces the toxicity of ergot alkaloids.

Toxicokinetics: Oral bioavailability of amino acid ergot alkaloids such as ergotamine is poor due to slow and incomplete absorption as well as high first pass metabolism. After absorption, ergotamine is distributed in various organs and is sequestered in tissues. It also effectively crosses blood-brain barrier and enters the brain. Ergotamine is metabolised in liver and largely excreted as metabolites (90%) in the bile. Traces of unmetabolised ergot compound can be found in urine and faeces. The plasma half-life of ergotamine is about 2 hours in some species (e.g. humans), but its vasoconstrictor action lasts for about 24 hours. This prolonged biological action occurs mainly because ergotamine is sequestered in tissues.

Mechanism of action: Ergot alkaloids are considered non-selective toxicological agents because they interact with numerous neurotransmitter receptors including adrenergic, serotonergic and dopaminergic receptors. All ergot alkaloids cause stimulation of smooth muscles, some being relatively selective for vascular smooth muscle and others acting mainly on uterus.

a. Ergot alkaloids act as partial agonist and antagonist at alpha-adrenergic receptors in vascular and other smooth muscles. Although they can reverse the pressor response of adrenaline due to alpha-adrenoceptor blockade (antagonistic action), they themselves are capable of producing stimulation of adrenergic receptors (agonistic action). The toxicological effects of ergot are produced mainly by continuous stimulation of adrenergic receptors in the vascular smooth muscles, which produces relatively persistent and sustained peripheral vasoconstriction. The vasoconstriction is often accompanied by damage to capillary endothelium. These actions initially result in reduced blood flow and eventually complete stasis with terminal necrosis of extremities due to thrombosis. The exact mechanism of gangrene formation is complex and not clearly understood, but the propensity of these alkaloids to cause gangrene of extremities appears to parallel the vasoconstrictor action. Of various natural ergot alkaloids, ergotamine has the greatest potency to produce vasoconstriction while ergometrine has little action.

b. Ergot alkaloids, particularly ergotamine, act as a partial agonist and antagonist at some serotonergic receptor subtypes. Although the role of serotonin receptors in ergot poisoning has not been defined, it is suggested that serotonin perhaps plays a role in vasoconstriction and development of thrombus.

c. Ergot alkaloids, especially ergometrine (ergonovine) has a potent oxytocic action. Ergot alkaloids produce CNS stimulation by interference with brain neurotransmitter functions especially the serotonin. Ergot alkaloids also mimic the action of dopamine in the central nervous system. Stimulation of D_2-dopaminergic receptors in CNS inhibits prolactin release from pituitary gland.

Clinical signs: Ergotism occurs in two well-defined syndromes: acute ergotism characterised by neurotoxicity and chronic ergotism characterised by gangrene of extremities. A third form characterised by hyperthermia has also been suggested.

Acute ergotism/Nervous ergotism: Acute or nervous ergotism occurs commonly in carnivores, horses and sheep, but only rarely in cattle. Onset of clinical signs may occur within 1 to 7 days and is characterised by combination of following signs: vertigo, weakness, recumbency, tremors, spasms, hyperexcitability, incoordination, ataxia or staggering gait, and drowsiness. There is nodding of head, exacerbation of tremors and incoordination by exercise or excitement, tonic convulsions with opisthotonos, and posterior paralysis. There may also be intermittent blindness and deafness and the skin may show alternating periods of increased and decreased sensitivity. Gangrene of extremities may also occur in this form of disease. The syndrome is terminated by either death or recovery in 10-14 days. Death may occur due to anoxia during convulsions.

Chronic ergotism/Gangrenous ergotism: The chronic or gangrenous form of ergotism occurs most commonly in cattle but may also affect other species including human beings. It is characterised by lameness, the first sign, which may appear 2-6 weeks or more after initial ingestion depending on the concentration of alkaloids in the ergot and the quantity of ergot in the feed. Associated with lameness are swelling and tenderness of the fetlock joint and pastern. There is development of sharply demarcated necrosis of feet, ear and tail ; in severe cases the hooves or feet and tail may be sloughed off leaving a clean surface that may ooze serum and become encrusted. This is due to prolonged constriction of the arteries which may lead to ischemia and dry gangrene. The condition is exacerbated in cold weather. Increased body temperature, increased pulse and respiration rates, diarrhoea and anorexia are also seen. Female swine, cattle and horses in late pregnancy have little or no udder development. Lactation does not occur after parturition as a result of ergot-induced inhibition of prolactin secretion. Occasionally abortion, foetal death and sterility may be seen.

Hyperthermic ergotism: In this form, there is hyperthermia (105-107°F), dyspnoea and hypersalivation. Milk production and growth rates are depressed. This syndrome is more severe in hot weather when affected animals seek water or shade.

Post-Mortem findings: Acute ergotism may not produce any gross lesion. However, there may be increased volume of CSF, incomplete rigor, empty arteries and some agonal changes attributable to convulsions. Ergot sclerotia may be found in the GI tract. In gangrenous form, the constant lesions at necropsy are in the skin and subcutaneous parts of the extremities. Subcutaneous haemorrhages and some oedema occur proximal to the necrotic area. Mammary glands of females in late pregnancy are small and flaccid, and there is no evidence of lacteal secretion. Microscopic lesions associated with gangrene include endothelial damage and coagulative necrosis.

Diagnosis: Diagnosis of ergot poisoning should be based on clinical signs, necropsy findings and chemical analysis. Findings of causative sclerotia in grains, hay, or pasture may provide important clues. Extraction and detection of ergot alkaloids may be done in suspected grain meals. Ergot alkaloids may be identified using thin-layer or gas chromatography or mass spectrometry.

Acute ergot poisoning is usually difficult to diagnose and may be confused with many other diseases that produce convulsions such as infectious disease, trauma, neoplasm, abscess or haemorrhage that affects the CNS. Chronic ergot poisoning should be differentiated from identical signs and lesions of lameness and sloughing of extremities seen in fescue foot in cattle, degnala disease, chronic selenosis and frost bite.

Treatment and management: There is no specific treatment for ergot toxicosis. Animals may be treated symptomatically.

a. If excessive ergot has been ingested, saline purgative (e.g. magnesium sulphate) may be used to eliminate the ingested poison.

b. Convulsions, tremors and behavioural aberrations may respond to treatment with chlorpromazine or diazepam.

c. Necrotic lesions may be treated with antibacterial agents. Flies and ectoparasites should be kept away from the lesions.

d. The animals should be kept warm to avoid cold-induced vasoconstriction in the extremities.

e. The offending feed or forage must be removed or fenced away from animals.

Prevention: Heavily ergotised grain or pasture fields containing ergotised grasses should not be used for animal feeding. Pasture fields may be grazed if the seed heads are mowed with the mower blade set high. Normally feed should not contain more than 0.1% of ergot infested heads.

2. Fescue

Fescue (*Festuca arundinacea*) is a widely used forage crop in some countries. Tall fescue is infected with a fungal endophyte, *Neotyphodium coenophialum* (formerly called *Acremonium coenophialum*) that produces several toxins including ergopeptide alkaloids (e.g. ergovaline) and peramine. Pregnant animals, particularly mares, are highly susceptible to the toxicity of fescue. Consumption of endophyte-infected tall fescue in mares increases the risk of spontaneous abortion, stillbirths, retained placenta, agalactia, laminitis, poor conception rates, prolonged pregnancy, and decreased prolactin and progesterone levels. Foals that survive *in utero* are generally larger than normal, have overgrown hooves, poor suckling reflexes, incoordination and lowered body temperatures. Foals may also have poor immunity due to lack of colostrum produced by the mare.

Fescue poisoning in cattle produces a disease commonly called "fescue summer toxicosis" characterized by decreased feed intake, poor weight gain, lower milk production, elevated body temperature, tachypnoea, rough hair coat, salivation and poor reproductive performance. Agalactia, due to decrease release of prolactin, is especially severe when cows graze tall fescue during the last trimester of gestation. Sheep are also affected by the fescue summer toxicosis with clinical signs of hyperthermia, poor wool production and reproductive problems as well as lowered feed intake and the resulting poor weight gains. The mycotoxin ergovaline, a potent vasoconstrictor, produced by fungus *Neotyphodium coenophialum* causes another syndrome in cattle and sheep commonly known as "fescue foot". Fescue foot occurs in winter, instead of summer, with lesions and clinical signs similar to gangrenous ergotism. Fescue poisoning has no effective treatment; supportive care is only recommended therapy.

B. BACTERIAL TOXINS

A large number of bacteria produce toxins, some of which cause food poisoning in humans and animals. The major factors contributing to bacterial contamination of food include improper storage, inadequate cooking, cross contamination between cooked and raw food, and inadequate cleaning of equipment and utensils. Bacterial toxins are relatively high molecular weight substances in the form of proteins, peptides and lipopolysaccharides. These bacterial toxins have diverse biological activities and some are highly lethal.

1. Botulinum Toxin

Botulism is an intoxication caused by serologically different but functionally similar toxins produced by strains of *Clostridium botulinum*. The *C. botulinum* proliferate in improper stored food/feed, in decomposing animal tissue and sometimes in plant materials such as decaying grass, hay and spoiled silage and elaborate a toxin called botulinum (or botulin) toxin. The botulinum toxin, a proteinaceous toxin, is among the most potent toxins known and occasionally causes heavy losses in animals that consume contaminated feed.

Classification: The botulinum toxin is two-chain polypeptide with a 100 kDa heavy chain joined by a disulphide bond to a 50 kDa light chain. There are seven serologically distinct botulinum toxin types, designated A through G. Out of all serotypes, types C and D have been most commonly implicated in domestic animals and poultry. Types A, B and E are of importance in human botulism, B in horses and cattle, C in dogs, cattle, horses, water fowl, wild ducks, pheasants and chickens, and D in cattle. Dogs are reportedly extremely sensitive to type E toxin. Only two outbreaks in humans have been caused by type F. Type G, which was isolated from soil in Argentina, is not known to have been involved in any outbreak of botulism either in man or in animals. The toxins are only slightly cross-reactive and can generally be regarded as immunologically specific.

Properties: *Clostridium botulinum, a* gram +ve spore forming anaerobic bacillus, occurs commonly in soil and in a suitable environment may contaminate feed stuffs and grow to produce toxin. Carcasses of decaying animals also form an anaerobic environment and the toxin may be present in maggots feeding on the contaminated tissues. Storage of meat by-products in metal drums, in which anaerobic conditions prevail, is an excellent medium for production of toxin. Intoxication in animals mostly occurs after ingestion of feed that already contains toxins or in some cases due to absorption of toxins elaborated in intestine. When *C. botulinum* grows in necrotic tissues of a living animal and produces toxin then the disease is called toxicoinfectious botulism.

In cattle, most botulism cases occur in South Africa where soil is deficient in phosphorus. The phosphorus-deficient cattle chew bones with accompanying tags of flesh contaminated from type D strains of *C. botulinum*. Approximately one gram of dried flesh from such a carcass may contain enough toxins to kill a mature cow. Such animals also become source of intoxication for other animals. Intoxication of waterfowl occurs around lakes and marshes where there is relatively shallow water with decaying vegetation. Dead invertebrates in such materials may be a major source of toxins for birds that feed in these areas. Occasional outbreaks occur due to drinking of water contaminated by carcass of dead animal. Dead rodents in haystacks or ensilage pits may provide a source of toxin. Chicken manure used as cattle feed or fertilizer, and chicken house litter used as bedding in cattle sheds also act as sources of toxin to cattle.

Toxicity: The incidence of botulism in animals is not known with accuracy, but is relatively low in cattle and horses, more frequent in chickens and high in water-fowls. Dogs, cats and pigs are relatively resistant to all types of botulinum toxin when taken by mouth. Botulinum toxin is the most potent toxicant known so far having LD_{50} of 10 ng/kg body weight in some experimental animals.

Mechanism of action: The botulinum toxin is a potent neurotoxin that inhibits release of acetylcholine and produces functional paralysis. The heavy chain of the toxin targets and attaches the toxin to specific cholinergic axon terminals. The botulinum toxin then enters the pre-synaptic membrane of cholinergic nerve endings via receptor mediated endocytosis. Thereafter, the light chain of the toxin leaves endocytotic vesicles and reaches the cytoplasm. The light chain of the toxin has protease activity, so the toxin proteolytically degrades and inactivates some surface proteins (e.g. synaptobrevin, syntaxin and SNAP) specifically involved in the process of exocytosis. Botulinum toxin thus prevents neuro-secretory vesicles from fusing with the nerve synapse plasma membrane and releasing the neurotransmitters. Failure of exocytosis or degranulation of synaptic vesicles in response to Ca^{++} leads to blockade of acetylcholine release at the neuromuscular junctions. This produces an essentially irreversible cessation of cholinergic transmission and a flaccid paralysis.

Clinical signs: Clinical signs of botulism usually appear 3-17 days after the animal gains access to the toxic material (incubation period decreases with increase in amount of toxin). In peracute cases, animal dies without showing prior signs of illness. In most cases, the disease is subacute. The signs are caused by muscle paralysis and include progressive motor paralysis affecting particularly the limb muscles and muscles of jaw and throat. The animal fails to remain standing for longer period and usually falls or sits with sternal and sometimes lateral recumbency. Reduced intestinal and rumen motility causes constipation, decreased urinary bladder motility produces urine retention, and difficulty in chewing and swallowing leads to dysphagia. Other signs of botulism may include disturbed vision, mydriasis, slow pupillary response to light, and generalised progressive weakness. Death is usually due to respiratory or cardiac paralysis.

In dogs, generalized weakness is followed by an ascending paresis and paralysis, but the poisoned animal remains alert and responsive. In birds, the disease is called limberneck due to paralysis of the neck. In toxicoinfectious botulism in foals (< 4 weeks), there is progressive symmetrical motor paralysis with signs of stilted gait, muscular tremors and inability to stand for longer than 4-5 minutes. As the disease progresses, dyspnoea with extension of head and neck, tachycardia and respiratory arrest occur. Death occurs most often 24-72 hours after the onset of clinical signs.

Post-mortem findings: In all species, the lesions are non-specific. The visceral organs may be congested, and sometime haemorrhages are seen in the central nervous system. The pathological changes may be ascribed to the general paralytic action of the toxin, particularly in the muscles of respiratory system. Aspiration pneumonia may be present. The urinary bladder is often distended with urine and rectum is filled with hard, mucus faeces. In toxicoinfectious botulism, most eminent necropsy findings are pulmonary oedema and congestion with excessive pericardial fluid which contain free-floating strands of fibrin.

Diagnosis: A presumptive diagnosis can be made from clinical signs and lack of significant post-mortem lesions. A positive diagnosis requires demonstration of the toxin in ingesta, serum or liver. The mouse inoculation test is becoming obsolete but may be used in some cases, especially in peracute intoxication. In this test, serum or filtrate of ingesta or liver from suspect animal or bird is injected into 2 sets of mice by I.P. route. One set of mice is protected by simultaneous injection of botulinum antitoxin of the suspected type or types. Positive test is manifested by a 'wasp-wasted' appearance with respiratory distress and progressive paralysis and death within 24 hours in most cases. In toxicoinfectious botulism, the organism may be cultured from tissues of affected animal.

Botulism should be differentiated from diseases and poisonings producing paralysis/paresis and dysphagia like tick paralysis, hypocalcaemia, parturient paresis, rabies, oesophageal or pharyngeal obstruction and leucoencaphalomalacia.

Treatment and management :

a. *Polyvalent antitoxin:* Specific or polyvalent botulinum antitoxin has been used for treatment with varying degree of success, depending upon the type of toxin involved and the species of animal. Treatment of ducks with type C antitoxin is often successful but not economical. Use of polyvalent antitoxin in horses early in course of the syndrome greatly enhances survival rates. Such treatments are less commonly used in cattle.

   Horses: 500 ml for adult and 200 ml for foal.

b. *Antibacterials:* Antibacterial therapy for eradication of causative *C. botulinum* should be started along with polyvalent antitoxin.

Crystalline penicillin G (sodium or potassium)

Dogs: 20,000 units/kg, IM, SC, or slow IV, 4 to 6 times daily.

: 40,000 units/kg, PO on an empty stomach, 4 times daily.

Horses: 25,000 – 50,000 units/kg, IM or IV, 4 times daily.

Ampicillin

Dogs: 10 – 20 mg/kg, PO on an empty stomach, 2 to 3 times daily.

: 5 – 10 mg/kg, IM or SC, 2 to 3 times daily.

Horses: 16 mg/kg, PO, 2 times daily.

: 5 – 10 mg/kg, IM, 1 to 2 times daily.

c. Treatment with guanidine hydrochloride (11 mg/kg body weight) has been reported to overcome some of the paralysis caused by the toxin; however, its use has not been extensive enough to determine the usefulness.

d. Fluid and electrolytes treatment and other supportive measures are advised. Artificial respiration may be a life saving measure.

e. Any dietary deficiency should be corrected and carcass disposed off, if possible. Decaying grass or spoiled silage should be removed from the diet.

f. Supportive care and nursing like provision of warm and dry environment, padding, and assistance in eating and drinking are very helpful.

e. Immunisation of cattle with types C and D toxoids is also successful.

Prognosis: Recovery of animal with thorough treatment and nursing may occur within 2 weeks or longer. Recovery of function occurs in the reverse order of loss of function during the development of syndrome.

2. Tetanus Toxin

Tetanus toxin is a highly potent neurotoxin produced by a gram positive, spore forming bacillus *Clostridium tetani* under anaerobic conditions. The *C. tetani* releases a neurotoxin when bacterial cells undergo autolysis in animal's body. The tetanus toxin causes tetanus, a highly fatal infectious disease, in all mammals.

Properties: *Clostridium tatani* spores are commonly present in faeces of animals, especially those of horses, and in soil contaminated by faeces. In most cases, the organism is introduced into tissues through deep puncture wounds and on getting suitable anaerobic conditions (i.e. necrotic tissue) at the original site of infection, it multiplies and releases a toxin commonly called tetanus toxin or tetanospasmin.

Factors affecting toxicity :

a. Horses and humans are most susceptible to tetanus toxin, while cattle, pigs and sheep are less susceptible. Dogs and cats are fairly resistant but are sometimes affected by tetanus. Birds are relatively resistant to the toxin.

b. Young animals like piglets and lambs are more susceptible to the toxin than adult animals.

c. Anaerobic conditions such as development of tissue necrosis at the site of infection facilitate production of toxin.

d. Tetanus generally occurs in individual animals, although outbreaks have been reported in cattle, young pigs and lambs.

Mechanism of action: Tetanus toxin is a protein containing two polypeptide fragments possessing a protease activity. The toxin is absorbed by the motor nerves and reaches the CNS through peripheral nerve trunks. It selectively binds to gangliosides at the presynaptic inhibitory motor nerve endings in the brain stem or spinal cord and is taken up into the axons by endocytosis. Once inside the inhibitory neurons, it appears to act by selective cleavage of a protein component of synaptic vesicles, the synaptobrevin. Inactivation of synaptobrevin and possibly some other proteins involved in exocytosis prevents release of inhibitory neurotransmitters glycine (mainly) and gamma-amino butyric acid. This causes excessive stimulation of spinal cord leading to spasmodic tonic contractions of skeletal muscles called tetany. The tetany, the predominant sign of tetanus, is characterised by sustained tonic contractions of muscles without twitching. Death occurs as a result of rigidity of the respiratory muscles and associated asphyxia.

Clinical signs: The clinical signs of tetanus are similar in all species, only their intensity varies. After an incubation period of one to several weeks (average 10-14 days), the affected animal displays initial signs of muscular stiffness accompanied by muscular tremors. The reflexes increase in intensity and the animal is easily excited into general spasms by external stimuli like noise, touch, etc. Spasms of head muscles cause difficulty in prehension and mastication of food. In horses, ears become erect, tail is stiff and there is prolapse of third eyelid. The animal assumes a "saw horse stance" due to spasms and stiffness of the neck, back and leg muscles. Animal cannot walk and falls on the ground. Tetanic convulsions begin which occur very frequently and spontaneously. There is profuse sweating and temperature may rise to 108—110°F. Involvement of autonomic nervous system causes cardiac arrhythmia, tachycardia and hypertension. The spasms affecting the larynx, diaphragm and intercostal muscles lead to respiratory failure and death.

Post-mortem findings: There are no specific lesions. Occasional signs of injury and fracture due to excessive struggling by the animal may be present.

Diagnosis: The clinical signs and history of recent trauma are usually adequate for the diagnosis of tetanus. It may be possible to confirm the diagnosis by demonstrating the presence of tetanus toxin in serum.

Differential diagnosis of the disease includes hypomagnesaemia encephalitis, eclampsia and strychnine poisoning.

Treatment and Management: The main purpose of tetanus treatment is to eliminate causative bacteria, to neutralise residual toxin and to relax muscle tetany to avoid asphyxia.

a. *Tetanus antitoxin:* Tetanus antitoxin should be administered, but is of little value once signs have appeared. Horses should receive 300,000 units 12 hourly for three injections. Local injections of the antitoxin around the wound should also be done.

b. Parenteral administration of penicillin in large doses is recommended to eliminate the organism.

c. A combination of chlorpromazine (0.4 mg/kg I.V. or 1.0 mg/kg I.M.) and phenobarbitone sodium may be used to decrease hyperaesthetic reactions and convulsions.

d. Affected animals should be kept as quite as possible in the dark room. Adequate bedding should be provided to avoid injury from convulsions.

e. In enzootic areas, all susceptible animals should be actively immunised with "tetanus toxoid", an alum-precipitated, formalin treated toxin.

f. Short-term prophylactic (for 10-14 days) passive immunity in horses can be achieved by injection of antitoxin at dose rate of 1500-3000 I.U.

Prognosis: The response to treatment is poor, if the animal is already recumbent. Horses and sheep generally respond less to tetanus therapy, while cattle frequently recover.

BIBLIOGRAPHY

Ballantyne B, Marrs T and Turner P (1995) General and Applied Toxicology. Macmillan Press Ltd., London.

Bartik M and Piskac A (1981) Veterinary Toxicology. Elsevier Scientific Publishing Company, Amsterdam.

Beasley V (1999) Veterinary Toxicology. International Veterinary Information Service, Ithaca NY (www.ivis.org).

Bommakanti AS and Waliyar F (2007) Importance of aflatoxins in human and livestock health. (http://www.aflatoxin.info/health.asp).

Booth NH and Mcdonald LE (1982) John's Veterinary Pharmacology and Therapeutics. 5th edn. Kalyani Publishjers, Ludhiana-NewDelhi.

Garg SK (2000) Veterinary Toxicology. CBS Publishers & Distributors, New Delhi.

Hartwig NR and Barnhart SK (2007) Nitrate toxicity. (http://www.iowabeefcenter.org/ content/newsrel/2001/701/nitrate_toxicity.htm)

Kadis S, Ciegler A and Ajl SJ (1972) Microbial Toxins. Academic Press, New York.

Lorgue G, Lechenet J and Riviere A (1996) Clinical Veterinary Toxicology. Blackwell Science Ltd., United Kingdom.

Luxsanakoses S (2007) Mycotoxicosis in animals. FAO Corporate Documentary Repository. (http://www.fao.org/docrep/X5036E/x5036E0b.htm).

Osweiler GD (1996) Toxicology. Williams and Wilkins, Philadelphia.

Pier AC, Richard JL and Cysewsky SJ (1980) Implications of mycotoxins in animal disease. *J. Am. Vet. Med. Assoc.* 176 : 719.

Puschner B (2002) Mycotoxins. *Vet. Clin. North Am: Small Anim Pract.* 32 : 409.

Radeleff RD (1970) Veterinary Toxicology. 2nd edn. Lea and Febiger, Philadelphia.

Raskova H (1971) International Encyclopedia of Pharmacology and Therapeutics. Section 71: Pharmacology and Toxicology of Naturally Occurring Toxins. Vol I and II. Pergamon Press, Oxford.

Rodostits O M, Gay C C, Blood D C and Hinchcliff K W (2000) Veterinary Medicine: A Textbook of the Diseases of Cattle, Sheep, Pigs, Goats and Horses. 9th edn. W. B. Saunders, London.

Shurtleff M (2003) Aflatoxin. In: Encyclopedia of Agrochemicals. Vol 1. Plimmer JR, Gammon DW and Ragsdale NN (Eds.). p 16. John Wiley &Sons, Inc., New Jersey.

Valdes JJ, Cameron JE and Cole RJ (1985) Aflatrem: a tremorgenic mycotoxin with acute neurotoxic effects. *Environ. Hlth. Perspect.* 62 : 459.

World Health Organization (1979) Mycotoxins: Environmental Health Criteria, 11, WHO, Geneva.

Wyllie TD and Morehouse LG (1978) Mycotoxic Fungi, Mycotoxins, Mycotoxicoses: An Encyclopedic Handbook. Vol 2: Mycotoxicoses of Domestic and Laboratory Animals, Poultry and Aquatic Invertebrates and Vertebrates. Marcel Dekker Inc., New York.

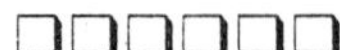

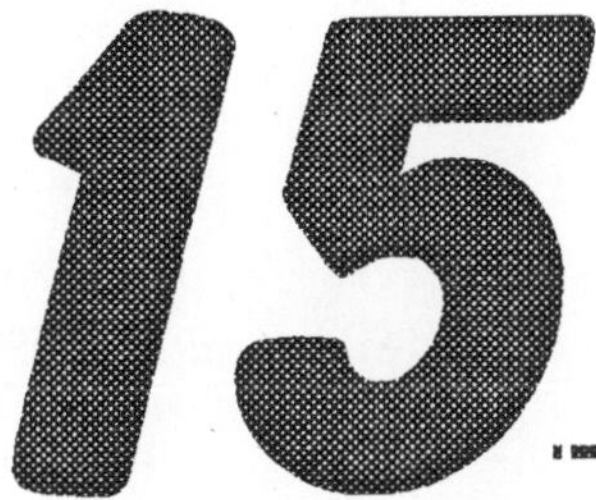

POISONOUS PLANTS

Poisonous plants are among the important causes of economic loss to the livestock industry. Poisonous plants affect animals in many ways viz. death, chronic illness and debilitation, decreased weight gain, abortion, birth defects, increased parturition interval, and photosensitization. Toxic plants are broadly of two types: plants containing toxic ingredients and are known to be toxic to animals and plants which are normally not toxic to animals but become so under unfavourable conditions. Animals are poisoned mostly when hunger or other conditions cause them to graze abnormally or when wrong managemental or/and agricultural practices are adopted in a farm.

1. Plants Containing Cyanide / Cyanogenetic Plants

Hydrogen cyanide or cyanide poisoning in animals occurs generally due to ingestion of certain plants which contain cyanogenetic (cyanogenic) glycosides. The cyanogenetic glycosides are present naturally in nearly 1000 species of plants, which yield hydrogen cyanide (hydrocyanic acid or prussic acid) upon acidic or enzymatic hydrolysis during digestive degradation or when crushed (chewed or chopped). Cyanide is one of the most rapidly acting and deadly toxicants that affect all mammals.

Properties: Hydrogen cyanide (HCN) is a colourless, readily volatile gas having a characteristic odour of bitter almond. A solution of hydrogen cyanide in water is called hydrocyanic acid or prussic acid. Hydrogen cyanide normally is not present as such in plants, but in a non-toxic organic form as cyanogenetic (cyanide producing) glycosides. The cyanogenetic glycosides are formed from nitrate and amino acids as part of normal plant metabolism. These cyanogenetic glycosides are located in epidermal cells (outer tissue) of the plant, while the enzyme β-glycosidase that enables hydrocyanic acid production is located in the mesophyll cells (leaf tissue). Any event that causes the plant cell to rupture allowing the cyanogenetic compound and the enzyme to combine will produce HCN. Plant cells can be ruptured by cutting, wilting, freezing, draught, crushing, trampling, chewing or chopping. Conditions in rumen also favour degradation of the glycoside to free HCN, mainly because the rumen microbes contain enzymes that metabolize cyanogenetic glycosides.

At least 1000 plants are known to contain cyanogenetic glycosides and have ability to release the cyanide, but relatively few of these plants are frequent causes of cyanide poisoning in humans or animals because they are infrequent food sources. Some important plants are sorghum, Sudan grass, Indian grass, corn, acacia, sugar cane leaves or tops, and linseed cake or meal (Table 15.1).

a. Bitter almond and wild cherry contain cyanogenetic glycoside amygdaline that liberates 250 mg of HCN/100 g.

Amygdaline → HCN + gentiobiose + benzaldehyde.

b. Sorghum (whole plant), millet, jwar and Sudan grass contain cyanogenetic glycoside dhurrin that liberates about 250 mg of HCN/100 g.

c. Linseed (Flax), velvet grass and wild clover contain cyanogenetic glycoside linamarin that releases about 10-300 mg of HCN/100 g.

d. Other plants releasing important cyanogenetic glycosides are: choke cherries and service berry leaves release prunasin, and arrow grass release triglochinin.

Other sources of cyanide poisoning: In addition to plants, cyanide poisoning in animals may occur due to careless and indiscriminate use of cyanide containing fumigants and rodenticides (Chapter 13) and drugs (e.g. nitroprusside). Other less common sources of cyanide poisoning are cyanide containing fertilizers (e.g. calcium cyanimide) and laboratory chemicals (e.g. sodium and potassium cyanide). Cyanide is used in various industrial processes such as in metal trades, mining, electroplating, jewellery manufacturing, photographic solutions and X-ray film recovery and could be a rare source of poisoning in animals. A number of synthesized (e.g. polyacrylonitrile, polyurethane, polyamide, urea-formaldehyde, melamine) and natural (e.g. wool, silk) compounds produce HCN when burned. These combustion gases are likely to contribute to the morbidity and mortality of smoke inhalation. Hydrogen cyanide is used as a chemical weapon and is commonly listed amongst chemical warfare agents which cause general poisoning.

Factors affecting toxicity :

a. *Species:* Ruminants are more susceptible to cyanide poisoning than other animals because mildly acidic to alkaline rumen pH (6.5-7.0), high water content, and rumen microfloral enzymes facilitate hydrolysis of cyanogenetic glycosides to HCN. Among ruminants, cattle are more susceptible than sheep.

b. *Plant factors:* Certain factors related to plants affect the levels of cyanogenetic glycosides. These factors include:

i. Plant species: Plant varieties differ in their potential for hydrogen cyanide

Table 15.1: List of selected cyanogenetic plants.

Common name	Botanical name	Common name	Botanical name
Acacia	*Acacia leucophloea*	Lotus	*Lotus sp.*
Almond, bitter	*Prunus amygdalus*	Maize	*Zea mays*
Apricot (seeds)	*Prunus armeniaca*	Peach	*Prunus persica*
Arrow grass	*Triglochin maritime*	Rosewood	*Heterodendrum oleifolium*
Bracken fern	*Pteridium aquilinum*	Star grass	*Cynodon spp.*
Elderberry	*Sambucus canadensis*	Sudan grass	*Sorghum sudanense*
Eucalyptus	*Eucalyptus spp.*	Sugarcane (leaves/tops)	*Saccharum spp.*
Indian grass	*Sorghastrum nutans*	Velvet grass	*Holcus lanatus*
Johnson grass	*Sorghum halepense*	Vetch seed	*Vicia sativa*
Lima bean	*Phaseolus lunatus*	Wild cherry	*Prunus avium*
Linseed or Flax (meal and cake)	*Linum usitatissimum*	White clover	*Trifolium repens*

poisoning. Plants most commonly associated with HCN poisoning are sorghums, sudangrass, Johnson grass and sorghum-sudangrass hybdrids. Grain sorghums are more toxic than forage sorghums or sudangrass.

ii. *Parts of plant:* Leaves contain more HCN than stems and stalks. Further, upper and newer leaves have more HCN than lower leaves. Contents of HCN in other parts of plant are variable with species of plant e.g. fodder plant seeds contain no or low HCN, while almond and flax seeds contain high HCN levels.

iii. *Age of plant:* Young rapidly growing plants contain high concentrations of cyanogenetic glycosides than the mature plants. New shoots and regrowth of plants after cutting often contain the highest levels of cyanogenetic glycosides. Cyanide content usually decreases after pollination.

iv. *Amount of degrading enzyme:* Plants containing high concentration of β-glucosidase enzyme release more of HCN.

c. *Injury to plant:* Wilted, injured or frost bitten plants have a transient increase in glycoside levels and also easily release HCN due to rupture of plant cells. Dead plants have less free prussic acid.

d. *Weather conditions:* Drought-stricken stunted plants contain high concentration of cyanogenetic glycosides because they fail to get mature and contain mostly leaves which are high in HCN. Rapidly growing plants after a period of draught contain dangerously high levels of HCN due to origin of new shoots and leaves. Toxicity is also more likely when periods of rapid growth are followed by cool, cloudy weather.

e. *Method of feeding:* Grazing may be the most dangerous method of feeding susceptible forage because cattle prefer to graze leaves and young shoots which tend to be high in HCN. Feeding the same material as green chop is usually safer than grazing since plant stems help dilute the high HCN content of the leaves.

f. *Time of cutting/grazing:* Cyanogenetic glycosides levels in plants are usually high during morning and low in the afternoon and evening. Therefore, toxicity is more likely when plants are fed / grazed in morning than in the evening.

g. *Use of fertilizers and pesticides:* Heavy use of nitrate fertilizers, especially in phosphorous deficient soils, and foliar herbicides (e.g. 2, 4-D) can increase HCN concentration in plants.

h. *Soil composition:* High soil content of nitrogen and low phosphorus is favourable for high HCN content in plants.

i. *Processing of material:* Drying or making of silage reduces HCN content in plant material. However, if the forage had extremely high concentration of HCN before cutting or if hay is not properly cured, dangerous amount of HCN may remain in the silage. Hay stored for two or more months gradually losses all its cyanide potential due to volatilization of the HCN.

j. *Gastric pH:* Acidic gastric pH decreases release of HCN and hence cyanide toxicity. Although gastric acid facilitates the release of HCN by hydrolysing cyanogenetic glycosides, yet at the same time it destroys the plant enzyme responsible for the release of HCN. Therefore, humans, horses, dogs and pigs that have a highly acidic stomach are less susceptible to HCN poisoning than ruminants.

k. In ruminants, chances of HCN release are more in full stomach as compared to empty stomach due to presence of more enzymes in ingested plants.

l. Rapid ingestion of plants causes rapid release of HCN gas from cyanogenetic glycoside. Therefore, hungry animals are more likely to get poisoned.

m. Water drunk after animals have eaten cyanogenetic plants enhances the hydrolysis of the glycosides and hence chances of poisoning.

n. Travelling stock and recently introduced stock are more likely to get poisoned as they are unaccustomed to local plants. Local animals due to frequent exposure to cyanogenetic plants can tolerate some higher amount of HCN.

Toxicity: Toxicity of cyanide varies with the type of salt, species, speed of ingestion and individual animal tolerance. Numerous forms of cyanide exist, including gaseous hydrogen cyanide (HCN), water-soluble potassium and sodium cyanide salts, and poorly water-soluble mercury, copper, gold, and silver cyanide salts. In addition, a number of cyanide-containing compounds, known as cyanogens, may release cyanide during metabolism. These include cyanogen-chloride and -bromide (gases with potent pulmonary irritant effects), nitriles (R-CN), and sodium nitroprusside, which may produce iatrogenic cyanide poisoning during prolonged or high-dose intravenous therapy. Hydrocyanic acid or its alkaline salts (potassium or sodium) are highly toxic having oral LD_{50} of 0.5 - 3.0 mg/kg in most of the species. In human beings, exposure to 150 ppm HCN for 30-60 min may cause death, while at a concentration of 300 ppm death may occur in few minutes. The plant material containing more than 20 mg of HCN/100 g is considered toxic to animals. Salts of cyanic acid (cyanates) have low while salts of thiocyanic acid (thiocyanates, rhodanide) have very low toxicity. Potassium ferrocyanide and potassium ferricyanide are practically non-toxic.

Toxicokinetics: Hydrogen cyanide is released rapidly from cyanogenetic glycosides when the ingested plant is macerated as in chewing. This mainly occurs due to damage to plant cell structures that allow the enzymes and the cyanogenetic glycosides to come into contact to release HCN. Rumen and intestinal microflora also cause decomposition of glycosides and release HCN. Once released, HCN is rapidly absorbed from GI tract and widely distributed to all organs and tissues of the body. It is also absorbed from lungs after inhalation. The cyanide ions are rapidly metabolised in liver and some other tissues. The principal excretion product is thiocyanate (Figure 15.1), production of which is catalysed by rhodanese, an enzyme widely occurring in most mammalian tissues. Minor metabolic routes of cyanide involve reaction with cysteine to produce a thiazoline and an oxidative pathway leading ultimately to CO_2 and formate. Some HCN is eliminated by exhalation from the lungs, giving a characteristic bitter almond smell to the exhaled air.

Mechanism of action: The toxic effects of cyanide are due to its affinity towards metalloporphyrin containing enzymes, more specifically towards cytochrome oxidase.

a. Cyanide has strong affinity for trivalent iron of the cytochrome oxidase molecule and acts by inhibiting its enzymatic activity and hence the cellular respiration. After gastrointestinal or respiratory exposure, cyanide ion is rapidly absorbed and readily reaches inside the cell. In the mitochondria, the CN^- radical combines with the ferric iron of cytochrome oxidase (cyt) and inhibits the electron transport system. The cytochrome oxidase enzyme is physiologically responsible for the transfer of oxygen and its utilization at cellular levels. Normally, O_2 combines with cyt_{a3}^{++} and oxidises it to cyt_{a3}^{+++}, which is reconverted to cyt_{a3}^{++} for the cycle to

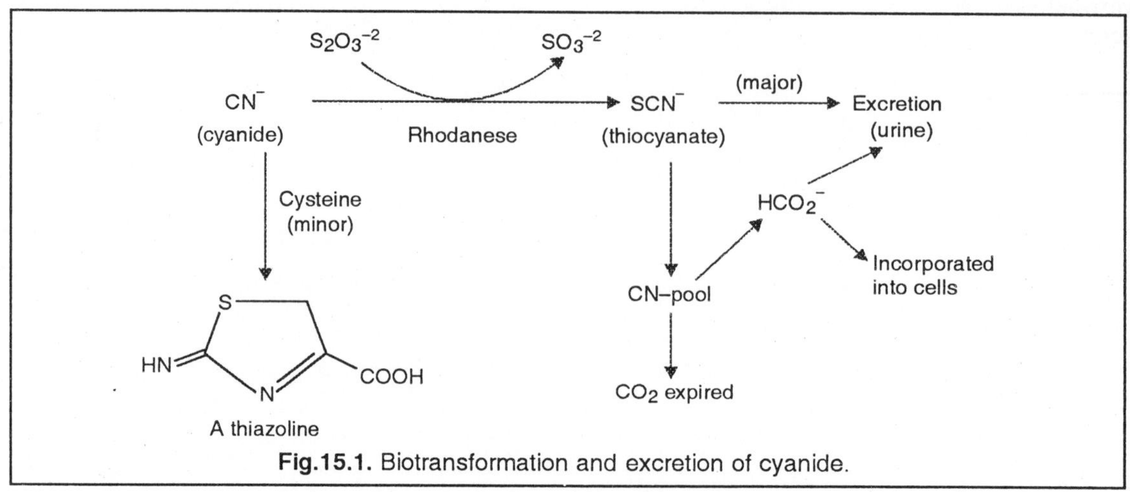

Fig.15.1. Biotransformation and excretion of cyanide.

continue. But when cyanide combines with cyt_{a3}^{+++}, it forms a stable complex called cyan-cytochrome oxidase. This complex does not allow conversion of cyt_{a3}^{+++} to cyt_{a3}^{++} and further combination of O_2 and subsequent re-formation of oxidised cyt_{a3}^{+++}. This results in blockade of electron transport system and hence respiration and cells die due to lack of oxygen. The electron transport chain and cellular respiration are inhibited despite large concentrations of oxygen in the blood stream. All tissues are susceptible but death is primarily from tissue anoxia in the brain. As oxygen of arterial blood cannot be utilised, venous blood retains the bright colour of oxyhaemoglobin.

b. Several other enzymes are alleged to be inhibited by cyanide, but their significance in acute cyanide poisoning is not clear. Cyanide also reacts with methaemoglobin to form cyanmethaemo-globin, but it is not much important.

Clinical signs :

Percute and acute toxicity: Cyanide is very rapidly acting poison, so there is always a peracute or acute toxicity. The clinical course of acute cyanide poisoning depends on the concentration of cyanogenetic glycoside in plant, amount of plant eaten, and rate and duration of consumption. Normally the ruminants are able to metabolise low levels of HCN without ill-effects, but when they consume larger amount of cyanogenetic glycosides in a short time, the high concentration of HCN overwhelms the animal's ability to metabolise and excrete the poison and hence the poisoning occurs.

In peracute cases, animal may be found dead or death may occur only in few minutes. In acute cases, clinical signs may occur within 15-20 min to few hours and include restlessness, laboured and quick breathing, stumbling gait and dyspnoea which develops shortly with tachycardia. Salivation, excessive lachrymation, mydriasis, and voiding of urine and faeces may also occur. Gum, sclera, and mucous membranes are bright red but become cyanotic terminally when tissues become depleted of oxygen. Muscle tremors and fasciculation are common and progress to generalised spasms and clonic convulsions. Regurgitation of rumen contents occurs when ruminants become recumbent and bloating ensues. Death occurs during severe asyphyxial convulsions due to respiratory paralysis. The heart may continue to beat for several minutes after breathing stops. The whole syndrome usually does not exceed 30-45 minutes. Most animals that survive for 2 hour after onset of clinical signs, usually recover.

Chronic toxicity: No chronic toxicity for cyanide has been described. However, some recent literatures have suggested that consumption of cyanide in lower concentrations for long periods may produce a neurotoxic syndrome similar to lathyrism. Low doses of cyanide are also goitrogenic in humans and animals.

Post-mortem findings: In acute or peracute cyanide toxicosis, blood may be bright cherry red initially but may become dark red if necropsy is delayed. Blood may clot slowly or not at all. Mucous membranes are pink initially, then become cyanotic when respiration ceases. The rumen may be distended with gas and the odour of "bitter almond" may be detected after its opening. The GI tract and lungs may have congestion and petechial

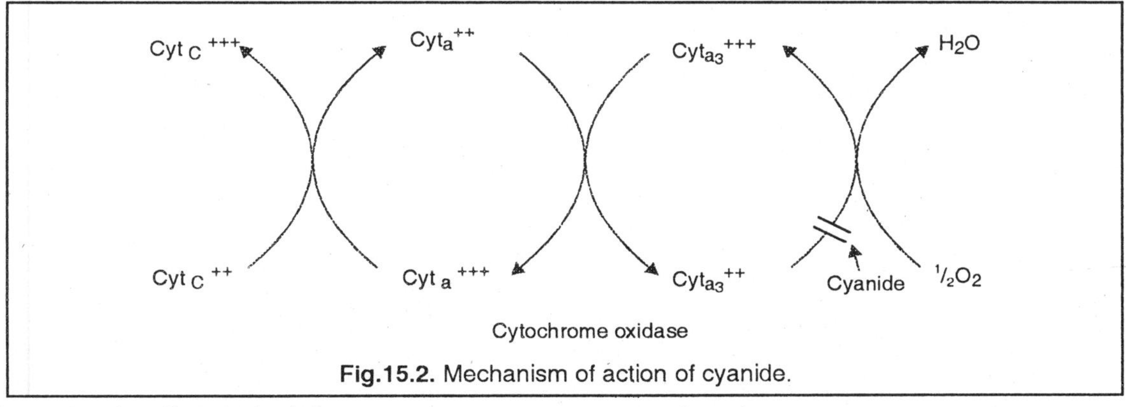

Fig.15.2. Mechanism of action of cyanide.

haemorrhages. There may be agonal haemorrhages on the heart. Some froth may also be detected in respiratory passages.

Diagnosis: The acute onset, bright red mucous membranes and blood, and odour of HCN are indicative of cyanide poisoning. Demonstration of HCN in rumen (stomach) contents or other diagnostic specimens support a diagnosis of cyanide poisoning. Specimens include rumen or stomach contents, heparinized whole blood, liver and muscles. Specimens should be collected as soon as possible after death and are refrigerated or frozen immediately. The samples should be submitted to the laboratory in frozen air-tight container as soon as possible because cyanide is rapidly lost from animal tissues. Plants containing 200 ppm or more of HCN are potentially toxic. Rumen contents and liver showing more than 10 ppm and 1.4 ppm of HCN, respectively, are indicative of cyanide poisoning.

Cyanide intoxication should be differentiated from the following poisonings:

a. *Carbon monoxide:* In CO poisoning, colour of blood is bright red but death is not so acute.

b. *Hydrogen sulphide:* Hydrogen sulphide causes rapid death by inhibition of cytochrome oxidase, but blood and tissues are dark brown in colour and smell of H_2S comes from tissues.

c. *Nitrate and Nitrite:* Nitrate and Nitrite cause rapid death but colour of blood is brown red.

d. *Urea:* Urea causes rapid death but main signs are colic, nervous and behavioural changes. Rumen gives off odour of ammonia.

Treatment and Management: Immediate treatment of cyanide poisoning is necessary to save the animal. The major objective of treatment is to re-establish oxygen transport at the cellular level.

a. *Sodium nitrite:* Sodium nitrite is used as an antidote to cyanide, often in conjunction with sodium thiosulphate. Sodium nitrite converts some haemoglobin (Fe^{++}) to methaemoglobin (Fe^{+++}) by process of oxidation. Methaemoglobin in turn reacts with lethal cyanide ion of cyan-cytochrome oxidase to produce cyan-methaemoglobin (Figure 15.3). This

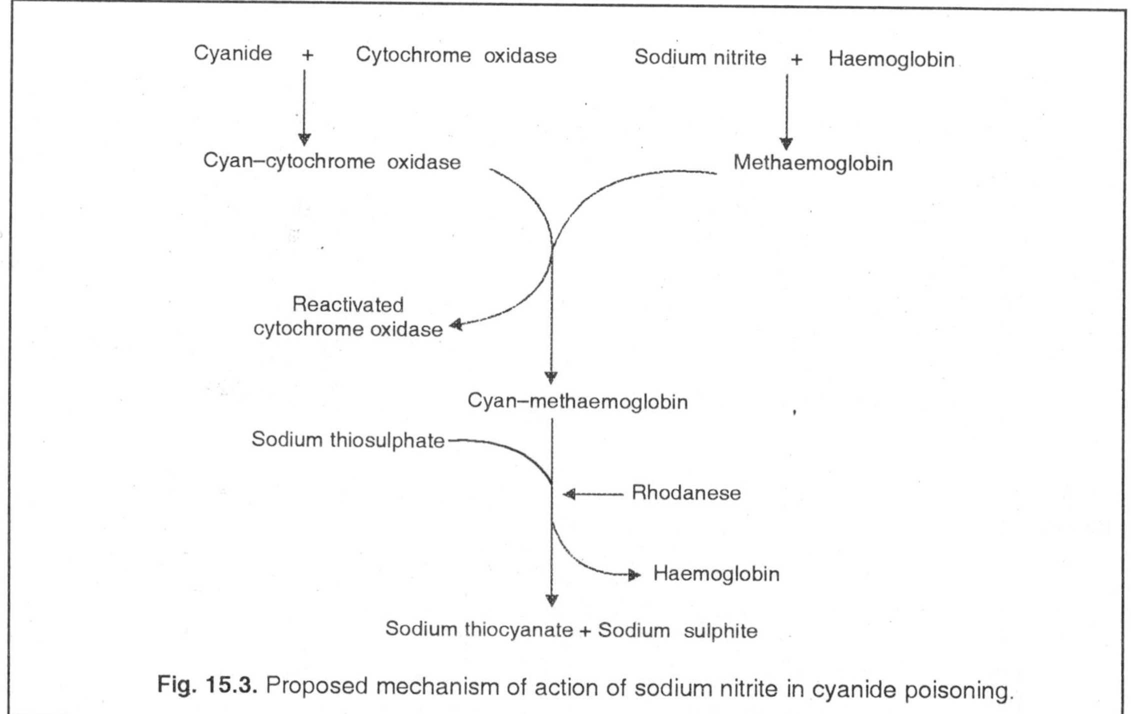

Fig. 15.3. Proposed mechanism of action of sodium nitrite in cyanide poisoning.

process reactivates the inactivated cytochrome oxidase enzyme. The cyan-methaemoglobin in the presence of enzyme rhodanese takes sulphur from the donor sodium thiosulphate (Na_2SO_3) and forms sodium thiocyanate (NaSCN) which is non-toxic and eliminated through urine. Haemoglobin (Fe^{++}) is released during the process. Sodium nitrite is a toxic substance due to its potential to produce methaemoglobinaemia, so its dose should be carefully regulated.

Cattle & sheep: 20 mg/kg, slow IV as 1% solution followed by sodium thiosulphate (500 mg/kg, slow IV as 25% solution).

Dogs & cats: 25 mg/kg, slow IV as 1% solution followed by sodium thiosulphate (1.25 g/kg, IV as 25% solution).

Horses: 16 mg/kg, slow IV as 1% solution followed by sodium thiosulphate (30-40 mg/kg, slow IV as 20% solution).

The sodium thiosulphate may be repeated as needed with little hazard. However, sodium nitrite therapy may be carefully repeated at dose rate of 10 mg/kg, at 2-4 hr or as needed.

b. *Sodium thiosulphate:* Sodium thiosulphate is often administered after systemic administration of sodium nitrite, but alone also is an effective antidote to cyanide poisoning. It may also be used in animals exposed to the poison source but not showing any clinical sign. Sodium thiosulphate hastens detoxification of cyanide by providing an exogenous source of sulphur to the enzyme rhodanese. The cyanide in presence of enzyme rhodanese takes sulphur from the donor thiosulphate and forms sodium thiocyanate, which is relatively non-toxic and is eliminated via the urine.

$$\underset{\text{(Cyanide)}}{CN^-} + \underset{\text{(Thiosulphate)}}{S_2O^{-2}} \xrightarrow{\text{Rhodanese}} \underset{\text{(Thiocyanate)}}{SCN^-} + \underset{\text{(Sulphite)}}{SO_3^{-2}}$$

Cattle & sheep: 500 mg/kg, slow IV as 25% solution plus 30 g/cow or 6 g/sheep, PO (to detoxify HCN in rumen if poisoning occurs through cyanogenetic plant ingestion).

Dogs & cats: 1.25 g/kg, IV as 25% solution.

Horses: 30 – 40 mg/kg, slow IV as 20% solution.

c. *Cobalt preparations:* Some cobalt preparations are reported to improve the clinical condition of intoxicated animals by forming a complex with cyanide in the circulation. Oral administration of 5 per cent solution of cobaltous chloride (10mg/kg) or large dose of hydroxocobalamin (Vitamin B_{12a}) or aquocobalamin (Vitamin B_{12b}) may be used in acute cyanide poisoning, mostly in combination with the primary therapy.

d. Other measures include cooling, diluting and acidifying the rumen contents by giving adult cattle 4 L of vinegar in 12-20 L of cold water to slow microbial hydrolysis of cyanogenetic glycosides.

Prevention: As with nitrate, most problems with HCN can be avoided with proper management of forage and animals. Appropriate steps should be taken to avoid exposing livestock to potentially cyanogenetic plants.

a. Do not graze or feed wilted, frosted or drought stressed plants. Keep livestock off fields for two weeks after a drought ends.
b. Do not graze or feed sorghum during early regrowth after the plants have been cut, when they are likely to be most toxic.
c. Select forage sorghum and other plant varieties that have been specifically developed for low cyanogenetic glycoside contents.
d. Do not graze or feed sorghum until plants are 18 to 24 inches high.
e. Acclimatise cattle to new pasture by grazing/feeding animals on native grass or hay during the day, and then graze sorghums in late after noon and evening.
f. Feed hungry cattle before allowing them to graze forages which may contain high levels of hydrocyanic acid.
g. When grazing, initially allow only a few low value cattle to pasture and observe them closely for two to three hours.
h. Chop or ensile plants high in hydrocyanic acid to reduce HCN level. However, do not feed young plants or regrowth as green

chop. Also do not feed for at least three to four weeks following ensiling.

i. Dry and cure the hay before baling. Well cured hay is rarely hazardous since HCN content declines during the curing process.

j. Thoroughly boil the linseed gruel to remove any free hydrocyanic acid.

k. Follow fertilizer recommendations to assure adequate soil phosphorus. Avoid high levels of soil nitrogen.

l. When in doubt, analyse all feeds and forages for cyanogenetic glycosides before grazing or feeding them to livestock.

Prognosis:. Prognosis of cyanide poisoning depends upon the time of institution of therapy. If the animal survives for a day, no further treatment is required.

2. Plants Producing Lathyrism

Lathyrism is a crippling disease of humans and domestic animals caused by eating legumes of the genus *Lathyrus* (wild pea, common Vetch). Outbreaks of lathyrism have occurred repeatedly throughout history with evidence provided by the Hippocrates (460-377 BC), who wrote about paralysis associated with consumption of peas. The disease is primarily restricted to Indian subcontinent, Ethopia, Russia, and some areas of Europe and North America and is seen mainly in draught conditions when people and animals are forced to eat large amount of *Lathyrus* spp. seeds. Two types of lathyrism are known to occur: osteolathyrism and neurolathyrism.

A. Osteolathyrism

Osteolathyrism is a disease seen in animals consuming various *Lathyrus* species viz. *L. odoratus* (sweet pea) *L. pusillius* and *L. latifolius.* The disease is characterised by skeletal deformities and aortic rupture due to defective synthesis of cartilage and connective tissue. Osteolathyrism is the most common form of lathyrism affecting the animals.

Toxic principles: Although many substances have been tested and found to have osteolathyrogenic activity, the lathyrogenic activity of *Lathyrus odoratus* seems to be restricted to a single substance, β-N-(γ-L glutamyl)-aminopropionitrile (BAPN). The lathyrogen is localized primarily in the pea or seed of the plant and affects the bones and connecting tissues, instead the nervous system. Once ingested, BAPN may be converted *in vivo* to β-aminoproprionitrile, which may also be responsible for the toxic effects. BAPN is heat labile and can be destroyed by cooking.

$$\begin{array}{l} HOOC-CH-CH_2-CH_2-CONH-CH_2-CH_2-CN \\ \quad\quad\;\; | \\ \quad\quad NH_2 \end{array}$$

Fig. 15.4. Chemical structure of β-N-(γ-L-glutamyl)-aminopropionitrile (BAPN).

Mechanism of action: BAPN exerts its toxic effect by inhibiting formation of elastic fibres in the walls of arteries by increased proliferation of fibroblasts and by causing irregularities in the synthesis of collagen fibres. Collagen cross-linking requires an initial oxidative deamination of peptide bound lysine, catalyzed by enzyme lysyl oxidase. The oxidised lysine residues combine with amino acids on adjacent peptide chains forming the insoluble cross-linked collagen. BAPN irreversibly inhibits lysyl oxidase, thus preventing the cross linkages between polypeptide chains in the collagen and elastin, thereby weakening the bones and blood vessels walls.

Clinical signs: Osteolathyrism is a syndrome affecting mainly cattle characterised by lameness of hind legs, exostoses, pain in feet and disinclination to rise. It appears to be caused by a neurological deficit. In experimental animals (rats, mice, chickens), osteolathyrism is characterised by severe connective tissues and skeletal abnormalities.

Treatment and management: Treatment of lathyrism is symptomatic and supportive. If large quantities of the *Lathyrus* seeds have been ingested, emesis or gastric lavage may be performed. Activated charcoal and a saline cathartic may also be useful in recent ingestion of poison.

B. Neurolathyrism

Neurolathyrism is a neurological disease affecting human beings, horses and cattle. This problem is mainly associated with long-term (>3 months) feeding of seeds of *Lathyrus sativus* (also known as *Grass pea* or *Khesari Dal*) and to a lesser degree with *L. cicera*, *L. ochrus* and *L. clymenum.* Neurolathyrism is less reported nowadays, but outbreaks of the disease may occur during famine or draught when people and animals consume large quantities of *Lathyrus sp.* seeds in their diet.

Toxic principles: The cause of neurolathyrism has been attributed to the neurotoxin, β-N-oxalyl-L-α, β-diaminopropionic acid (ODAP) (Synonym: β-oxalylaminoalanine or BOAA), which is a structural analogue of the neurotransmitter glutamate. It is isolated from *L. sativus* and is suspected to produce neurolathyrism in both humans and animals. The toxin can be destroyed by boiling the peas and by allowing them to ferment thoroughly.

Another toxic ingredient, L-α, γ-diaminobutyric acid isolated from *L. clymenum,* produces tremors, convulsions and death in rats.

$$\begin{array}{l} HOOC - \underset{\displaystyle NH_2}{\underset{|}{CH}} - CH_2 - NH - CO - COOH \end{array}$$

Fig. 15.5. Chemical structure of β-N-oxalyl-L-α-β-diamino propionic acid (ODAP).

Toxicity: Different species of domestic animals vary considerably in susceptibility to neurolathyrism. The humans and horses are highly susceptible to the toxicity and are affected most often. A diet of exclusively *L. sativus* seeds may produce signs of neurolathyrism in horses in about 10 days.

Mechanism of action: The mechanism by which ODAP exerts its toxic effect on nervous system has not been fully established. However, there are increasing evidences that ODAP bring neuronal damage to the motor cells of the thoracic and lumbar spinal nerves through its excitatoxic action on the glutamate receptors. Symmetrical axonal degeneration of both crossed and uncrossed pyramidal tracts in the spinal cord is the principal pathological change observed. In addition, the ODAP may cause free radical damage to the brain. A direct neurotoxic action of ODAP has also been suggested.

Clinical signs: The onset of neurolathyrism may be either sudden or gradual with weakness of legs. There is muscular weakness, shifting of weights from one leg to another, stiffness or stilted gait or both, paralysis of legs, paralysis of bladder and rectum muscles and finally paralysis of laryngeal muscles leading to dyspnoea and roaring. Respiratory problems generally lead to death. Horses are more severely affected than cattle.

In humans, important clinical signs include muscular rigidity, weakness, and paralysis of legs that may result in patient actually crawling around his knees. The neuronal damage is mostly permanent.

Post-mortem findings: Post-mortem lesions in the acute stage of neurolathyrism are very rare. In chronic toxicity, there may be complete demyelination of posterior one-half to one-third of the lateral white columns on both sides in the spinal cord.

Treatment and management: There is no specific treatment of neurolathyrism. Symptomatic and supportive care with skeletal muscle relaxants may help.

3. Plants Producing Thiamine Deficiency / Bracken Fern Poisoning

Certain fern plants including *Pteridium aquilinum* (Bracken fern) contain thiaminase enzyme that catalyses thiamine and produces vitamin B_1 deficiency in animals. A similar thiaminase enzyme is also found in some other plants including the horsetail (*Equisetum arvense),* Australian nardoo fern (*Marsilea drummondii*) and rock fern (*Cheilanthes sieberi*). Ingestion of significant quantities of bracken fern produces signs of acute poisoning related to thiamine deficiency in monogastric animals and bone marrow depletion (aplastic anaemia) in ruminants.

Properties: Ferns are pteridophytes and mostly distributed in hilly areas of the world. Types of fern vary according to the altitude, rain fall, soil type and climate of the area. The genus *Pteridium* has probably the widest distribution of any fern genus in the world, being found on all continents and in all environments except for hot and cold deserts. *Pteridium aquilinum* (Bracken or Common Bracken) is the most common species with a cosmopolitan distribution, occurring in temperate and subtropical regions. Bracken fern is primarily a natural plant of dry to wet forest areas, but also occurs in pasture meadows, sandy soils, roadsides, lake-shores, bogs, and burned areas. It has horizontal branching root system with triangular leaves extending up to 2 metres in height. The whole plant (both fresh and dried plants) material is toxic, but the newly emerging fiddleheads and fronds of bracken fern are about five times more toxic than other parts and are more common cause of poisoning. Most acute poisonings are seen after periods of draught when grazing is scarce or when contaminated hay is fed to animals.

Toxic principles:

Bracken fern contains a number of toxic factors, some of which are not yet fully characterised:

a. *Thiaminase:* Thiaminase is a methyl-transferase that produces thiamine (Vitamin B_1) deficiency in non-ruminants.

b. *Aplastic anaemia factor:* Ptaquiloside, a norsesquiterpene glycoside, produces bone marrow suppression and anaemia in cattle and sheep. Ptaquiloside is also a suspected carcinogen

c. *Haematuria factor:* Enzootic haematuria with haemorrhages is associated with this factor.

d. *Quercetin*: Quercetin acts a co-carcinogen.

Toxicity: All parts of the *Pteridium aquilinum* plant including the fronds and rhizomes (most toxic) are toxic. The toxic effects appear to be cumulative and require 1-3 months to develop depending on the species of animal, quantity of plant consumed, time of year and other factors. Horses and cattle are primarily affected by bracken fern, although the syndromes in two species differ. In horses, it produces mainly neurological signs but no anaemia is seen. In cattle, bracken causes bone marrow depression leading to aplastic anaemia. Urinary bladder neoplasms are also reported in cattle consuming bracken fern for long period of time.

Mechanism of action :

a. Toxicity of *Pteridium aquilinum* (Bracken fern) and *Equisetum arvense* (Horsetail) in non-ruminants has been ascribed to the presence of thiaminase in the fern which splits thiamine into two inactive components thiazole and pyrimidine (Figure 15.6) in the alimentary tract and results in deficiency of vitamin B_1 (thiamine). Thiamine is essentially required for conversion of pyruvate to acetyl-coenzyme A and oxidation of α-ketoglutarate to succinyl coenzyme A in the citric acid cycle. Deficiency of thiamine thus results in impaired pyruvate utilization as a result of which blood pyruvate levels rise and animal suffers from abnormal energy metabolism due to inadequate ATP production. Decreased energy production affects primarily the central nervous system with neuronal dysfunction and damage often characterized by CNS depression and polioencephalomalacia.

Thiamine deficiency is generally not a problem in ruminants since the vitamin is synthesized in the rumen. However, polioencephalomalacia associated with impaired thiamine metabolism occurs in

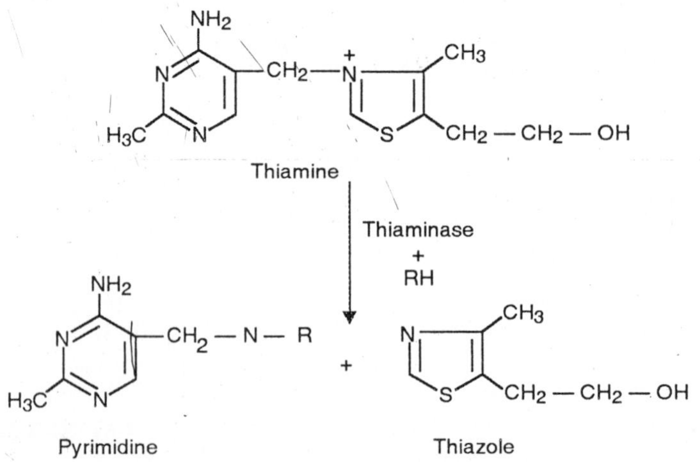

Thiamine

Thiaminase + RH

Pyrimidine + Thiazole

Fig. 15.6. Proposed mechanism of action of thiaminase containing bracken fern. RH = Nucleophilic agent like aromatic amines, heterocyclic amines or sulphur containing amino acids.

sheep. Horses and pigs are most susceptible to the effects of thiaminase.

b. The toxicity of bracken fern in ruminants is ascribed mainly to presence of the aplastic anaemia factor ptaquiloside. The aplastic anaemia factor causes death of precursor cells in the marrow and affects production of newer blood cells. The toxic effect is first seen on cells with shorter life span. There is granulocytopenia and thrombocytopenia with resultant susceptibility to infections and tendencies for spontaneous haemorrhages.

Cattle appear to be most susceptible to the effects of ptaquiloside; sheep are minimally affected and horses are resistant.

c. Long-term consumption of bracken fern leads to development of tumours in the urinary bladder and possibly parts of the digestive tract. Cattle are most susceptible to the carcinogenic effects of bracken fern because they have alkaline urine and under these alkaline conditions the ptaquiloside is converted to the active carcinogen dienone that alkylates DNA leading to tumour formation. Formation of small polyp-like tumours in the bladder often leads to multiple bleeding tumour masses (haemangiomas) that causes formation of red urine (enzootic haematuria and red water disease).

d. In cattle, the compound quercetin acts as a co-carcinogen with papilloma virus to produce malignant tumours in the mouth, oesophagus and rumen. A variety of different tumours in human beings have been associated with carcinogens in bracken fern.

Clinical signs :

Non-ruminants: In horses, clinical signs of bracken-induced thiamine deficiency (bracken staggers) generally occur after consumption of fern for 1-2 months. Important signs include emaciation, lethargy, anorexia, weight loss, incoordination and staggering gait. Animal stands with feet well spread and back arched. There is recumbency followed by muscular tremors, cardiac irregularity, clonic spasms and opisthotonos. Horses may also show colic, haemoglobinuria, severe anaemia, hyperthermia and tachycardia. Haemolytic crisis may occur rarely. If the animal remains untreated, death may occur in 2-10 days or in some cases up to 30 days.

In pigs, signs of thiamine deficiency are less distinct and resemble heart failure. Affected animals show anorexia, depressed growth rate and weight loss. Death may occur suddenly following terminal recumbency and dyspnoea.

Ruminants: Bracken fern poisoning in ruminants may be seen in various forms depending on the quantity and duration of exposure to the plant.

In acute or subacute bracken poisoning, cattle develop severe bone marrow depression that results in thrombocytopenia, anaemia, leucopenia and prolonged clotting time. There is often bleeding from body orifices such as urogenital tract, nostrils, mouth and intestinal tract. The anterior chamber of the eyes may be filled with blood (hyphema). Affected animals are weak, anorexic, pyrexic (106-110°F) and have pale mucous membrane with petechiae and clots of blood in the faeces. Secondary bacterial infections often result from the depressed bone marrow and decreased circulating neutrophils. The disease is mostly fatal with death occurring at 7-8 weeks after first access to the fern. In calves, the poisoning often takes a laryngic form with depression and excessive mucous discharge from mouth and nostrils. Oedema of throat region may occur with difficult breathing. No gross or internal bleeding may be seen. In sheep, haemorrhagic syndrome is similar to cattle.

Consumption of bracken fern for longer time results in chronic enzootic haematuria in cattle characterised by intermittent haematuria and ultimate death due to anaemia. Cattle with enzootic anaemia are often first noticed when voiding red-coloured urine, which over time leads to severe blood loss and anaemia. A variety of tumour types including haemangioma, haemangiosarcomas, papillomas, fibromas, adenomas and transitional cell carcinomas have been associated with bracken fern carcinogenicity. In sheep, a bright blindness may occur due to progressive retinal atrophy that is characterised by permanent blindness. The pupils respond poorly to light and the sheep adopt a characteristic alert attitude. The blindness in sheep is permanent.

Post-mortem findings: In horses, no specific lesions are seen. Acute bracken poisoning in cattle shows multiple haemorrhages throughout the carcass. Necrotic ulcers may be present in the GI tract. In chronic enzootic haematuria in cattle, the bladder contains small haemorrhages, dilated vessels or tumours, which can be vascular, fibrous, or epithelial. In many cases, a mixture of lesions is found.

Diagnosis: Diagnosis of bracken fern poisoning is made from history, clinical signs and lesions. Blood thiamine level in non-ruminants decreases to 2.5 μg/dl from an average normal of 8.5 μg/dl, while blood pyruvate level increases to 8.5 mg/dl from a normal of 2.0 mg/dl.

Differential diagnosis of bracken fern poisoning in non-ruminants can be made from other plants which induce thiamine deficiency like horse tail (*Equisetum arvense*) and turnip (*Beta vulgaris*). In cattle, acute haemorrhagic syndrome should be differentiated from acute septicaemias including anthrax and mycotoxins or sweet clover poisoning. Chronic enzootic haematuria should be distinguished from haemoglobinaemia of babesio' is.

Treatment and management :

Non-ruminants: In non-ruminants, treatment of thiamine deficiency is highly effective, if diagnosis is made early. Thiamine (0.1% solution) is given at dose rate of 5 mg/kg body weight, initially I.V. at 3 hr interval followed by I.M. route for several days. Oral supplementation may be required for an additional 1-2 weeks, although S.C. injection of 100-200 mg daily for 6 days is also successful.

Cattle: No specific antidote is available for the bone marrow suppression and aplastic anaemia.

a. DL-Batyl alcohol is given 1 g in 10 ml olive oil for 5 days by S.C. route. However, it has limited value.

b. Antibiotics should be given to check secondary infections.

c. Blood or platelet transfusions from a healthy donor may be appropriate.

d. Animals should be removed from contaminated areas and provided high-quality diets to aid convalescence.

e. The other syndromes are essentially untreatable and must be controlled by denying access to the fern.

Prevention:

a. Keep animals out of bracken fern-infested pastures, especially during dry periods.

b. Eliminate all bracken fern from pastures and hayfields.

c. Do not use hay from bracken infested meadows for feeding or bedding.

d. Reduce the size of large infestations of bracken fern by pulling or mowing the fronds at least twice a year (in June and August) or by limiting infested areas.

Prognosis: Prognosis in advanced stages of bracken poisoning is poor.

Public health concern: Some epidemiological evidences suggest that regular consumption of untreated milk from cattle with access to bracken fern may be associated with an increased risk of human oesophageal or gastric cancer, but is still under investigation.

4. Plants Producing Oxalate Poisoning

Oxalate poisoning of livestock, household pets and people is of great importance throughout world. Oxalate poisoning in animals from pure substances is rare, but it usually occurs after ingestion of oxalate containing plants. As these plants are palatable, they may sometimes form a large part of a ruminant's diet. The principal oxalate containing plants belong to genera Halogeton (*H. glomeratus*), Sarcobatus (*S. vermiculatus* or grease wood), Oxalis (*O. pescaprae* or soursob), Rheum (*R. rhaponticum* or rhubarb) and Beta (*B. vulgaris* or sugar beat). Of various plants, *Halogeton glomeratus* and *Oxalis pescaprae* are two important oxalate producing plants of the world. Certain grasses and fungi also accumulate harmful amounts of oxalates (Table 15.2) and contribute to the occurrence of poisoning.

Properties: Oxalates occur in plants primarily as salts of calcium, sodium, ammonium, potassium and magnesium. The calcium and magnesium oxalates are insoluble, so less absorbed from the GI tract. The sodium and potassium oxalates (more common in plants), being soluble, are free to be absorbed or to react with the calcium in the GI tract to form insoluble salts. *Halogeton glomeratus* contains oxalic acid (HOOC-COOH) as soluble sodium and potassium oxalates, while *Oxalis pescaprae* contains oxalic acid as acid-potassium oxalate. Therefore in *Halogeton* sp., only acute intoxication has been described, while with *Oxalis*

Table 15.2: List of selected plants containing oxalates.

Common name	Botanical name	Common name	Botanical name
Bassia	*Bassia hyssopifolia*	Oak	*Quercus* spp.
Buffel grass	*Cenchrus ciliaris*	Philodendron	*Philodendron* sp.
Calla lily	*Zantedeshia aethiopica*	Pigweed	*Amaranthus* spp.
Dieffenbachia	*Dieffenbachia* sp.	Pulslane	*Portulaca oleraceae*
Elephant grass	*Panicum* sp.	Rhubarb	*Rheum rhaponticum*
Grease wood	*Sarcobatus vermiculatus*	Russian thistle	*Salsola* spp.
Halogeton	*Halogeton glomeratus*	Sorrel	*Rumex crispus*
Kochia	*Kochia scoparia*	Soursob	*Oxalis pescaprae*
Kikuyu grass	*Pennisetum clandestinum*	Sugar beet	*Beta vulgaris*

pescaprae all forms of toxicity i.e. chronic, subacute and acute have been described. Halogeton contains about 34% soluble oxalates on dry matter basis and *Sarcobatus* (greasewood) contains 10 to 20% oxalates. In *H. glomeratus*, about 30% oxalate is present in leaves, 10% in seeds and 3% in stems. Halogeton is dangerous at all times, but it becomes more toxic as the growing season advances, reaching a peak of toxicity at maturity. *Aspergillus*, an oxalate-producing fungus, may elevate oxalate content to toxic level in some mouldy feeds.

Toxicity: Toxicity of oxalate producing plants depends largely on species of animal, type of plant, form of oxalate present in plant, and duration of exposure. Ruminants, especially cattle, can consume large quantities of oxalate-containing plants without apparent ill-effects because these animals are more effective in producing insoluble calcium oxalate from free oxalate than the simple stomach animals. Toxicity in ruminants mostly occurs when large quantities of soluble potassium and sodium oxalates are eaten that overwhelms the rumen's ability to metabolize the oxalates. In general, oxalate poisoning is commonest in sheep and also occurs in cattle and horses. Up to 450 g of sodium oxalate given orally produces fatal effects in horses, whereas cattle and buffalo can tolerate as much as 685 g of oxalic acid without harmful effects. Death in sheep can occur on pasture containing as little as 2% soluble oxalate. Gradual low feeding of halogeton plants usually show less toxic response than abrupt high feeding because in former case, rumen bacteria get time to become conditioned to degrade oxalates. Pregnant and lactating animals are more susceptible than others.

Toxicokinetics: When oxalate is consumed by a ruminant, it may undergo different pathways: it may be degraded by rumen bacteria to form non-toxic metabolites, it may be combined with calcium or magnesium in rumen to form insoluble salt that is excreted in faeces and/or it may be absorbed from rumen into blood stream. Once absorbed from the GI tract, soluble oxalates readily combine with blood calcium and magnesium to produce hypocalcaemia and hypomagnesaemia, respectively. Soluble oxalate also interferes with various body processes. The insoluble oxalate salts may accumulate in various tissues, especially the rumen wall and kidneys. Oxalates are metabolized to formate and then to CO_2 and excreted from the body. Oxalates are also detoxified in the rumen and get converted to carbonate and bicarbonate, which in excess can produce severe alkalosis.

Mechanism of action: Once the soluble oxalate ($C_2O_4^-$) has been absorbed into the body, it may produce toxicity by number of ways:

a. Oxalate forms a complex with serum calcium to form calcium oxalate. This depletes ionized calcium and causes hypocalcaemia resulting in impairment of normal cellular functions.

   i. Hypocalcaemia interferes with electrical activity of the heart, muscles, and nerves. This leads to muscular weakness, CNS depression and cardiovascular collapse leading to death.

   ii. Hypocalcaemia impairs the blood clotting mechanism and causes enhanced bleeding.

   iii. Hypocalcaemia upsets calcium metabolism in the body and interferes with milk production and bone growth in lactating and pregnant animals.

iv. Hypocalcaemia impairs normal cell membrane functions.

b. Oxalate interferes with the cellular energy metabolism that contributes to acute death of affected animals.

c. Insoluble oxalate crystals accumulate in various organs and produce direct organ damage.

i. Deposition of insoluble calcium oxalate crystals in the renal tubules causes severe renal tubular necrosis called oxalate nephrosis. If the poisoned animal does not die from the acute effects of hypocalcaemia and impaired cellular energy metabolism, death results from kidney failure.

ii. In some cases, oxalates get crystallize in brain tissues and cause symptoms of paralysis and other CNS disorders.

iii. Accumulation of large quantities of oxalate crystals in rumen epithelial lining causes haemorrhages in the ruminal wall.

iv. Crystallization and deposition of insoluble salts in the blood vessels cause damage to vessels.

d. Continued low-level dosing of oxalate in sheep may cause ruminal dysfunctions due to changes in pH of its content and interference with cellulose digestion. Oxalates are readily detoxified in the rumen and get converted to carbonate and bicarbonate, which in excess can produce severe alkalosis.

e. Oxalic acid is corrosive and its direct contact may cause skin and gastrointestinal irritation.

Clinical signs: Onset of clinical signs in sheep and cattle is noted within 2-6 hours of ingestion of oxalate containing plants. Early clinical signs include dullness, reluctance to move, slobbering, lowering of head, loss of appetite, stasis of rumen motility and bloat. In acute poisoning, there is salivation, progressive weakness, incoordination, prostration, laboured respiration, dilatation of pupil, twitching of muscles, tetany, convulsions and coma. Death mainly occurs due to shock within 9-12 hours of the onset of clinical signs. These signs are mainly due to oxalate induced hypocalcaemia. Azotemia, oliguria, hyperkalaemia and cardiac failure may occur due to renal tubular necrosis. In swine, there is diarrhoea and animal may bleed to death from severe GI haemorrhages.

In subacute poisoning, there is stiff gait, frequent attempts to urinate and recumbency. Urine may be red-brown in colour. Chronic poisoning primarily results from renal damage resulting in uraemia (increased serum creatinine and urea nitrogen levels). As animals become uraemic, they develop severe depression, stop eating and after a few days become comatose and die. Albuminuria and sometimes haematuria may be observed.

Post-mortem findings: Lesions of oxalate poisoning include oedema and haemorrhages of the rumen wall in ruminants and gastrointestinal haemorrhages in swine. In acute poisoning, the kidneys may be oedematous and dark in colour, whereas in chronic poisoning the kidneys may be pale and smaller in size. On examination of the cut surface of kidneys, oxalate crystals can be seen in the renal tubules. Calculi may be found in urethral process of ram and sigmoid flexure of bull and ram. Lungs may be filled with blood and are of dark red or purplish colour. Various tissues may show cyanosis. Microscopic studies show urinary tubules virtually filled with crystals of calcium oxalate, many of the tubules may be found ruptured and some may show degenerative changes.

Diagnosis: Diagnosis of oxalate poisoning should be based on history of feeding oxalate containing plants, clinical signs (hypocalcaemic syndrome) and lesions. Demonstration of calcium oxalate crystals in the kidneys and rumen epithelium histologically is diagnostic of oxalate poisoning. Suspected plants should be analysed for oxalate content. Packed cell volume decreases but BUN and blood potassium level may increase.

Treatment and management: There is no specific treatment for oxalate poisoning. Only supportive therapy is advised for treating nephrosis.

a. Calcium salts: Administration of calcium for correcting hypocalcaemia may be helpful, but not always effective in reversing the toxic effects of oxalate. This is mainly because irreversible oxalate nephrosis and impaired cellular energy metabolism are more detrimental to the animal than hypocalcaemia. In early stages, calcium borogluconate (300-500 ml as 25% solution by I.V. or S.C. in cattle) has been found beneficial. Treatment of hypocalcaemia with calcium salts and prevention of toxicosis by feeding calcium containing mineral supplements such as dicalcium phosphate may not be successful.

b. Excessive and forceful administration of water has some success in flushing out the oxalate from the system. However, it may not be practicable under field conditions.

c. Administration of lime water ($Ca[OH]_2$) orally may help to prevent further absorption of soluble oxalate.

Prognosis: Prognosis is poor, if advanced signs of oxalate intoxication have occurred.

5. Plants Producing Photosensitization

Photosensitization is a syndrome of abnormal sensitivity of the lightly pigmented areas of skin to sunlight due to presence of photodynamic agent(s) in the peripheral circulation and skin. Photosensitization, a form of severe dermatitis, occurs in many countries of the world and at one time or another in all species of farm animals and human beings mainly due to ingestion of certain plants, fungi or drugs. Among farm animals, it is most common in cattle and sheep.

Types of photosensitization: Photosensitization produced by plants and some other exogenous substances is of two major types: primary photosensitization and secondary photosensitization.

a. Primary photosensitization: Primary photosensitization occurs when a photodynamic agent is directly ingested or when an agent is biotransformed to a photodynamic metabolite which reaches the skin and reacts with UV light to cause photosensitization. The photodynamic substances producing primary photosensitization include hypericin (from *Hypericum* spp.) and fagopyrin (from *Fagopyrum* spp.) present in plants, and phenothiazine, sulphonamides, tetracyclines and acridine dyes used as drugs.

b. Secondary photosensitization: Secondary or hepatogenous photosensitization occurs due to ingestion of some substances that give rise to liver dysfunctions and/or obstruction of the bile duct. These hepatotoxins themselves have no photodynamic activity but damage to liver by them causes plant pigments normally eliminated in bile to reach peripheral circulation and give rise to the photosensitization. Secondary photosensitization is caused by several plants (e.g. *Senecio* spp. and *Lantana camara),* mycotoxins (e.g. sporidesmin) and drugs (e.g. carbon tetrachloride and phenanthridium).

Plants producing photosensitization:

a. Primary photosensitization: A large numbers of plants containing polyphenolic pigments are capable of producing primary photosensitization in animals. The photodynamic pigments are present at highest concentration in the green plant and are readily absorbed from GI tract to circulate in the peripheral blood. In the non-pigmented skin they react with UV light to produce dermatitis and photosensitization. Two important plants associated with primary photosensitization are *Hypericum perforatum* (Saint John's wort) that contains photodynamic substance hypericin, and *Fagopyrum esculentum* (buckweed) that contains fagopyrin. Other plants capable of producing primary photosensitization include plants in the families of Umbelliferae and Rataceae that contain photoactive furocoumarins (psoraleus) and cause photosensitization in livestock and poultry. *Ammi majus* (Bishop's weed) and *Cymopterus watsonii* (spring parsley) have produced photosensitization in cattle and sheep, respectively. Species of *Trifolium, Medicago* (clovers and alfalpha), *Erosium* and *Brassica* have been suspected to cause primary photosensitization, but the phototoxins have not been fully identified.

b. Secondary (Hepatogenous) photosensitization: The secondary or hepatogenous photosensitization is by far the most frequent type of photosensitization in livestock and is caused by the photosensitizing agent "phylloerythrin", a bacterial breakdown product of chlorophyll. Normally phylloerythrin is removed by liver and is excreted in bile, but if the liver is severely damaged or if the bile duct is occluded, the pylloerythrin accumulates in the peripheral blood to cause photosensitization. Several plants are capable of producing secondary photosensitization (Table 15.3). These include pyrrolizidine alkaloids containing plants blue-green algae (*Microcystis* spp.), horse brush (*Tetradymia glabrata*) and Lantana (*Lantana camara*). Some mould toxins which are icterogenic (e.g. sporidesmin) also produce secondary photosensitization.

i. Plants causing liver damage: A variety of plants, especially those containing pyrrolizidine alkaloids (e.g. *Senecio* spp., *Crotolaria* spp., and *Heliotropium* spp.) can cause liver damage and produce secondary photosensitization. So far, more than 100 pyrrolizidine alkaloids have been isolated from various plants and their levels range from traces to 5% of dry weight of the plant. After ingestion of such plants, the pyrrolizidine alkaloids are readily absorbed from GI tract and are bioactivated to toxic pyrroles and possibly other reactive metabolites by the liver mono-oxygenases system. The active pyrroles presumably alkylate macromolecules in the hepatocytes, principally DNA, and impair cell division. The cells continue to grow although unable to divide resulting in hepatomegaly and karyomegaly and eventually in cell death. With the death of large number of hepatocytes, the necrosis triggers a regenerative response accompanied by bile duct proliferation. Therefore at high doses pyrrolizidine alkaloids cause hepatocellular necrosis, while at lower doses necrosis is less severe allowing time for the pathological changes of megalocytosis, bile duct hyperplasia and fibrosis to occur. Pigs are most susceptible to pyrrolizidine alkaloid poisoning followed by poultry, cattle, horses, goats and sheep. Some pyrrolizidine alkaloids in addition to being hepatotoxic are potent carcinogen, mutagen, teratogen and abortifacient.

ii. Plants causing biliary occlusion: Some plants produce secondary photosensitization by causing obstruction of the biliary system rather than the liver disease. Although the principle toxin(s) responsible for photosensitization from many plants have not been identified,

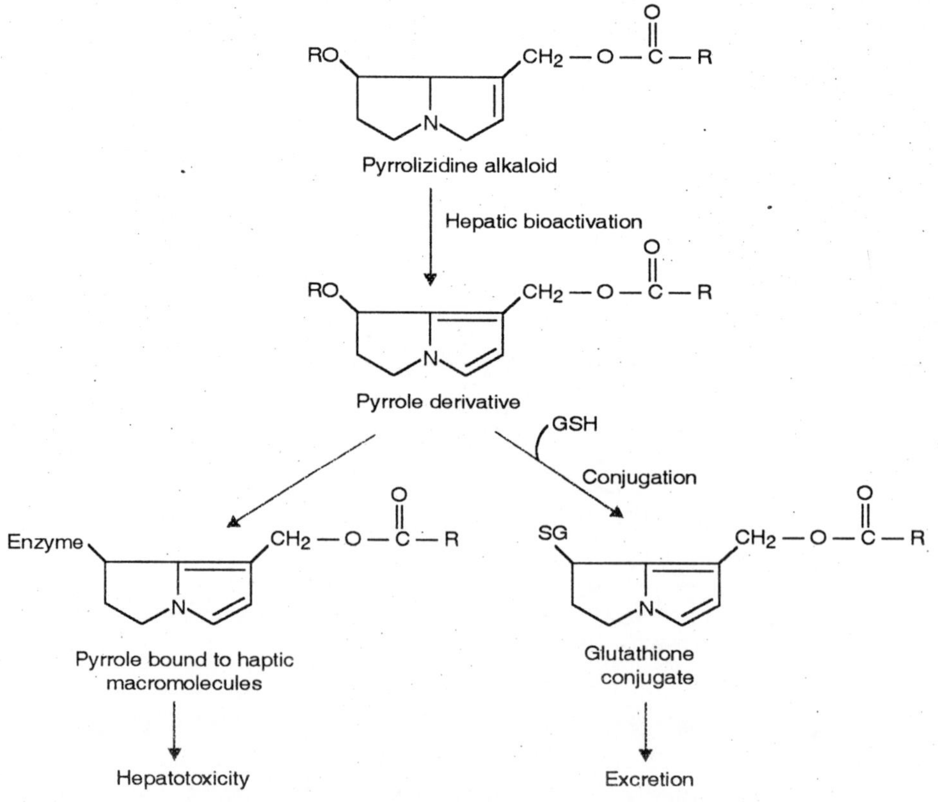

RO — CH_2—O—C(=O)—R
Pyrrolizidine alkaloid
Hepatic bioactivation
RO — CH_2—O—C(=O)—R
Pyrrole derivative
GSH
Conjugation
Enzyme — CH_2—O—C(=O)—R
SG — CH_2—O—C(=O)—R
Pyrrole bound to haptic macromolecules
Glutathione conjugate
Hepatotoxicity
Excretion

Fig. 15.7. Proposed hepatotoxic action of pyrrolizidine alkaloids.

saponins present in some plants have been suggested to cause inflammation and obstruction of the biliary duct. When bile cannot be excreted normally by the liver, the phylloerythrin and other photodynamic compounds accumulate in the animal's bloodstream and result in photosensitization (See for detail Sporidesmin, Chapter 14). Plants producing photosensitization through biliary obstruction include puncture vine (*Tribulus terrestris*) and Kleingrass (*Panicum colaratum*). Agave poisoning (*Agave lecheguilla*) is induced by plant saponins that forms crystals in the bile duct and occlude the biliary system. *Lantana camara,* an ornamental plant, causes photosensitization due to presence of two polycyclic triterpenes - Lantadene A and Lantadene B, which cause damage to liver and bile ducts. Among various varieties of *Lantana camara*, the red flowered variety is considerably toxic. Animals generally eat this plant in drought conditions. Sheep is most susceptible species; however, cattle, goats and camels are also susceptible to Lantana toxicity.

Mechanism of action: Three factors contribute to the development of photosensitization: presence of a photoactivating (photodynamic) substance in skin, exposure to UV light and lack of skin pigment which enables more light to penetrate the skin. It is suggested that when the molecules of a photodynamic substance comes into the peripheral circulation (irrespective of cause, primary or secondary), they are energized by certain wavelengths of ultraviolet light thereby causing the molecules to attain a high-energy state. When the molecules of the photodynamic agent return to less energized state, they release energy which is transferred to receptor molecules to initiate chemical reaction in the skin. Tissue injury results probably from the production of reactive oxygen intermediates, which causes cellular membrane damage and alters cell membrane permeability. Tissue destruction causes release of histamine from mast cells that initiates local inflammatory reactions i.e. erythema, oedema, vesicles and bullae, intense pruritus, and eventual necrosis. Damage to epidermal cell nucleic acid by activated photodynamic molecules and oxidation of essential amino acids in the skin's cells may contribute to cellular dysfunction and tissue destruction. The cells die in the photosensitization process and the affected skin eventually sloughs off.

Clinical signs: The photosensitization syndrome has similar clinical signs regardless of the cause. Photosensitive animals are photophobic when exposed to sunlight. Animal feels discomfort and scratches or rubs lightly pigmented exposed areas of skin. Frequently the skin around ears, eyelids, muzzle and coronary band of hooves is most severely affected because in these areas skin is heavily vascularised and poorly protected by hair or wool. White skin on the face, back, udder and legs of animals are equally prone to photosensitization. Affected skin rapidly becomes reddened, painful and oedematous. If exposure to light ceases at this stage, the lesions soon resolve; if exposure is prolonged, there is marked serum

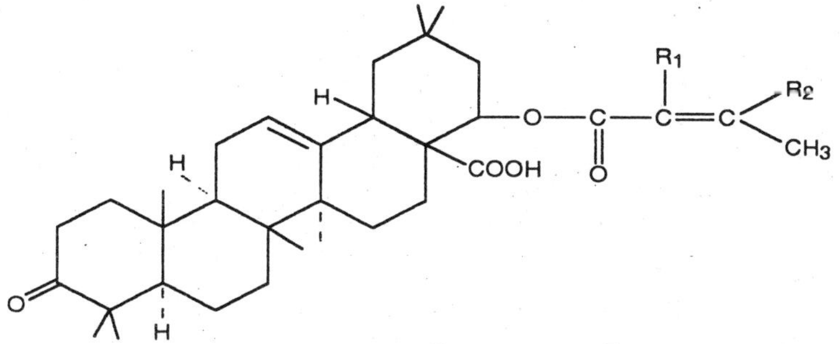

	R_1	R_2
Lantana A :	$-CH_3$	$-H$
Lantana B :	$-H$	$-CH_3$

Fig. 15.8. Chemical structures of lantadenes.

Table 15.3: List of selected photosensitizing plants.

Common name	Botanical name	Common name	Botanical name
		Primary Photosensitization	
Alfalfa	*Medicago sativa*	Parthenium	*Parthenium hysterophorus*
Bishop's weed	*Ammi majus*	Rain lily	*Cooperia pedunculata*
Buckwheat	*Fagopyrum esculentum*	Rape, kale	*Brassica* spp.
Clovers	*Trifolium* spp.	Spring parsley	*Cymopterus watsonii*
Giant hog weed	*Heracleum mentegazzianum*	St. John's wort	*Hypericum perforatum*
Dutchman's britches	*Thamnosma texana*	Knottweed	*Polygonum fagopyrum*
Perennial rye grass	*Lolium perenne*		
		Secondary Photosensitization	
Agave	*Agave lecheguilla*	Horsebrush	*Tetradymia glabrata*
Blue-green algae	*Microcystis* spp.	Kochia	*Kochia scoparia*
Blue weed	*Echium vulgare*	Kleingrass	*Panicum colaratum*
Bog asphodel	*Narthecium ossifragum*	Lantana	*Lantana camara*
Fiddle neck	*Amsinckia* spp.	Puncture vine, caltrope	*Tribulus terrestris*
Giant hog weed	*Heracleum* spp.	Ragwort, groundsel	*Senecio* spp.
Heliotrope	*Heliotropium spp.*	Rattle box	*Crotolaria* spp.

exudation, scab formation and skin necrosis. After 2-3 weeks, the necrotic skin becomes dry and parchment-like, and the hair and skin slough leaving ulcerated areas that may develop secondary bacterial infections. In cattle, exposure of the tongue while licking may result in glossitis with ulceration and deep necrosis. Lameness is common in horses, which develop photosensitization of skin over joints and coronet.

If photosensitization is of hepatic origin (secondary photosensitization), the affected animal shows depression, anorexia, weight loss, and jaundice. Other signs of liver disease like abdominal distension, ascites and diarrhoea may also be present. Neurological signs may develop in some cases due to accumulation of toxins in the brain. In lantana poisoning, animal becomes sluggish, faeces are soft and may contain blood, and there is paralysis of limbs (in some cases). Death mostly occurs in a few days due to extensive liver damage.

Post-mortem findings: Fatal cases usually result from the hepatogenic form of the disease. Necropsy lesions include superficial necrosis on the unpigmented skin and on the tender parts of pigmented surfaces. Extensive necrosis may be found around eyes, muzzle, ears and other areas. The carcass may be emaciated and dehydrated and visible mucous membranes are usually icteric. The body tissues may show the yellow colour of icterus. Liver may be enlarged and cirrhotic with abnormally thin margins, gall bladder is usually distended, and there may be proliferation of bile ducts. The kidneys may show degenerative changes. Ascites may be present with gastroenteritis. Histologically, hepatomegaly, karyomegaly, hepatic necrosis, cirrhosis and bile duct proliferation may be found.

Diagnosis: Dermatitis limited to areas of non-pigmented skin presents well recognised clinical signs of photosensitization. Identification of photosensitizing plants in the animal's environment and food may substantiate the diagnosis. Liver biopsy to confirm the presence of hepatomegaly, fibrosis and biliary hyperplasia are optimal test for diagnosis of hepatogenous photosensitization. Serum analysis for liver function enzymes and examination of blood, faeces and urine for porphyrin should be considered.

Early or mild cases of photosensitization are similar to the primary effects of sunburn. Photosensitization differs from sunburn, in which (sunburn) lightly pigmented skin slowly becomes inflamed following exposure to ultraviolet rays. Photosensitization should also be differentiated from mycotic dermatitis on the basis that photodynamic substance removal in photosensitization causes quick recovery.

Treatment and management: Treatment of photosensitization is only supportive. Primary photosensitization responds well to treatment, but success of secondary photosensitization is usually doubtful.

a. Animal should be immediately removed from plants or photodynamic substances and provided with shelter from sun or preferably housed and fed inside.

b. Corticosteroids, if given parenterally in the early stages, may be helpful.

c. Secondary skin infections and suppurations should be treated and flies strike must be prevented.

d. In hepatogenous photosensitization, appropriate supportive therapy may be started such as fluid and electrolyte therapy.

Prognosis: The prognosis and eventual productivity of an animal is related to the site and severity of primary lesion and to the degree of resolution. The skin lesions heal remarkably well, even after extensive necrosis. The prognosis of secondary photosensitization is mostly poor because the liver disease is generally irreversible and affected animals eventually die from liver failure.

6. Datura (Dhatura) and Related Plants Poisoning

Certain genera of the *Solanaceae* (Nightshade) family have been associated with poisoning in animals and humans since ancient times. These include *Datura stramonium* (jimson weed, thornapple), *Atropa belladonna* (deadly nightshade), *Hyoscyamus niger* (black henbane), *Solanum nigrum* (black nighshade) and *Physalis virginiana* (ground cherry). Various genera consisting of large number of species contain alkaloids or glyco-alkaloids, which cause almost similar pharmacological and toxicological actions. Datura and related plants commonly occur in India and several other parts of world and are source of malicious and accidental poisoning.

Properties: *Datura* exists in more than dozen varieties e.g. *D. stramonium*, *D. metal*, *D. tatula*, *D. fastuosa*, *D. meteloides*, *D. quercifolia*, *D. alba*, and *D. niger*. They are large, vigorous annual plants or short-lived perennial plants, growing to 1-3 m tall. *Datura stramonium* is a foetid annual plant with large, long, and white flowers which ripen into thorny capsules. *Datura alba,* a white flowered plant, and D. niger, a black or deep purple flowered plant, are indigenous to India and grow commonly on waste places all over the country. They have bell shaped flowers and contain more or less spherical fruits which are covered with sharp spinous projections with yellowish brown seeds. The toxins (alkaloids) are present in the entire plant, but are more concentrated in seeds. Most poisonings in animals occur when *Datura* seeds that contaminate cereal grains are fed to animals. The tops and roots give off a very unpleasant smell and are seldom the source of poisoning.

Toxic principles: *Datura* spp. and related plants contain tropane alkaloids like hyoscine (scopolamine), atropine (dl-hyoscyamine), hyoscyamine, daturine (mixture of atropine and hyoscyamine) and solanine (glycoalkaloid). Tans, nitrites, fatty acid glycerides, etc. are also present.

Toxicity: Datura and related plants poisoning is not frequent in animals because many of these plants are unpalatable. Poisoning occurs mainly when hungry animals ingest the plant or when a large amount of the toxic plant is present in hay. Seeds which heavily contaminate small grains may be a greater hazard than green plants. Seeds are sometimes taken as a drug of abuse by some persons for their potential hallucinogenic effects, and small animals and birds may accidentally gain access to the seeds. Dogs are often target of deliberate poisoning. Oral toxic or lethal doses are not known in all species. Pigs appear to be very sensitive to datura seeds with 2.2-2.7 mg/kg/day causing toxic signs.

Mechanism of action: Toxicity from plants containing tropane alkaloids manifests as classic anticholinergic poisoning. Tropane alkaloids (e.g. atropine, hyoscine) of datura plant interact with and inhibit all muscarinic receptors in the body. Therefore, their primary action is blockade of the action of neurotransmitter acetylcholine at muscarinic receptor sites and hence the response of parasympathetic nervous system. High doses of atropine may also block nicotinic receptors at the autonomic ganglia and neuromuscular junctions.

Clinical signs: Toxic signs of datura and related plants are similar to effects of overdosage by atropine. Signs usually occur 30-60 minutes after ingestion and may continue for 24-48 hours because tropane alkaloids delay gastric emptying and absorption. Toxic manifestations include dryness of mouth and throat, dysphagia and difficulty in swallowing. These are followed by staggering gait, incoordination, dry-hot skin with a rise in body temperature, photophobia, dilated pupils, cycloplegia, urine retention, tachypnoea and tachycardia. Bloat and rumen atony in cattle and colic in horses may be observed. Animal becomes restless, markedly excited and apprehensive. Behavioural changes like disorientation and hallucination (in man) may also occur. Very high doses produce coma, skeletal muscle paralysis and death from respiratory failure.

Post-mortem findings: Necropsy lesions of datura poisoning are not specific. Datura seeds or their fragments may be found in the stomach and intestine. The oesophagus, stomach, duodenum and other organs are mostly congested. In some cases, mucous membranes of the stomach may be inflamed. Haemorrhages in brain, stomach and upper intestine may be observed.

Diagnosis: Diagnosis of datura poisoning may be made from history, clinical signs and lesions. Analysis of datura alkaloids in body fluids and tissues may help in the diagnosis. Placing a drop of urine from poisoned animal in the eye of a cat or any other animal may cause mydriasis.

Treatment and management: No specific antidote is available; only symptomatic and supportive care is advised.

a. Physostigmine: Parasympathomimetic drug physostigmine should be used to stimulate cholinergic secretions and activities. It competitively inhibits cholinesterase enzyme and increases acetylcholine concentration, which compete with atropine for the cholinergic receptor sites. Overdosage and frequent repetition of physostigmine should be avoided.

Cattle: 0.02 mg/kg, slow IV over 5 minutes. Dose may be repeated, if required.

Dogs: 0.05 mg/kg, slow IV over 5 minutes.

Horses: 0.1-0.6 mg/kg, IM or slow IV over 5 minutes.

b. If marked excitement is present and more specific treatment is not available, diazepam should be used for sedation and control of convulsions. Large doses should be avoided.

c. Other supportive and detoxification therapy should be instituted e.g. cold water or ice-packs to reduce fever, artificial respiration to restore respiration, general gastrointestinal detoxification to remove recently ingested poison, etc.

Contraindications

Phenothiazine tranquilizers should not be used for sedation and controlling CNS excitation because they possess anticholinergic action and often aggravate the datura intoxication.

Prognosis: Prognosis of datura and related plants poisoning depends on the early treatment and other supportive measures.

7. Oleander and Related Cardiotoxic Plants Poisoning

A large number of plants contain toxic glycosides and have direct effect on the heart. These include *Nerium odorum* (white oleander), *Digitalis purpurea* (foxglove plant), *Convallaria majalis* (lily of the valley), *Apocynum cannabinum* (dogbane), *Asclepias* spp. (milkweed), *Taxes* spp. (yew) and *Urginea* spp. (squill). Out of various plants, oleander is widely cultivated as ornamental plant in India and some other countries and its poisonous effect has been well known for centuries. Most poisonings in livestock occur when animals ingest the stem or leaves of oleander plant during drought or when the cuttings of the plant get mixed with green fodder or hay.

Properties: Oleander (*Kaner*) is an evergreen vigorously growing ornamental shrub, occasionally a small tree (12-25 feet). It is draught tolerant and is extensively used in landscaping along highways or as a potted house plant. *Nerium odorum* (white or sweet scented oleander) and *Cerbera thevetia* or *Thevetia nerifolia* (yellow oleander) are native of India, whereas *Nerium oleander* grows in subtropical climates of U.S.A. and some other countries. *Nerium odorum* has lanceolate leaves and a two follicled fruit which contains seeds. All parts of plant are toxic. *C. thevetia* has large and yellow bell shaped flowers and a green globular fruit containing a single nut. The plant is highly poisonous and the milky juice which exudates from all parts of the plant contains high concentration of toxic principles.

Toxic principles: Oleander is one of the highly toxic plants which contain many cardio-active glycosides including nerioside, oleandroside, oleandrin, nerin, folinerin, and digitoxigenin. *Nerium odorum* contains one toxic glycoside nerin ($C_{35}H_{50}O_{10}$) and *Cerbera thevetia* contains two active glycosides namely thevitin ($C_{27}H_{84}O_{12}$) and cerberin ($C_{20}H_{38}O_{14}$). *Nerium indicum* contains odoroside, a steroidal glycoside. The cardiotoxic glycosides are found in all plant parts, but growing tops and leaves are the most toxic. All glycosides have similar actions and produce mainly cardiotoxicity.

Toxicity: Oleander is toxic to all animals and many birds, but poisoning is mostly seen in horses, cattle and sheep. Many cases of poisoning have been noted in human beings, particularly in children. Toxic doses are approximately 0.005% of body weight in horses and cattle, and 0.015% in sheep. Mature cattle and horses may be killed after eating 30-50 g of oleander leaves. One leaf can kill an adult human and 2-3 leaves can kill an adult sheep. Dry leaves are about as toxic as the green ones. Livestock are usually poisoned when they are allowed to graze in places where oleander is abundant or when pruning are carelessly thrown into animal pens.

Mechanism of action: The oleander glycosides have action on heart similar to digitalis. They inhibit the Na^+/K^+-ATPase enzyme system (sodium-potassium pump) resulting in increased intracellular sodium and serum potassium concentrations. This results in progressive decrease in electrical conductivity through the heart causing conduction block and eventual asystole. In low doses, they may have beneficial therapeutic effects like digitalis by increasing the force of contraction, slowing heart rate and enhancing cardiac output, but in toxic doses most cardiac glycosides cause a variety of arrhythmias and conduction disturbances that result in decreased cardiac output and death. There is also initial stimulation followed by paralysis of vagus nerve.

Clinical signs: The clinical signs of oleander and related plants poisoning are similar in all species and related mainly to heart and GI tract. In peracute toxicity, cattle and less often horses are often found dead because of profound cardiac effects of the plants. In less severe cases, onset of clinical signs may take few hours after ingestion of the toxic plant. The affected animal shows signs of weakness with rapid pulse, tachycardia, and arrhythmias. Nausea, vomiting, anorexia, abdominal pain, colic, and sweating (horses) may be observed in some animals. Blood often appears in the faeces in terminal stages. Other signs include cold extremities, dilated pupils, muscular weakness, slowed pulse (late stages), ataxia, hypotension, and hypothermia. These are followed by tetanic spasms, drowsiness, unconsciousness, coma and death. Death usually occurs within 24 hours after clinical signs appear from peripheral circulatory failure.

Post-mortem findings: Necropsy findings of oleander poisoning are not definitive. There may be severe catarrhal or haemorrhagic gastroenteritis with congested patches in the stomach and upper portion of the small intestine. Agonal haemorrhages are commonly seen on heart and serous and mucous membranes. In less acute but fatal poisoning, multifocal myocardial degeneration and necrosis is often present.

Diagnosis: Diagnosis of oleander and other cardiotoxic plants poisoning is made from history or evidence of plant consumption, clinical signs and lesions. Presence of plant material in stomach or rumen may help in diagnosis. Detection of cardiac glycosides in serum, urine, tissues and stomach contents is possible using high-performance liquid chromatography. Oleander glycosides cross-react with digoxin radioimmunoassay. Hyperkalaemia is a common feature of oleander poisoning.

The clinical signs and lesions of oleander poisoning closely mimic poisoning due to monensin, a feed additive in cattle ration.

Treatment and management: Oleander poisoning has no specific therapy.

a. Early and active gastro-intestinal detoxification should be followed by administration of activated charcoal and osmotic cathartics.

b. In ruminants known to have eaten oleander, a rumenotomy to remove all traces of plant from rumen may be life-saving.

c. Cardiac irregularities may be controlled by appropriate use of antiarrhythmic drugs such as procainamide and lignocaine.

d. Other supportive measures including intravenous fluids may be instituted.

e. Poisoned animals should be kept away from stressful conditions to avoid further stress on the heart.

Contraindications

Intravenous fluids containing calcium should not be used in oleander and related plants poisoning because calcium augments the toxic effects of cardiac glycosides. Use of potassium in IV fluids should also be avoided due to existing hypercalcaemia.

Prognosis: Prognosis in oleander poisoning is usually poor and treatment is generally unrewarding in later stages.

8. Plants Containing Toxic Lectins / Castor Bean and Rosary Pea Poisoning

A group of unrelated plants including *Ricinus communis* (castor bean) and *Abrus precatorius* (rosary pea, jequirity bean) contain highly toxic glycoprotein (toxalbumin) compounds called lectins. Lectins are capable of causing severe poisoning in humans and animals including cattle, goats, horses, poultry and dogs. Lectins are concentrated in seeds and produce poisoning when seeds are crushed and fed to animals without detoxification. For centuries castor beans and rosary peas have been used for malicious poisoning and criminal activities.

Properties: The castor bean (*Ricinus communis*) is an ornamental plant and is commonly found in jungles and wastelands in tropical areas. It is also cultivated in India and other tropical countries for castor oil. The castor seeds are about 8-15 mm long, 6-9 mm wide and 4-8 mm thick. All parts of the plant are toxic, but the seeds are particularly rich in the toxin. The phytotoxin is absent in the expressed oil but the cake is rich in ricin which makes it unfit for use as animal feed. *Abrus precatorius* (Rathi) is a trailing, twinning perennial vine, 3-6 metres long, using other plants for support. It grows in tropical locations with yellow or red flowers and pod like fruits containing oval, shiny red and black seeds. The seeds are particularly rich in the toxic lectin. The seeds of both castor and rosary peas have a tough outer coating hence the seeds pass through the digestive system without being digested, unless they are disrupted through chewing or crushing.

Toxic principles: The principal toxins in castor beans and rosary peas are the lectins (called toxalbumins) ricin and abrin, respectively. Both toxins consist of two peptide chains (chain A and chain B) joined by sulphide bonds. The castor seeds and rosary peas also contain several other toxic and non-toxic proteins and alkaloids, some of which have not been clearly defined. For example, castor beans contain a toxic alkaloid ricinine, an irritant and purgative ricinoleic acid, and a powerful haemagglutinin RCA (*Ricinus communis* agglutinin). Poisoning by ingestion of the castor bean is due to ricin, not RCA, because RCA does not penetrate intestinal wall and does not affect red blood cells unless given intravenously. If RCA is injected into blood, it will cause the red blood cells to agglutinate and burst by haemolysis. Both ricin and abrin toxins are plant proteins, so they are heat labile and destroyed by heating. Aging also reduces toxicity of phytotoxins.

Toxicity: Ricin and abrin are some of the most poisonous plant compounds known. All species of animals are susceptible to ricin and abrin poisoning, but humans and horses are more susceptible than goats, cattle and dogs. Castor beans at 0.01% of body weight cause toxicosis in horses and at about 0.02% of body weight may cause poisoning in cattle. In humans poisoning has been seen with as little as 1 mg ricin or 1-3 beans. Abrin is much more toxic than ricin. One seed of rosary peas, approximately 0.5 cm in diameter, can kill a small child or medium sized dog. Toxicity is unlikely if the seeds are ingested as such because toxins are released only when seeds are broken, crushed or chewed and then ingested. Castor oil is not poisonous, but untreated cakes are toxic.

Mechanism of action: The exact mechanism of toxic action of ricin and abrin is not clearly known, but inhibition of protein synthesis appears to be the primary action of lectins. The inhibition of protein synthesis causes severe cytotoxic effects on many organ systems.

a. The ricin and abrin toxins consists of two protein subunits, termed A and B, linked by a disulphide bond. The chain B of the lectin binds to galactosyl (galacto-lipid and galacto-protein) components in cell membrane and causes internalization of chain A. Once inside the cell, the chain A prevents protein synthesis by inactivating the ribosomes. The reported mechanism for ricin is enzymatic de-adenylation of ribosomal RNA (removal of adenine base from ribosomal RNA) by chain A and thus inactivation of 60 S ribosome. Some studies have suggested that the primary action of ricin is via a ribonuclease activity. The abrin prevents protein synthesis possibly by inactivating the 26 S subunit of the ribosome. One molecule of abrin may inactivate up to 1,500 ribosomes per second. As the process of inhibition of protein synthesis is slow, the ricin and abrin have relatively slow onset of toxic action.

For inhibition of protein synthesis both chains A and B are essentially required. Many plants such as barley have the chain A but not the chain B, therefore they are virtually non-toxic to animals.

b. Lectins are known to cause severe irritation and damage to the gut epithelium, resulting in defective digestion and absorption and increased permeability of intestinal mucosa. Lectins also attack the lining of liver and kidneys and induce hepatitis and nephritis.

Clinical signs: The clinical signs of castor bean and rosary pea poisoning begin after a lag period of few hours to several days (usually 12-48 hours) after the consumption of a toxic dose of lectins. The signs in different species are characterised by nausea, vomiting, gastrointestinal irritation, abdominal pain, diarrhoea (often bloody diarrhoea), ruminal atony, anorexia, weakness, excessive thirst and muscular twitching. Rapid loss of water and electrolytes through the diarrhoea results in dehydration and hypovolaemic shock. In some animals there may be ulcerative lesions in mouth and oesophagus. In later stages, there may be incoordination, dyspnoea, hyperpyrexia, haemolytic anaemia, convulsions, opisthotonos, paralysis and coma followed by death. Renal failure with oliguria and sometimes uraemia may be seen in acute cases. Death usually occurs in 1-10 days from hypovolaemic shock and/or paralysis of respiratory centre. Non-fatal cases may proceed to secondary infections.

In horses, additional signs may include trembling, sweating, cold extremities, weak pulse and shivering. In dairy cattle, lactation stops abruptly. Hallucinations have been recorded in human beings. Depression, roughened feathers, droopy wings, greyish wattles and combs and decreased egg production may be observed in poultry.

Post-mortem findings: Important lesions of lectins poisoning include inflammation and ulceration of stomach and intestine, and fatty degeneration necrosis of liver and kidneys. Contents of the gut are fluid or semi-fluid. Haemolytic anaemia and generalized petechial haemorrhages may be found throughout the body. Severe congestion, oedema and emphysema may be observed in lungs; trachea and bronchi may be filled with frothy oedematous fluids.

Diagnosis: Diagnosis of castor bean and rosary pea poisoning can be difficult to confirm unless animals are observed eating the seeds. Clinical signs and post-mortem lesions with history of feeding ricin containing feed stuffs may help in diagnosis. Increases in serum liver enzymes, creatinine and urea nitrogen may suggest liver and kidney damage.

Treatment: There is no specific therapy for castor bean and rosary pea poisoning. Treatment is directed at removing the seeds from the digestive tract and providing the supportive therapy.

a. Emesis and gastric lavage should be followed by administration of activated charcoal.

b. Demulcents should be given to decrease pain and GI tract irritation.

c. Appropriate fluid and electrolyte therapy should be given to correct dehydration and electrolyte imbalance.

d. Anti-ricin serum from a previously hyperimmunized animal may be used in castor bean poisoning, if readily available.

Prognosis: Prognosis depends on the early treatment. Mostly it is guarded to grave.

9. Ipomoea Poisoning

Ipomoea plants belong to the family Convolvulaceae and there are over 500 species viz. *Ipomoea turpethum* (Indian Jalap or white turpeth), *I. orizabensis, I. violacea, I. carnea, and I. purga*

(Jalap). Many species are known as morning glory, a name shared with some other related genera. Livestock do not graze on Ipomoea, but in fodder scarcity they feed on these plants and succumb to toxicity.

Properties: The genus *Ipomoea* occurs throughout tropical and subtropical regions of the world and comprises annual and perennial herbaceous plants, shrubs and small trees. Many species climb naturally on fences and trellises. Ipomoea plants have heart-shaped leaves with showy, trumpet-shaped white, blue or violet flowers. Both the root and bark contain toxic principles but root is more important. In some species, seeds are also toxic. A resinous mixture from the dried root of *I. orizabensis* is available as a brownish, translucent bright mass or powder with favourable odour and acrid taste for cathartic purposes.

Toxic principles: The active principles in Ipomoea plants are mostly resins. In *I. orizabensis,* the resin is scammonin (jalapin), in *I. turpethum* (Indian jalap) is turpethin and in *I. hederaceae* is pharbitisin. The resins are strong irritants and produce cathartic action. The seeds of *I. violacea* contain lysergic acid and other indole alkaloids which have hallucinogenic actions. *Ipomoea carnea* leaves are known to contain toxic saponins. Ipomoea species also accumulate very high concentrations of nitrates from the soil.

Clinical signs: Clinical signs of Ipomoea depend upon the amount of plant ingested. In lower doses there is diarrhoea and in higher doses there is drastic purgation. In toxic doses, signs may include nausea, salivation, mydriasis, incoordination, ataxia, staggering gait, hallucinations, decreased reflexes, severe diarrhoea, prostration, paralysis of limbs, hypotension and death. Bizarre behaviour, barking and disorientation may occur in dogs.

In subacute poisoning, which appears to be more common in filed conditions, there may be weakness, anaemia, leucopenia, and enhanced erythrocytic fragility.

Post-mortem findings: Lesions of Ipomoea poisoning are not specific. Degenerative changes in liver, congestion of kidneys, oedema of lungs and haemorrhages in heart may be observed.

Diagnosis: Diagnosis may be made from history of animal grazing near Ipomoea hedges, clinical signs and lesions. Presence of plant material in stomach may confirm the diagnosis.

Treatment and management: There is no specific treatment for Ipomoea poisoning; only detoxification and supportive therapy is advocated. Suspected plant material should be removed from digestive tract by using gastric lavage or saline purgative. Rumenotomy may be undertaken in case of ruminants. Appropriate fluid therapy should be administered to overcome dehydration and electrolyte imbalance.

10. Cottonseed Poisoning / Gossypol Poisoning

Cotton (*Gossypium* spp.) is used for soft fibre and its seeds are often used in animal feed as high protein materials. The seeds contain a yellow polyphenolic binaphthalene pigment called gossypol, which is toxic to animals. Gossypol is found in the glands of cottonseed in both bound (non-toxic) and free (toxic) forms and is released when the glands are ruptured. Gossypol contents vary with species of plant and method of extraction and may range from 0.002% to more than 6%. The free gossypol content of cottonseed meal generally decreases during processing or heating, but in some cases it may be retained to significant concentrations to cause toxicosis. Cotton seed cake containing up to 0.01% of gossypol is considered to be safe.

Gossypol is lipid soluble and readily absorbed from the digestive tract. It binds strongly to proteins and amino acids (especially lysine and methionine) rendering them unavailable during the digestive process. It chelates iron (e.g. ferrous sulphate) in the body and makes it unavailable for heme synthesis resulting in anaemia. Gossypol also acts as an inhibitor for several dehydrogenase enzymes and reversibly blocks calcineurin and binds to calmodulin. Inhibition of testicular lactic dehydrogenase (LDH) enzyme, in particular, has significant effect on the male reproductive performance. Gossypol also inhibits glutathione-S-transferase, impairing the liver's ability to metabolize several xenobiotic compounds. The acute toxicity of gossypol is generally low with the oral LD_{50} of 5 g/kg body weight. However,

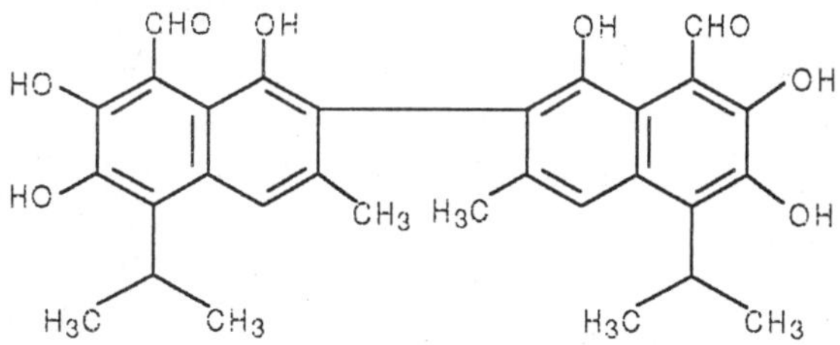

Fig. 15.9. Chemical structure of gossypol.

continuous ingestion of small amounts of cottonseed cake or cottonseed meal over long times leads to toxicity. Therefore, cattle should not be fed this cake in daily ration higher than 1 kg, and after 2-3 months its administration should be interrupted for 3-4 weeks. Various species including cattle, horses, swine, poultry and dogs are considered to be susceptible to gossypol poisoning. Cattle are not very susceptible to gossypol, except young calves, because microorganisms in the rumen have ability to detoxify gossypol. However, this ability can be overcome at very high levels of cottonseed feeding. Use of gossypol in swine and poultry diets is restricted because of its potential toxicity to monogastric animals.

The onset of first clinical signs occurs within 10-30 days (1-2 days, if intake is large) depending upon the amount of cake in the feed and the content of gossypol in the cake. There is loss of appetite, restlessness, gastroenteritis, diarrhoea, laboured and shallow breathing, and spasms. In acute cases, death may occur during the first few days. In chronic poisoning, the disease lasts for several weeks, being manifested by weakness, loss of weight, and growth retardation in young animals. Protein malnutrition and reduced weight gain may occur as a result of protein binding. Gossypol appears to interrupt pregnancy by exerting a luteolytic action on the ovary. In males, there are spermatozoal abnormalities and infertility due to inhibition of enzymes necessary for steroid synthesis in testicular Leydig cells. In layers, excessive gossypol has shown to affect weight gain, feed intake and efficiency, egg production and quality, and hatchability. The necropsy findings depend on the course of poisoning. Most frequent lesions are gastritis, hepatitis and inflammation of the kidneys. Degeneration of cardiac muscles and pulmonary oedema may also be seen. Straw-coloured to red-tinged fluids may occasionally be found in the thorax and abdomen.

Treatment of gossypol poisoning involves detoxification processes like addition of iron or calcium carbonate in the diet, which helps to inactivate free gossypol. Supportive measures like high quality diet supplemented with lysine, methionine and fat soluble vitamins should be instituted. High protein intake is protective against the effects of gossypol.

11. Nux Vomica Poisoning

Strychnos nux vomica tree belongs to family of Loganiaceae and grows in jungles in some parts of India and some other countries. Its ripe fruit contains nux vomica seeds which are poisonous. The seeds are disc shaped and nearly flat and covered with short satin like hair.

Strychnos nux vomica seeds contain two major alkaloids viz. strychnine and brucine. The major alkaloid is strychnine and normally the seeds contain not less than 1-2 per cent of the same. The bark, wood and leaves contain brucine but no strychnine. In addition to toxic alkaloids, nux vomica contains a glycoside loganin and an acid caffeotannic acid. Toxicity of nux vomica is due to alkaloid strychnine.

Toxicity, clinical signs, post-mortem findings and line of treatment of nux vamica poisoning have been discussed in strychnine poisoning (see Rodenticides, Chapter 13).

12. Other Toxic Plants

Thousands of other toxic plants exist all over the world and can cause sickness or death if ingested or come into contact with animals. The toxicology of many of these plants is well documented in literature, but is beyond the scope of this book. The important features of selected toxic plants that are abundantly found in India or some other countries and not discussed in the present chapter are given in Table 15.4.

Table 15.4. Important features of miscellaneous toxic plants.

Common name (Botanical name) Important species.	Toxic part(s)	Toxic principle(s)	Susceptible species	Mechanism of action	Important clinical signs	Treatment and management
Aconite/ Monkshood (*Aconitum* spp.) *A. columbianum* *A. napellus* *A. lutescens*	All parts, especially roots, seeds and new leaves.	Diterpene alkaloids–aconitine (Most important), aconine, mesaconitine, and napelline	Most species	Neuromuscular blockade; blocks tetrodotoxin-sensitive sodium channels	Irritation, nausea, vomiting, muscular weakness, bloat, frothy salivation, dyspnoea, slow and weak heart beats, arrhythmias, ventricular fibrillation and paralysis. Death from asphyxia.	No specific treatment. Cardiac stimulants and symptomatic and supportive therapy.
Avocado (*Persea*) *P. americana*	Fruits, leaves, bark, skin and seeds	Fatty acid derivative–persin	Many species including cattle, horses, goats, dogs, cats, birds, fish	Poorly defined; direct action on myocardium and mammary tissues.	Gastrointestinal irritation, vomiting, diarrhoea, oedema of lips, mouth, eyelids, head, neck and brisket, followed by respiratory distress. Lactating animals develop non-infectious mastitis.	Symptomatic and supportive care.
Brassica *B. hirta* (Yellow mustard) *B. kaber* (Wild mustard) *B. napus* (Rape) *B. oleracea var. acephala* (Kale) *B. oleracea var. capitata* (Cabbage) *B. oleracea var. botrytis* (Broccoli) *B. rapa* (Turnip)	All parts, especially seeds	Glucosinolates or their breakdown products (e.g. isothiocyanate, thiocyanate, nitrile, S-methyl cysteine sulphoxide, goitrin)	Many species, mainly poultry and swine	Isothiocyanate - severe gastroenteritis; S-methyl cysteine sulphoxides - haemolysis; Goitrin - interference with iodine incorporation and secretion.	*Acute* : Severe gastroenteritis, scouring, rumen stasis, jaundice, anaemia. *Chronic* : Goitre, poor conception, poor growth.	Symptomatic and supportive care. Intravenous fluid or bood transfusion, if required.
Daffodil (*Narcissus*) *N. pseudonarcissus*	All parts, especially bulb	Alkaloids–narcissine and narcipoietin	Most species	Poorly defined	Severe gastroenteritis, vomiting, diarrhoea, lethargy, tremors or convulsions and hypotension. Death in severe cases.	Symptomatic and supportive care. Emetics, activated charocoal, saline cathartic, gastric demulcents and IV fluids

Contd....

Common name (Botanical name) Important species.	Toxic part(s)	Toxic principle(s)	Susceptible species	Mechanism of action	Important clinical signs	Treatment and management
Horsechestnut (*Aesculus*) *A. hippocastanum* *A. indica*	All parts, especially young sprouts, fruits and leaves	Glycosides – aesculin and fraxin	Cattle, sheep, horses, pigs and poultry	Poorly defined	Vomiting, colic, dullness, incoordination, staggering, hyperesthesia, followed by trembling, recumbency, paralysis, coma, and convulsions. Death from respiratory paralysis.	Symptomatic and supportive care. Gastric demulcents, fluids, and sedatives.
Hyacinth (Hyacinthus *spp.*) *H. orientalis* *H. litwinowii*	Bulb	Calcium oxalate raphides	Dogs, cats, cattle, pigs	Gastrointestinal and skin irritant	Nausea, vomiting, colic, and diarrhoea.	Symptomatic and supportive care.
Larkspur (*Delphinium* spp.) *D. barbeyi* *D. occidentale* *D. bicolor*	All parts	Polycyclic diterpene alkaloid methyllyca–conitine	Mostly cattle	Neuromuscular blockade (curare-like action)	Sudden death; hyperirritability, tremors, stiffness, constipation, bloat, collapse, convulsions. Death from respiratory paralysis or bloat.	Physostigmine, saline cathartic, activated charcoal.
Lily (*Lilium spp. and Hemerocallis* spp.) *L. longiflorum (Easter lily)* *L. tigrinum (Tiger lily)* *H. flava (Day lily)*	All parts	Unknown	Cats	Poorly defined, necrosis of renal tubular epithelial cells	Vomiting, anorexia, depression, renal casts in urine	Symptomatic and supportive care. Diuresis with IV lactated Ringer's solution.
Lupin/Bluebonnet (*Lupin* spp.) *L. leucophyllus* *L. argenteus* *L. caudatus*	Foliage and seeds	Several quinolizidine (e.g. teratogenic anagyrine) and piperidine alkaloids	Sheep, cattle and other herbivores; occasionally small animals	Poorly understood	Two syndromes: a. Teratogenicity: crooked calf disease with misaligned joints and twisted bones; vertebral column malformation (scoliosis, kyphosis, torticolis). b. Nervous syndrome: muscle tremors, labored breathing, convulsions, coma and death	Symptomatic and supportive care, activated charcoal, saline purgative, haloperiodol, diazepam.

Contd....

Common name (Botanical name) Important species.	Toxic part(s)	Toxic principle(s)	Susceptible species	Mechanism of action	Important clinical signs	Treatment and management
Marijuana/Hemp (Cannabis) *C. sativa*	All parts, especially leaves, flowering parts, sap and resinous secretions.	Resins called canabinoids, mainly tetrahydrocannabinol (THC)	Cattle, horses, pigs and dogs; rarely cats	Stimulation of dopamine pathway in brain.	Hyperexcitability followed by depression, vomiting salivation, muscle tremors, ataxia, mydriasis, stupor, coma and death	Symptomatic and supportive care, activated charcoal, saline purgative, haloperiodol, diazepam,
Oak (Quercus spp.) *Q. gambelii* *Q. havardii*	Leaves, bark, acorns	Gallotannin (combination of tannic and gallic acid)	Cattle, sheep, horses and pigs	Denaturation of cell proteins	Anorexia, depression, intestinal and ruminal stasis, excessive thirst, abdominal pain, hard faeces initially followed by black tarry diarrhoea terminally.	Symptomatic and supportive care. Gastrointestinal demulcents, oral calcium hydroxide solution, and intravenous fluids.
Onion and garlic (*Allium* spp.) *A. sepa (Cultivated onion)* *A. canadensis* (Wild *onion)* *A. validum* (Wild onion) *A. ampeloprasum* (Garlic)	All parts	N-Propyl disulphide	Dogs, cattle most susceptible; horses and sheep moderately susceptible; goats less susceptible.	Haemolysis secondary to oxidant-associated effects.	Weakness,haemoglobinuria, jaundice, rapid breathing, tachycardia, characteristic onion odour. Death in severe cases due to haemolytic anaemia.	Symptomatic and supportive care. Blood transfusion, IV fluids.
Senna (*Cassia*) *C. fasciculate* *C. occidentalis*	Seeds	Anthraquinones; specific toxic principle not identified	Many species including cattle, sheep, goats, horses, pigs and chickens	Poorly defined, possibly strong binding to cell membranes and muscle degeneration.	Severe diarrhoea, abdominal pain, tenesmus followed by muscle degeneration in few days causing weakness and recumbency. Myoglobinuria from acute muscle degeneration. Death occurs from renal and hepatic failure	Symptomatic and supporitve care. Intravenous fluid and nutritious diet.

Contd....

Common name (Botanical name) Important species.	Tcxic part(s)	Toxic principle(s)	Susceptible species	Mechanism of action	Important clinical signs	Treatment and management
Tobacco (*Nicotiana* spp.; *Lobelia* spp.) *N. tabaccum* (Cultivated tobacco) *N. trigonophylla* (Wild tobacco) *L. inflata* (Indian tobacco)	All parts	Pyridine alkaloids - a. Nicotine (*Nicotiana* spp.) b. Lobeline and lobilidine (*Lobelia* spp.)	All species, espcially sheep, cattle and goats.	Nicotine and lobeline initially stimulate than inhibit nicotinic cholinergic sites in autonomic ganglia and myoneural junctions.	Excitement, salivation, hypertension, vomiting, diarrhoea followed by depression, constipation, staggering, collapse, irregular heat beats, and coma. Death occurs from respiratory paralysis.	Symptomatic and supportive care.
White snakeroot (Eupatorium spp) *E. rugosum* *E. adenophorum* *E. riparium*	Greer plant	Alcohol - tremetol (Tremetone).	All species, especially cattle, horses, sheep and goats.	Poorly defined.	Listlessness, lethargy, depression, muscle tremors, colic, blood in faeces, acetone odour to breath, recumbency, coma and death. Consumption of milk from sick animal produces a disease in humans called milk sickness.	Symptomatic and supprotive care. Parenteral administration of sodium lactate, glucose, and hypotonic Ringer's solution.

BIBLIOGRAPHY

Albertsen JC (2000) Evaluation of castor bean toxicosis in dogs : 98 cases (1987-1997) *J. Am. Vet. Med. Assoc.* 213 : 99.

Allison CD and Baker RD (2002) Prussic acid poisoning in livestock. Cooperative Extension Service, New Mexico State University. (http://cahe.nmsu.edu/pubs/_b/B-808.pdf).

Bartik M and Piskac A (1981) Veterinary Toxicology. Elsevier Scientific Publishing Company, Amsterdam.

Beasley V (1999) Veterinary Toxicology. International Veterinary Information Service, Ithaca NY (www.ivis.org).

Booth NH and Mcdonald LE (1982) John's Veterinary Pharmacology and Therapeutics. 5th edn. Kalyani Publishjers, Ludhiana-NewDelhi.

Bradley D (2007) Ptaquiloside - the Poison in Bracken. (http://www.chm.bris.ac.uk/motm/ptq/ptqh.htm).

Brown D (2007) Cornell University Poisonous Plants Information Database. (http://www.ansci.cornell.edu/plants/).

Bull LB, Culvenor, CCJ and Dick AT (1968) The Pyrrolizidine Alkaloids. North Holland Publishing Company, Amsterdam.

Burrows GE (1981) Cyanide intoxication in sheep. *Vet. Hum. Toxicol.* 23 : 22.

Burrows GE and Way JL (1979) Cyanide intoxication in sheep: Enhancement of efficacy of sodium nitrite, sodium thiosulphate and cobaltous chloride. *Am. J. Vet. Res.* 40 : 613.

Byass TD (1986) Antidotal effect of vitamin K against warfarin induced anticoagulation in horses. *Am. J. Vet. Res.* 47 : 2309.

Cheeke PR (1998) Natural Toxicants in Feeds, Forages and Poisonous Plants. Interstate Publishers, Danville.

Clarke ECG and Clarke ML (1967) Garner's Veterinary Toxicology. 3rd edn. Williams and Wilkins, Baltimore.

Cran HR (1985) Suspected hydrocyanic acid poisoning in cattle. *Vet Rec.* 116 : 349.

Crawford RF, Kennedy WK and Davison KL (1966) Factors influencing the toxicity of forages that contain nitrate when fed to cattle. *Cornell Vet.* 56 : 1.

Garg SK (2000) Veterinary Toxicology. CBS Publishers & Distributors, New Delhi.

Hartwig NR (2007) Cyanide toxicity. (http://www.iowabeefcenter.org/content/toxic.htm).

Hooper PT (1978) Pyrrolizidine alkaloid poisoning. Pathology with particular reference to differences in animal and plant species. In: Effects of Poisonous Plants on Livestock. Keeler RF, Kampen KRV and James LF (Eds.) p 161. Academic Press, New York.

James LF (1970) Locomotor disturbance in cattle grazing *Halogeton glomeratus*. *J. Am. Vet. Med. Assoc.* 156 : 1310.

James LF (1972) Oxalate toxicosis. *Clinc. Toxicol.* 2 : 231.

James LF, Ralphs MH and Nielsen DB (1990) The Ecology and Economic Impact of Poisonous Plants on Livestock Production. International Book Distributors, Dehradun.

Keeler RF, Kampen KRV and James LF (1978) Effects of Poisonous Plants on Livestock. Academic Press, New York.

Kirk J, Adaska J and Blanchard (2007) Oleander poisoning in cattle. (http://www.vetmed.ucdavis.edu/vetext/INF-DA/INF-DA_Oleander.html).

Knight AP and Walter RG (2002) A Guide to Plant Poisoning of Animals in North America. International Veterinary Information Service, Ithaca NY (www.ivis.org).

Lorgue G, Lechenet J and Riviere A (1996) Clinical Veterinary Toxicology. Blackwell Science Ltd., United Kingdom.

Mandial RK (1996) Clinico-biochemical, pathological and therapeutic studies on *Lantana camara* toxicosis. Ph.D. Thesis, Punjab Agricultural University, Ludhiana.

Mclean EK (1970) The toxic actions of pyrrolizidine (Senecio) alkaloids. *Pharmacol. Rev.* 22 : 429.

Michael PW (1959) Oxalate ingestion studies in the sheep. *Aust. Vet. J.* 35 : 431.

Muth OH (1968) Tansy ragwort (*Senecio jacoba*), a potential menance to livestock. *J. Am. Vet. Med. Assoc.* 153 : 310.

Norton S (1996) Toxic effects of plants. In: Casarett & Doull's Toxicology: The Basic Science of Poisons. 5th edn. Klaassen CD (Ed.) p 841. Mcgraw Hill Companies Inc., New York.

Osweiler GD (1996) Toxicology. Williams and Wilkins, Philadelphia.

Parker AJ, Mehta T, Zarghami NS, Cusick PK and Haskell BE (1979) Acute neurotoxicity of *Lathyrus sativus* neurotoxin, L-3-oxalylamino-2-aminopropionic acid, in the squirrel monkey. *Toxicol. Appl. Pharmacol.* 47 : 135.

Plumlee KH (1995) Photosensitization in ruminants. *Vet Med.* 90 : 605.

Radeleff RD (1970) Veterinary Toxicology. 2nd edn. Lea and Febiger, Philadelphia.

Radostits OM, Blood DC and Gay CC (1994) Veterinary Medicine: A Textbook of the Diseases of Cattle, Sheep, Pigs, Goats and Horses. Bailliere Tindall, London.

Rebhun WC (1995) Miscellaneous toxicities and deficiencies. In: Disease of Cattle. p 503. Williams & Wilkins, Baltimore.

Roberts C and Adrae J (2004) Tall fescue toxicosis and management. (http://www.plantmanagementnetwork.org/pub/cm/management/2004/toxicosis/).

Robson S (2007) Photosensitization in stock. *Primefact* 449. (http://www.dpi.nsw.gov.au _data/assets/pdf_file/0016/111157/photosensitisation-in-stock.pdf).

Robson S (2007) Prussic acid poisoning in livestock. Primefact 417. (http://www.dpi.nsw.gov.au/__data/assets/pdf_file/0013/111190/prussic-acid-poisoning-in-livestock.pdf).

Rodostits O M, Gay C C, Blood D C and Hinchcliff K W (2000) Veterinary Medicine: A Textbook of the Diseases of Cattle, Sheep, Pigs, Goats and Horses. 9th edn. W. B. Saunders, London.

Rumbeiha WK and Oehme FW (1995) Veterinary toxicology. In: General and Applied Toxicology. Ballantyne B, Marrs T and Turner P (Eds.) p 1157. Macmillan Press Ltd., London.

Shepherd S and Lydon TJ (2005) Plant poisoning: Phytophototoxins. eMedicine. (www.emedicine.com/emerg/topic446.htm).

Smith BP (2001) Large Animal Internal Medicine. 3rd edn. Mosby, St. Louis.

Smith MC (2007) Photosensitization. (http://web.vet.cornell.edu/CVM/HANDOUTS/plants/Photosens. html).

Stanton TL and Whittier J (2007) Prussic acid poisoning. Colorado State University Extension – Agriculture. (http://www.ext.colostate.edu/pubs/livestk/01612.html)

Stoltenow C and Lardy G (1998) Prussic acid poisoning. (http://www.ag.ndsu.edu/pubs/ansci/livestoc/v1150w.htm)

Vallachira A (1998) Veterinary Materia Medica. Jaypee Brothers, New Delhi.

Wagner RA and Keim SM (2005) Plant poisonings, alkaloids – Tropane. eMedicine. (www.emedicine.com/emerg/topic438.htm).

Way JL (1984) Cyanide intoxication and its mechanism of antagonism. *Ann. Rev. Pharmacol. Toxicol.* 24 : 451.

Young JA and James LF (1990) Oxalate poisoning. In: The Ecology and Economic Impact of Poisonous Plants on Livestock Production. James LF, Ralph MH and Nielsen DB (Eds). p 261. International Book Distributors, Dehradun.

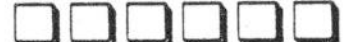

POISONOUS ANIMALS

Poisonous insects
- Honeybees, wasps and hornets
- Ants

Poisonous arachnids
- Spiders
- Scorpions
- Ticks

Poisonous amphibians
- Toads.

Poisonous reptiles
- Snakes
- Lizards

Poisonous fishes
- Tetrodotoxic fish
- Ciguatera
- Scombroid fish

Poisons of animal origin include a broad range of toxic agents that are possessed by thousands of animal species. Intoxication of livestock by animal poisons does not occur very frequently but their characteristics are specific and should be mentioned. As it is difficult to classify and characterise vast number of poisonous and venomous animals, they are reviewed by discussing representative animal species.

Venomous animal: A venomous animal can produce venom in specialized glands or cells and deliver it either by biting or stinging or in some cases by squirting or spitting.

Poisonous animal: A poisonous animal possesses a toxin(s) within its tissue that can have deleterious effects when ingested.

Considerable differences exist within the animal kingdom with respect to the venom apparatus, mode of envenomation and constituents of venom. The venom of most species is unique but complex proteinaceous mixture. The biochemical and pharmacological properties of most venoms are incompletely understood because of their complexity, difficulties of obtaining sufficient venom and extracting individual components.

Classification of poisonous animals

I. Poisonous insects e.g. bees, hornets, wasps and ants.

II. Poisonous arachnids e.g. spiders, scorpions and ticks.

III. Poisonous amphibians e.g. marine toads.

IV. Poisonous reptiles e.g. snakes and lizards.

V. Poisonous fishes e.g. tetrodotoxic fish, ciguatera and scombroid fish.

I. POISONOUS INSECTS

Insects (Class Insecta) are a major group of arthropods (Phylum Arthropoda) and the most diverse group of animals on the Earth. The Class Insecta includes several orders of veterinary and human importance, but the order Hymenoptera that contains greatest numbers of poisonous insect species is the most important order from toxicology point of view. Poisonous insects of order Hymenoptera belong to three important families: Apidae (e.g. honey bees), Vespidae (e.g. wasps and hornets) and Formicidae (e.g. ants). These insects possess true stingers and can bite or sting humans, pets, livestock and wildlife.

1. Honeybees, Wasps and Hornets

Honeybees, wasps and hornets, the flying insects of order Hymenoptera, are distributed world wide and are significantly hazardous to human beings and animals. They are found in greater numbers in mild climates and are usually located in secluded places. Exposure to these insects most commonly occurs when animal unintentionally disturbs a nest or a swarm. Being social, these insects usually attack as a group and may continue to sting until they sense that the perceived or real danger has passed. The most dangerous and life-threatening encounter is when some of these insects attack with multiple stings.

Properties: The Vespidae is a large (nearly 5,000 species), diverse, cosmopolitan family of inesects consisting of all wasps, hornets and yellowjackets. These insects are social insects, building colonies out of paper like material and are generally more aggressive and attack vigorously, if disturbed. Their stinging apparatus consists of a modified oviposter that is connected to a venom sac. They grasp the victim's skin with their claws and then insert their stinger into the skin. Vespids are generally able to withdraw their stingers and are capable of stinging again. The Apidae are a large family of bees, comprising the common honey bees, stingless bees, bumblebees, and various other less important groups. The stinger of honey bees is barbed so the stinger and venom sac remain attached to victim's skin when the bee flies away resulting in the insect's death. The stinger's injection of the toxin into the victim is accompanied by release of alarm pheromones, a process which is accelerated if the bee is fatally injured. Release of alarm pheromones near a hive or swarm may attract other bees to the location.

Toxic components of venom: The toxins of Hymenoptera are not well characterised. The venom may contain histamine, serotonin, kinins, hyaluronidase, phospholipases A and B, peptides and formic acid. In addition bee venom has mellitin, a specific protein, and formaldehyde. Venom may also contain toxic substances from plants e.g. bees collect toxins from plants like oleander, rhododendron, azalea, etc.

Toxicity: All animals are susceptible to the toxic effects of insect sting. The flying insects are capable of injecting up to 50 μl of venom with each sting. Wasps can often be seen in the settlements of people or animals, so a wasp sting is a common poisoning.

Toxicokinetics: A single sting usually has localised action and venom remains at the site of stinging. If the animal is stung many times at once, then sufficient venom is absorbed into systematic circulation and may produce systemic toxicity.

Mechanism of action: Toxicity from insect stings may include an adverse response ranging from exaggerated local effects to anaphylaxis and death. In mild cases, multiple constituents of sting venom produce localized pain, irritation and swelling. In severe cases due to multiple stings, the systemic absorption of venom constituents (e.g. histamine, kinins and proteins) produces vasodilation, hypotension, bronchoconstriction, and inflammation and oedema of tissues. The acute allergic-like response is followed by delayed effects such as haemolysis, rhabdomyolysis and renal failure.

In allergic individuals, the toxic response is mediated by IgE or indirect complement activation. The venom components circulating in the body combine with antibodies that are associated with mast cells resting on vital organs. The mast cells release histamine and other biologically active substances. This results in leakage of fluid out of blood and into body tissues. Blood pressure drops dangerously low, fluid builds up in lungs, and bronchospasm and laryngospasm start. If this response is not reversed within short time, the patient could die of anaphylactic shock.

Clinical signs: Bee, wasp or hornet stinging may include both localised and systemic toxicity signs. Clinical signs can begin immediately following the sting or up to 30 minutes later and might last for hours.

Localised toxicity: Clinical signs include mild to severe pain, heat and swelling around the sting. The swollen area may be pinkish-red in colour and produces itching. The pain usually disappears over a few hours but in some cases, especially when there is a large local reaction to the insect sting, the swelling, redness, and pain may persist for up to a week. Areas adjacent to the site of skin may also be involved in the large local reaction.

Systemic toxicity: The incidence of systemic toxicity in humans vary from 0.5-4 per cent of total stinging exposure. Systemic allergic reactions may range from mild, primarily dermatological manifestations, to life threatening anaphylaxis. In human beings, there is giddiness, sense of constriction in chest, urticaria, tachycardia, unconsciousness, jerky breathing, cold and clammy skin, involuntary passage of urine and faeces, sometimes haemoglobinuria, and peripheral neuritis. Laryngeal oedema, bronchospasms and hypotension may be life threatening in severe cases. Death may occur from shock. In people who are allergic to insect stings, there may be a dangerous anaphylactic reaction that is potentially deadly.

In animals, systemic toxicity due to multiple stinging may cause redness or swelling at sites on body distant from the site of sting such as lips/ muzzle, eyelids, tongue, and vulva. Pain and swelling may result in pronounced excitement. In severe cases in horses, there may be diarrhoea, haemoglobinuria, jaundice, tachycardia, tachypnoea, sweating and prostration. Animals attacked about the head may show dyspnoea because of severe local swelling. Sometimes the reaction can be severe with closing of airway and perhaps shock. In rare cases, the attack is fatal.

Post-mortem findings: Lesions of bee, wasp or hornet stinging are usually localized and include small puncture sites, with possible intercalation of a stinger in the epidermis or dermis. There is redness, swelling, heat and eosinophilic accumulation in 0.5 to 2 cm region around the sting. In systemic toxicity, lesions may be variable like allergic encephalitis, angio-oedema, generalised urticaria, and erythema. There may be haemorrhages and oedema of all connective tissues and intestinal wall.

Diagnosis: History, clinical signs and lesions may help in the diagnosis. Laboratory evaluation is of little value in insect sting, except that stress related leucocytosis may be present.

Treatment and management: Specific antidotes for venomous insects are not available.

a. The stinger may be removed (if it remains) by scrapping across the site with a blunt-edged object such as a post-card. The stinger should not be grabbed and pulled out as squeezing the venom sac may inject more venom.

b. The stinged area should be washed well with soap and water. Normal local reactions can be managed by applying ice to reduce the swelling, oedema and pruritus. Local application of a weak solution of ammonia or sodium bicarbonate also helps.

c. The affected area should be rubbed with an anti-histaminic cream.

d. Large local reactions may be helped by administering an analgesic as well as a glucocorticoid such as prednisone.

e. Combined use of H_1- and H_2 -histamine receptors antagonists has been suggested to decrease the severity of late phase cutaneous reactions.

f. Adrenaline is the drug of choice for systemic sting reactions. Subcutaneous administration is adequate in mild to moderate cases. In severe hypotension, adrenaline may be used intravenously.

g. Intravenous fluids and aggressive cardio-pulmonary resuscitation should be provided, if adrenaline therapy alone is not adequate.

2. Ants

Ants are wingless members of the order Hymenoptera and belong to the family Formicidae. Thousands of ant species are distributed world-wide, some of which can inflict painful venomous sting. Not all venomous ants sting, some such as carpenter and weaver ants of subfamily Formacinae bite their prey and then spray venom into the wound. Fire ant envenomation is a significant health hazard in the southern U.S.A.

Properties: Ants mostly use their sting as a mean of defence to subdue the prey. The fire ant uses its mandibles to grasp its victim and arches its body and drives an abdominal stinger into the skin to release the venom. If not quickly removed, it then moves around its mandibles and inflicts further stings in a circular pattern. Unlike other hymenoptera, ants sting slowly and may inject venom for seconds to minutes. With each sting, an ant injects from 0.05 to 0.1 μl of venom.

Toxic components: Formic acid, a potent cytotoxin, is the primary constituent of ant venom. In addition venom contains some proteins. Fire ant venom contains primarily dialkylpiperidine alkaloids (haemolytic factors) and very less protein. The fire ant venom contains some allergenic proteins, measuring about 1.5% by dry weight. Four major allergenic proteins called Soli 1- 4 induce immunoglobulin E (IgE) responses, including anaphylaxis, in allergic patients.

Mechanism of action: Toxicity associated with ant envenomation is normally limited to the site of sting. Some studies indicated that venom has haemolytic and cytotoxic actions. The dialkylpiperidine alkaloids also called haemolytic factors induce the release of histamine and other vasoactive amines from mast cells, resulting in a sterile pustule at the sting site. These alkaloids are not immunogenic, but their toxicity to the skin is believed to form the pustules.

Clinical signs: The local response to ant envenomation includes an initial weal and flare reaction. There is pain, irritation and swelling at the site of sting, which develop over hours into pruritic, oedematous and erythematous lesions that persist for up to 72 hours. Development of vesicles and pustules may also occur at the site of sting. Large local reactions may also occur which may be immunologically mediated.

Systemic allergic reactions characteristic of those caused by other Hymenoptera species may also occur (See bees, wasps, and hornets). Anaphylaxis may result in up to 1 per cent of stings. With fire ant stings, neurological sequelae including seizures and neuropathy have also been reported in few cases. Bites from aggressive fire ants (*Solenopsis invicta*) can cause focal necrotic ulcers of the cornea and conjunctiva of new born calves. Weak calves are more likely to be injured.

Treatment and management :

a. First aid for fire ant envenomation should be provided primarily through washing the sting site with soap and water.

b. Application of a cold compress may help to relieve some swelling and discomfort.

c. Large local reactions and systemic allergic reactions should be managed as described previously for bees, wasps and hornets.

II. POISONOUS ARACHNIDS

Arachnids are chiefly terrestrial arthropods having an exoskeleton, a two-part segmented body, and 8 jointed legs. The Class Arachnida comprises of some 65,000 to 73,000 named species including spiders, scorpions, ticks, and mites. Arachnids are aggressive predators and many are venomous. They secrete poison from specialized glands to kill prey or enemies and are often the source of poisoning in humans and animals.

1. Spiders

Spiders are arthropods of the order Arachnidae. Thousands of venomous spiders are distributed world-wide but only few possess the attributes necessary to cause clinical envenomation in mammals i.e. mouth parts of sufficient size to allow penetration of skin and toxin of sufficient quantity and/or potency to produce consequential morbidity. Of various poisonous spiders, black widow spider, brown recluse spider, red widow spider, red-legged spider, desert violin spider and cobweb spider have been implicated in bites of human beings. Black widow spider is most toxic and cause considerable morbidity and mortality in both animals and humans.

Properties: Black widow spider (*Lactrodectus mactans*) is indigenous to the eastern and south-western United States. The female spiders are 1-1½ inch in size and shiny black in colour with a red hourglass mark on the abdomen. The male spiders are only ½ inch and they do not have an hourglass mark. The female often eats the male after they mate; that is why the female is called a "widow". The black widow spider has claw-like hollow fangs which are connected to two venom glands in its cephalothorax. Generally these spiders are non-aggressive and bite defensively only when threatened or disturbed. The brown recluse spider (*Loxosceles recluse*) is somewhat smaller than the black widow and has a characteristic fiddle or violin marking on its back. Its back and belly are brown.

Toxic components: Black widow spider venom contains several biologically active components including proteins. Of various toxic proteins, α-lactrotoxin (α-latrotoxin), a labile neurotoxin is the most important and potent toxin. The venom also contains high contents of isoleucin and leucin, lipoproteins and hyaluronidase. The venom of brown recluse spider is rich in hyaluronidase, proteases, sphingomyelinase D, esterases and haemolysin.

Toxicity: Both female and male black widow spiders are toxic, but only the female is large enough to envenomate an animal. The venom of the black widow spider is one of the most potent biological toxins. The venom gland contains just less than 0.2 mg of venom. The median lethal dose of black widow spider venom in various animal species ranges from 0.005 to 1.0 mg/kg body weight. The black widow spider characteristically produces a systemic reaction because its venom is a neurotoxin.

In contrast, the brown recluse spider venom produces a necrotic local lesion at the site of bite but can also cause systemic reaction such as DIC.

Mechanism of action :

Black widow spider :

a. The alpha-lactrotoxin acts at the neuromuscular junctions and causes the release of acetylcholine from pre-synaptic nerve fibre. The release of acetylcholine continues till there is complete depletion of the neurotransmitter. The release and subsequent depletion of acetylcholine result in severe painful cramping of all large muscle groups, which account for most of the clinical signs.

b. The neurotoxins bind to glycoproteins or gangliosides on neuromuscular synaptic membranes and allow opening of cationic channels. Calcium-channel binding increases the membrane's permeability to calcium and enhances depolarization. Enhanced calcium influx also causes calcium-dependent release of neurotransmitters.

Brown recluse spider: The venom of brown recluse spider is primarily cytotoxic to endothelial cells. The venom components trigger disseminated intravascular coagulation (DIC) and microthrombi formation within capillaries. This is followed by capillary occlusion, haemorrhage and necrosis. Polymononuclear leucocytes and complement play important roles in potentiating the response to envenomation. The brown recluse spider bite is very slow to heal.

Clinical signs :

Black widow spider: Clinical signs of black widow spider sting occur almost immediately after the bite. There is dull-numbing pain, which gradually spreads from the region of bite to the muscles of entire body. The pain becomes severe and other signs appear such as restlessness, vomiting, anxiety or apprehension, muscle cramps, and rapid, shallow and irregular respiration. In later stages, there may be abdominal rigidity and/ or tenderness, muscle fasciculation, tonic-clonic convulsions, sweating, hypersalivation, flaccid paralysis and shock. Death may result from respiratory or cardiovascular failure.

Brown recluse spider: Clinical signs of brown recluse spider sting may occur in two forms: cutaneous and viscerocutaneous forms. In cutaneous form, signs begin as pain and oedema at the sting site and progresses to an ulcerated wound. The viscerocutaneous form is more severe and produces systemic signs of haemolytic anaemia, haemoglobinuria, jaundice and hyperthermia. Complications associated with intravascular haemolysis may include kidney damage. Most skin lesions resolve within 1-3 weeks. Some skin lesions are permanent and may need skin grafting.

Post-mortem findings: The lesions of spider envenomation are not conclusive or distinctive except for venous congestion.

Diagnosis: Unless there is a history of a spider bite, diagnosis must be based on clinical signs. Laboratory analysis is not useful.

Treatment and management: Most spider envenomations are self limiting and clinical signs resolve within few hours.

a. A specific black widow spider antivenin that reduces pain and brings relief within 15 minutes of its intravenous administration is available in humans and has also been used in small animals.

b. Muscle-relaxants (e.g. methocarbamol), analgesics (e.g. meperidine) and sedatives (e.g. diazepam) may be used to control muscle spasms and pain.

c. Atropine can be used to reduce salivation.

d. Therapy of shock (e.g. corticosteroids and fluid) should be instituted in severe cases.

e. Antihistamines and respiratory stimulants may be administered, if required.

f. In brown recluse spider envenomation, haemolytic anaemia should be corrected with blood transfusion.

Prognosis: Prognosis of black widow spider envenomation is reasonably good in dogs, but may be guarded in cats. Recovery in severe cases may be prolonged, and weakness and even paralysis may persist for several days.

2. Scorpions

True scorpions are arachnids of the order Scorpionida. There are approximately 650 species of scorpion distributed world-wide, some of which are of significant toxicological importance. Almost all of these toxic scorpions, except the *Hemiscorpius* species, belong to the scorpion family called the Buthidae. The lethal members of the

Buthidae family include the genera of Buthus, Parabuthus, Mesobuthus, Tityus, Leiurus, Androctonus, and Centruroides. Black bark scorpion (*Centruroides exilicauda*) found in Mexico and southwest America and *Leiurus quinquestriatus* found in Asia and Africa cause severe poisoning in humans and animals.

Properties: Scorpions are eight legged arthropods. They possess a hard exoskeleton and three primary body parts: a cephalothorax to which are attached a pair of pincers, an abdomen, and a tail that ends in a telson which contain stinging apparatus. The telson contains two venom glands which lead via independent ducts to the stinger. The scorpion uses its pincers to grab its prey and then arches its tail over its body and head to inject venom, sometimes repeatedly. Scorpions also have an ability to regulate the amount of venom to be injected with each sting using striated muscles in the stinger, the usual amount being between 0.1 and 0.6 mg. Scorpions are nocturnal and take shelter during the day under rocks, piles of debris or may hide inside house in clothing and shoes. Scorpions primarily inhabit deserts and semi-arid regions.

Toxic components: Scorpion venom is a heterogeneous mixture of toxic chemicals. It is composed of varying concentrations of neurotoxins, cardiotoxins, nephrotoxins, haemolysin, agglutinins, coagulins, phosphodiesterases, phospholipases, hyaluronidases, glycosamino-glycans, histamine, serotonin, tryptophan, and cytokine releasers. The most potent is the neurotoxins comprising of a variety of long-chain and small chain polypeptides. The various constituents of the venom may act directly or indirectly and individually or synergistically to manifest their effects. In addition, differences in the amino acid sequence of each toxin account for their differences in the function and immunology.

Toxicity: All scorpion species possess venom, but the toxicity varies in severity, depending on the species of scorpion, the amount of poison actually injected and the site of stinging. The venom of some species produces only mild signs, while that of others may produce death within an hour. If the venom is deposited into a venous structure, it is distributed rapidly into body tissues and causes more rapid onset of systemic signs. *Leiurus quinquestriatus* is one of the most dangerous scorpions with very potent venom (Subcutaneous LD value in mice 0.16 - 0.50 mg/kg). This species causes several deaths each year in human beings.

Mechanism of action: The venom of all scorpions, except a few, is primarily neurotoxic in nature. The long-chain polypeptide neurotoxins interact with voltage-dependent sodium channel and stabilize it in the open position, leading to continuous, prolonged, repetitive firing of the somatic, sympathetic, and parasympathetic neurons. This repetitive firing causes excessive release of various neurotransmitters such as acetylcholine, noradrenaline and adrenaline from their storage sites causing autonomic and neuromuscular over-excitation signs. The over-excitation may be followed by inhibition of normal nerve impulse transmission. The short polypeptide neurotoxins also play an important role in neuronal over-excitation by blocking the potassium channels. The binding of these neurotoxins to their target sites is reversible, but different neurotoxins have different affinities.

Clinical signs: The clinical signs of scorpion sting are characterised in human beings. The sting causes local pain, numbness, hyperesthesia, skin discolouration, salivation, agitation, wheezing, tachycardia, hypertension and muscle spasms. In severe cases, cranial nerve and somatic motor abnormalities such as eye movement disorders, blurred vision, tongue fasciculation, convulsions, impaired pharyngeal muscle control and jerking of extremities may develop. Death may result from respiratory or cardiac failure.

Post-mortem findings: Toxic myocarditis, disseminated intravascular coagulation, acute pancreatitis and pulmonary oedema have been reported in various cases of scorpion stinging.

Treatment and management :

a. Specific antivenin therapy is available in some parts of world, but its safety, efficacy and specificity are not clear.

b. Cold compresses can be applied to help relieve pain and inflammation, if present.

c. Atropine sulphate may be indicated to control excessive parasympathetic manifestations. If required, β-adrenoceptor blockers (e.g. propranolol) may be used to antagonise action on adrenergic receptors.

d. Calcium gluconate may be given intravenously to relieve muscle spasms.

e. First aid consisting of good local wound care including thorough cleansing and tetanus prophylaxis must be provided.

Contraindications

Morphine and meperidine hydrochloride should not be used in scorpion envenomation because they generally worsen the respiratory depression produced by most scorpion venoms.

3. Ticks

Ticks are important arachnoid ectoparasites of mammals, birds and reptiles throughout the world and have been associated with transmission of some important diseases. In addition, a number of tick species have been reported to secrete toxins and cause a disease commonly known as "tick paralysis". There are several genera of ticks worldwide that may cause tick paralysis, but poisoning is more common with *Dermacentor* spp., *Ixodes* spp., *Amblyomma* spp., *Rhipecephalus* spp. and *Ornithodorus* spp.

Properties: There are two major families of tick, the Ixodidae or hard ticks and Argasidae or soft ticks. Hard ticks have a thick outer shell made of chitin just behind the mouthparts, whereas soft ticks do not have the hard shield but a membranous outer surface. One of the most frequently encountered hard ticks is American dog tick or wood tick (*Dermacentor variabilis*) that feed on humans and medium to large mammals such as dogs. Another hard tick *Ixodes holocyclus*, commonly called Australian paralysis tick, infest mammals, birds and reptiles and causes the most severe form of paralysis. *Rhipecephalus sanguineus* (brown dog tick), one of the most widely distributed ticks in the world, is known to occur on a number of hosts. Unfed males and females of various tick species are smaller in size, whereas the engorged females after feeding may become bigger to many times their normal dimensions. It is during the feeding on host blood that a female tick injects the toxic saliva and produces the tick paralysis.

Toxic components: The ticks secrete a neurotoxin from the salivary gland when feeding on the host. Specific toxin has not been identified.

Toxicity: Tick poisoning varies with genus, species, life-cycle stage and gender of tick, and age of animal. Poisoning is also affected by seasonal activity of ticks in a given geographical area. It is generally the adult female tick that causes paralysis, although the larval and nymphal stages of some tick species also elaborate small amounts of toxin. Adult male ticks might produce toxin but they do not engorge on host so the toxin is not of toxicological importance. Most mammals including dogs (most susceptible), cats, cattle, sheep, goats, pigs, horses, and humans are susceptible to tick poisoning. Young and immature hosts of larger species are more susceptible to poisoning than the adult animals. Although tick poisoning is mostly caused by large infestation of ticks, in some cases a single tick is enough to cause clinical signs. Tick paralysis is commonly seen during spring and summer when tick infestation is highest. Four to ten adult female *Ixodes holocyclus* ticks are sufficient to produce paralysis within 6-13 days.

Mechanism of action: The exact mechanism of tick toxin is not known. The neurotoxin affects the lower motor neurons perhaps by inhibiting depolarization of motor nerves and/or by blocking release of neurotransmitter acetylcholine at the neuromuscular junction. *Dermacentor* toxin is reported to block axonal sodium channels in motor neurons, whereas *Ixodidae* toxin mainly decreases release of acetylcholine from presynaptic motor nerve terminal. The nerve conduction blockade in both cases leads to hypotonia and hyporeflexia ultimately resulting in paresis or paralysis.

Clinical signs: Clinical signs of tick poisoning are usually observed 3-7 days after attachment of the ticks; however, the period preceding the onset of signs appears to depend on the rate of engorgement of ticks rather than on a fixed time period. The early signs of poisoning include lethargy, loss of appetite, anxiety, apprehension, retching, regurgitation, groaning when lifted, altered voice/bark, weakness in limbs and ataxia. Paresis begins in the pelvic limbs and ascends. The signs may become generalized in 2-3 days with quadriplegia and paralysis of different body systems or organs. Respiratory paralysis can occur within 5 days and saliva accumulates in dilated pharynx leading to gagging or choking sensation with drooling of saliva. Loss of voice, dyspnoea and secondary aspiratory pneumonia are observed in dogs and some other species. Difficulty in voiding urine and faces may be observed in some dogs and cats. There are usually no sensory deficits. Death occurs due to paralysis of respiratory muscles.

Post-mortem findings: Tick poisoning has no specific lesions. Trachea and bronchi may be filled with frothy fluid. Histologically, congestion may be observed in different organs including blood vessels, lungs, liver and kidneys.

Diagnosis: Diagnosis of tick poisoning is made from finding feeding female ticks on the host and clinical signs. Recovery upon removal of ticks and lack of occurrence in their absence confirms the diagnosis. There are no blood tests for toxin detection yet available.

Treatment and management: Tick poisoning has no specific antidote or treatment.

a. Ticks may be removed either manually or by using an appropriate ectoparasiticide. Removal of ticks normally results in marked improvement in animal's condition within 1-2 days.

b. Hyperimmune serum, if available, may be administered in dogs. Tick antiserum acts to neutralise the toxin at neuromuscular junction of skeletal muscle.

c. Sedatives such as benzodiazepines (e.g. diazepam) and opioid analgesics (e.g. morphine or buprenorphine) may be used either alone or in combination to calm the patient.

d. Other symptomatic and supportive treatment may be administered, if required.

Prognosis: Prognosis of tick poisoning depends on the stage of treatment. Complete recovery occurs if animal is treated early, whereas death may occur in untreated animal.

III. POISONOUS AMPHIBIANS

Amphibians are a diverse group of animals that have evolved numerous different adaptations to their environments. Most amphibians, if not all, often secrete fluids from secretory glands in the skin to prevent desiccation, control bacterial infection and discourage predator. These secretory glands are distributed throughout the skin of amphibians and are a source of poisoning in animals and humans. Although there are over 2,600 species of amphibians including frogs, toads and salamanders, the most important toxicologically being the toads belonging to family Bufonidae (true toads).

1. Toads

True toads belonging to family Bufonidae comprise large number of genera, with Bufo being the most widespread and known genus containing over 200 species. The Bufo toads inhabit a diverse range of environment conditions and occur natively on every continent except Australia and Antarctica. All toads belonging to the genus *Bufo* are considered toxic, but only some such as *Bufo marinus* (marine toad, giant toad), *B. alvarius* (river toad), and *B. vulgaris* (common toad) are commonly involved in poisoning of animals and human beings. The true toads have two lumps on either side of the back of their head, called the parotoid glands, and produce venom as methods of warding off intruders and predators.

Properties: Marine toad (*Bufo marinus*) is a large, lethargic toad that is indigenous to South and Central America. It can grow to 9 inches in length and about 1 kg in weight. Marine toads prefer developed areas, where they use man-made canals and ponds for spawning and collect under electric lights to feed on insects. Toad venom is thick, creamy-white, highly irritating substance secreted by glands located dorsal and posterior to the eyes and other dermal structures including warts. It is expelled quickly by contraction of periglandular muscles in the skin, especially when toads are threatened. The venom of marine toad is highly poisonous and harmful when ingested by small animals.

Toxic components: Toad venom contains a mixture of different classes of toxic chemicals. The concentrations of each of the different chemicals in toad venom (and therefore the toxicity of the venom) vary from species to species.

a. The first class of chemicals in toad venom includes the cardiac glycosides called bufodienolides. The bufodienolides comprises of two subgroups - bufogenins and their derivative bufotoxins. The cardiac glycosides in the venom are known for their effects on the cardiovascular system, including the heart and blood vessels.

b. The second class of chemicals in toad venom includes phenethylamines and their derivatives. These include catecholamines such as dopamine, noradrenaline and adrenaline. This class of chemicals are not as prominent as bufodienolides in producing the quick adverse effects in animals, but it is thought that they probably contribute to vasoconstriction.

c. The third class of chemicals consists of tryptamines and their derivatives. These include serotonin (5-hydroxytryptamine) and 5-hydroxy dimethyltryptamine (5-hydroxy DMT, bufotenine). This class of chemicals in toad toxin is thought to have oxytocic action and frequently a marked pressor effect. The 5-MeO-DMT (5-methoxy-N,N-dimethyltryptamine), a tryptaminergic derivative present only in the venom of *Bufo alvarius*, has significant hallucinogenic and/or psychoactive effect.

d. The fourth class of chemicals in toad venom includes non-cardiac sterols. These contain cholesterol, provitamin D, ergosterol, and gamma sitosteral. Their exact role in toxic effects is not clear.

Toxicity: The venom is produced by all toads, but its potency varies with species. *Bufo vulgaris* is least toxic and *Bufo marinus* is most toxic to animals. Most toad poisonings occur in dogs (mainly), cats and children. In dogs, severity of poisoning depends on the size of dog and the amount of toxin absorbed into blood stream. Puppies and small breed dogs such as Dachshunds, Mini-Pins, Jack Russell Terriers and miniature Schnauzers are more seriously affected because they get "more poison per kg body weight" than a large breed dog. Exposure to toad usually occurs when dogs attack or mouth the large, slow-moving toad. In children, handling the toad with naked hands and placing the contaminated fingers in their mouth causes poisoning. Bufo toads are most active in the spring and summer months when the environment is warm and moist. They are also nocturnal; therefore most poisonings occur in the evening, late-night or early-morning hours. A dog can die following one exposure to *B. marinus* toxin.

Mechanism of action: When a dog mouths or bites a Bufo toad the toxin is released and rapidly absorbed across the mucus membranes of the mouth. After absorption of the venom, the bufodienolides bind to a specific receptor site on the cardiac cell membrane and inhibit the Na^+/K^+ ATPase pump. Normally the Na^+/K^+-ATPase pumps sodium into the cell and potassium out of the cell. However when this pump is inhibited, the cell relies on the Na^+/Ca^{2+} pump to maintain its sodium gradient, which pumps sodium out and calcium in. This results in increased intracellular calcium concentration in cardiac cells and hence excessive cardiac stimulation and ventricular fibrillation. Failure of the Na^+/K^+-ATPase pump also results in an increased extracellular potassium concentration, resulting in hyperkalaemia Death occurs rapidly from heart failure. The overall action of bufodienolides is believed to be similar to that of digitalis.

Clinical signs: Signs of toad poisoning are variable and range from local effects to systematic effects. Local effects in dogs are immediate and include profuse and sometimes frothy salivation, vigorous head shaking, pawing at mouth and retching. These are due to extremely irritant nature of the venom. With more severe intoxication, cardiac arrhythmias, dyspnoea, diarrhoea, incoordination or stiff gait, cyanosis, apparent blindness, convulsions, prostration and collapse are characteristic. Ventricular fibrillation precedes death from heart failure. In general, morbidity rates are high.

Post-mortem findings: Distinctive lesions are not present in toad poiosning.

Diagnosis: Diagnosis of toad poisoning is usually based on seeing a dog or cat mouthing a toad, or finding a toad or toad pieces in vomitus, if symptoms have already occurred. Circumstantial evidences and clinical signs may also help in the diagnosis. Haematological and clinical chemistry changes in toad poisoning include increase in packed cell volume (PCV), blood glucose, blood urea nitrogen, potassium and calcium levels.

Treatment and management: There is no specific antidote for Bufo-toxin and treatment consists mainly of supportive care.

a. The mouth of dog should be immediately and thoroughly flushed with water from a slow-moving stream from a garden pipe/hose. The toxin is very sticky, so it may need to be gently rubbed off of the mucus membranes of mouth.

b. Detoxification with activated charcoal and an osmotic cathartic is recommended.

c. A large dose of propranolol (up to 2 mg/kg) may be used to control cardiac arrhythmia and potential fibrillation. Any other β_1- adrenoceptor blocker may also be used.

d. Atropine may help to control salivation and potential bronchoconstriction.

e. CNS excitation, if present, should be controlled by pentobarbitone or diazepam, or a combination of the two.

Prognosis: Prognosis of toad poisoning is good to guarded, if prompt intervention and detoxification are followed by appropriate supportive therapy.

IV. POISONOUS REPTILES

Reptiles are cold-blooded vertebrates of the class Reptilia, comprising a large number of animals such as snakes, crocodiles, alligators, lizards, and turtles. They inhabit every continent except for Antarctica, although their main distribution comprises the tropics and subtropics. Poisonous reptiles of veterinary or medical importance include snakes and lizards. Wide spread problems in domestic animals are more frequently associated with the poisonous snakes and less with lizards.

1. Snakes

Snakes are long, slender, reptile of order Serpentes. Snakes are probably the most recognised of all venomous animals. Snakes and snakebites have been extensively studied because of the vast number and complexity of these species and their venoms. Most of the cases of snakebite have been reported in dogs and horses, although other species of animals are also affected.

Types of snake and properties: Snakes may be poisonous and non-poisonous. It is essential to differentiate the two types for effective understanding of snake envenomation.

a. Venomous/Poisonous snakes: There are more than 3500 different species of snakes out of which about 600 species have been found to be poisonous. The tail of venomous snakes are usually compressed and flat, and the scales on the head are

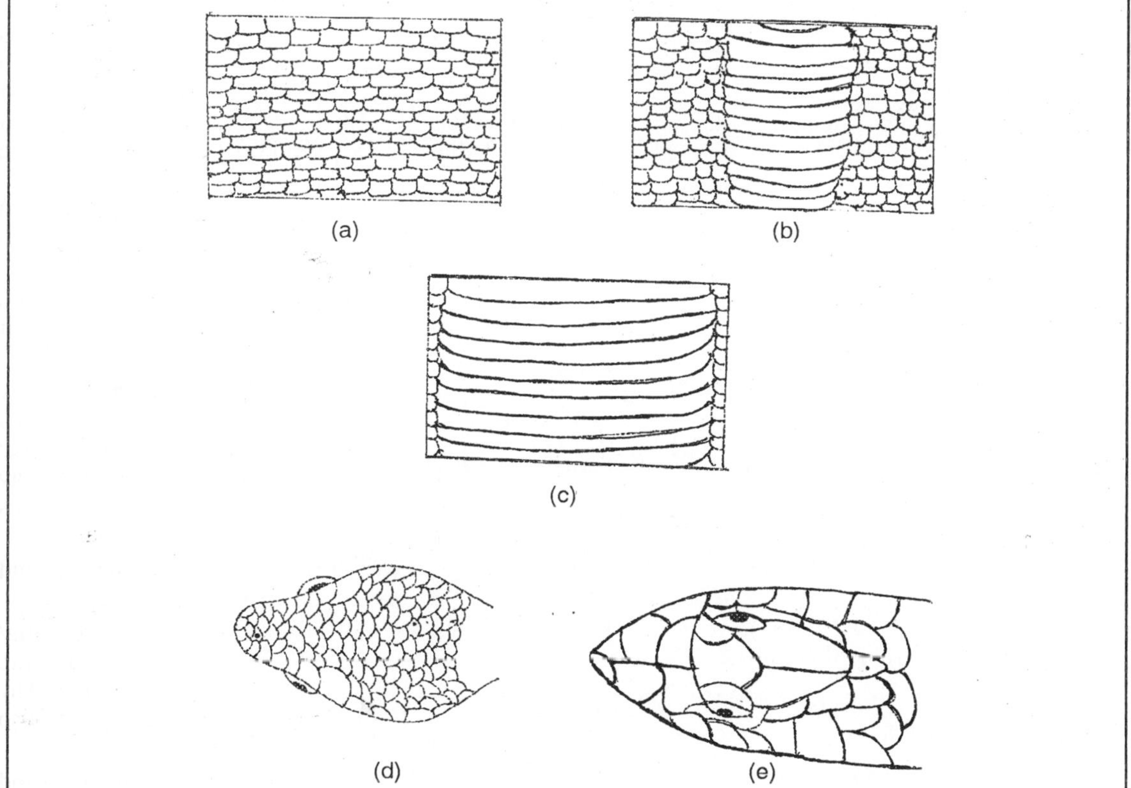

Fig.16.1. Identification of poisonous and non-poisonous snakes.

Belly upwards :

a. If the belly scales are small like those on the back, the snake is not poisonous.

b. Moderately large belly scales that do not cover the entire breadth suggest that snake is not poisonous.

c. Large belly scales that cover the entire breadth suggest that snake may be poisonous or non-poisonous.

Top of the head :

d. Small scales on the head suggest that snake is poisonous and one of the vipers.

e. Large scales on the head suggest that snake may be non-poisonous or poisonous.

small (e.g. vipers) or large. The venomous snakes possess two grooved or tubular fangs or poison teeth. Bite marks usually show clear puncture wounds of fangs with or without small marks of other teeth.

b. Non-venomous/non-poisonous snakes: There are several species of non-venomous snakes. Their tails are not markedly compressed and in most of varieties the belly is covered with transverse plates that, however, do not extend completely across it. They possess several small teeth attached to a short maxillary bone and have no long and grooved fangs like the poisonous variety. Their bite leaves a semicircular set of teeth marks. At the site of bite, there is absence of oedema even after many hours.

Venomous snakes: Venomous snakes belong to several families of snakes such as Elapidae, Crotalidae, Viperidae, Hydrophiidae and Colubridae, but for toxicological purposes they have been grouped into two main classes: elapines and viperines.

i. *Elapines:* The elapines belong mainly to the family Elapidae or cobra family and include cobra (nag), mambas, kraits and coral snakes. Elapine snakes have short fangs and tend to hang on and "chew" venom into their victims. Their head is of about the same width as that of the neck and the pupils of their eyes are circular. Their third labial touches the eye and nasal shields (see figure 16.2). Their venom is mainly neurotoxic and results in paralysis of the respiratory centre. Animals that survive their bite seldom have any sequelae.

ii. *Viperines:* There are two types of viperines: the true vipers/pitless vipers belonging to family Viperidae (e.g. puff adder and Russell's viper) and the pit vipers belonging to the family Crotalidae (e.g. rattlesnakes and copperhead). Pit vipers are those which have a pit or a deep depression on each side of the head between the eye and the nostrils. Pitless vipers are those which have no pit on the head. Viperine snakes have broad plates on the belly extending right across and the pupil is like vertically elliptical slits. The vipers have long and strong fangs, so that they can easily bite through the clothes unlike elapines which have short fangs that cannot bite through clothes. The elapines must close the lower jaw before they can inject venom, whereas the vipers can do so without closing the lower jaw. Viperine venom is typically haematotoxic, necrotising and anticoagulant, although a neurotoxic component is also present in the venom of some species.

The venom glands are homologues of the parotid glands and situated below and behind the eyes, one on each side. The two grooved or tubular fangs or poison teeth communicate by means of

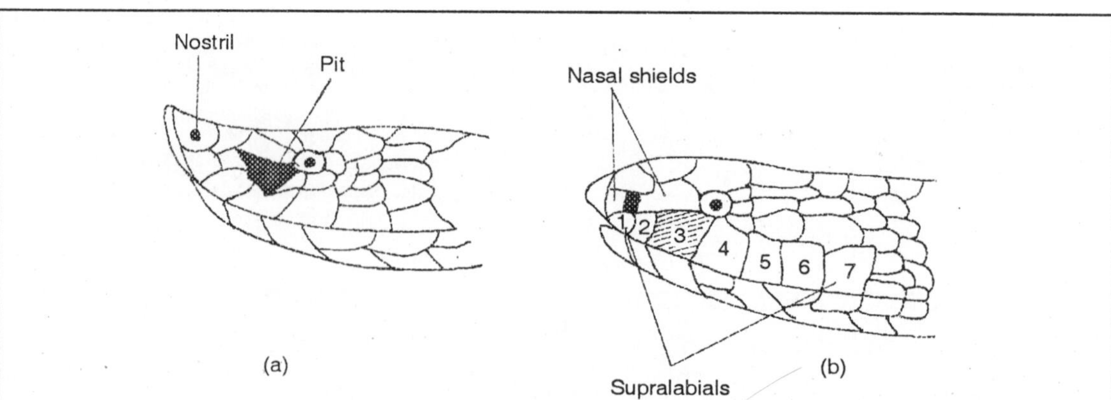

Fig.16.2. Identification of pit vipers and other snakes.

a. If there is a conspicuous opening or 'pit' between the eye and the nostril, it is poisonous and one of the pit vipers.

b. If the 3rd labial touches the eye and nasal shields, it is poisonous, being a cobra or a coral snake.

duct with the racemose glands secreting venom, a secretion meant for digestion. The whole mechanism is so arranged that all the venom secreted by glands is discharged without any leakage when the fangs penetrate the skin.

Toxic components: Snake venom is highly concentrated clear amber coloured digestive juice of the snake. It is a complex mixture of amino acids, proteins, enzymes, biogenic amines, metals and other inorganic substances. The venom of some species may contain up to 20 or more different components. However, relatively little is known about the composition of most venoms.

Proteins : Large numbers of enzymatic and non-enzymatic proteins occur in snake venom.

a. *Enzymes:* Snake venom contains about 26 enzymes. However, no single venom contains all of these. Some enzymes are usually present in all types of venoms. Others are scattered in different families and genera.

i. Proteolytic enzymes (e.g. proteases): They digest tissue proteins. Proteases are also implicated in the anticoagulation events.

ii. Hyaluronidase: It solubilises glycosidic bonds and dissolves intercellular gel of the connective tissue and thus helps in the rapid spread of venom.

iii. Phosphodiesterases: These interfere with the prey's cardiac system, mainly by lowering the blood pressure.

iv. ATPases: These metabolise ATP to disrupt the prey's energy fuel use.

v. Acetylcholinesterase: It hydrolyses acetylcholine and interferes with neurotransmission in neuromuscular junction. Neuromuscular blockade make the prey lose control of its muscles.

vi. Phospholipases A, B and C : They hydrolyse phospholipids and release saturated and unsaturated fatty acids. Phospholipase A is a strong haemolytic and mycotoxic agent that contributes to cardiotoxicity.

vii. Lipases: They cause hydrolysis of lipids, thus destroying membranes.

viii. Collagenase: It digests collagen.

ix. Ribonuclease: It acts against ribonucleic acids (RNA).

x. Deoxyribonuclease: It acts against deoxyribonucleic acids (DNA).

xi. Ophio-oxidase : It helps in autolysis and putrefaction.

xii. Thrombin like enzyme : It causes fibrinogen clot formation.

xiii. L-Amino acid oxidase : It gives yellow colour to the venom and catalyses oxidation of L-α-amino and α-hydroxy acids. It also triggers some other enzymes.

b. *Non-enzymatic proteins:* Several low molecular weight peptides or polypeptides with no enzymatic activity also occur in snake venom. These include neurotoxins, haemorrhagins, cardiotoxins, myotoxins, cytolisins, and toxalbumins. The neurotoxicity mainly occurs due to presence of certain peptides, amides, or polypeptides. Haemorrhagins present in the crotalid venom are vasculotoxic causing haemorrhage and shock. Myotoxins cause muscle necrosis and myoglobinurea and cytolisins cause tissue necrosis.

Non-protein toxins: In addition to proteins, large numbers of other components like lipids, steroids, glycoproteins, amines, metals (Na, Ca, K, Mg, Zn, Co, Ni, Fe, etc.) have been identified in the snake venom and may play important roles in the envenomation.

Factors affecting toxicity:

a. Snake venom envenomation is more common in people and animals living in regions inhabited by venomous snakes.

b. Severity of envenomation depends on the species of snake involved, its age and size, number and depth of bites, and total quantity of venom injected.

c. Fatal snake bites are common in dogs due to their relatively small size and their nature of attacking snakes. It is less common in cats as cats avoid snakes. Horses and cattle seldom die (except when bitten on head or neck) as a direct result of snake bite due to their large size. However on the basis of per kg body weight, horses are more susceptible to venom than any other species. Pigs are less susceptible due to poor absorption of venom through layers of subcutaneous fat.

d. Snake bite near the head region (i.e. muzzle, lips, neck) is more toxic than other parts of body. In large animals (horses and cattle), bite near head and neck results in excessive swelling and dyspnoea which may be fatal.

e. Snake venom injected directly into the blood stream is more toxic than injected into relatively non-vascular areas (e.g. fat).

f. Not all bites by snakes result in envenomation: so called "dry bites" may range from 30-70% of total bites depending upon the species and conditions. The amount of venom injected is regulated by the snake.

g. If there has been a previous bite, the victim develops some degree of humoral immunity and is less vulnerable to the toxic effect of the venom.

Toxicity: Snake bite occurs most often when animals graze, hunt or play in infested areas. Small animals are usually bitten on head, body or extremities (i.e. muzzle and legs). Large animals are generally bitten on legs and muzzle. Toxicity of viperine venoms can vary substantially e.g. less than 2 mg/kg body weight in rattlesnake venom and more than 10 mg/kg in copper head venom. A large rattlesnake can yield more than 500 mg of venom, compared to copperheads which may yield less than 75 mg of venom. Elapine snake venom is required in less than 1 mg/kg to produce envenomation, however venom yield is usually small (i.e. less than 6 mg per snake). Incidence of snake bite is highest in summer.

Toxicokinetics: The venom is deposited with help of fangs by the snake into the victim's body. Once deposited, it is rapidly distributed in the body. If the venom is deposited directly into a vein, toxicological effects ensue very rapidly. Snake venom is biotransformed to variable amounts and largely excreted via the kidneys.

Mechanism of action: The mechanism of action of snake venom is complex and has not been fully understood. The action also varies with the types of toxin present in the venom. The effects of venom include neurotoxicity, haematotoxicity, myotoxicity, nephrotoxicity, and necrotoxicity (local tissue damage). The venom of elapine snakes is primarily neurotoxic, whereas that of viperines is mostly haematotoxic. Some snakes contain venom having combinations of both neurotoxins and haematotoxins.

Neurotoxicity: Venoms often contain different neurotoxins that work synergistically to cripple the nervous system. Death from neurotoxins results from the paralysis of respiratory muscles or respiratory centre in the medulla. The neurotoxins can be further classified according to their site of action: post-synaptic neurotoxins and pre-synaptic neurotoxins.

i. Post-synaptic neurotoxins primarily bind to cholinergic receptors in the neuromuscular junctions and antagonise action of acetylcholine on skeletal muscles. These post-synaptic neurotoxins produce curare-like effects and cause paralysis. Some venoms, in addition, contain acetylcholinesterase enzyme that destroys neurotransmitter acetylcholine, which might compete with the toxin for receptor binding. The post-synaptic neurotoxins are found only in elapids and sea snakes (*Hydrophiidae*).

ii. Pre-synaptic neurotoxins inhibit the release of acetylcholine at the myoneural junctions and block neurotransmission. The venom of elapids such as banded krait contains such pre-synaptic neurotoxins. In many-banded krait, the pre-synaptic toxin is β-bungarotoxin, while the post-synaptic toxins are α- and κ-bungarotoxins.

Haematotoxicity: Haematotoxic venom attacks the circulatory system and muscle tissue causing coagulopathies, cardiotoxicity, and haemolysis. Haematotoxic bites are the most painful due to rapid death of tissues.

a. *Coagulopathies:* Both anticoagulant and procoagulant properties have been identified but bleeding disorders due to defective coagulation occur most commonly.

i. Anticoagulation: Anticoagulation results from various constituents of snake venom that may:

- Interfere with activation of clotting factors.
- Have fibrinolytic and fibrinogenolytic factors.

- Directly or indirectly activate plasminogen.
- Directly act on phospholipids.

ii. Procoagulation : Some constituents of snake venom promote clotting of blood.

- Snake venom constituents may interact at various points of the coagulation cascade to activate clotting factors or even prothrombin directly. Significant amounts of thrombin-like enzymes have been identified in the venom of viperine snakes. Disseminated intravascular coagulation (DIC) may complicate severe cases.
- Some venoms have ability to coagulate pure fibrinogen in *vitro* without calcium ions, tissue extract and prothrombin. Proteolytic enzymes in them convert fibrinogen into fibrillar gel, while other venoms cannot coagulate fibrinogen but convert prothrombin to thrombin.

b. *Cardiotoxicity:* Cardiovascular shock is a common cause of death in snake bite. Shock results from increased capillary permeability and intravascular volume depletion. Reduced cardiac output secondary to venom-induced cardiac changes as well as the release of mediators such as bradykinin, histamine and serotonin may contribute to haemodynamic compromise.

c. *Haemolysis:* Haemorrhagins that cause haemolysis of the blood corpuscles, haemohagines that cause decomposition of the mucous membranes, and leucolysins that cause disintegration of the white blood cells are other modes of producing haematotoxicity.

Local toxic effects: Envenomation by viperine (mainly) and elapine snakes may result in significant local toxic effects. Pain, swelling and oedema occur soon after the bite. Vesicles may also appear which are usually filled with clear fluid but may be filled with blood in severe cases. Local necrosis and gangrene formation may occur due to either direct effect of venom enzymes or interruption of blood supply due to haematotoxic effects.

Other effects: Numerous other systemic effects have been associated with snake bites. A direct nephrotoxic effect of the venom is postulated as the primary cause of renal failure in viperine envenomation. Respiratory distress syndrome may develop in severe cases. The aetiology is unclear, but shock and disseminated intravascular coagulation are postulated.

Clinical signs :

Viperines: Typical pit viper bites are characterised by severe local tissue damage and pain that spreads rapidly from the bite site. Severe pain generally causes restlessness, anxiety and excitement, which is followed by incoordination of movement and lameness. Marked discolouration of tissues occurs within few minutes and dark, bloody fluid may ooze from the fang wounds, if not prevented by swelling. Frequently, the epidermis sloughs when the overlying hair is clipped or merely parted. The skin becomes cold, pupils are dilated which responds poorly to light, and animal does not respond to external stimuli like pinching and pricking. This is followed by unconsciousness and collapse. In small animals, there may be vomiting, hypotension with tachycardia, pulmonary oedema, salivation, diarrhoea, convulsions, renal failure and shock. Death is due to respiratory or circulatory failure. If the animal survives for a few days, then there is extensive local suppuration, sloughing and gangrene, and malignant oedema or tetanus may supervene. Death in such cases may occur from septicaemia. In large animals, death may not occur directly from venom (except when bitten on head or neck region) due to insufficient toxin injection, but from a serious secondary bacterial infection that sets up in the local swelling.

Elapines: In elapine snakebites, the pain and swelling are minimal but systemic neurological signs predominate. There is muscular weakness developing into paralysis. As the swallowing becomes difficult, the viscid saliva and food collects in mouth. Pharyngeal paralysis can result in aspiration pneumonia. Consciousness is usually retained till end. In a bite from krait, violent abdominal pain and convulsions may precede death. In calves, effects of the neurotoxin are manifested by marked pupillary dilatation, excitement, incoordination and later paralysis. In dogs, there is vomiting, salivation, defecation, tremors, and convulsions. Death is due to respiratory paralysis. Death usually occurs within 6 hours in elapine and 2-4 days in viperine snake bite. However, if the venom is injected directly into a vein death may occur very soon.

Post-mortem findings: Lesions resulting from snake bite are two lacerated punctures i.e. fang marks about 1.25 cm deep in elapines and about 2.5 cm deep in case of viperines. Many times fang marks are visible only with lens. There is acute swelling, oedema, ecchymotic to suffusion haemorrhages, and haematomas in the affected area. Necropsy may reveal haemorrhagic interstitial nephritis, toxic proliferative glomerulitis, intracerebral haemorrhages, and necrosis of liver.

Diagnosis: Diagnosis of snake bite is often difficult unless the snake has been seen. Recognition of fang marks also helps in diagnosis, but is difficult to find in animals having long fur, hair or wool. In suspected cases, history, circumstantial evidences, clinical signs and lesions may be carefully considered for proper diagnosis. An immunoassay diagnosis for the detection of snake bites has been developed in human medicine, but is not freely available in animals. Owner should be instructed, when ever possible, to bring the dead snake along with the bitten animal and they should be warned not to mutilate the snake's head since identification may depend on the head's morphology. Many bites are made only by non-poisonous snakes. Laboratory findings are not specific but may include elevated plasma creatine kinase released from degenerated muscles (it may be normal in too early or too late cases), extended clotting time, haemoglobinuria, or myoglobinuria.

Snake bite should be carefully differentiated from tick paralysis, botulism, anthrax, black leg and polyradiculoneuritis.

Treatment and management: Treatment should be instituted as soon as possible because irreversible effects of venom begin immediately after the snake-bite.

Specific therapy

Antivenin: Antivenin therapy is the most important point in therapy. The choice of antivenin depends on the species of snake involved and available form of antivenin. Antivenin may be monovalent (activity against one species) or polyvalent (activity against two or more species of snakes). If available, monovalent antivenin is preferable when offending species of snake is known with certainty. A polyvalent horse-serum-origin antivenin is available against all cases of substantial pit envenomation. The dose of antivenin is dependant on the species of snake, the particular antivenin and the severity of envenomation. Antivenin should be administered as soon as possible after the bite as delayed administration often diminishes its effect. As antivenins are derived from hyper-immunised horse serum and contain concentrated purified immunoglobulin, so chances of immediate or delayed immune reaction may occur in some patients. So this therapy must be pre-tested or potential risks and benefits from the therapy must be weighed and if required 0.5-1 ml of 1 : 1000 adrenaline should be administered subcutaneously.

In smaller animals, dose of antivenin per kg body weight basis is more as they also receive more venom per kg body weight. Total dose in small dogs is up to 100 ml of which 5-10 ml may be injected into the tissues around the bite and remainder is given by I.V. route.

Supportive therapy: This includes number of agents and measures. The supportive therapy involves many controversial points:

a. The animal should be kept calm and quiet. Tranquilization in horses may be required.

b. The bitten limb or extremity should be immobilised to retard the absorption and distribution of venom in the body. In animals, immobilisation of a part can be done with the help of sand bags or splints.

c. Spread of venom from the bitten area may be minimized by tying a piece of cord, bandage or strip of cloth at some distance above the site of wound, if the bite is on an extremity, to stop lymphatic circulation in the affected part. However, the knot must be slackened for a few seconds at regular intervals of ten minutes and should not be kept for more than half an hour. This is useful in the management of elapine snake bite but contraindicated following bites by snakes that cause tissue necrosis such as viperines. Icepacks are also used locally but are contraindicated in viperine snake bite.

d. Incisiòn and suction at the bite is generally impractical and potentially dangerous by mouth. It may be beneficial in a few select cases when it can be performed within a few minutes (maximum up to 1 hour) by an expert using appropriate equipment i.e. breast pump or any other cupping device. Incision if incorrectly done can lead to spread of venom and may exacerbate tissue damage and introduce infection.

e. Fluid therapy (e.g. lactated Ringer's solution) may be required to prevent or control shock especially in pit viper envenomation.

f. Rapid acting corticosteroids may be useful to control shock, protect against tissue damage and minimise likelihood of allergic reactions to antivenin. However, use of corticosteroids in snake bite is controversial.

g. Anti-histamines are contraindicated where local tissue damage is evident but some agent like diphenhydramine (10-25 mg I.V. or S.C. for dogs) are frequently used to reduce anxiety and to prevent allergic reactions associated with antivenin.

h. Tetanus antitoxin should be administered to avoid clostridial infection after snake bite.

i. Blood transfusion should be instituted in case of haemolytic or anticoagulant venoms.

j. Analgesics should be used to control severe bite pain.

k. Broad-spectrum antibiotics should be given to prevent wound infection and other secondary infections. Antibiotics should be continued until all superficial lesions have healed.

Contraindications

a. Application of chemicals (e.g. potassium permanganate) to the incised bite area is of no value and may exacerbate tissue damage.

b. Alcohol should not be used to clean the wound because it causes vasodilation and would promote uptake and spread of venom.

Prognosis: Prognosis depends upon the area of bite, size of animal, time since envenomation has occurred, type of snake and level of supportive care. If the animal survives initial few hours and is not in shock condition, the prognosis is favourable.

2. Lizards

The only poisonous lizard known is the Gila Monster or Beaded Lizard (*Heloderma suspectum*) found in the desert regions of south-western United States and northern Mexico. Gila Monsters are identified by their beaded skin (as opposed to scales), distinct colour banding of black and red or black and yellow/orange and big size (up to 2 feet long). These animals are heavy, slow moving lizard, which spend about 80% of their life underground but become more active at the surface during spring season. The Gila Monster bites with its teeth rather than fangs and the venom enters the bite wound by dripping down grooves in the teeth. Unlike venomous snakes, these lizards tend to hang on to their victims, making them hard to remove once they have bitten. The venom of Gila Monster is mainly neurotoxic, which is secreted into the lizard's saliva. Poisonous lizards do not generally bite unless they are handled or disturbed.

The jaws of Gila Monster are strong, so their bite can cause a crushing or compression injury. These injuries can cause severe swelling and may damage underlying tissues, blood vessels, nerves, joints, or bones. Symptoms at the site of bite may include moderate to severe bleeding, swelling, and severe throbbing or burning pain. The localized signs may be followed by generalized weakness, nausea, vomiting, and dyspnoea. The venom also contains several pathogens, which may produce secondary infection. Treatment of poisonous lizard bite includes only supportive care as followed in a general snake bite. The Gila Monster bite is rarely reported in humans and animals.

V. POISONOUS FISHES

There are several species of venomous fish, which are capable of producing poisoning in humans and animals. The fish produce poisoning in one of three ways: by attacking and biting (e.g. sharks and barracudas), by injecting toxic venom through their venomous spines or tentacles (e.g. stingrays), and through eating fish whose flesh is toxic (e.g. puffer fish). The fish venoms injected through spines or bites cause intense pain and are potentially fatal. However, the danger of actually encountering one of these dangerous fish is negligible in animals. Fish poisoning in animals mostly occur when dogs and certain other animals and birds are being fed fish or fish meal in their feed.

1. Tetrodotoxic Fish / Pufferfish Poisoning

Tetrodotoxic fish contain a potent marine neurotoxin tetrodotoxin (TTX) and cause a syndrome commonly called tetrodotoxication. The members of the tetrodotoxic fish belong to the order Tetraodontiformes (*tetras*-four and *odontos*-tooth) or the tetraodon pufferfish and include the genera *Tetraodon* (*T. fahaka, T. miurus and T. mbu*), *Fugu* (*F. flavidus, F. poecilonotus* and *F. niphobles*) and *Takifugu* (*Takifugu rubripes*). Some other marine and terrestrial animals that can store TTX include starfish, certain crabs, molluscs, toads, salamanders and algae. Tetrodotoxin poisoning has been reported in pet animals (carnivores) and human beings eating the toxic fish

Properties: The pufferfish, belonging to order Tetraodontiformes and family Tetraodontidae, contain more than 120 species in 19 genera, some of which are potentially toxic. They are mostly found in coastal regions though some are oceanic or live in deep sea. Pufferfish are named for their ability to inflate themselves to several times their normal size by swallowing water or air when threatened. These fish are equipped with four large teeth that are nearly fused, forming a beak-like structure used for crushing the shells of molluscs and crustaceans, their natural prey. In some pufferfish, a powerful neurotoxin is present in the internal organs, mainly as a defence chemical used to subdue or kill the predators. This neurotoxin is found primarily in the ovaries and liver, although smaller amounts exist in intestines and skin as well. The meat of pufferfish is considered a delicacy in Japan and Korea, when prepared carefully by an expert by removing the toxic organs.

Toxic components: Pufferfish contains a potent toxin called tetrodotoxin (anhydrotetrodotoxin 4-epitetrodotoxin, tetrodonic acid) with a molecular formula of $C_{11}H_{17}O_8N_3$ (Figure 16.3). The oxygen link between C_5 and C_{10} in tetrodotoxin seems to be essential, if the derivatives are to be toxic. The puffer fish do not make tetrodotoxin in their body; instead this toxin is produced within the pufferfish by certain bacteria such as *Pseudoalteromonas tetraodonis* and some species of *Pseudomonas* and *Vibrio*, which are acquired through food. Saxitoxin, the cause of PSP (paralytic shellfish poisoning), can also be found in pufferfish.

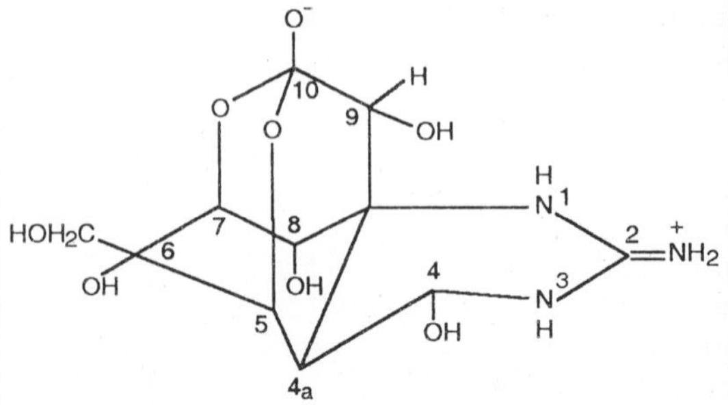

Fig.16.3. Chemical structure of tetradotoxin.

Toxicity: Pufferfish poisoning usually occurs as a result of accidental consumption of fish or meat tainted with pufferfish and is mostly seen in carnivores and humans. Weight-for-weight, tetrodotoxin is considered ten times as deadly as the venom of many snakes, 10 to 100 times as lethal as black widow spider venom and more than 1200 times deadlier than cyanide. The LD_{50} of tetrodotoxin in mice by I.V. route is 10 μg/kg, which is almost the same as for saxitoxin. However, tetrodotoxin when taken orally is absorbed much better than that of saxitoxin. Its fatal dose in humans is about 1-2 mg which is approximately equivalent to 1 g of the ovary from a highly toxic species captured during winter (it is more toxic in winter). It is estimated that a single pufferfish has enough poison to kill 30 adult humans. However, toxicity varies between species of pufferfish and at different seasons and geographic localities. The flesh of many pufferfish may not usually be dangerously toxic.

Mechanism of action: Tetrodotoxin is a potent neurotoxin that acts by blocking neurotransmission in the central and peripheral (i.e. autonomic, somatic, sensory nerves) nervous systems. The toxin rapidly reaches the voltage-gated Na^+-channels on the surface of nerve membranes and strongly binds at the pore opening (mouth) of the channel. It is proposed that this binding results from the interaction of positively charged guanidino group on the tetrodotoxin and negatively charged carboxylate groups on the side chains in the mouth of channel. This binding blocks the sodium channels as a result of which sodium movement is completely shut down and the action potential along the nerve membrane is stopped. The toxin also blocks the fast Na^+ current in myocytes (contractile cells of heart), thereby inhibiting their contraction. The pufferfish itself has immunity to the poison due to a mutation in the protein sequence of the sodium channel pump on cell membranes.

Clinical signs: The first clinical signs of tetrodotoxin intoxication may appear between 20 minutes to three hours after eating the poisonous pufferfish. The toxicity has been well described in human beings and includes numbness of lips, tongue and fingers followed by nausea, vomiting, epigastric pain, muscular paralysis of extremities, ataxia, and respiratory distress. Speech is affected and the victim usually exhibits dyspnea, cyanosis, and hypotension. Paralysis increases and convulsions, mental impairment, cardiac arrhythmia and unconsciousness may occur. Death usually occurs within 4 to 6 hours from respiratory paralysis..

Post-mortem findings: Tetrodotoxin poisoning has no specific lesions.

Diagnosis: Diagnosis of tetrodotoxin can be made from history of eating fish, circumstantial evidence and clinical signs.

Treatment and management: Tetrodotoxin is not antigenic so no antiserum is available. Treatment consists of only intestinal detoxification with gastric lavage and activated charcoal and supportive care (e.g. artificial respiration). Case reports suggest that anticholinesterase agents such as edrophonium may be useful; however, their efficacy is not certain. Treatment is mostly unsuccessful.

2. Ciguatera

Ciguatera is a fish-borne poisoning of humans and pets caused by eating certain marine fish that bioaccumulate a toxin called ciguatoxin (CTX) synthesized by certain marine micro-organisms, especially the micro-algae *Gambierdiscus toxicus* living in tropical water. The fish commonly associated with ciguatera poisoning include over 400 species of reef fish (fish living in warm tropical waters), particularly the predator species near the top of food chain such as barracuda, moray eel, red snapper and grouper.

Ciguatoxin is a lipid soluble and very heat resistant toxin, so it is not destroyed by temperature, gastric acid or cooking method. Presence of toxin does not affect odour, colour, or taste of the fish. In mice, CTX is lethal at 0.45 μg/kg, IP. Oral intake of as little as 0.1 μg ciguatoxin can cause illness in humans. Ciguatoxin produces toxic effects by causing opening of voltage dependant sodium channels in cell membranes which induces membrane depolarization. The toxic signs of ciguatera in human beings are gastrointestinal distress (nausea, vomiting and diarrhoea) followed by neurological symptoms such as headache, muscle ache, numbness, ataxia, and hallucination. Severe cases of ciguatera can also result in hot-cold reversal, in which hot and cold sensations seem reversed. The toxic symptoms can last from weeks to months and in extreme cases for many years, but the poisoning is rarely lethal. Ciguatoxin has been found to be excreted in milk and can be transmitted sexually. Although not completely reliable, an immunoassay and a mouse biological assay are available for detection of ciguatoxin in affected fish.

Treatment of ciguatera has been to a large extent symptomatic. Gut emptying and decontamination with charcoal is recommended in acute cases, although the severe ongoing vomiting and diarrhoea may prevent it. A variety of agents including vitamins, antihistamines, anticholinesterases, steroids and tricyclic antidepressants have been tried with limited results. Intravenous mannitol (1 g/kg) has been found effective when administered within 72 hours of exposure. Avoidance of consumption of all reef fish is the only sure way to avoid exposure to the toxin.

3. Scombroid Fish / Scombroid Poisoning

Scombroid poisoning is a type of food borne illness caused by the consumption of scombroid and scombroid-like marine fish species that have begun to spoil with the growth of particular types of bacteria. Fish most commonly involved are members of the scombridae family (tunas and mackerels) and few non-scombridae fish (bluefish, dolphin or mahi-mahi, and amberjack). Scombroid poisoning has been attributed to the histamine produced by bacterial decarboxylation of the amino acid histidine, concentration of which is high in fish. Histamine concentrations can reach up to 5 mg/g in fish. As ingestion of pure histamine has low toxicity in humans and animals (histamine is rapidly destroyed in GI tract), it is suggested that other substances in fish such as putrescine and cadaverine trigger the toxicity of histamine.

Clinical signs of scombroid poisoning can become evident within few minutes to two hours following consumption of contaminated fish and generally resemble allergic reactions due to histamine. Initial signs include nausea, vomiting, diarrhoea, dizziness and abdominal pain. These initial signs can advance to skin rash, hives, oedema, urticaria, tachycardia, hypotension and respiratory stress. The poisoning usually runs its course within 16 hours with no lasting ill effects. Fatalities are very rare. Treatment of scombroid poisoning is mainly supportive in the form of IV fluids and oxygen. Administration of H_1- and H_2- receptor antagonists provides some success.

BIBLIOGRAPHY

Banerji P (1985) Handbook of Snake-bite. International Books and Periodical Supply Service, New Delhi.

Bartik M and Piskac A (1981) Veterinary Toxicology. Elsevier Scientific Publishing Company, Amsterdam.

Beasley V (1999) Veterinary Toxicology. International Veterinary Information Service, Ithaca NY (www.ivis.org).

Benzer TI (2007) Toxicity, tetrodotoxin. eMedicine. (http://www.emedicine.com/emerg/topic576.htm).

Berger RS (1984) Management of brown recluse spider bite. *J. Am. Med. Assoc.* 251 : 889.

Clarke ECG and Clarke ML (1967) Garner's Veterinary Toxicology. 3rd edn. Williams and Wilkins, Baltimore.

Dunn TJ (2002) Snake bites and dogs. Dog World magazine. (http://www.thepetcenter.com/ exa/sb.html).

Fenner PJ, Williamson JA and Skinner RA (1989) Fatal and non-fatal stingray envenomation. *Med. J. Aust.* 151 : 621.

Fischer N (2006) Tick Poisoning in Animals – In Depth. (http://www.tickalert.org.au/paraldet.htm).

Garg SK (2000) Veterinary Toxicology. CBS Publishers & Distributors, New Delhi.

Gopalakrishnakone P and Tan CK (1987) Progress in Venom and Toxin Research. National University of Singapore, Singapore.

Hardy DL (1986) Fatal rattlesnake envenomation in Arizona. 1969-84. *J. Toxicol. Clin Toxicol.* 24 : 1.

Harvey AL (1991) Snake Toxins. Pergamon Press, New York.

Hashimoto Y (1979) Marine Toxins and other Bioactive Marine Metabolites. Japan Scientific Societies Press, Tokyo.

Hoffman DR, Doover DE and Jacobson RS (1988) Allergens in hymenoptera venom. *J. Allergy Clin. Immunol.* 82 : 828.

Johnson J (2002) Tetrodotoxin: An ancient alkaloid from the sea. (http://www.chm.bris.ac.uk/motm/ttx/ttx.htm).

Narahashi T (1972) Mechanism of tetrodotoxin and saxitoxin on excitable membrane. *Fed. Proc.* 31 : 1124.

Osweiler GD (1996) Toxicology. Williams and Wilkins, Philadelphia.

Rodostits O M, Gay C C, Blood D C and Hinchcliff K W (2000) Veterinary Medicine: A Textbook of the Diseases of Cattle, Sheep, Pigs, Goats and Horses. 9th edn. W. B. Saunders, London.

Russell FE (1996) Toxic effects of animal toxins. In: Casarett & Doull's Toxicology: The Basic Science of Poisons. 5th edn. Klaassen CD (Ed.) p 801. Mcgraw Hill Companies Inc., New York.

Tu AT (1973) Neurotoxins of animal venoms: Snakes. *Ann. Rev. Biochem.* 42 : 235.

Tu AT (1977) Venoms: Chemistry and Molecular Biology. John Wiley and Sons, New York.

Wedin GP (1995) Poisons of animal origin. In: General and Applied Toxicology. Ballantyne B, Marrs T and Turner P (Eds.) p 1243. Macmillan Press Ltd., London.

Wikipedia (2007) Snake venom. (http://en.wikipedia.org/wiki/Snake_venom).

World Health Organization (1984) Aquatic (Marine and Freshwater) Biotoxins. WHO Publications Center U.S.A. Albany, New York.

❑❑❑❑❑❑

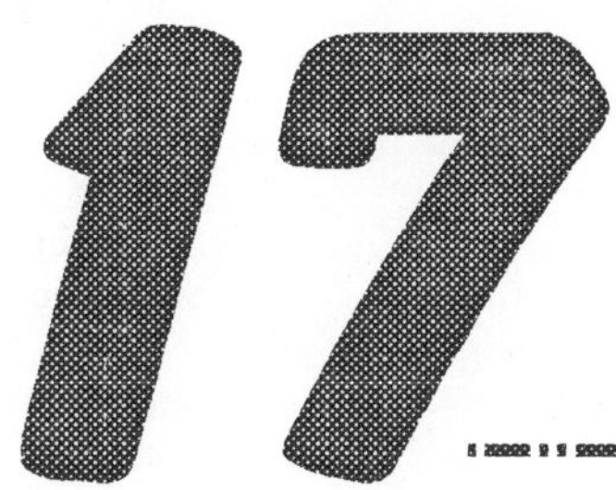

ENVIRONMENTAL POLLUTANTS

Air pollutants
- Primary pollutants
  - Carbon monoxide
  - Carbon dioxide
  - Sulphur dioxide gases
  - Nitrogen oxide gases
  - Smoke and other particulate matter
  - Hydrocarbons
  - Pesticides
- Secondary pollutants
  - Ozone
  - Peroxyacetyl nitrate

Water and soil pollutants
- Organic pollutants
  - Polychlorinated biphenyls
  - Polybrominated biphenyls
  - Polycyclic aromatic hydrocarbons
  - Trihalomethanes
  - Pesticides
- Inorganic pollutants
  - Heavy metals
  - Non-metals

Food and feed contaminants
- Organic compounds
  - Dioxins
  - Polychlorinated and polybrominated biphenyls
  - Pesticides
- Inorganic pollutants
  - Metals
  - Non-metals
- Other toxicants

Pollution may be defined as the state of being contaminated or the act or process of contaminating soil, water, or atmosphere by the discharge of harmful substances. Pollution of the environment has been an undesirable part of man's activity since ancient times. Man dug coal from the ground and used it to heat his clustered dwellings, thus creating an atmosphere of sulphurous smoke and filth above the cities. Industrialization and technologic development added a second dimension to pollution of the environment with numerous power plants (burn fossil fuel to generate electricity), oil refineries, metal industries, etc. Automobiles further added to the pollution of atmosphere. All these environmental pollutants can harm ecosystems, plants and animals and cause health problems in humans and animals. Some of them such as mercury, PCBs and dioxins have been spread throughout the world and tend to accumulate in living organisms. The concentrations of chemicals in the air, food and water are usually below the levels that can produce acute poisoning, but often they are sufficient to cause chronic adverse effects.

Types of pollutant

Humans and animals are mostly exposed to environmental chemicals by the air they breathe, the water they drink and the food they eat. Accordingly, the environmental pollutants have been divided into three broad categories:

A. Air pollutants.

B. Water and soil pollutants.

C. Food and feed contaminants.

A. AIR POLLUTANTS

Air pollutants originate from geographical, biological and man-mad sources and enter the body predominantly through the lungs. There are numerous air pollutants, but some such as oxides of carbon, nitrogen and sulphur, organic compounds and particulate matter are ubiquitous and account for maximum air pollution. After inhalation, many of these chemicals are absorbed into blood, some are retained in lungs and others are eliminated by the respiratory system. Particles of 5 μm or larger diameter are usually deposited in the upper airway, 1 to 5 μm are deposited in the terminal airways or alveoli and less than 1 μm particles reach the alveolar zone of lungs where they may be readily absorbed.

Types of air pollutant: Air pollutants, depending on their release, can be classified as either primary or secondary. Primary pollutants are directly produced and released in atmosphere by various natural or man-made processes such as ash from a volcanic eruption or carbon monoxide gas from a motor vehicle exhaust. Secondary pollutants, in contrast, are not directly emitted but are formed in the air when primary pollutants react or interact e.g. ozone and peroxyacetyl nitrate (PAN). Some pollutants may be both primary and secondary i.e. they are both emitted directly and formed from other primary pollutants. The man-made primary pollutants are more of health concern and account for almost 98% of air pollution. These include mainly 5 pollutants namely carbon monoxide (52%), sulphur oxides (18%), hydrocarbons (12%), particulate matter (10%) and nitrogen oxides (6%). The concentration of other primary pollutants such as metal oxides (especially those of lead, cadmium, copper and iron), pesticides, silicon, and other substances vary considerably from one place to another.

Adverse effects of air pollution: There is a wide range of pollutants whose nature and concentration vary from one area to another and hence their incidence of poisoning. Chronic exposure of air pollutants are more common and mainly cause respiratory diseases e.g. chronic bronchitis, chronic obstructive ventilatory disease, pulmonary emphysema, bronchial asthma and cancer. However, from time to time some situations arise when the level of air pollutants rises to concentrations that are definitely hazardous to human beings and animals. In rare instances, some incidents occur where the accidental release of a specific chemical into air proves fatal for large population e.g. accidental release of chlorine, ammonia or other poisonous gases from industrial plants (i.e. methyl-isocyanate in Bhopal) or natural release of poisonous gases from volcanic eruptions. Though large proportion of population is exposed to air pollutants, yet morbidity and mortality is mostly very small. Insignificant physiological changes are not taken as adverse effects (Fig. 17.1).

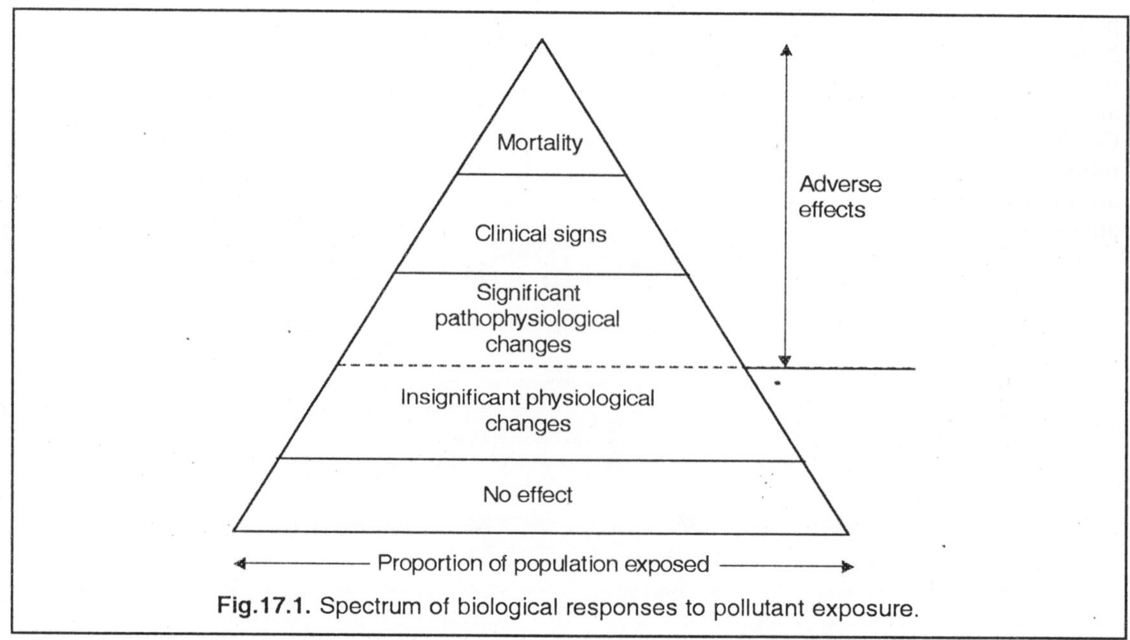

Fig.17.1. Spectrum of biological responses to pollutant exposure.

I. PRIMARY AIR POLLUTANTS

1. Carbon Oxide Gases

Carbon Monoxide

Carbon monoxide (CO) is the most notorious and abundant pollutant present in the lower atmospheric air. It is produced by incomplete combustion of hydrocarbon fuels; therefore it is mainly generated by fires in closed spaces. It is a highly poisonous gas, which causes a large number of accidental and suicidal deaths in human beings. Poisoning in veterinary species is not common, but occurs occasionally in animals in confined quarters heated by petroleum fuels.

Properties: Carbon monoxide is a colourless, odourless, tasteless and non-irritating gas which results from incomplete combustion of organic matter. The normal average concentration of CO in atmosphere is about 0.1 ppm (mainly produced by atmospheric oxidation of methane, forest fires, ocean micro-organisms) which is maintained by efficient natural sinks like reaction with ambient hydroxyl radicals to form CO_2, the upper atmosphere, soil, etc. However in areas having high numbers of furnaces or automobiles, this concentration may increase many fold. Under ordinary conditions, CO is less dense than air but during fires it accumulates on the ground that enhances chances of poisoning.

Sources of toxicity: Carbon monoxide is produced by both natural and man-made sources. Natural sources such as atmospheric oxidation of methane, forest fires, terpine oxidation and ocean are responsible for about 90% of the atmospheric CO. Human activities like municipal incinerators, refineries, blast furnaces, lime kilns, coal mines and automobiles produce the remaining 10% of atmospheric CO.

a. *Fire:* Carbon monoxide is a major and ubiquitous component of fire or heating atmosphere. In the early phase of burning carbon monoxide is produced along with other components like sulphur dioxide, carbon dioxide and water, but as the fire progresses to smouldering phase and oxygen become depleted (in closed spaces) more and more of toxic gases like CO and SO_2 are produced. Burning of man-made polymeric material (e.g. Polyvinyl chloride and polyurethane foam) releases mainly CO and other toxic gases (e.g. HCN). Confined animals are often poisoned accidentally by CO emitted from improperly adjusted or vented fuel heaters or fires.

b. *Incinerators and furnaces:* Carbon monoxide is the most significant gaseous pollutant emitted by municipal incinerators. The CO in furnaces is the result of incomplete burnout of gaseous pyrolysis products and of char in the fuel bed.

c. *Automobiles:* Automobiles are the greatest source of CO in urban areas. In metropolitan cities, the concentration of CO in heavy traffics and underground garages and tunnels may reach >100 ppm and in residential areas >20 ppm. Dogs in trunks of cars with faulty exhaust system or in enclosed garages are often affected by CO. The automobile exhaust fumes can be greatly reduced by catalytic converters in the exhaust system.

d. *Smoking:* Carbon monoxide is a toxic metabolite of dihalomethanes that are found in cigarette. Non-smoking human adults do not have more than 1% of their total circulating haemoglobin in the form of carboxyhaemoglobin, but heavy smokers may show these values as high as 5 to 10 percent saturation.

e. *Endogenous production:* Carbon monoxide is also generated endogenously in normal humans or animals by catabolism of heme proteins, particularly haemoglobin. The average rate of CO production (0.4 ml/h) is increased in haemolytic diseases.

f. *Industries:* Carbon monoxide is a major industrial gas that has many applications in bulk chemicals manufacturing.

g. *Volcanic eruptions:* Carbon monoxide occurs dissolved in molten volcanic rock at high pressures in the earth's mantle and is released as a product of volcanic activity. Carbon monoxide contents of volcanic gases vary from less than 0.01% to as much as 2% depending on the volcano.

h. *Other sources:* Carbon monoxide is generated in large amount (up to 8%) when gunpowder or dynamite is exploded and when explosion of gases occur in coal mines. It is found in the proportion of 30 to 40 percent in water which is obtained by blowing steam through red hot coal or coke. It is also present in natural sources of gases present in illumination.

Factors affecting toxicity :

a. *Concentration of gas:* High concentration of CO in the inspired gas produces rapid toxicity due to rapid formation of carboxyhaemoglobin.

b. *Duration of exposure:* Long duration of exposure facilitates toxic effects of CO.

c. *Respiratory rate:* Animals having higher respiratory rate may be more susceptible to CO toxicity due to rapid accumulation of gas in the blood.

d. *Species:* The incidence of CO poisoning is more common in humans than other species due to their frequent and excessive exposure to the gas.

e. *Pregnancy:* The toxicity of CO is more significant on the foetus than the adults because foetal haemoglobin has higher affinity for CO than adult haemoglobin and also because elimination of carbon monoxide is slower in the foetus leading to its accumulation in tissues.

f. *Pathological conditions:* Pre-existing cerebral, respiratory or cardiovascular diseases, reduced cardiac output and anaemia increase risk of CO poisoning.

g. *Environmental conditions:* High altitude, high humidity and high temperature aggravate CO poisoning.

h. *Interactions:* Carbon monoxide has strong interactions with certain other gases. Carbon monoxide and hydrogen cyanide often co-exist in a fire and act synergistically by reducing the availability of oxygen to tissues.

Toxicity: Carbon monoxide is a highly toxic gas, although animals may demonstrate varied clinical manifestations with different outcomes even under similar exposure conditions. Carbon monoxide is life-threatening to humans, animals and all other forms of air-breathing life, as inhaling even relatively small amounts of it can lead to hypoxic injury, neurological damage and possibly death. A concentration of as little as 0.04% (400 parts per million) carbon monoxide in the air can be fatal. Serious toxicity is often associated with carboxyhaemoglobin (COHb) levels above 25% and risk of fatality with levels over 60%, although a consistent dose response relationship between COHb levels and clinical effects has not been established in animals. The CO is especially dangerous because it is not easily detected by animal senses and produces drowsiness and loss of consciousness, which allow still more inhalation of the toxic gas.

Toxicokinetics: Carbon monoxide is efficiently absorbed across the respiratory tract and rapidly distributed through the body. In blood, it binds avidly with the haemoglobin (Hb) of red blood cells to form a relatively stable compound called carboxyhaemoglobin (COHb). After termination of exposure, recovery from COHb is rapid. The half-recovery time in terms of blood carboxyhaemoglobin is approximately 4 hours. The CO is excreted mostly unchanged via lungs. A small amount of CO is also oxidised to carbon dioxide. Carbon monoxide rapidly crosses the placenta and combines with foetal haemoglobin, which has 10% to 15% higher affinity for CO than adult haemoglobin. Elimination of carbon monoxide is comparatively slower in the foetus than in the adults.

Mechanism of action: The precise mechanisms by which toxic effects are induced by CO are not fully understood, but binding with haemoglobin, myoglobin and mitochondrial cytochrome oxidase is thought to be the primary action.

a. *Haemoglobin:* The toxicity from carbon monoxide is mainly due to its combination with haemoglobin and formation of carboxyhaemoglobin (COHb). Carbon monoxide combines with haemoglobin at the same site of molecule as does the oxygen. Haemoglobin in this form cannot carry oxygen and hence tissues die from oxygen starvation. The affinity of haemoglobin for carbon monoxide is about 200–250 times greater than its affinity for oxygen. Therefore, CO displaces haemoglobin bound oxygen and increases the concentration of carboxyhaemoglobin. In addition to reducing the capacity of blood to transport oxygen, CO causes oxyhaemoglobin (O_2Hb) to dissociate at lower rate. A reduction in unloading of oxygen is particularly serious in tissues such as myocardium, where 60-70 per cent of the oxygen from blood is usually extracted in comparison to 25% in many tissues. Net result of CO exposure and COHb formation is tissue hypoxia. Tissue hypoxia results in lactic acidosis and cell death. Because brain and heart are the organs with the greatest oxygen demand and the highest metabolic rates, so they are most sensitive to hypoxia.

b. *Myoglobin:* Carbon monoxide also has high affinity for myoglobin. It exerts a direct toxic effect by binding to myoglobin, which reduces the oxygen storage capacity. This action of CO may impair cardiac output and result in cerebral ischemia.

c. *Cytochrome oxidase:* Carbon monoxide binds to mitochondrial cytochrome oxidase and inhibits the cellular respiration. However, CO affinity for cytochrome oxidase is less than its affinity for oxygen. This binding interferes with aerobic metabolism and efficient adenosine triphosphate (ATP) synthesis and may contribute to hypoxia induced by formation of COHb. Cells respond by switching to anaerobic metabolism, causing anoxia, lactic acidosis and eventual cell death.

d. *Other effects:* The delayed actions of CO involve lipid peroxidation and demyelination in the CNS. Carbon monoxide causes release of nitric oxide (NO) from the endothelial cells and helps in formation of oxygen free radicals. In the brain, this causes lipid peroxidation capillary leakage, leukocyte sequestration, and apoptosis. Demyelinization of white matter, oedema of CNS and focal areas of necrosis within the brain are common sequelae of CO exposure. The brain damage occurs mainly during the recovery period and results in neurological deficits, cognitive defects (especially affecting memory and learning) and movement disorders.

Clinical signs

Acute toxicity: The signs and symptoms of acute CO poisoning are characteristic of hypoxia and depend upon the concentration of CO inhaled. High exposure to CO may produce rapid death without significant clinical signs. In low to moderate concentrations, varying degree of toxic signs may be displayed by the poisoned animal including drowsiness, incoordination, weakness, increased respiration and pulse, involuntary urination and defecation, and unconsciousness. Carbon monoxide poisoning may also produce myocardial ischemia, atrial fibrillation, pneumonia, pulmonary oedema, hyperglycaemia, muscle necrosis, acute renal failure, skin lesions, and visual and auditory problems. In moderately high concentrations (>60%), there may be intermittent convulsions, depressed cardiac functions, collapse, coma, respiratory arrest and death. The skin and mucous membranes give a characteristic cherry-red colour due to the high concentration of carboxyhaemoglobin in blood. Permanent deafness has been reported in dogs and cats following CO poisoning.

Pregnant sows and ewes held in buildings with fossil fuel heaters may develop levels of carboxyhaemoglobin significant enough to cause foetal anoxia leading to near-term abortions and stillbirths. Carbon monoxide adversely affects the surviving foetus with functional neurological deficits and mental retardation. The level of foetal morbidity and mortality in acute carbon monoxide poisoning is significant, even when the mothers do not suffer acutely.

Chronic toxicity: Repeated exposure to sublethal concentrations of CO may result in various adverse health effects. This type of toxicity is mostly seen in humans working in gas houses, workshops and garages and in traffic police. Persons or animals living in ill-ventilated rooms in which fire is burning may suffer neurological or behavioural disorders. In humans there may be headache, dizziness, under-performance of skilled tasks, decreased reaction time, decreased exercise tolerance, dementia, and disturbance of vision.

Post-mortem findings: The post-mortem lesions are characteristic of hypoxia and depend on the survival time. If death occurs rapidly, no significant changes except the congestion of meningeal vessels and some other organs and petechial haemorrhages in white matter may be observed. The blood is usually fluid and of bright cherry-red colour. The internal organs in acute poisoning are hyperaemic and bright red owing to the colour of blood. Sometimes there may be bronchial dilation and distension of major blood vessels. Microscopically, there may be necrosis of cortex and brain stem, haemorrhages in brain and demyelination.

Diagnosis: Diagnosis of CO poisoning may be facilitated by circumstantial evidence, clinical signs and post-mortem lesions. A final diagnosis depends upon demonstration of COHb in the blood. Putrefaction has very little effect on COHb, which may be detected in blood several days after death.

Carbon monoxide poisoning should be differentiated from following poisonings/ conditions:

a. *Cyanide:* Cyanide produces severe respiratory distress and hypoxia and colour of blood is bright-red, but the tissues give smell of bitter almond.

b. *Nitrite:* Nitrite causes rapid death, but colour of blood is brown-red.

c. *Haemolytic agents:* They reduce oxygen carrying capacity of the blood by rupturing erythrocytes. The haemolysis can be detected in fresh plasma.

d. *Hydrogen sulphide:* Hydrogen sulphide causes rapid death, but blood and tissues are dark brown in colour and smell of H_2S comes from tissues.

e. *Alcohol:* In humans, COHb concentration in the range of 15-30% may cause symptoms similar to drunkenness. Careful chemical analysis may differentiate the alcoholic intoxication.

Treatment and management :

Specific therapy

a. *Oxygen:* Oxygen is the specific antagonist to carbon monoxide. Artificial respiration (90-95% oxygen with 5-10% carbon dioxide) should be administered with positive pressure. Recovery occurs quickly or not at all depending upon the severity and duration of toxicosis. Risk of oxygen poisoning in the form of pulmonary oedema and haemorrhage must be kept in mind while administering oxygen.

Supportive therapy

a. Intoxicated animal should be immediately removed into fresh air and kept in horizontal position.

b. Whole blood transfusion may be provided to maintain the normal haemoglobin levels.

c. Mannitol (20%) or glucose (50%) may be administered intravenously to reduce cerebral oedema.

d. Systemic corticosteroids may be used to reduce the systemic effects of CO.

e. Systemic antibiotics may be used to avoid lung and other systemic infections.

f. Correction of hypotension, acidosis and cardiac dysfunctions may be taken appropriately, if needed.

Prognosis: Recovery of intoxicated animal occurs quickly or not at all depending on severity and duration of toxicosis. Some degree of neurological impairment occurs, if the patient recovers from acute CO induced coma.

Carbon Dioxide

Carbon dioxide (CO_2) is a heavy, colourless, odourless gas having a slightly acid taste. Carbon dioxide is a constituent of atmospheric air in which it exists to an extent of 0.4 per cent. It is given off in the process of respiration, combustion, fermentation and putrefaction of animal matter. It is also evolved in neighbourhood of lime kilns or coal mines. Being heavier than air, it tends to accumulate at the bottom of old wells, mine shafts, grain pits and ship's holds. It is commercially used in fire extinguishers, foundry works, refrigeration and arc welding. Poisoning from carbon dioxide in humans and animals is not commonly seen because its concentration in air rarely approaches dangerous level. Accidental exposure to high concentration of gas may produce acute poisoning in animals. Mild intoxication may occur in humans or animals living in poorly ventilated and overcrowded rooms.

Carbon dioxide at a concentration of 5 percent in air may produce increased respiration, nausea, giddiness, anxiety and weakness of muscles. At concentration of 10 percent in air it causes tachypnoea, muscular tremors, sweating, visual disturbances, staggering gait and loss of consciousness. A concentration of 25 to 30 per cent CO_2 may produce cyanosis, convulsion and death from cortical excitability. Very high concentration (>60 per cent) produces immediate insensibility followed by death from glottis spasms causing suffocation. Carbon dioxide poisoning produces no specific necropsy lesions. The body heat is retained for a longer period after death. Brains and lungs are deeply congested and other tissues and blood are dark in colour. Treatment of carbon dioxide poisoning involves immediate removal of patient to fresh air and provision of artificial air, if needed. After breathing is established, body temperature and blood pressure should be maintained.

2. Sulphur Oxide Gases

Sulphur dioxide (SO_2) and sulphur trioxide (SO_3) are industrial atmospheric effluents, constituting about 18% of total air pollutants. The SO_2 often accompanies smoke and other suspended particulates produced from sulphur impurities in coal and oil. Sulphur trioxide is formed when sulphur dioxide reacts with water in the air. Heavy smog is likely to contain these gases in combination with sulphuric acid and other pollutants. Sulphur dioxide and sulphur trioxide are potentially fatal gases and are of significant environmental concern.

Properties: Sulphur dioxide (SO_2) is a colourless gas with a pungent burnt match-like smell and it mainly comes from burning of coal and oil. In the air it can be converted to sulphuric acid, sulphur trioxide and sulphates. Sulphur trioxide (SO_3), also called sulphuric oxide and sulphuric anhydride, is generally a colourless liquid but also exists as a gas. When SO_3 is exposed to air, it rapidly takes up water and gives off white fumes. It can also react with water to form sulphuric acid. Both SO_2 and SO_3 are important air pollutants, being the primary agents in acid rain.

Sources of toxicity: The main source of sulphur oxide gases are combustion of sulphur compounds such as coal and petroleum. The main natural sources of sulphur dioxide are volcanoes, forest fires and oceans. It is released in considerable quantities in the manufacture of sulphuric acid, liquid sulphur dioxide and cast iron, and in petroleum refining, bleaching, disinfecting and paper production. It is also found as a contaminant in the production of cellulose, sugar and superphosphates. Sulphur dioxide is often added as a preservative in pre packaged pet meats and fish to give the product a longer life. Sulphur dioxide neutralizes the odour of meat and also improves the colour to create an impression of freshness.

Toxicity: Sulphur oxide gases are highly toxic gases and their exposure at high levels can be fatal. Exposure to 100 parts of sulphur dioxide per million parts of air (100 ppm) is considered dangerous to human life and health. Exposure of grazing animals to a SO_2 concentration of 500 ppm for 1 hour is considered dangerous. Daily exposure of rats to SO_2 at 10 ppm for 1-2 months thickens the mucous membrane in trachea about 5 fold. Although the cilia beat with normal frequency, the thick mucous membranes retard the clearance of mucus. Mucosal irritation also causes reflex bronchoconstriction which may be more prominent in asthmatic individuals even at sufficiently lower concentrations (0.25 ppm). Exposure of pigs to 40 ppm SO_2 for 8 hours can cause pulmonary fibrosis within 160 days as a delayed effect. Sulphuric acid mist (present in smog) is more toxic than SO_2; a 22 ppm concentration may kill a guinea pig after exposure of 3 hours.

Toxicokinetics: Sulphur dioxide enters the body via the respiratory tract or by swallowing after dilution in the saliva where it enters the gastro-intestinal tract in the form of sulphurous acid. After absorption, the sulphur dioxide is rapidly distributed throughout the body due to its high solubility. In the blood sulphur dioxide forms sulphuric acid that is further metabolized to sulphates, which are excreted in the urine. Sulphur trioxide enters the body via respiratory tract, is metabolized to sulphate in blood and eliminated in urine in the same way as sulphur dioxide.

Mechanism of action: Sulphur dioxide enters the body via respiratory tract and acts as a local irritant and general toxic agent. The mechanism of action of sulphur trioxide is almost similar to sulphur dioxide.

a. Sulphur dioxide is an irritant gas and its effect is mainly due to the formation of sulphurous and sulphuric acids on contact with moist mucosae. The irritant action of SO_3 is more pronounced than the SO_2.

b. Sulphur dioxide and its metabolic products (e.g. sulphuric acid) produce metabolic acidosis with a reduction in blood alkali reserve and compensatory elimination of ammonia in the urine and alkali in the saliva.

c. Sulphur dioxide produces protein and carbohydrate metabolism disorders, vitamins B and C deficiency, and oxidase inhibition. Sulphur dioxide toxicity due to prolonged intake of preserved pet foods causes thiamine deficiency that can affect brain function and cause brain damage.

d. It is probable that absorption of large quantities of sulphur dioxide has a pathological effect on the haematopoietic system and may produce methaemoglobin.

Clinical signs:

Acute toxicity: Though high concentration of sulphur oxide gases is not really breathable and will be avoided by animals, if possible, yet animals confined to areas near smelters, power plants or factories burning sulphur-rich coal may be acutely poisoned by the toxic gases. Clinical signs of acute SO_2 poisoning include intense irritation and reddening of mucous membranes of conjunctiva and upper respiratory tract, lachrymation, salivation, coughing and irregular respiration. Severe dyspnoea develops from bronchoconstriction, pulmonary oedema, haemorrhage and emphysema. Cyanosis occurs that is followed rapidly by consciousness disorders. Death may ensue as a result of suffocation due to reflex spasm of larynx, sudden circulatory arrest in lungs, or shock.

Sulphur dioxide also causes skin irritation which is aggravated by perspiration. This may be attributed to the conversion of sulphur dioxide to sulphurous acid from contact with sweat.

Chronic toxicity: The chronic effects are observed mainly in occupational workers and consist primarily of bronchopulmonary disease which, after several years, may be complicated by emphysema and bronchiectasis. Sulphur oxide gases irritate the mucous membranes and produce obstructive reactions and chronic bronchitis. The mouth can be affected with dental caries, peridontal and gingival disorders, and enamel striation and yellowing. Both behavioural and nervous system disorders may occur, probably due to the general toxic effect of sulphur dioxide on the body. In pets eating SO_2 preserved foods, the signs may include turned or tilted head, disorientation and wobbly legs, which may progress to paralysis and seizures.

Post-mortem findings: The necropsy findings of sulphur oxide gases poisoning may include cyanosis, pulmonary oedema, hyperaemia, emphysema, atelectasis and haemorrhages.

Diagnosis: Diagnosis of sulphur oxide gases poisoning is based on history, circumstantial evidence, clinical signs and post-mortem lesions.

Treatment and management: Sulphur oxide gases have no specific therapy or antidote. Removal of animals from the contaminated area and breathing of fresh air may help to prevent severe consequences of small exposures.

Prognosis: The initial upper and lower respiratory tract symptoms may regress with suitable treatment and removal from the exposure source; however, the prognosis is poor for the advanced stages, especially when accompanied by bronchiectasis.

3. Nitrogen Oxide Gases

Nitrogen oxide gases constitute a mixture of oxides of nitrogen including nitrogen dioxide (NO_2), nitrogen tetroxide (N_2O_4) and nitric oxide (NO). The nitrogen oxide gases constitute about 6% of the total air pollutant gases and are considerably toxic to humans and animals. The nitrogen dioxide and nitrogen tetroxide gases readily convert to one another, but the relative amount of NO_2 is more at higher temperature. Inhalation of nitrogen dioxide produced from silage of nitrogen rich forages produce a disease commonly called "Silo-filler's disease or Silage gas poisoning" in agricultural workers and animals.

Properties: Nitric dioxide, nitrogen tetroxide and nitrogen oxide almost always occur together; hence, the terms oxides of nitrogen and nitrogen oxides (NOX) are used in literature to refer to these molecules. Nitrogen dioxide is reddish-brown gas with a characteristic sharp odour, whereas the nitrogen tetroxide and nitric oxide are colourless and odourless gases. The nitrogen oxide gases are formed from nitrogen and oxygen during high-temperature combustion, incomplete reduction of nitrates and microbial digestion of organic matter. Nitrogen dioxide is formed largely from nitric oxide (NO), which makes up the majority of the nitrogen oxides emitted by combustion processes such as from automobiles, diesel engines, thermal power plants, boilers, kerosene lamps, un-vented gas stoves and heaters, and burning of industrial wastes. Forages rich in nitrates (e.g. alfalfa) favour production of nitrogen dioxide, especially when nitric oxide in fresh silage comes in contact with oxygen in the air. In smog, sunlight converts NO and oxygen to NO_2 and ozone (O_3), which is also an irritant. Nitrogen tetroxide has received much attention as a rocket fuel, so missile industry has potential of giving off the toxic nitrogen oxide gases.

Toxicity: Nitrogen dioxide and nitrogen tetroxide are in chemical equilibrium and both contribute to the production of toxicosis. Inhalation of NO_2 and N_2O_4 in a concentration of 100 ppm in air is dangerous for humans, even for a short time, and 200 ppm may be fatal. The safety limit for prolonged exposure in humans is 0.6 ppm. Animals have been acutely exposed to 25 ppm without ill-effects, but long exposures to only a few ppm can lower resistance to respiratory infections. Toxicosis in agricultural workers and sometimes animals living near silos is seen shortly after silo pits have been filled (highest concentration in first 48 hours). The nitrogen oxide gases are as dense as air and, therefore, can flow into animals' quarters or houses from the silo pits. The risk is highest when feedstuffs are high in nitrates as in draught years. In water, nitrogen dioxide and nitrogen tetroxide gases form nitric acid (HNO_3) and nitric oxide (NO). When these gases dissolve in atmospheric moisture, the result can be acid rain which can damage both trees and forest ecosystems.

Mechanism of action :

a. Nitrogen dioxide and nitrogen tetroxide dissolve in water on respiratory mucosa to form a mixture of nitric and nitrous acids, both of which are very irritating and corrosive to the mucous membranes. Thus, nitrogen dioxide-nitrogen tetroxide gases irritate mucous membrane of respiratory tract and produce lung lesions. Damage to the lower respiratory tract, especially the type I pneumocytes and ciliated airway cells, is more where the duration of contact and the amount of moisture are greater. The nitrogen oxide gases have a shorter residency time in the upper respiratory tract; therefore damage to organs in the upper respiratory tract is less severe.

b. Nitrogen dioxide has ability to initiate free radicals generation in the terminal bronchioles, resulting in protein oxidation, lipid peroxidation, and subsequent cell membrane damage. Vitamin E deficiency increases susceptibility to the nitrogen dioxide poisoning.

c. Nitric oxide synthesised from inhalation of NO_2 is absorbed through lungs and binds to haemoglobin, forming nitrosyl haemoglobin. This complex is readily oxidized to methaemoglobin, which produces methemoglobinaemia. Methemoglobinaemia aggravates the pre-existing hypoxemia induced by nitric oxide gases.

d. Nitrogen dioxide alters the macrophage and immune function, which suppresses immunity and impairs the resistance to infection.

Clinical signs :

Acute toxicity: The clinical manifestations of acute poisoning vary according to the concentrations of gases and the period of exposure. Pulmonary signs are the most common manifestations of nitrogen oxides poisoning, which may appear within few minutes, hours or days after exposure. Clinical signs of acute poisoning in cattle include coughing, choking, wheezing, panting or irregular respiration, reddening of mucous membranes, lachrymation and salivation. There is inappetence, wasting, dehydration and cyanosis. Dyspnoea soon appears which becomes severe as pulmonary oedema develops. Fluid sounds may be auscultated in the lungs. Death from anoxemia occurs 3-25 days after exposure.

Chronic toxicity: In chronic exposure to small concentrations of nitrogen gases for longer time, signs of respiratory distress develop which are intensified by bacterial pneumonia and other lung lesions.

Post-mortem findings: Necropsy findings usually correspond to the degree of exposure to nitrogen oxide gases. Lesions may reveal pulmonary oedema, hyperaemia and haemorrhagic lesions with fibrin deposits in the inflamed bronchioles. In addition, cyanosis, methaemoglobinaemia, necrosis of skeletal muscle, and dark red kidneys are manifested. Emphysema may occur in chronic cases.

Diagnosis: Diagnosis is mostly based on history, circumstantial evidence, clinical signs and lesions. Nitrogen dioxide usually is seen as a yellow-brown haze, whose presence may be further confirmed by using potassium iodide starch paper which turns dark when exposed to NO_2 gas. Methaemoglobin levels may be increased after exposure to NO_2.

Treatment and management: Nitrogen oxide gases have no specific treatment. Some of the symptomatic and supportive therapy may be used, but success would be doubtful in advanced cases.

a. Oxygen and artificial respiration must be administered immediately, if required.

b. Corticosteroids have been found useful in relieving the pulmonary oedema.

c. Animal quarters that develop the irritant odour of NO_2 – N_2O_4 or contain a yellowish haze in air must not be entered.

d. Silage from a silo giving off nitrogen oxide gases should not be fed to animals.

Prognosis: Prognosis depends on the stage of poisoning. Exposure to large concentrations of NO_2–N_2O_4 concentration that leads to development of oedema is not treatable and prognosis is poor.

4. Smoke and Other Particulate Matters

Suspended particulate matter is a generic term used for finely solid or liquid particles that are small enough to remain in suspension for periods of hours or days, being capable of travelling long distances during that time. The suspended particulate matter causing air pollution may include both organic and inorganic materials of different diameters.. In general, their effective diameter is less than 1 μm, but it may extend up to 5 or 10 μm. Black smoke is one component of suspended particulates, produced in complete combustion of coal or oil. Other components of suspended particulates include inorganic ash largely from coal-burning, fine dusts from some industrial processes, acid sulphates or nitrates formed as secondary pollutants by atmospheric reactions, and residues of lead compounds from leaded petrol. Fluoride is also an important by-product of coal combustion and is released in large quantities entirely in gas phase. Suspended particulate matters usually constitute about 10% of total air pollutants. The particulate matters generally are inhaled with air and get deposited in the upper and to lesser extent in the lower respiratory tract.

Smoke: Smoke inhalation, such as that occurs in a stable or house fire, is an acute form of inhalation toxicosis. The smoke consists of a mixture of gases (Table 17.1) and various particulates produced by the combustion, but the exact composition (and thus the potential lesions) is determined by the specific substances being burnt.

The smoke inhalation can cause damage to the body in three different ways: thermal injury, asphyxiation and pulmonary irritation. Thermal injury is limited to the oropharyngeal area and is caused by the hot air that may actually cause burns and laryngospasm. Asphyxiation mostly occurs either from inhalation of toxic gases such as carbon monoxide and hydrogen cyanide, or by suffocation. Pulmonary damage occurs due to inhalation of various irritants in the smoke that may cause direct tissue injury and activation of the body's inflammatory response system. Such pulmonary injuries by smoke components mostly occur in two phases: the initial cellular and exudative phase and the terminal repair and proliferation phase. The first phase is characterized by activation and influx of neutrophils, production of inflammatory mediators, elaboration of oxygen-free radicals and proteolytic enzymes, and liberation of complement degradation products and the second phase is characterized by cellular hyperplasia and fibrosis. Smoke

Table 17.1. Gases found in fire smoke.

Irritants	Asphyxiants
Acrolein	***Simple asphyxiants****
Aldehydes	Carbon dioxide
Ammonia	Methane
Chlorine	Nitrogen
Hydrogen chloride	***Chemical asphyxiants*****
Isocyanides	Carbon monoxide
Nitrogen oxide	Hydrogen cyanide
Phosgene	
Sulphur dioxide	

* Simple asphyxiants are physiologically inert agents that when present in high concentration simply displace the oxygen in the atmosphere. Animals exposed to them will suffer from lack of oxygen.

** Chemical asphyxiants are agents that interfere with the body's ability to utilise oxygen. They either prevent oxygen delivery or inhibit utilization of oxygen by the cells.

components can cause atelectasis by destroying lung surfactant, increasing pulmonary vascular resistance, and contributing to pulmonary oedema. The location of pulmonary injury by smoke components depends on the lipid solubility of the substances. Low lipid-solubility substances such as acrolein, sulphur dioxide, ammonia and hydrogen chloride cause injury to the upper airway, intermediate solubility substances such as chlorine and isocyanates cause both upper and lower respiratory tract injury, and high-lipid solubility substances such as phosgene and oxides of nitrogen cause diffuse parenchymal injury.

Clinical manifestations of smoke inhalation may vary depending on the extent of exposure and duration of smoke inhalation. In severe smoke poisoning, animal may rapidly die from suffocation, bronchospasm or carbon monoxide poisoning. Thermal injury by smoke burns is more common in the upper airways and may be seen as mucosal damage with erythema, ulceration, blistering, oedema and soot deposition in the nose or mouth. Dyspnoea and respiratory distress often develop several hours after thermal injury. In less severe non-burn cases, inhalation of smoke may initially cause hyperventilation, hypoxia and decreased pulmonary compliance followed by decreased cardiac output and a severe lung injury with airway and alveolar inflammation, epithelial damage and pulmonary oedema. Secondary bacterial infection develops after 24 hours and death may occur from lung failure. Smoke inhalation injury can be diagnosed from exposure to smoke, circumstantial evidence and clinical signs. Pulmonary function testing can confirm obstructive or restrictive ventilatory defects.

Treatment of smoke inhalation involves immediate removal of animal from the toxic environment. Supportive treatments of acute smoke inhalation are directed at improving the lung function and preventing the shock and secondary sepsis. However, not all of these measures are always beneficial. Glucocorticoids and antibiotics have been recommended to help control the serious circulatory shock and secondary infection, respectively. Fluids may be carefully administered to avoid overhydration that may aggravate lung oedema. Prognosis in absence of bacterial pneumonia is good.

Other particulate matters: A large number of particulate matters are present in the air and are inhaled by the animal. These may include acids (such as nitrates and sulphates), organic chemicals, metals, and soil or dust particles. The toxicology of these substances varies considerably depending on the nature and size of the particle. In general, inhalation of high concentration of particulate matters hinders the normal mucociliary mechanism resulting in gradual build up of particles in the lungs. This may lead to deposition of particles in alveoli, epithelial hyperplasia, dyspnoea, chronic cough and various pulmonary disorders. Secondary infections of respiratory tract are common sequelae of particle deposition in lungs. Dusts of silicon and asbestos in human beings produce respiratory diseases commonly called silicosis and asbestosis (a form of pulmonary fibrosis), respectively. Many other occupational pulmonary diseases are caused by the long-term inhalation of dusts containing minerals and organic matters.

5. Hydrocarbons

Hydrocarbons are a heterogeneous group of organic substances that are primarily composed of carbon and hydrogen molecules. Number of hydrocarbons including solvents and vapours are a common part of our environment and constitute about 12% of the total air pollutants. The hydrocarbons are produced from both natural and anthropogenic sources including vegetation, microbial decomposition, natural gases, solvents, incomplete combustion of fossil fuels, and evaporative emissions from automobiles. Although toxicity to organic solvents is usually associated with occupational exposure in human beings, their accidental inhalation or ingestion by animals may produce acute toxicity.

The toxicity of hydrocarbons is directly related to their physical properties, specifically the viscosity, volatility, surface tension and chemical activity of the side chains. Many hydrocarbons produce harmful effects by direct action of various body systems, but some produce secondary toxic compounds from atmospheric reactions with other pollutants in air. In general, short incidental exposure to low concentrations of solvent vapours such as gasoline, lighter fluids, aerosol sprays and spot removers may be relatively less toxic but exposure to others like paint removers and solvents in home and industry may be dangerous. Some such as olefins and dienes tend to polymerise via free radical formation to form polycyclic aromatic hydrocarbons (PAH), which are potent carcinogens and mutagens. Motor vehicle hydrocarbons contribute significantly to the formation of ground-level ozone.

Hydrocarbons affect many systems in the body but their inhalation in polluted air most commonly affects the lungs. As lipids in the cell membrane are vulnerable to the solvent characteristics of organic molecules, many organic solvents "defat" the membranes and produce irritation of pulmonary tissues and membranes. Inhalation of hydrocarbons decreases the surfactant production and directly alters the pulmonary function. The end result of hydrocarbon inhalation or aspiration is interstitial inflammation, congestion, intra-alveolar haemorrhage, pulmonary oedema and bronchial necrosis. Important clinical signs include coughing, choking, tachypnoea, haemoptysis, wheezing sounds and cyanosis. Many of the hydrocarbons are highly lipophilic, so they easily cross the blood-brain barrier and directly affect the CNS. The most common CNS signs include lethargy, weakness, fatigue and CNS depression. Prolonged exposure to hydrocarbons can result in white matter degeneration (leucoencephalopathy) and in some cases (e.g. n-hexane or methyl-n-butyl ketone) in peripheral neuropathy. The chlorinated hydrocarbons, in particular carbon tetrachloride, are quite hepatotoxic and chronic exposure to some others like toluene, an aromatic hydrocarbon, can result in distal renal tubular acidosis. Some hydrocarbons such as benzene have been proven to cause bone marrow damage, leukaemia, and lymphomas in human beings.

6. Pesticides

Residues of pesticides i.e. insecticides, herbicides, fungicides, rodenticides, etc. have been detected in the air after aerial sprays, anti-mosquito fogging and drifts from agricultural applications. Concentration of pesticides in air is normally more in rural areas than urban areas. Normally much of the pesticidal material that finds its way into the air is returned to earth in the same general area. However, strong winds can take it to an area hundreds of kilometres away. DDT, DDE, chlordane, heptachlor, dieldrin, 2, 4, 5-T and ronnel dusts have been collected from different parts of world and have also been measured in rain water. In most instances, the collections were made in agricultural or urban areas where the residues found might be of local origin. World wide distribution of pesticides in air is indicated by a report which found traces of DDT in water melted from Antarctic snow. The toxicology of pesticides has been discussed earlier in Chapter 13.

II. SECONDARY AIR POLLUTANTS

1. Ozone

Ozone (O_3) is a natural component of the Earth's stratosphere (1-10 ppm) and helps in absorbing harmful ultraviolet radiation and preventing it from reaching the earth. However, near the Earth it is considered as an important secondary pollutant formed by chemical reactions between reactive organic gases and oxides of nitrogen in the presence of sunlight. It is also produced from various man-made sources (e.g. electric arc welding, electroplating, mercury vapour lamps, photoengraving, electrostatic air cleaners, and high voltage electrical equipment) and has number of uses (e.g. purification and disinfection of drinking water, disinfection and odour control of industrial and municipal wastewater and sewage, food preservative, bleaching and in various industrial processes). Ozone is strongly oxidizing and is considered the highest concentration of oxidant present in polluted environment. Inhalation of even small concentrations of ozone can be harmful to the upper respiratory tract and the lungs. It also damages plants.

Properties: Ozone is a colourless gas near the ground at low concentrations, but appears blue at higher concentration (>15%). It has characteristic odour of freshly mown hay. Ozone is a powerful oxidizer and is dangerously reactive; on contact with combustible materials it may cause fire or explosion. Normally in the ozone-oxygen cycle occurring in atmospheric stratosphere, the ozone is continuously created and destroyed primarily by ultraviolet radiation as molecules of oxygen (O_2) are split to form atomic oxygen (step i) and the atomic oxygen produced reacts immediately with other oxygen molecules (step ii) to form ozone (O_3) molecules. These ozone molecules subsequently reform oxygen (step iii), so the ozone-oxygen cycle will not lead to net production of ozone. In upper atmosphere, ozone is not regarded as a pollutant because it is produced naturally.

$$O_2 + \text{UV light} \longrightarrow 2O \quad \text{(i)}$$
$$O + O_2 \longrightarrow O_3 \quad \text{(ii)}$$
$$O_3 + \text{UV, visible light} \longrightarrow O + O_2 \quad \text{(iii)}$$

In polluted environment near the ground, the ozone is produced by a different process. It is formed by the major atmospheric pollutant nitrogen dioxide (NO_2), which absorbs UV light and produces nitric oxide (NO) and atomic oxygen (iv). This atomic oxygen as usual combines with molecular oxygen and produces ozone (v). The nitric oxide generated by petrol and engines may combine with ozone and is oxidised to NO_2 (vi). Normally these reactions also do not form much of ozone due to its rapid formation and inactivation. However under certain conditions such as in traffic congested metropolitan cities (i.e. excess NO_2) where warm conditions and intense solar radiation are present (e.g. intensification of UV light at the earth's surface), the reactions (steps iv and v) are intensified and there is more production of ozone. Simultaneously in polluted atmosphere, there is less inactivation of ozone as more of oxygen molecules react with hydrocarbons (due to their more concentrations in polluted air), especially olefins and substituted aromatics, resulting in oxidised compounds and free radicals that react with NO to produce more NO_2. Thus in hot sunny weather in polluted urban areas, there is more production of ozone but at the same time it's less degradation resulting in an overall build up of ozone in the air.

$$NO_2 + \text{UV light} \longrightarrow NO + O \qquad \text{(iv)}$$

$$O + O_2 \longrightarrow O_3 \qquad \text{(v)}$$

$$NO + O_3 + \text{UV, visible light} \longrightarrow NO_2 + O_2 \qquad \text{(vi)}$$

Toxicity: Toxicity of ozone depends on both the concentration of ozone and the duration of exposure. Even very low concentrations of ozone can be harmful to the upper respiratory tract and lungs. Severe and permanent lung injury or death could result from even a very short-term exposure to relatively low concentrations of ozone. In human beings, increased bronchial responsiveness has been observed following 7-hour exposure to 0.1 ppm (with moderate exercise) or 1-hour exposure to 0.35 ppm ozone. Exposure to approximately 11 ppm for 15 minutes may cause severe respiratory irritation and a 30-minute exposure to 50 ppm is considered potentially lethal. The LC_{50} of ozone in rats is 7.4-8.2 ppm and in mice is 5.9-6.8 ppm (4-hour exposure). In mice, gross pulmonary oedema has been observed at concentrations above 2 ppm. Literature on ozone poisoning in domestic animals is lacking.

Mechanism of action: Ozone is a strong oxidizing agent and an irritant. Exposure to extremely low concentrations of ozone initially increases the reactivity of airways to other inhaled substances (bronchial hyper-responsiveness) and causes an inflammatory response in the respiratory tissue. In higher concentrations, it produces intense irritation and causes desquamation of epithelium and degenerative changes through out the ciliated airways. Severe irritation of lung is capable of causing death from pulmonary oedema. Long-term exposure to ozone may cause thickening of the terminal respiratory bronchioles. Chronic bronchitis, fibrosis and emphysematous changes are observed in a variety of species. A small amount of inhaled ozone is absorbed into the blood and reacts with proteins and lipids, particularly within the biological membranes. Also when ozone breaks down to dioxygen it gives rise to oxygen free radicals, which are highly reactive and capable of damaging many organic molecules.

Clinical signs: Exposure to ozone mainly produces respiratory signs including coughing, shortness of breath, dyspnoea, dry throat and wheezing. At higher concentrations (>1 ppm), more severe signs such as reduced lung function, extreme fatigue, cyanosis, bronchitis, pneumonia and pulmonary oedema have been reported. Death occurs mainly from pulmonary oedema and lung failure. Exposure to ozone also enhances susceptibility to bacterial infections of the respiratory system, which aggravates the respiratory problems. Individuals with asthma are more sensitized to the effects of other irritants. Ozone is also irritating to the eyes and skin.

Long-term exposure to ozone can impair lung functions, cause structural changes in lungs, and may influence pulmonary clearance of other hazardous substances.

Diagnosis: Diagnosis of ozone poisoning is made from history, circumstantial evidence and clinical signs.

Treatment and management: Ozone has no specific treatment. Removal of patient from the polluted environment and provision of general supportive measures is indicated.

2. Peroxyacetyl Nitrate

Peroxyacetyl nitrate, commonly abbreviated as PAN, is an important secondary pollutant that contributes significantly to the phenomenon of photochemical smog. PAN forms in the atmosphere through a series of complicated chemical reactions deriving from hydrogen peroxide, hydrocarbons, and nitrogen oxides emitted from sources of urban pollution such as power plants, oil refineries, automobiles, and aircrafts. The concentration of PAN tends to be greater during the night than during the day because in colder temperatures PAN remain stable.

Peroxyacetyl nitrate is a strong oxidizing agent and an irritant. At concentrations of only a few parts per billion it can cause eye irritation. At higher concentrations it may cause extensive damage to respiratory mucosa. Both PAN and its chlorinated derivates are said to be mutagenic and they can be a factor causing skin cancer. Due to its highly oxidizing nature, PAN is also injurious to plants in any concentration greater than 50 ppb. The catalytic converter in automobile exhaust systems reduces production of PAN and other air pollutants by oxidizing hydrocarbons to CO_2 and H_2O and, to a lesser extent, converting nitrogen oxides to N_2 and O_2.

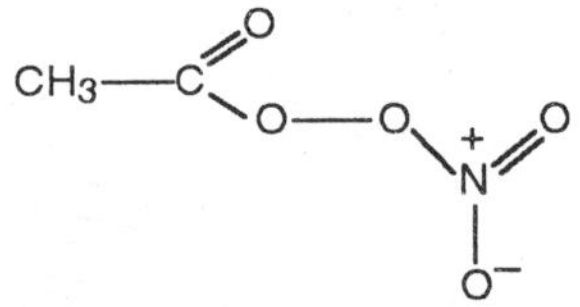

Fig.17.2. Chemical structure of peroxyacetyl nitrate.

B. WATER AND SOIL POLLUTANTS

Water is the earth's most abundant and most neglected natural resource. Water and soil act as the ultimate sinks for most chemicals produced and used by man. Water and soil get contaminated from industrial, agricultural, domestic and urban disposal of chemicals or due to naturally occurring toxicants such as minerals and plants. Contaminated water is more important a source of toxicity than the soil because it directly affects the health of man and animals. Residues of chemicals in soil are rarely an important source of direct exposure to people or animals, but ordinary pollutants in the soil constitute a reservoir from which water, crops and air may acquire toxic compounds. All residues in soil may be subject to run off in the presence of heavy rain and some are subject to leaching; both sources may contaminate water bodies. Some of these chemicals in soil are also absorbed by the plants or evaporate into the air from where they may condense on plants; in such cases soil becomes a source of poisoning to herbivores eating the toxic plants. Overall, both water and soil contaminations are important and pose serious health hazards to the local population.

Water

Contaminated water is an important direct source of toxicity and diseases to human beings, domestic animals and wild-life. In addition, contaminated water is the major contributor to the contamination of food chain of humans and animals. There are two important sources of water pollution: point source and non-point source. Point source of pollution occurs when harmful substances are emitted directly into water bodies such as rivers, lakes, ponds and sea. The point source water contamination mainly occurs from untreated discharges of municipal sewage, industrial units, and thermal plants, and from oil spill. A non-point source delivers pollutants indirectly through environmental changes. An example of this type of water pollution is when fertilizers and pesticides added to a field are carried into a stream by rain in the form of run-off. Pollution arising from non-point source accounts for majority of the contaminants in streams and lakes.

Quality of water: Quality of water is influenced by a number of factors which affect its pH, hardness, salinity, conductivity, total dissolved solids (TDS), etc.

a. Quality of water is affected by constituents dissolved in water which gives its TDS value. TDS content of 1000 mg/L poses little or no hazard to livestock and poultry, 1000-5000 mg/L may produce transient diarrhoea or reduced water intake in animals, 5000-7000 mg/kg may produce toxic effects in ruminants and horses, and 7000 mg/L TDS is unfit for animal consumption.

b. Of all the constituents dissolved in water, calcium, magnesium, sodium, bicarbonate, chlorine, silicate and sulphate make major constituents (10-1000 mg/L); boron, iron, potassium, strontium, fluoride, nitrate and phosphate are secondary constituents (0.1—10.0 mg/L); and arsenic, cadmium, copper, lead, molybdenum and zinc are minor constituents (<0.1 mg/L). Large increase in concentration(s) of one or more of the constituents may affect the quality of water.

c. Hardness of water (calcium and magnesium salt contents >120-180 mg/L) affects the quality of water.

d. Elevated pH of water (> 9.0) due to high ammonia affects the quality of water and may be highly toxic to fish. Heavily polluted water, fresh domestic sewage, or treated effluents may contain 1-10 mg/L ammonia in water (recommended safe levels <0.5 mg/L).

e. Sediment (undissolved materials) carried as suspension in water may adsorb or transport variety of organic and inorganic toxicants that are not soluble in water (e.g. pesticides and heavy metals).

f. Extreme salinity reduces water intake by animals. Decreased feed intake often accompanies decreased water intake.

g. Bacterial count is a common laboratory measure of water quality. Generally coliform (*E. coli*) levels greater than or equal to 5000/100 ml should be avoided.

Types of water pollutant: Advanced analytical methods have detected a vast spectrum of chemical compounds in water that had been previously gone unnoticed. Depending on the nature, the water pollutants are of three types: Physical pollutants, biological pollutants and chemical pollutants. Physical pollutants primarily constitute mud, girt, stone lime, ash, animal and human waste, and mining wastes. These results in turbidity and decreased solubility of oxygen in water making it unfit for human or animal consumption. Aquatic fauna such as algae, bacteria, viruses, parasites and plants contribute towards biological pollution, which may produce a number of diseases in animals. The chemical pollutants include a large number of organic and inorganic chemicals released into water from various natural and anthropogenic sources. These chemical pollutants are toxicologically more important due to their potential to produce serious adverse effects on human and animal health. The adverse effects of some of the common water pollutants have been described in the present chapter.

I. ORGANIC POLLUTANTS

Over 400 organic chemicals have been identified in drinking water supplies, over 300 of which have been identified in treated drinking water. The toxicity of most of these chemicals is unknown and uncharacterised at present. Sources of the organic contaminants in drinking water include mainly agricultural and urban run off, discharges from industry and domestic sewage treatment plants, and chlorination practices.

1. Polyhalogenated Biphenyls

Polychlorinated Biphenyls

Polychlorinated biphenyls (PCBs) is a generic term used to describe a number of chlorinated derivatives of biphenyls. Polychlorinated biphenyls that are available commercially are a mixture of several major and minor components; the major ones being biphenyl compounds with varying degrees of chlorination e.g. arochlor 1242, a proprietary PCB compound, has 42% chlorine and arochlor 1248 has 48% chlorine. The minor components are contaminants such as halogenated dibenzofurans or dibenzodioxins. Polychlorinated biphenyls are widely distributed in environment and are considerably toxic. Contaminated water and feed-stuffs are responsible for most exposures of animals.

Properties: Polychlorinated biphenyls (PCBs) are a class of organic compounds with 1 to 10 chlorine atoms attached to biphenyl and a general chemical formula of $C_{12}H_{10-x}Cl_x$. Most of the 210 congeners of PCB are colourless and odourless crystals, but the commercial mixtures are mostly clear viscous liquids. Polychlorinated biphenyls are unusual organic molecules because they are highly stable, lowly volatile, and resistant to acids, bases, water, high temperatures and electrical currents. Therefore, they were previously widely used as insulating fluids in electrical transformers and capacitors, as well as in hydraulic fluids where resistance to high temperature was required. They have been extensively used in industry in plasticizers, paints, lubricants, insulating tapes, fireproofing materials, printing inks, sealants,

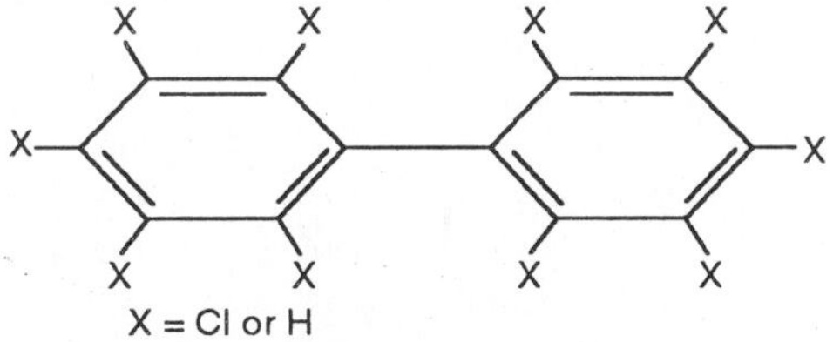

X = Cl or H

General structure

Fig.17.3. Chemical structure of polychlorinated biphenyls (PCBs).

carbon-less copy paper and pesticide preparations. Now their production has been banned in many developed countries and the PCB compounds are destroyed or discarded. However because of their stability, high lipid solubility, and resistance to microbial breakdown and biotransformation, several million tonnes of PCBs still exist in some form in the environment e.g. in lakes, ponds and marine water and have bioaccumulated in the food chain. In water, a small amount of PCBs may remain dissolved, but most stick to organic particles and bottom sediments. PCBs also bind strongly to soil and can travel long distances in the air and be deposited in areas far away from where they were released. Polychlorinated biphenyls in soils are reported to cause plant contamination, animal residues or both.

Toxicity: Polychlorinated biphenyls are highly toxic due to their high lipid solubility and stability. The stability and hence their persistence in environment and animal body vary with the pattern and extent of halogenation. A group of PCBs, known as non-ortho PCBs or coplaener PCBs (i.e. PCBs 77, 126, 169, etc), tend to have dioxin-like properties and generally are among the most toxic congeners. All species of animals can accumulate PCBs in their tissues, but their susceptibility and potential to suffer clinically varies. The toxicity of PCBs also varies to some extent with the age and sex with young animals and females being more susceptible. Among domestic animals, the ranch mink appears to be most susceptible with a dietary level of only 1 ppm PCB causing decreased litter size and viability of offspring. Swine appear to be somewhat tolerant clinically, but high doses of PCB produce toxic effects. The reproductive performance of swine is affected when 20 ppm arochlor 1242 is fed throughout the gestation period resulting in increased number of mummified foetuses. Fish are highly susceptible to toxic effects of PCBs with concentrations of 20 and 50 ppb lethal to catfish and bluegill when exposed for several weeks. Some species of fish are killed by concentration as low as 1 ppb. Fish and fish-eating wild life are the primary biological magnifiers and contain very high concentrations of PCBs in tissues.

Toxicokinetics: Polychlorinated biphenyls are highly lipid soluble compounds, so they are extensively absorbed (> 90%) from GI tract, widely distributed in body and stored primarily in adipose tissues. Dermal exposure of PCBs also results in very rapid absorption. These compounds are relatively less metabolised in body and are excreted as such. Once exposure to PCBs stops, they show two-phase elimination kinetics: the initial rapid elimination with half-life of 6 days followed by terminal slow elimination with half-life of 68 days. The PCBs are easily excreted in milk and have ability to cross the placenta. Weight loss, parturition, lactation and other metabolic changes mobilize body fat stores and therefore increase the rate of biotransformation and excretion of PCBs.

Mechanism of action: The exact mechanism of action of most PCB compounds is not clearly known. Some of the important actions are given below:

a. Some PCBs bind to specific receptors and enter into the nucleus. In the nucleus, they interact with DNA and initiate transcription of a number of proteins. These proteins may include some P-450 enzymes (e.g. arylhydrocarbon hydroxylase), which cause liver enlargement. Induction of cytochrome P-450 enzymes alters metabolism of a number of endogenous substances including steroids and hormones.

b. Some PCBs are potent acnegenic and are capable of producing hyperkeratosis and hyperpigmentation of skin in various species.

c. Several PCBs act as endocrine disruptors and produce abnormal changes in body. Their anti-oestrogenic or oestrogenic effects alter the sex (e.g. feminization of male foetus) and sexual functioning. Some components possess significant antithyroid effects.

d. PCBs affect the synthesis of certain biogenic amines and neurotransmitters. Inhibition of dopamine synthesis/ concentration in brain has been documented after exposure to PCBs.

e. High doses of some PCBs (e.g. lower halogenated PCBs) may induce hepatic dysfunction with subsequent abnormalities in heme synthesis. This results in accumulation of large quantities of dermatitis-inducing porphyrin.

f. PCBs interact with various components of immune system and alter the immune response. Increased susceptibility to diseases has been observed following exposure to PCBs in some species.

g. Some PCBs are teratogenic in nature. In pregnant animals, they easily cross placenta and produce foetus malformation.

Clinical signs: Polychlorinated biphenyls toxicosis in human beings produces clinical signs such as dark pigmentation of nails and skin, acne, swelling of limbs, lachrymation, conjunctivitis, jaundice, peripheral neuropathy, fever, headache, vomiting and diarrhoea. Infants born to mothers exposed to excessive levels of PCBs during pregnancy are "cola coloured". In cattle and some other species, acute poisoning is rarely seen (only at high PCB concentration) with clinical signs of decreased milk production, anorexia, lachrymation, salivation, dehydration, diarrhoea, alopecia, hyperkeratosis, behavioural alterations and terminal recumbency. Low concentrations of PCBs in feed may produce weight loss, anorexia, decreased feed convertibility, abortions, embryonal resorption and decreased fertility. In pregnant sows, depression, septicaemia, mummification of foeti, smaller litter size and increase in stillbirths also occur. These compounds are also carcinogenic as their long-term feeding to female rats result in liver tumours.

In birds, PCBs produce a clinical condition commonly called "Chick oedema" characterised by loss of body weight, anorexia, ascites, subcutaneous oedema, hydropericardium, enlarged kidneys and dermatitis. PCBs may also produce decreased fertility and egg production, reduced hatchability of eggs, and reduced chick viability.

Post-mortem findings: Post-mortem findings of PCBs poisoning are not specific, but may include lesions of gastric irritation and hyperaemia. With higher exposures, mucoid hyperplasia, mucosal oedema, gastric/abomasal ulceration and thickening of gall bladder may be present. In cattle, there may be dehydration, emaciation, enlarged pale kidneys, enlarged liver and dermal hyperkeratosis. Microscopically, there may be fatty degeneration, dilatation of sinusoids and rarely centrilobular necrosis in liver. In chicks, necropsy lesions may include hydropericardium, enlarged kidneys, centrilobular hepatic necrosis, spleenic atrophy and occasional enteritis with intestinal haemorrhages.

Diagnosis: PCB poisoning is difficult to diagnose from clinical signs and lesions. Diagnosis is primarily aimed at detecting PCBs in milk and body fat, liver, feed and other suspected samples with help of gas chromatography.

Treatment and management: There is no specific effective therapy for PCBs toxicosis. Efforts should concentrate on identification of contaminated animals and environments to prevent further contamination. The long-term residue problems and potential for permanent effects often make the treatment uneconomical in livestock.

Polybrominated Biphenyls

Polybrominated biphenyls (PBBs) are chemically and toxicologically similar to that of polychlorinated biphenyls (PCBs), but they contain bromine instead of chlorine in their structure. They have fire retardant properties and are added to plastics used in products such as home electrical appliances, textiles, plastic foams etc. to make them difficult to burn. While once widely used commercially, PBBs are now controlled substances. They can enter the air, water, and soil during their manufacture, use, and disposal and from accidental spills and leaks during their transport. Similar to PCBs, they persist in the environment in aquatic sediments, landfills, food chains and in adipose tissues of animals. Although their distribution is less widespread compared to PCBs, they are still a cause of environmental concern due to high stability, persistence and lipid solubility. A toxic syndrome associated with PBBs contaminated feed to dairy cattle was reported in 1974 in U.S.A. which caused heavy losses.

Polybrominated biphenyls, similar to PCBs, contain several isomers with major and minor components; the major components with varying degrees of bromination. These are believed to activate RNA synthesis in the cell nucleus and lead to the induction of monooxygenases. Generally PBBs appear more potent than comparable PCBs in inducing microsomal enzymes and altering metabolism of endogenous substances, but their toxicity potential appears to be comparatively less than the PCBs. Toxicosis in dairy cattle is likely at dosages exceeding 50 mg/kg body weight for 60 days. They accumulate in adipose tissues of animals and their clearance from body below 1 ppm may not occur during a normal life time of the animal.

Clinical signs of PBBs poisoning in dairy cows include anorexia, depressed milk production, frequent urination, lachrymation, lameness, excessive hoof growth, infertility, abortion, early embryonic resorption, prolonged gestation, alopecia and wrinkling, and thickening of skin. Because of immunosuppression, there are increased chances of infectious diseases. These agents have no specific and satisfactory treatment. Disposal of the contaminated animals and decontamination of the premises are the only available course of action. Accidental contamination of the animal feed supply by PCBs and PBBs is a potential source of contamination of the human food supply, so any incidence of toxicity in animals should be closely monitored.

2. Polycyclic Aromatic Hydrocarbons

Polycyclic aromatic hydrocarbons (PAHs) are a class of very stable organic molecules made up of only carbon and hydrogen. There are more than 100 different PAHs, generally occurring in nature as complex mixtures. The typical PAHs include benzo(a)pyrene, benzo(a)anthracene, benzofluranthrene and chrysene. These compounds can be point source pollutants (e.g. oil spill) or non-point source pollutants (e.g. atmospheric deposition) and occur widely in the environment in water, soil dust, air and in many foods. Levels of PAHs in soil can be quite high and levels of these substances decrease with increased distance from industrialized centres and highways.

Properties: Polycyclic aromatic hydrocarbons are organic compounds that consist of fused aromatic rings and do not contain heteroatoms or carry substituents. They are stable lipophilic organic compounds that are primarily formed by incomplete combustion of carbon-containing fuels such as wood, coal, diesel, gas, garbage, or other organic substances such as fat or tobacco. They can also be found in substances such as crude oil, coal tar pitch, and creosote and in sewage sludge. PAHs usually occur naturally, but they can be manufactured as individual compounds for research purposes and a few are used in medicines and to make dyes, plastics and pesticides. PAHs enter the environment mostly as releases to air from forest fires, residential wood burning, volcanoes and exhaust from automobiles and are carried in air to long distances before returning to earth in rainfall or particle settling. They can also enter surface water through discharges from industrial plants and waste water treatment plants, and can be released to soils at hazardous waste sites if they escape from storage containers. Some PAHs evaporate into the atmosphere from surface waters, but most stick to solid particles and settle to bottoms of rivers or lakes. Plants and animals living on the land or in water can bioaccumulate PAHs and may contaminate the food chains. Breakdown of PAHs in soil and water occurs very slowly over weeks to months and is caused primarily by the action of microorganisms.

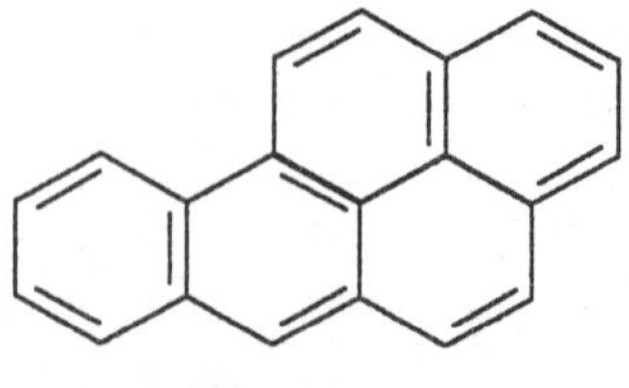

Benzo(a)pyrene

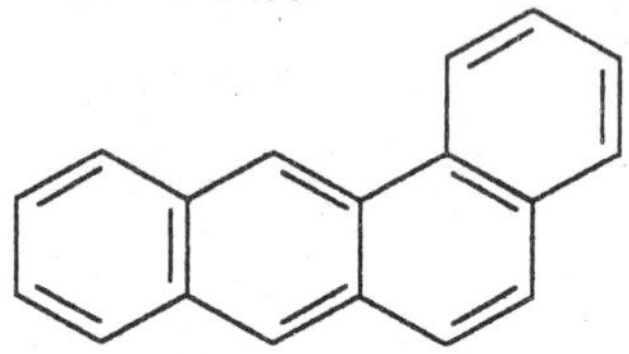

Benzo(a)anthracene

Fig.17.4. Chemical structures of some important polycyclic aromatic hydrocarbons.

Toxicity: Toxicity of PAHs depends on the chemical structure, with isomers varying from being nontoxic to being extremely toxic. Benzo(a)pyrene (BP), a common PAH, is shown to cause lung and skin cancer in laboratory animals, but other PAHs are not known to have this effect. A diet containing 25 ppm of benzo(a)pyrene for 140 days in mice produces leukaemia, lung adenoma and stomach tumour. Skin tumours develop in many rats, if they are treated topically with benzo(a)pyrene. Exposure via inhalation is considered more toxic due to better absorption of PAHs than by ingestion or dermal exposure.

Toxicokinetics: Polycyclic aromatic hydrocarbons can enter the body through lungs when the contaminated air is inhaled or through drinking water and food that contain these chemicals. They could also enter the body via dermal exposure, especially when the skin comes directly in contact with contaminated soil or products (e.g. crankcase oil or creosote) that contain PAHs. The rate of absorption of PAHs from different routes is variable and can be influenced by presence of other compounds. After absorption, PAHs are rapidly distributed to all tissues that contain fat. They tend to get stored mostly in the kidneys, liver and fat with smaller amounts in other organs such as spleen, adrenal glands and ovaries. PAHs are metabolized in body to different degrees to both active and inactive metabolites. Some of the active metabolites are more harmful than the parent compounds. Results from animal studies show that most PAHs that enter the body are excreted within a few days, primarily in faeces and urine.

Mechanism of action: The PAHs produce their action in different ways, some of which have not been clearly defined.

a. Some PAHs including benz(a)anthracene and benzo(a)pyrene are mutagenic and highly carcinogenic. It is suggested that benzo(a)pyrene is not mutagenic or carcinogenic by itself, but it is pro-carcinogen and pro-mutagen that produces an active metabolite benzo(a)pyrene diolepoxide, which reacts with various components in the cells including DNA to produce mutagenicity and carcinogenicity. The active metabolite benzo(a)pyrene diolepoxide mainly intercalates in DNA by covalently binding to the nucleophilic guanine nucleobases at the N-2 position. This can disrupt the normal process of copying DNA and may lead to cancer. This mechanism of action is similar to that of aflatoxin which binds to the N-7 position of guanine.

b. Similar to PCBs, PBBs and dioxins, the benzo(a)pyrene induces cytochrome P450 and some other proteins. It first binds to certain cytosolic receptors (e.g. arylhydrocarbon receptor), which translocate it to the nucleus. In the nucleus it binds to DNA and increases transcription of certain genes, notably cytochrome P4501A1 (CYP1A1), followed by increased protein production.

c. Some PAHs including benzo(a)pyrene produce reproductive problems and teratogenic effects if given during pregnancy.

d. Some studies in animals have also shown that PAHs can cause harmful effects on immune system after both short- and long-term exposures. The exposed animals were found more susceptible to infections.

Clinical signs: Polycyclic aromatic hydrocarbons mostly produce chronic toxicity; acute poisoning in animals is rarely reported except in accidental exposure to large amount. Acute and chronic exposure to benzo(a)pyrene generally leads to reproductive system abnormalities and bone marrow toxicity. However, it is unlikely that noncarcinogenic adverse health effects would be caused at the levels of benzo(a)pyrene currently found in the environment. The benzo(a)pyrene and some other PAHs are primary carcinogenic and produce various types of tumour.

Diagnosis: Diagnosis of PAHs poisoning is difficult. Many PAHs can be detected in blood or urine soon after exposure, but tests for these compounds are not routine and can only be performed using special equipment.

Treatment and management: There is no specific effective therapy for PCBs toxicosis. Efforts should concentrate on identification of contaminated animals and environments to prevent further contamination.

3. Trihalomethanes

Trihalomethanes (THMs) are chemical compounds containing three halogen atoms substituted for the three hydrogen atoms normally present in a methane molecule. The THMs are mostly formed as by-products of the water treatment process when chlorine or bromine added to disinfect water reacts with natural organic matter such as the decaying vegetation, commonly found in lakes and reservoirs. The THMs of clinical importance include chloroform, bromoform, bromodichloromethane and dibromochloromethane. Chloroform is also formed in swimming pools which are disinfected with chlorine or hypochlorite in the haloform reaction with organic substances like urine, sweat and skin particles. Exposure to low concentrations of chloroform in water can irritate the skin, nose and eyes and can cause nausea, dizziness, fatigue and confusion. Higher levels of chloroform may be able to cause a rash or a burning feeling and repeated skin contact may produce dermatitis. Absorption of chloroform through intact skin may also occur to produce some systemic effects. Scientific studies have linked some THMs (e.g. dichlorobromomethane) to increased risk of cancer. Other studies have linked increased chlorination by-products to reproductive problems and damage to CNS, heart, lung, kidney and liver. To avoid their adverse effects on health, many countries have set the permissible limits of THMs in drinking water.

4. Pesticides

The increasing use of insecticides and herbicides in agriculture has substantially increased their concentrations in the surface water (e.g. streams and ponds) as well as in the ground water due to run off from field or leaching. The concentration of these chemicals may be much more in non-potable water where pesticides are added purposely to control insects, especially vectors of diseases breeding in it. Such compounds may involve organochlorine insecticides (e.g. DDT, DDE, BHC and heptachlor) and many organophosphorus compounds (e.g. fenthion). These biocide chemicals can cause various types of adverse effects in humans, domestic animals and wildlife including nervous, circulatory and respiratory disorders (See for detail Chapter 13).

II. INORGANIC POLLUTANTS

1. Heavy Metals

The environmental metals of greatest concern are lead, mercury, arsenic and cadmium followed by nickel, cobalt, tin, manganese, copper, etc. Epidemiological studies have demonstrated associations between several diseases and consumption of heavy metal contaminated water. Danger to the food chain from metals may result when plants are grown nearby contaminated water or when contaminated water is used directly for irrigation of crops. Danger to animals drinking the contaminated water also exists. Toxic amounts of arsenic and lead, for instance, have been found in certain domestic waters and toxic effects were noted in human beings and animals. An outbreak of mercury poisoning in Minimata and Niigata in Japan have been traced to the methyl mercury contents of the fish from nearby heavily polluted water. The detailed toxicology of heavy metals has been discussed separately (see Metals, Chapter 11).

2. Non-Metals

The use of nitrogen fertilizers and modern feed-lot practices can cause significant increase in the size of nitrogen pool and, thereby, increase in levels of nitrogen materials in soil, water and food crops. Of particular concern are high levels of nitrates and nitrites in drinking water. Nitrates in water tend to occur in the nitrate (NO_3^-) oxidation state which produces nitrite (NO_2^-) in the presence of nitrate-reducing bacteria. Nitrite can react with secondary amines to form nitrosamines. Nitrosamines have been identified in the air and water. Based on both field and experimental evidences, less than 300 ppm nitrate in water is acceptable for drinking purposes.

High sulphate in drinking water may be associated with industrial processes or pyrite oxidation (associated with acid mine drainage) and oxidation of sulphides to sulphates. Sulphates as a component of saline water are associated with a purging or diarrhoeic effect similar to the effects from saline cathartics (e.g. sodium or magnesium sulphate). However, the response to saline-sulphate water is usually transient and animals adapt to the sulphate intake after 3-7 days. Field observations have led to recommendations that water containing more than 1000 ppm sulphates should be used cautiously, especially in weanling pigs.

C. FOOD AND FEED CONTAMINANTS

Food and feed contaminants are substances that have not been intentionally added to food and are also not a part of food. These substances may be present in food as a result of various stages of its production, packaging, transport or storage. They also might result from environmental contamination. Their number is numerous and their knowledge is incomplete. They mostly come from the environment or, in some cases, are produced in the food due to bacterial or fungal contamination. Many plants result in production and accumulation of abnormal and, in some cases, toxic metabolites when subject to a variety of stress conditions. Recent introduction of genetically modified food is also referred to some extent as a form of food contaminants. This chapter addresses the environmental contamination of foods, as opposed to microbiological or plant contamination that has been taken earlier in Chapters 14 and 15. Residues of pesticides, fertilizers, industrial chemicals, growth-promoting substances, antibiotics and radioactive substances are examples of environmental food contaminants.

I. ORGANIC COMPOUNDS

1. Dioxins

Dioxins are a large class of natural and synthetic halogenated organic compounds that contain oxygen atoms held in ether linkages to carbon atoms generally with in a six-membered ring. One sub-group of these substances, the polychlorinated dibenzodioxins, is of significant toxicological importance. The most notorious of the dibenzodioxins is tetrachlorodibenzodioxin (TCDD). Although TCDD has 22 different isomers that generally occur in mixtures in the environment, the 2, 3, 7, 8-tetrachloro isomer has unusual degree of toxicity. The dioxins have been shown to bioaccumulate in humans, animals and wildlife due to their lipophilic properties.

Properties: The term dioxin is often used to denote compounds that are actually polychlorinated dibenzodioxins (PCDDs) and less commonly polybrominated dibenzodioxins (PBDDs) and polychlorinated dibenzofurans (PCDFs). The basic structure of PCDDs comprises two benzene rings joined by a double or a single oxygen bridge. Chlorine atoms are attached to the basic structure at any of 8 different places on the molecule, positions 1–4 and 6–9. The polychlorinated dibenzodioxins are mainly formed as contaminants during manufacturing of chlorophenol compounds such as trichlorophenol, pentachlorophenol and hexachlorophenol and bleaching fibres for paper or textiles. Contaminants of trichlorophenol and herbicides such as 2,4-dichlorophenoxyacetic acid (2,4-D) and 2,4,5-trichlorophenoxyacetic acid (2,4,5-T) include tetrachlorodibenzodioxin and that of pentachlorophenol include hexachlorodibenzodioxin and octachlorodibenzodioxin. Dioxins are also produced in small concentrations when organic material is burned in the presence of chlorine or organochlorine compounds (e.g. Coal fired utilities, metal smelting, diesel vehicles, land application of sewage sludge and burning of treated wood). The dibenzodioxins after synthesis are released into the environment and enter food chain. They accumulate in food chains in a fashion similar to other chlorinated compounds and produce adverse effects. Accordingly, dioxin-containing products such as pentachlorophenol and chlorinated phenoxy herbicides (especially 2, 4, 5-T) and antibacterial hexachlorophene soaps are not used currently.

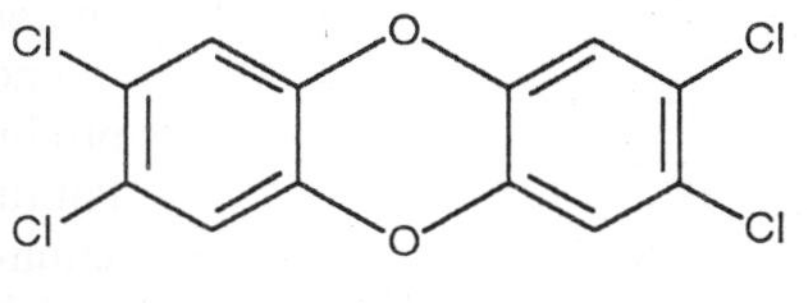

Cl Cl O Cl Cl O

Fig.17.5. Chemical structures of 2,3,7, 8-tetrachloro dibenzo-p-dioxin (TCDD).

Toxicity: Dioxins are among the most toxic substances known to man, with the 2,3,7,8-tetrachlorodibenzo-*p*-dioxin being the most toxic of the congeners. The toxicity of TCDDs varies greatly with the type of compound, isomer of compound, and species of animal. For example, the isomer 2,3,7,8-TCDD is 3-100 times as toxic as other TCDDs. Other dioxins are relatively less toxic, but vary widely in producing toxicity. Among different species, guinea-pig is the most sensitive species to 2,3,7,8-TCDD with an oral LD_{50} 0.6 μg/kg and hamster the least sensitive species with oral LD_{50} >10,000 mg/kg. Chronic toxicity of TCDDs is of greater concern than acute toxicity. Dosages of 1 μg/kg/day of 2,3,7,8-TCDD for 90 days cause death in mice. TCDDs can produce a wide range of biological effects in humans and experimental animals.

Toxicokinetics: Toxicokinetic data on dioxins in animals are not sufficient. TCDDs are readily absorbed orally or dermally but less by inhalation. They bioaccumulate primarily in fatty tissues over time; therefore even small exposures may eventually reach dangerous levels. TCDD has a half-life of approximately 7 years in humans, but at high concentrations the elimination rate is enhanced by metabolism.

Mechanism of action: It is believed that dioxins such as the 2,3,7,8-TCDD bind to a cytosolic enzyme and are transferred into the nucleus and thereafter, regulate gene expression for protein production. Similar to PCBs and PBBs, the TCDDs induce hepatic cytochrome P-450 enzymes and alter metabolism of several endogenous substances. Dioxins affect adrenocortical functions, thyroid functions and immunocompetence. Cell-mediated immunity is altered more than humoral immunity.

Clinical signs: Clinical signs and lesions of TCDDs are similar for various isomers. Important signs in domestic animals include listlessness, chronic weight loss, emaciation, alopecia, liver damage, abortion and reproductive problems. In horses, additional signs may include unsteady gait, laminitis, subcutaneous oedema, ascites, diarrhoea, colic, haematuria, polydipsia and jaundice. In dogs and cats, there may be chronic respiratory infections and oral and nasal lesions. Drop in milk production is often seen in dairy animals. In poultry, hydropericardium, oedema and ascites are prominent. Chloracne is the most obvious and initial effect in humans. Other signs that develop with increased exposure in humans include a general sense of fatigue, polyneuropathy especially affecting legs, anaemia and thrombocytopenia. Pancytopenia and widespread haemorrhages occur in monkeys. Death may occur in severe cases in all species.

The 2,3,7,8-TCDD is a potent carcinogen and teratogen. Teratogenesis includes cystic kidneys and cleft palate in mice and absence of eyelids in hamsters. TCDDs can produce immunosuppression with exposures too low to produce clinical signs or pathological changes.

Post-mortem findings: Important necropsy findings of TCDDs in animals may include hepatic necrosis, haemorrhages in different organs and renal degeneration. In horses, there may also be lymphoid atrophy, skin and oral ulcerations, hepatic portal cirrhosis and biliary proliferation. Hypertrophy of all squamous epithelia including the skin may be observed in some species.

Diagnosis: Diagnosis of dioxin poisoning is difficult from clinical signs or post-mortem lesions.

Treatment and management: There is no specific effective therapy for dioxin toxicosis. Efforts should concentrate on identification of contaminated animals and environments to prevent further contamination.

2. Polychlorinated Biphenyls and Polybrominated Biphenyls

Polychlorinated biphenyls (PCBs) and polybrominated biphenyls (PBBs) occurrence in food and feed stuffs may result in harmful effects in animals and human beings. Their detailed toxicity has been discussed earlier in water and soil pollutants.

3. Pesticides

In recent years, contamination of food by pesticides has been recognised as a serious and growing problem in the world. Different crops require different pesticide in their production and may vary in their retention. While many pesticides degrade rapidly in the environment or bind tightly to the soil, some are stable and persist in crops. So residues of pesticides often remain on produce and animals are exposed to low levels of the pesticides. In addition, numerous incidents of acute poisoning from pesticides have resulted from eating food that was grossly contaminated during storage, transportation, etc. A large number of pesticides present in food and feed are chlorinated hydrocarbons (e.g. DDT, BHC, heptachlor) followed by other groups such as herbicides, OP insecticides and fumigants.

II. INORGANIC COMPOUNDS

1. Metals

The problem of toxicity by metals and metallic compound in foods is very complex because a number of metals are dietary essentials and all foods contain at least trace quantities of many metals. Lead has been detected in all foods examined, even those grown far away from the industrialised areas. In general, plant foods grown in industrialised areas and near highways contain significantly higher level of lead and other metals than food grown in remote areas. Seeds treated with mercurial fungicides constitute an important source of mercury entering the food chain. Several other metals like selenium and molybdenum are present in high concentrations in fodder plants and crops grown on metal rich soils and pose danger to the animals.

2. Non-metals

Heavy use of nitrogenous fertilizers and herbicides such as 2,4-D increases the nitrate/nitrite content of the soils and plants making them unsuitable for animals. Several cases of acute poisoning have been reported following ingestion of plants, feed or water containing excessive amounts of nitrate.

III. OTHER TOXICANTS

Several different types of toxicants and chemicals may contaminate food and feed products. These include petroleum products, antibiotics, antiparasitic drugs, growth and performance enhancers, dyes, solvents, household chemicals and detergents. Such contaminations usually occur due to inadvertent and accidental mixing of these compounds with food and it is difficult to ascertain their toxic effects. Presence of antibiotic residues in milk and foods of animal origin is a serious medical problem and is creating drug-resistance in animals and humans. More recently, concern has been focused on possible release of vinyl chloride monomer from polyvinyl chloride (PVC) wrappers and containers. Vinyl chloride has been shown to be carcinogenic in rats and other experimental animals and results in liver tumour in man.

BIBLIOGRAPHY

Awang R (2005) Inhaled poisons. Pusat Racun Negara, Universiti Sains Malaysia. (www.prn2.usm.my/mainsite/bulletin/1995/prn5.html).

Bartik M and Piskac A (1981) Veterinary Toxicology. Elsevier Scientific Publishing Company, Amsterdam.

Beasley VR (1990) Smoke inhalation. *Vet. Clin. North Am: Small Anim Pract.* 20 : 545.

Beasley V (1999) Veterinary Toxicology. International Veterinary Information Service, Ithaca NY (www.ivis.org).

Bjorseth A (1983) Handbook of Polycyclic Aromatic Hydrocarbons. Mercel Dekker, New York.

Costa DL and Amdur MO (1996) Air pollution. In: Casarett & Doull's Toxicology: The Basic Science of Poisons. 5th edn. Klaassen CD (Ed.) p 857. Mcgraw Hill Companies Inc., New York.

Davis MS and Foster WM (2002) Inhalation toxicology in the equine respiratory tract. In: Equine Respiratory Diseases. Lekeux P (ed.) International Veterinary Information Service, Ithaca, NY. (www. ivis.org).

EPA (2001) Principal air pollutants. (http://www.epa.nsw.gov.au/envirom/princairpol.htm).

Folinsbee LJ (1989) Human health effects of exposure to airborne acid. *Environ Hlth Perspect.* 79 : 195.

Garg SK (2000) Veterinary Toxicology. CBS Publishers & Distributors, New Delhi.

Guidotti TL (1978) The higher oxides of nitrogen: Inhalation toxicology. *Environ. Res.* 15: 443.

Hazucha MJ (1987) Relationship between ozone exposure and pulmonary function changes. *J. Appl. Physiol.* 62 : 1671.

Hughes WW (1996) Essentials of Environmental Toxicology. Taylor & Francis, Washington.

Johnson RL, Gehring PJ, Kociba RJ and Schwertz BA (1973) Chlorinated dibenzodioxins and pentachlorophenol. *Environ. Hlth. Perspect.* 5 : 171.

Kalf GF (1987) Recent advances in the metabolism and toxicity of benzene. *CRC Crit. Rev. Toxicol.* 18 : 141.

Kinney PL and Ozkaynak H (1991) Associations of daily mortality and air pollution in Los Angeles County. *Environ. Res.* 54 : 99.

Kinney PL, Ware JH and Spengler JD (1988) A critical evaluation of acute ozone epidemiological results. *Arch. Environ. Hlth.* 43: 168.

Klaassen CD (1996) Casarett & Doull's Toxicology: The Basic Science of Poisons. 5th edn. Mcgraw Hill, New York.

Klaassen CD (2001) Non-metallic environmental toxicants: Air pollutants, solvents and vapours, and pesticides. In: Goodman & Gilman's The Pharmacological Basis of Therapeutics. 10th edn. Hardman JG, Limbird LE and Gilman AG (Eds.) p 1877. The McGraw-Hill Companies Inc., New York.

Lu FC and Kacew S (2002) Lu's Basic Toxicology: Fundamentals, Target Organs and Risk Assessment. Taylor & Francis, New York.

Maynard RL and Waller RE (1995) Air pollution. In: General and Applied Toxicology. Ballantyne B, Marrs T and Turner P (Eds.) p 1097. Macmillan Press Ltd., London.

Osweiler GD (1996) Toxicology. Williams and Wilkins, Philadelphia.

Peterson JS, Miller SM and Charles BC (2005) Toxicity, nitrous dioxide. (www.emedicine.com/emerg/topic847.htm).

Plunkett ER (1976) Handbook of Industrial Toxicology. Chemical Publishing Company, Inc., New York.

Poland A and Knutson J (1982) 2,3,7,8-Tetrachlorobnezo-p-dioxin and related halogenated aromatic hydrocarbons : examination of the mechanism of toxicity. *Ann. Rev. Pharmacol. Toxicol.* 22 : 517.

Polson CJ and Tattersall RN (1980) Clinical Toxicology. 2nd edn. Pitman Medical, London.

Prakash R (1989) Recent Trends in Toxicology. Environmental Series Vol. II. Society of Biosciences, Muzaffarnagar.

Sielken R Jr. (1987) Quantitative cancer risk assessment for 2,3,7,8-tetrachlorodibenzo-p-dioxin (TCDD). *Food Chem. Toxicol.* 25 : 257.

Sodergren A (1972) Chlorinated hydrocarbon residues in airborne fallout. *Nature (London)*. 236 : 395.

Spencer WF (1975) Movement of DDT and its derivatives into the atmosphere. *Res. Rev.* 59 : 91.

Stewart RD (1975) The effects of carbon monoxide on humans. *Ann. Rev. Pharmacol.* 15 : 409.

Teofilo L. Lee and Chiong Jr. (1999) Smoke inhalation injury. *Postgrad. Med. Online*. 105. (http://www.postgradmed.com/issues/1999/02_99/chiong.htm).

Wikipedia (2007) Air pollutants. (http://en.wikipedia.org/wiki/Air_pollution).

World Health Organization (1990) Environment Health Criteria 104: Principles for the Toxicological assessment of Pesticide Residues in Food. WHO, Geneva.

❑❑❑❑❑❑

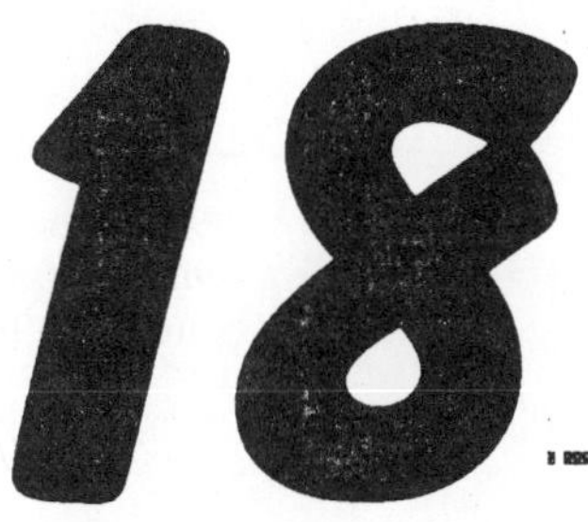

FOOD AND FEED ADDITIVES

- **Food additives**
  - Anticaking agents
    - Sodium aluminosilicate
  - Antioxidants
    - Ascorbic acid (Vitamin C)
    - Propyl gallate
  - Colouring agents
    - Amaranth
    - Tartrazine
    - Other colouring agents
  - Flavouring and flavour enhancing agents
    - Methyl anthranilate
    - Safrole
    - Monosodium glutamate
  - Non-nutritive sweeteners
    - Saccharin
    - Sodium cyclamate
    - Aspartame
  - Preservatives
    - Benzoic acid
    - Sorbic acid and its salts
- **Feed additives**
  - Growth and performance enhancers
    - Ionophore antibiotics
    - Zinc bacitracin
    - Tylosin
  - Non-protein nitrogen compounds
    - Urea and ammonium compounds
    - 4-Methylimidazole
  - Miscellaneous feed additives
    - Sodium chloride

FOOD ADDITIVES

Food additives may be defined as non-nutritive substances added intentionally to food, generally in small quantities, to improve its appearance, texture or storage properties. The practice of adding substances or chemicals to food is very old. These additions are usually made during production, processing, storage and/or packaging. Today as many as 2500 substances are being added to foods for various purposes.

Purpose of Food Additives

Food additives are added for specific purposes like:

a. To facilitate handling, distribution and preparation of food stuffs.

b. To control chemical, physical and microbial changes so as to lessen wastage, hazards from microorganisms, and to preserve quality over extended period.

c. To facilitate modification and synthesis of standard food contents to meet special dietary needs and to offer many novelties and convenient foods.

d. To improve sensory and nutritive properties.

Numbering and Classification

Numbering: Each food additive is assigned a unique number to regulate its use, to protect health of consumers and to ensure fair practices in the international food trade. These numbers are prefixed by "E" in European countries and without "E" by some other countries. For example, benzoic acid is written as E210 on products sold in Europe, but is simply known as additive 210 in some other countries. This numbering scheme has been adopted by the Codex Alimentarius Committee to internationally identify all additives, regardless of whether they are approved for use. The Codex Alimentarius is a collection of internationally recognized standards, codes of practice, guidelines and other recommendations relating to foods, food production and food safety under the aegis of consumer protection. Officially, it is maintained by the Codex Alimentarius Trade Commission and their laws are adopted by the Food and Agriculture Organization (FAO) and the World Health Organization (WHO).

Classification: Food additives are usually classified according to their use, rather than chemical structure. The most commonly used categories are based on their intended functions.

I. *Anticaking agents:* These agents are added to finely powdered or crystalline foods to prevent caking or lumping e.g. sodium aluminosilicate and calcium silicate.

II. *Antioxidants:* These agents retard deterioration, rancidity and discolouration due to oxidation e.g. ascorbic acid, triethyl citrate and propyl gallate.

III. *Colouring agents:* These agents impart, preserve or enhance the colour e.g. amaranth, tartrazine and erythrosin.

IV. *Emulsifying agents:* These agents modify surface tension (maintain a desired consistency), especially to keep oil in water mixtures e.g. cholic acid, desoxycholic acid and gum tragacanth.

V. *Flavouring agents:* These agents impart or help to impart an aroma in food e.g. methyl anthranilate, safrole and maltol.

VI. *Non-nutritive sweeteners:* These agents have less than 2% of the caloric value of sucrose per equivalent unit of sweetening capacity e.g. saccharin, sodium cyclamate and aspartame.

VII. *Nutrient supplements:* These agents provide additional essential nutrients e.g. vitamins and amino acids.

VIII. *Preservatives:* These agents prevent growth of microorganisms such as fungi and increase shelf life of food e.g. benzoic acid, sorbic acid and salicylic acid.

IX. *Sequestrants:* These agents combine with polyvalent metal ions to form a soluble metal complex to improve the quality and stability of products e.g. calcium acetate, sodium citrate and tartaric acid.

X. *Stabilisers and thickeners:* These agents improve consistency or stabilise emulsions e.g. acacia and agar-agar.

XI. *Miscellaneous additives:*

   i. *pH control agents/buffers:* These agents maintain the required pH of the food e.g. phosphoric acid.

   ii. *Drying agents:* These agents absorb excessive moisture in the food e.g. bisulphites.

   iii. *Hemectants:* These agents retain essential moisture in the food e.g. glycerine.

The margin of safety for most food additives mentioned above is many times the normal intake, but in some instances their level in food is likely to exceed the toxic threshold, especially when diet is restricted or unlimited use of food additive is permitted. However, food additives are usually not involved in animal poisonings; therefore the present chapter gives only a brief review of some important agents.

I. ANTICAKING AGENTS

Anticaking agents are added to finely powdered or crystalline foods such as table salt to keep the product from forming lumps, making it better for packaging, transport and use by the consumer. The anticaking agents include sodium aluminosilicate, calcium silicate and dimethyl polysiloxane.

1. Sodium Aluminosilicate

Sodium aluminosilicate (sodium silicoaluminate, silicic acid; E554) is a white crystalline solid. It is often added as an anticaking agent to various products including table salt and other food products, and powders to prevent formation of large crystals or lumps. It is also used for some non-food purposes like in silicated soaps and fabric washing powders, for dishwashers, etc. In recommended concentrations as a food additive, sodium aluminosilicate is non-toxic by ingestion; however, accidental intake of high amounts may cause mouth and throat irritation, nausea, gastro-intestinal disturbances and abdominal pain. It produces mild irritation to skin and eye on contact. Inhalation of sodium aluminosilicate produces irritation to respiratory tract and lungs. Prolonged inhalation may lead to mucous membrane irritation, dizziness, nausea, chest pain, coughing, difficulty of breathing, severe lung irritation or damage, and pneumoconiosis.

II. ANTIOXIDANTS

One of the most common food deterioration is the undesirable change in colour or flavour of food caused by the oxygen in air (oxidative deterioration). Oxidation also decreases the nutritional value of food and sometimes even produces toxic materials. Several agents such as vitamin C inhibit such adverse effects of oxygen on food and act as anti-oxidant and food preservative.

1. Ascorbic Acid (Vitamin C)

L-Ascorbic acid or vitamin C (E300) is an essential nutrient required in small amounts to carryout some essential metabolic reactions in animals and plants. It is not only an important nutrient needed as a coenzyme in some enzymatic reactions but also an antioxidant that protects the body against oxidative stress. Therefore, it is often added to food as an antioxidant to prevent adverse effects of oxygen. Ascorbic acid is readily oxidised in body to dehydroascorbic acid, which is reduced by glutathione in the blood. Ascorbic acid in recommended concentrations is safe and its toxicity as food additive has not been reported. However, ingestion of relatively large doses of vitamin C may cause indigestion, particularly when taken on an empty stomach. In very large doses in human beings, it may cause diarrhoea, perspirations, nervous tension and lowered pulse. The risk of urinary oxalate stones may also be increased. Ascorbic acid is an irritant and may cause irritation of skin and eyes on contact and respiratory tract on inhalation. Repeated intravenous injections of 80 mg dehydroascorbic acid were reported to have diabetogenic effects in rats. World Health Organization (WHO) has recommended that its daily intake should be less than 0.25 mg/kg body weight.

2. Propyl Gallate

Propyl gallate (n-propyl-3, 4, 5-trihydroxybenzoate, gallic acid; E310) is a fine, white to nearly white, odourless powder having slightly bitter taste. It is slightly soluble in water and freely soluble in alcohol and ether. Propyl gallate is made from natural gallic acid by condensation of gallic acid and propanol. It exhibits excellent antioxidant activity in food and vegetable oils, especially in combination with ascorbyl palmitate. It is also used as antioxidant in cosmetics, hair products, adhesives and lubricants. As a food additive, it may be added to edible fats, oils, butter, baked goods, candy, dried meat, fresh pork sausage and dried milk. It protects against oxidation by hydrogen peroxide and oxygen free radicals in a catalytic manner similar to the superoxide dismutase. Based on the oral LD_{50} values, propyl gallate is of low acute oral toxicity (LD_{50} mice 1.7 g/kg and rabbits 2.7 g/kg). Ingestion of large doses of propyl gallate may produce harmful effects, but on contact or inhalation it has mild toxicity. Propyl gallate at a concentration of 1.2% or 2.3% in feed of rats produces loss of weight. In one study, when it was given for 10-16 months at 2-3% level, 40% of the rats died within first month and the remainder showed severe growth inhibition. Dietary levels of 5% over 14 days are lethal to mice. Necropsy of rats indicated kidney damage.

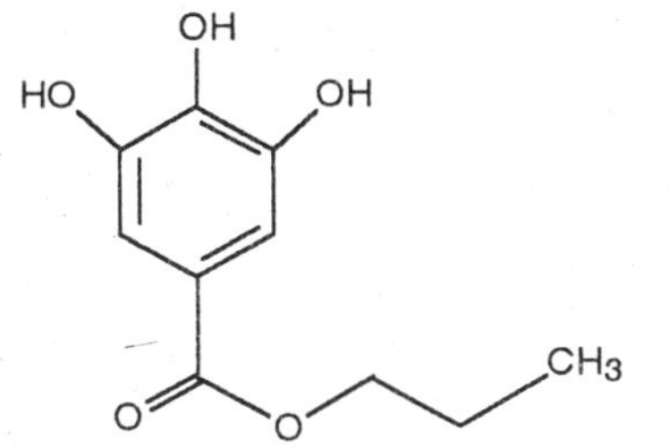

OH, HO, OH, CH_3, O, O

Fig.18.1. Chemical structure of propyl gallate.

III. COLOURING AGENTS

Colouring agents have been used to make food more attractive since ancient times. The number of colouring agents, currently permitted as food additives, is much fewer than previously and is still being reduced due to their adverse effects.

1. Amaranth

Amaranth (FD & C Red No. 2; E123) is chemically 1-(4-sulpho-1-naphthylazo)-9-naphthol-3, 6-disulphonic acid, trisodium salt and is an azo dye. It exists as dark, reddish-brown powder mainly used for dying wool and silk and in photography. FDA and several countries have banned the use of amaranth in foods, drugs and cosmetics following indications that it induces malignant tumours in rats, but its use continues,

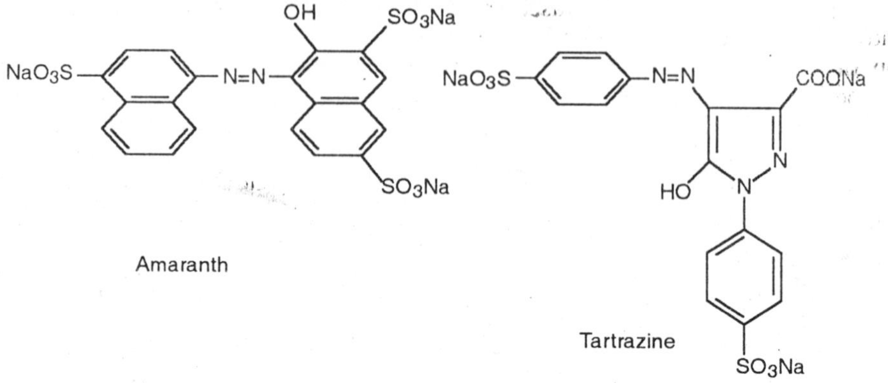

Fig.18.2. Chemical structures of some important colouring food additives.

legally or illegally, in many countries for providing a reddish or brownish colour in food. Amaranth is metabolised into amine derivatives *in vivo*. Amaranth is reduced by D-fructose and D-glucose at elevated temperatures to form a mixture of hydrazo and amine species, which may have toxicological significance. In one study, it produced liver damage, including vacuolisation and fatty degeneration accompanied by a rise in serum albumin and β-globulin when fed to rats for 18 months at 0.12% in the diet. The FAO/WHO special committee determined its acceptable daily intake (ADI) as 0-1.5 mg/kg.

2. Tartrazine

Tartrazine (FD & C Yellow No. 5; E102) is chemically 5-hydroxy-1-p-sulpho-phenyl-4-(p-sulpho phenyl azo)-pyrazol-3-carboxylic acid, trisodium salt and is a coal tar derivative dye. It is a yellow powder and has been used as a food colouring additive since 1916. Large number of food products and drugs contain tartrazine including soft drinks, flavoured chips, custard powder, soups, sauces, ice cream, candy, chewing gum, jam, jelly, pickles and other pickled products, certain brands of fruit squash, medicinal capsules, antacids and vitamins. Certain non-food products such as soaps, hair products and moisturizers also contain tartrazine. It is known to be least toxic colouring agent among synthetic colouring compounds. The oral acute LD_{50} of tartrazine in mice is 12-17 g/kg. Human sensitivity to tartrazine has been reported with some frequency and has been estimated to occur in 1 in 10,000 persons. Anaphylactic shock, potentially life threatening, has been reported but symptoms more cited are urticaria, asthma and purpura (blue or purple spots on skin or mucous membranes). Clinical signs from tartrazine sensitivity can occur by either ingestion or cutaneous exposure to a substance containing tartrazine. Food and Drug Administration (FDA) has set its ADI at 0-7.5 mg/kg.

3. Other Colouring Agents

Many synthetic colouring agents are toxic, if used in large amounts, and many are suspected carcinogens as well. Caramel (E150), which gives a light brown colour, contains carcinogenic benzo(a)pyrene in small amounts. Curcumin (E100), which gives yellow colour, is 15 times as toxic as tartrazine. Erythrosine (E127), a cherry-pink coal based fluorone food dye, can cause photosensitivity and it may be carcinogenic. Orange Yellow S (FD&C Yellow 6; E110), added to foods to induce a colour change, has the capacity for inducing an allergic reaction. Beet juice, turmeric, and saffron are other colourants used in food.

IV. FLAVOURING AND FLAVOUR ENHANCING AGENTS

A. FLAVOURING AGENTS

In addition to wide variety of spices, natural extractives, oleoresins, and essential oils used in processed foods, many synthetic flavours have been developed to increase the acceptability of food. The compounds used to produce artificial flavours are almost identical to those that occur naturally, but are prepared in laboratory by chemists using one or more chemicals. Presently over 3000 synthetic chemicals are used as flavour ingredients. These are used extensively in small amounts ranging from few parts per million to 300 ppm. Although it has been assumed that the flavouring agents are not health hazards, still their chronic toxicity should be carefully reviewed.

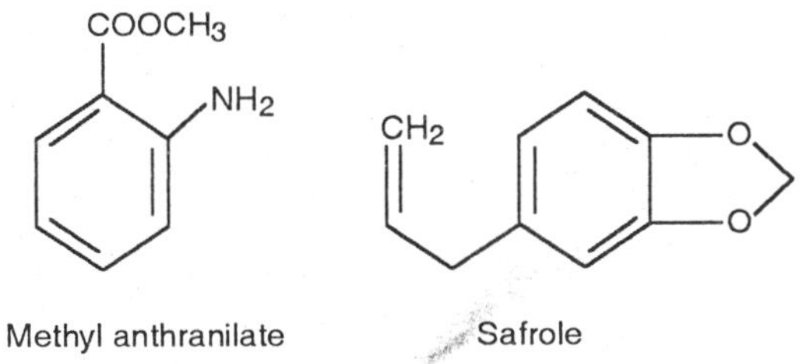

$COOCH_3$ NH_2 CH_2 O O

Methyl anthranilate Safrole

Fig.18.3. Chemical structures of some important flavouring food additives.

1. Methyl Anthranilate

Methyl anthranilate (O-Aminobenzoic acid methyl ester, MA) is a colourless liquid that has a sweet, fruity, grape like flavour. It is found in the essential oils of orange, lemon and jasmine and has been used by the food and drug industry for more than forty years to flavour candy, sodas, gums, and drugs. Its oral LD_{50} in mice and rats has been calculated to be 3900 and 2910 mg/kg body weight, respectively. Methyl anthranilate promotes some allergic reactions on human skin and may cause skin and eye irritation, so is being prohibited for use in cosmetic industries. Methyl anthranilate is classified as a "Generally Recognized as Safe (GRAS)" compound.

2. Safrole

Safrole (3, 4-Methylene dioxallyl benzene) is a colourless or slightly yellow oily liquid possessing a sweet, warm-spicy flavour. It is typically extracted from the root-bark or the fruit of sassafras plants in the form of sassafras oil, or synthesized from other related methylenedioxy compounds. Oil of Sassafras, which contains 80% safrole, has also been used as a spice. Safrole has a characteristic "candy-shop" aroma and was once widely used as a food additive; however, the Food and Drug Administration (FDA) has barred its use after it was shown to be mildly carcinogenic. Safrole and sassafras oil are not freely available because they are being used in the illicit manufacture of MDMA (ecstasy), a drug of abuse.

B. FLAVOUR ENHANCING AGENTS

Flavour enhancing agents or Flavour enhancers are food additives used to enhance the food's existing flavour, even though they do not directly contribute to flavour. They may be extracted from natural sources or created artificially and are commonly added to commercially produced food products. Monosodium glutamate and table salt (sodium chloride) are well known flavour enhancers.

1. Monosodium glutamate

Monosodium glutamate (2-aminopentanedioic acid, MSG; E621) is a sodium salt of glutamic acid, popularly marketed as a "flavour enhancer". It is suggested that part of the flavour-enhancing effect of tomatoes, yeast extracts, and fermented or hydrolyzed protein products (e.g. soy bean paste) is due to the presence of free glutamate; therefore glutamate or MSG promote the natural flavour. MSG stimulates specific receptors located in taste buds such as the amino acid receptor or glutamate receptor and induces the taste known as umami, one of the five basic tastes. Monosodium glutamate (MSG) is commonly added to canned vegetables, soups and processed meats. Although the Food and Drug Administration (FDA) has classified MSG as a food ingredient that is "generally recognized as safe," the use of MSG in food remains controversial. Some individuals are susceptible to short-term reactions to MSG commonly known as MSG symptom complex. The signs of MSG ingestion include headache, flushing, sweating, sense of facial pressure or tightness, numbness, tingling or burning in or around the mouth, rapid fluttering heartbeats (heart palpitations), shortness of breath and drowsiness. The symptoms are usually mild and don't require treatment. When MSG is added to food, the regulatory agencies including FDA require that "monosodium glutamate" be listed on the food label.

V. NON-NUTRITIVE SWEETENERS

A non-nutritive or non-sugar sweetener is a food additive which attempts to duplicate the effect of sugar in taste, but often with less food energy. The sugar substitute sweeteners include saccharin, sodium cyclamate, aspartame, sucralose, neotame and acesulfame potassium. These compounds are all high intensity sweeteners i.e. their sweetness is many times that of sucrose, so they are required in much less quantity and thus the energy contribution is often negligible. The use of non-nutritive sweeteners is useful for diabetic patients and for those who wish to limit carbohydrate calorie intake.

1. Saccharin

Saccharin (E954) is the oldest artificial sweetener, discovered in 1879. Saccharin is about 300 times as sweet as sucrose but has an unpleasant bitter or metallic aftertaste, especially at high concentrations. It is one of the most commonly used artificial sweeteners. Saccharin is not sufficiently water-soluble, but its sodium or calcium salts are water soluble and hence are often used as food additive. Saccharin is mostly used together with other non-nutritive sweeteners (e.g. cyclamate or aspartame) mainly to mask/compensate other's weaknesses/after-taste. After ingestion, saccharin is absorbed as such without being digested. In the body it does not affect blood insulin levels and has effectively no food energy.

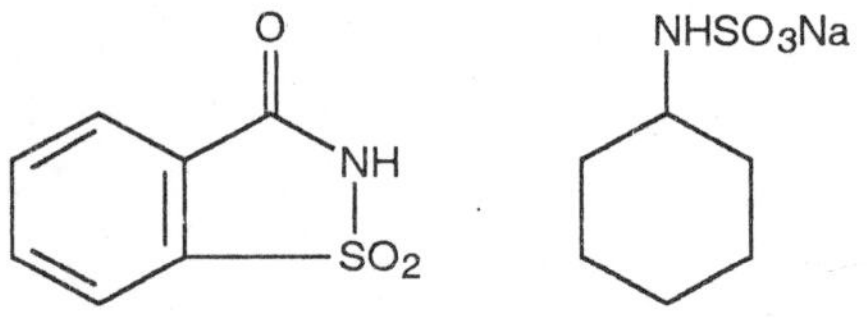

O
NH
SO_2
$NHSO_3Na$

Saccharin | Sodium cyclamate

Fig.18.4. Chemical structures of some important sweetener food additives.

The oral LD_{50} of sodium saccharin in mice and Webster rats is 17.5 and 14.2 g/kg body weight, respectively. Sodium saccharin induces bladder tumour in male (but not female) rats when administered at high doses for life-time. It induces epithelial hyperplasia in the urinary bladder of rats. However, various studies have failed to show any relationship between saccharin and incidence of cancer in humans at normal doses. Consequently, saccharin is approved in more than 100 countries around the world and has been determined safe by the Joint Expert Committee on Food Additives (JECFA) of the World Health Organization and the Scientific Committee for Food of the European Union.

2. Sodium Cyclamate

Sodium cyclamate (E952) is the sodium salt of cyclamic acid (cyclohexanesulfamic acid). It exists as an odourless, white crystalline powder and is used as non-nutritive sweetener in some countries. It is about 30 times as sweet as sucrose in dilute solution, making it the least potent of the commercially used artificial sweeteners. It has an unpleasant aftertaste, but less than that of saccharin. Sodium cyclamate is often used synergistically with other artificial sweeteners, especially saccharin; the mixture of 10 parts cyclamate to 1 part saccharin masks the off-tastes of both sweeteners. Its oral LD_{50} in mice and rats is 10 and 12-17 g/kg body weight, respectively. In the body, sodium cyclamate is converted to cyclohexylamine which is more toxic (oral LD_{50} in rat 157 mg/kg). In 1968, the FDA discovered teratogenicity and carcinogenicity (urinary bladder tumour) of sodium cyclamate in rats and put a ban on this sweetener. However, more than 50 countries have now approved or reapproved the use of the sweetener due to lack of clear cut relationship between cyclamate and adverse effect on health in humans.

3. Aspartame

Aspartame (E951), a dipeptide of aspartic acid and a methyl ester of phenylalanine, is a non-carbohydrate sweetener approved for use in pharmaceutical products and is being used increasingly in chewable tablets and sugar-free formulations. It is approximately 180 times sweeter than sugar in typical concentrations without the high energy value of sugar. The taste of aspartame is not identical to that of sugar as its sweetness has a slower onset and longer duration than that of sugar. Like many other peptides, aspartame may break down into its constituent amino acids under conditions of elevated temperature or high pH. Upon ingestion, aspartame breaks down into several residual chemicals including aspartic acid, phenylalanine, methanol and further breakdown products including formaldehyde and formic acid. Some studies have indicated that aspartame induces brain tumours, brain lesions and lymphoma in experimental animals. Therefore there is lot of controversy regarding the safety of aspartame as food additive. Further investigation into connections between aspartame and diseases such as tumours are required.

VI. PRESERVATIVES

Some of the oldest and most common preservatives such as acids, salt, sugar and wood smoke are the ones still most commonly used. Use of antibiotics as preservatives is generally discouraged as they pose danger of developing resistant strains of pathogens. Nowadays, many synthetic chemicals are available which are widely used as food preservatives.

1. Benzoic Acid

Benzoic acid is a colourless crystalline solid and the simplest aromatic carboxylic acid. This weak acid is mostly used as an important precursor for the synthesis of many other organic substances. Benzoic acid (E210) and its sodium salt sodium benzoate (E211) have long been used as food preservatives. Benzoic acid inhibits the growth of mould, yeast and some bacteria by lowering the intracellular pH to 5 or less and thereby decreasing the anaerobic fermentation of glucose. The effectivity of benzoic acid and benzoate is thus dependent on the pH of the food. The use level of benzoic acid in food ranges from 0.05% to 0.1%. The sodium salt is preferred because of low aqueous solubility of the free acid. *In vivo,* the salt is converted to acid, which is the more toxic form.

The acute oral LD_{50} of sodium benzoate in rats, rabbits and dogs is 2700, 2000 and 2000 mg/kg body weight, respectively. Large oral doses of benzoic acid are moderately toxic and may cause abdominal pain, sore throat, nausea and vomiting. Skin contact may cause irritation with redness and pain. Inhalation of benzoic acid or its salts may cause irritation of the respiratory tract (nose and throat) with coughing and sore throat. Studies on the subacute toxicity of benzoic acid in mice have indicated that ingestion of benzoic acid or its salt may cause weight loss, diarrhoea, irritation of internal membranes, internal bleeding, enlargement of liver and kidney, hypersensitivity and paralysis followed by death. Chronic toxicity studies, however, did not reveal deleterious or harmful effect of benzoic acid following daily feeding of 0.5% and 1% in diet. Concerns have been expressed that benzoic acid and its salts may react with ascorbic acid (vitamin C) in some foods, forming small quantities of benzene, which is toxic.

2. Sorbic Acid and Its Salts

Sorbic acid (2,4-Hexadienoic acid; E200) is a tasteless organic acid found naturally in the fruit of mountain ash (genus *Sorbus*) or is prepared synthetically. Sorbic acid and its mineral salts such as sodium sorbate, potassium sorbate and calcium sorbate are antimicrobial agents often used as preservatives in food and drinks such as wine, soft drinks, animal feeds, bread and cheese. They have broad-spectrum activity against mould, yeast and fungi, but are less active against bacteria. In general the salts are preferred over the acid form because they are more soluble in water. Sorbic acid is practically non-toxic with oral LD_{50} in rats more than 10.5 g/kg body weight. Ingestion of large amount of sorbic acid produces burning sensation and abdominal pain. Exposure to eyes or skin produces irritation. It has negligible subacute toxicity. Chronic toxicity of sorbic acid among various animals has shown that neither sorbic acid nor its potassium salt induces malignant growth in animals. Overall sorbic acid and its salts are generally recognised as safe food additives.

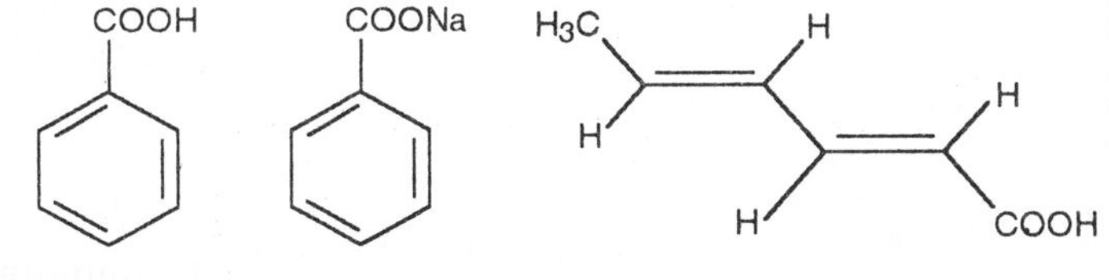

COOH | COONa | H_3C H H H H COOH

Benzoic acid | Sodium benzoate | Sorbic acid

Fig.18.5. Chemical structures of some important preservative food additives.

FEED ADDITIVES

Feed additives are substances used in animal nutrition for purposes of improving either the quality of feed and food from animal origin or the animals' performance and health. Large numbers of feed additives are available in market including the growth and performance enhancers, non-protein nitrogen compounds, vitamins, amino acids and other nutrients. Although feed additives are approved only after scientific evaluations demonstrate that they do not have harmful effects on the human and animal health and on the environment, toxicosis may still be possible when these agents are mixed or formulated into the basic feedstuffs of livestock and birds.

I. GROWTH AND PERFORMANCE ENHANCERS

Growth promoters (Growth promotants) are agents that increase the growth rate and feed conversion ability of animals. These agents are often used in food animals in which high conversion of feed into animal tissues is required at short time. When used judiciously, growth promoters improve live-weight gain, enhance feed conversion ability, and increase efficiency of production. These include antibiotics, probiotics and hormones. Most of these agents require strict regulation and must be used in animals on a high nutrition diet and under good husbandry conditions.

A. ANTIBIOTICS

Antibiotics are mostly used in therapeutics for their antimicrobial purposes, but some ionophore (e.g. monensin) and non-ionophore (e.g. zinc-bacitracin) antibiotics are used for growth promoter and production-enhancing properties in domestic animals. These agents are often used as feed additives in pig and poultry diets and also in rations for intensively reared cattle and animals bred for fur such as rabbits and minks. Ionophore antibiotics are highly toxic to animals, so they are discussed in detail.

1. Ionophore Antibiotics

Ionophore antibiotics (Polyether antibiotics) are fermentation products of *Streptomyces* species. Initially ionophores were developed as anticoccidial drugs, but some agents such as monensin, lasalocid, and salinomycin have found their use as growth promoter in food producing animals. Horses and some other species are highly susceptible to toxic effects of ionophore antibiotics.

Properties: Ionophore antibiotics are either monovalent (e.g. monensin and salinomycin) or divalent (e.g. lasalocid) polyether antibiotics obtained from *Streptomyces* spp. These agents are widely used in therapeutics for their anticoccidial action at 100 g/ton of poultry feed. In addition, they increase feed conversion efficiency and live-weight gain by primarily acting on microflora of the rumen and altering rumen fermentation. They enhance the microbial production of gluconeogenic fatty acid propionate and to some extent acetate, at the cost of butyrate. The beneficial effect may also be achieved by suppression of pathogenic organisms and harmful bacterial metabolites. They are used in feed lot cattle at 5-30 ppm of finished ration to improve feed efficiency by 10-20%.

Toxicity: Toxicity of ionophore antibiotics vary with the species of animal and the dose of compound. Horses are at the greatest risk with oral LD_{50} of 2-3 mg/kg (monensin), 21.5 mg/kg (lasalocid) and 0.6 mg/kg (salinomycin). Acute oral LD_{50} of monensin in sheep, dogs, cattle and chickens is 12, 20, 22 and 200 mg/kg, respectively. In cattle, clinical signs have been observed at 3-5 times the recommended feeding level of monensin. Toxicity in animals mainly occurs due to improper mixing or use of therapeutic doses for food animals in susceptible species. Equines and turkeys are highly susceptible to ionophores, even at very low doses. Therefore, accidental ingestion of poultry or cattle rations containing the ionophores like monensin is often fatal in horses.

Toxicokinetics: The detailed toxicokinetics of polyether antibiotics in domestic animals is not available. These agents are rapidly absorbed from the GI tract and metabolized by hepatic cytochrome P-450 enzymes. Metabolites are mainly excreted in bile and faeces. Monensin has short half-life in animals.

Mechanism of action: The primary action of ionophore antibiotics is due to their ability to form complexes with cations. In the cells, they may also block the secretion of glycoproteins.

a. The ionophore antibiotics have affinity for the cations, principally sodium, potassium, and/or calcium, and form lipophilic complexes with them. The ionophore-cation complex renders cell membrane permeable to cations allowing their excessive entry inside the cell. Different ionophores may have different affinities for cations i.e. monovalent ionophores form complexes primarily with Na^+ or K^+, while divalent ionophores form complexes with Ca^{++}; some ionophores may have affinity for both types of cation.

i. The high intracellular cation concentrations interfere with certain mitochondrial functions (e.g. substrate oxidation) and ATP hydrolysis. This diminishes cellular energy production and produces cell death.

ii. High intracellular sodium leads to secondary intracellular calcium overload in cardiac and skeletal muscles. This leads to mitochondrial swelling, catecholamine release and increased myocardial cell and diaphragm cell contractility. These actions result in initial positive ionotropy followed by terminal

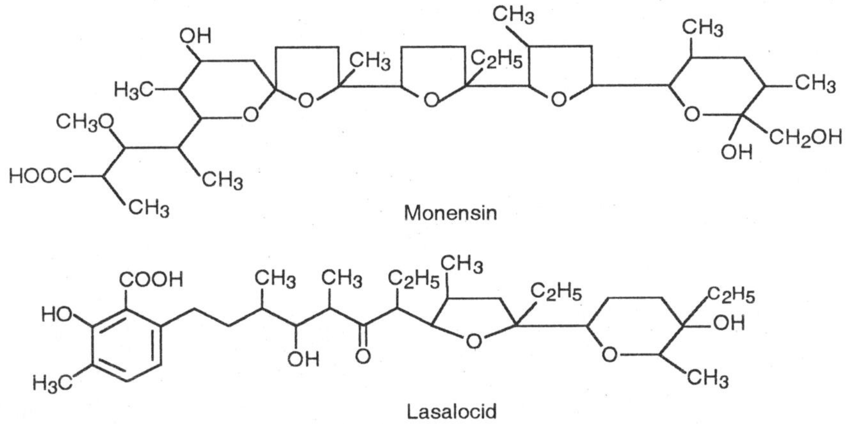

Monensin

Lasalocid

Fig. 18.6. Chemical structures of some important ionophore antibiotics used as feed additives.

negative ionotropy and skeletal muscle contractility leading to death.

iii. Alterations in membrane integrity and internal osmolality induced by ionophores may upset the osmotic balance of cells affecting various cellular reactions that depend on the specific ion balance.

iv. Proton exchange for sodium results in acidosis and potassium loss.

b. It is suggested by some *in vitro* studies that ionophore antibiotics like monensin also inhibit intracellular protein transport and block the secretion of glycoproteins. Incubation of cells in culture with monensin leads to blockade of protein transport to the Golgi complex (GC) and accumulation of proteins in the endoplasmic reticulum (ER). *In vitro* activation of cells results in enhanced detection of intracellular cytokines.

Clinical signs: Type and onset of clinical signs of ionophore antibiotics vary with the species and other host factors like age and diet. Important clinical signs in different species may include anorexia (12-36 hours post-exposure), depression, weakness, ataxia, dyspnoea and diarrhoea. Animals recovered from acute toxicosis may experience collapse and death during periods of exertion or high environmental temperatures. In horses, additional signs may include loose watery diarrhoea, colic, sweating and renal tubular damage. Myoglobinuria may be observed in dogs, sheep and swine. Death may occur either suddenly due to cardiovascular collapse and shock or weeks after apparent recovery due to cardiac fibrosis. Permanent cardiac damage is possible in sublethal cases.

Signs of subacute toxicosis are indicative of reduced cardiac function and congestive heart failure.

Post-mortem findings: Post-mortem lesions include mild haemopericardium, epicardial and pericardial haemorrhages, and pale myocardium. Hydrothorax, ascites and pulmonary oedema may also be present. Lesions of skeletal muscle damage may be evident. Sanguinous tracheal exudates and myocardial enlargement and pallor are observed in poultry. Histologically, there are lesions of myocardial necrosis and secondary lesions associated with heart failure.

Diagnosis: Diagnosis of ionophore antibiotic poisoning should be made from history, clinical signs and necropsy lesions. Analysis of feed samples and stomach/rumen contents are useful for laboratory diagnosis, but tissues samples (e.g. liver and kidneys) may not be very useful in detecting poisoning due to half-life of these drugs.

Ionophore antibiotics poisoning should be differentiated from white muscle disease and white snakeroot poisoning.

Treatment and management: There is no specific antidote or treatment to ionophore antibiotics poisoning. Treatment mainly includes detoxification (activated charcoal, saline cathartic, etc.) and supportive therapy. Administration of intravenous fluids for shock and bicarbonate for acidosis is useful. Stress to the poisoned animal should be minimized.

Prognosis: Prognosis of ionophore antibiotic poisoning in advanced stages is generally poor, especially when cardiac related signs are present due to possibility of permanent cardiac damage.

2. Non-Ionophore Antibiotics

Non-ionophore antibiotics include compounds from several antibiotic groups. These agents selectively modify the microbial population of animals to improve the production efficiency. They maintain normal health of animal by controlling low-level infections, particularly in intensive systems. Some of the commonly used non-ionophore antibiotics are zinc-bacitracin, tylosin, flavomycin and virginiamycin.

Zinc Bacitracin

Bacitracin is a topically used polypeptide antibiotic obtained from a strain of *Bacillus subtilis*. Zinc bacitracin (also bacitracin, bacitracin methylenedisalicylate and bacitracin manganese) is permitted for veterinary use as a feed additive for growth promotion purposes. As a growth promoter, it is given in feed to young ruminants, piglets and pigs, broiler and laying hens, and fur-bearing species excluding rabbits. In recommended oral doses, zinc-bacitracin is hardly absorbed from the GI tract, so its distribution to tissues and organs is negligible. The oral acute toxicity of zinc-bacitracin is low with LD_{50} values greater than 1200 mg/kg for rabbits, 3750 mg/kg for mice and 9500 mg/kg for dogs. It is contraindicated to use bacitracin zinc simultaneously with other feed additives or growth promoters. It should not be used in lactating cows.

Tylosin

Tylosin is a macrolide antibiotic obtained from a strain of *Streptomyces fradiae*. It is structurally and pharmacologically related to erythromycin and is used for growth promotion in pigs. After oral administration, tylosin is absorbed quickly and distributed widely in the organs (mainly concentrated in lung, liver, kidney, spleen and gallbladder). The oral LD_{50} of tylosin in different species is: rats 500 mg/kg, mice 6200 mg/kg, dogs 400 mg/kg and pigs 5000 mg/kg. Similar to erythromycin, tylosin may induce severe diarrhoea if administered orally to ruminants or by any route to horses. Therefore, tylosin is not recommended in adult horses. Although the lethal dose of tylosin is higher in pigs, but its overdosage in this species may produce adverse effects including oedema of rectal mucosa and mild anal protrusion with pruritis; erythema and diarrhoea. Shock and death have been reported in baby pigs overdosed with tylosin.

II. NON-PROTEIN NITROGEN (NPN) COMPOUNDS

Urea, biurate, dicyanodiamide, glutamine and some ammonium salts are often added to ruminant ration as a source of non-protein nitrogen (NPN), a cheap protein substitute in the diet. The normal feeding rate for NPN products is 3% of the grain ration or 1% of the total ration. Toxicosis from urea and ammonium compounds occurs when their large quantity is mixed in ration or when animal accidentally ingests ammoniated fertilizers.

1. Urea and Ammonium Compounds

Urea and ammonium compounds (diammonium phosphate and monoammonium phosphate) are cheap source of NPN. The urea, ammonia and ammonium salts are also widely used as nitrogen fertilizers on crop and pasture fields. In addition, urea is used as a substitute for common salt in melting of snow and ice in snow clad residential areas and roads. Accidental exposure to high concentration of urea or ammonium compounds in diet or as fertilizers can cause heavy mortality in animals. Sometimes urea is in the proper concentration in the ration but the animal is not accustomed to ingesting urea (abrupt change of diet from natural protein to urea or other NPN sources), which may also result in poisoning. Ammonium nitrate and urea if excessively used as fertilizers may produce nitrate poisoning through soil and plants.

Properties: Urea (Carbamide, carbonyl diamide, carbonic acid diamide) is a simple compound that contains 46.7 percent nitrogen. It is naturally found in many plants and is a normal end product of protein metabolism in mammals. Urea is not necessary in the diet of ruminant animals, but is fed as a replacement for a part of the protein in the ration. One gram of pure urea furnishes as much nitrogen as 2.92 grams of protein (protein equivalent of 292 percent). The feed grade of urea, however, has other ingredients that lower the protein equivalent, depending on the amount of material added. The amount of urea, ammonium salts or other ammoniated products in a ruminant animal depends on the digestible energy or total digestible nutrients (TDN) content of the ration. In feedlot cattle consuming a high concentrate ration, no more than 0.2 to 0.5 kg urea per head per day should be fed.

When urea from feed sources enters the rumen, it is rapidly dissolved and hydrolyzed to ammonia and water by bacterial urease. The rate of ammonia production depends primarily on the amount of urea ingested, the amount of urease present in ruminal contents or diet (plants) and the pH (alkaline) of ruminal contents. The ammonia once released can then be utilized as nitrogen source by rumen bacteria for the synthesis of amino acids required for further protein synthesis and their growth. For proper utilization of ammonia for protein synthesis, soluble carbohydrates in form of starch and glucoses are essential. When ammonia is produced rapidly in the rumen in concentration more than required by rumen bacteria, it is absorbed directly into the bloodstream, reconverted to urea in the liver, and excreted through the kidneys in urine. Production of ammonia in very high concentration beyond handling capacity of liver results in urea poisoning. The ability to recycle and utilize urea differs among various species of ruminants and hence the urea toxicity.

Factors affecting toxicity :

a. Toxicosis of urea and other NPN compounds is related to their ability to liberate ammonia.

b. Alkaline pH increases the release of ammonia from urea. Liberation of ammonia from urea will further make the rumen more alkaline which in turn hastens release of ammonia. This way, the release of ammonia from urea goes on unabated with higher and higher intensity due to self-releasing process.

c. Ruminants are more susceptible to urea poisoning because urease enzyme is also present in the plants taken as fodder. Monogastric animals are less susceptible than ruminants because neither alkaline pH nor urease enzyme exists in the stomach.

d. Young ruminants can tolerate more amount of urea than adults due to less development of rumen and rumen microflora.

e. Diets low in energy and high in fibre are more commonly associated with NPN poisoning because full utilisation of ammonia does not occur with low energy diets. Therefore, urea can be highly toxic to sheep and cattle when given without feed.

f. Urea can be highly toxic when consumed rapidly in sufficient quantity to produce a marked rise in rumen ammonia concentration.

g. Animals which are adapted to ingesting urea in diet, can tolerate more quantity of urea without showing ill-effects than animals which are not used to it. Tolerance is reduced by starvation and by a low protein diet.

h. Malnutrition and liver damage can increase susceptibility to urea poisoning. Dehydrated animals are more susceptible to urea poisoning as when there is insufficient water supply.

Toxicity: Toxicity of NPN compounds depends on the type of compound, species of animal, and some other factors like tolerance and diet. In ruminants unaccustomed to urea, ingestion of 0.3-0.5 g urea/kg may be toxic, whereas cattle accustomed to urea can ingest up to 1 g urea/kg/ day. In general, oral LD_{50} of urea in cattle and sheep is 1-1.5 g/kg and in horses is 4.0 g/kg weight. Pigs are mostly unaffected by large doses of urea unless they are deprived of water or have developed caecal flora that produces urease enzyme. Monogastric animals are more susceptible to poisoning by inorganic ammonium salts (toxic oral dose 1.5 mg/kg) but not very susceptible to oral urea toxicity. Most cases of urea poisoning are due to poor mixing of feed or to errors in calculating the amount of urea to be added to the ration. Accidental over-consumption of urea-containing supplements also has resulted in some cases of urea toxicity. Thus urea should be uniformly mixed with cereal grains, molasses or similar low-protein feeds before it is fed.

Toxicokinetics: After ingestion, urea is hydrolysed to ammonia in rumen (ruminants) or caecum (horses). The release and absorption of ammonia from NPN sources depends on the pH of rumen. In normal rumen (pH 6.0-6.2), ammonia liberated from NPN sources is in the form of ammonium ion (NH_4^+) which is ionized and water soluble and hence cannot cross the ruminal wall. Therefore at normal or low rumen pH, the ruminants are able to withstand large urea doses. When pH of rumen is 9, both ammonium ion (ionized) and ammonia (unionized) are produced in equal amounts (ratio of NH_4^+ : NH_3 is 1) and significant amount of ammonia is absorbed. However, when the rumen pH is elevated to 11.0 or so, more and more of ammonia will be released and will be rapidly absorbed.

Once in systemic circulation, the blood buffer systems attempt to maintain blood pH at about 7.4. At this pH (7.4), most of the ammonia (not all) is again in the form of charged ammonium ion (NH_4^+) which is unable to cross the cell membrane. At lower concentration, ammonia in blood is detoxified in liver by its conversion to urea (in urea cycle) or formation of glutamic acid and glutamine. However when the concentration of ammonia in blood is more, as in NPN poisoning, it is not fully detoxified and can cross blood brain barrier and other tissues at a rate dependent on the speed of dissociation from NH_4^+ at the level of cell membrane.

Mechanism of action :

The toxicity of urea and other non-protein nitrogen sources is due to ammonia absorbed from the stomach. When the hepatic urea and glutamine synthesising mechanisms are saturated, the hyperammonemia develops. Ammonia acts primarily by inhibiting the tricarboxylic acid (TCA) cycle, but the exact mechanism by which it blocks the TCA cycle is not clear. Inhibition of TCA cycle results in decrease in energy production and cellular respiration. These result in increase in anaerobic glycolysis, blood glucose and blood lactate levels with development of metabolic acidosis. Cellular energy and respiration deficits cause ultrastructural damage and then degenerative changes in different organs. Central nervous system responds first to the energy deficit because of large requirement of energy. Liver dysfunction increases susceptibility to the poisoning.

Clinical signs: The onset and severity of clinical signs of urea and other NPN substances poisoning is related to rate and amount of ammonia released and absorbed into the blood. In peracute toxicity, the intoxicated animal may be found dead without typical signs of urea toxicosis. In acute toxicity, onset of signs may take 10-15 minutes to several hours and a spectrum of clinical signs is seen. Early signs in various species may include uneasiness, frothy salivation, grinding of teeth, muscle tremors (especially of face and ears), polyuria and abdominal pain. In ruminants, there is also rumen atony followed by ruminal tympany, violent struggling, bellowing and kicking at abdomen due to colic. There is marked jugular pulse, incoordination, severe twitching and tonic convulsions which are elicitable by external stimuli. As death nears, animal becomes cyanotic, dyspnoeic, anuric and hyperthermic. Blood pH decreases from 7.4 to 7.0. Recumbency indicates advanced toxicosis. Regurgitation may occur especially in sheep. Death related to excess NPN usually occurs within 2 hr in cattle, 4 hr in sheep and 3-12 hr in horses. Survivors recover in 12-24 hours with no sequelae.

Post-mortem findings: In urea poisoning, there may be no characteristic lesions. Carcass of animal appears to bloat and decompose rapidly. Pulmonary oedema, congestion and petechial haemorrhages may be observed frequently. Liver may be enlarged, pale and friable and there may be mild bronchitis and catarrhal gastro-enteritis. The odour of NH_3 may or may not be apparent in ingesta. A ruminal or caecal pH ≥ 7.5 from a recently dead animal is highly suggestive of NPN poisoning. The rumen pH remains stable for several hours after death under most circumstances, but continues to rise in NPN toxicosis.

Diagnosis: Non-protein nitrogen poisoning is suggested by signs, lesions, history of acute illness and dietary exposure. Laboratory analysis for the ammonia nitrogen in both ante- and post-mortem specimens and for urea or other NPN compounds in suspected feeds and other dietary sources helps in the diagnosis. Specimens for ammonia-nitrogen include ruminal-reticular fluid, serum, whole blood and urine. All specimens should be frozen immediately after collection and thawed only for analysis. Alternatively, ruminal-reticular fluid may be preserved with a few drops of saturated mercuric chloride solution to each 100 ml of specimen. Animals dead more than few hours in hot temperature or 12 hours in moderate climate probably have undergone too much autolysis to be of diagnostic value. Diagnostic values are: blood ammonia 1-4 mg/100 ml and rumen ammonia 80 mg/100 ml of rumen liquor. Decreased blood pH due to acidosis is characteristic of toxicosis.

Elevated levels of blood glucose, blood lactate, blood urea nitrogen (BUN), aspartate aminotransferase (AST), serum potassium, etc. may be seen in urea toxicosis.

Urea toxicosis should be differentiated from following toxicoses:

a. *Arsenic and other heavy metals:* They cause severe colic with bloody diarrhoea without any behavioural, nervous or motor signs. In urea toxicosis, there is colic but without diarrhoea.

b. *OP insecticides toxicosis:* Organophosphorus insecticide toxicosis may mimic aspects of urea toxicosis. Treatment with atropine alleviates OP insecticides toxicosis signs but will have no effect on urea toxicosis.

c. *OC insecticides toxicosis:* Organochlorine insecticides toxicity cause high rise in body temperature with intermittent convulsions of clonic-tonic nature.

d. *Other toxicoses:* Other conditions that can be differentiated from urea toxicosis include grain engorgement, nitrate and cyanide poisoning and encephalic diseases.

Treatment and management: Examination and treatment of urea toxicosis may be difficult because of violent behaviour of animals. Animals that are recumbent and moribund usually do not respond favourably to treatment.

a. *Acetic acid/Vinegar:* Ruminal infusion of 5% acetic acid/vinegar in sufficient quantity of cold water helps to lower the ruminal pH and hence the concentration and absorption of unionized ammonia. Acetic acid also inactivates existing NH_3 in the GI tract and rapidly forms ammonium acetate which can be utilised by rumen microflora. Ruminal-reticular fluid specimen should be taken before acetic acid therapy to ascertain the rumen pH. Administration of acetic acid may be repeated, if affected animals again show clinical signs.

   Cattle: 2-8 litres, intra-ruminally.

   Sheep and goats: 0.5-2 litres, intra-ruminally.

b. *Iced-water:* Ruminal infusion of iced (0-4°C) water, often concomitantly with acetic acid/vinegar, is helpful in lowering the rumen temperature and diluting the rumen ingesta and reacting media which slows urease activity.

   Cattle: Up to 40 litres in adult cattle (proportionally less in sheep and goats), intra-ruminally.

c. Rumen tympany, if present, should be corrected and a trochar may be installed to prevent recurrence.

d. Supportive therapy such as isotonic saline solution should be given by I.V. route to correct dehydration.

e. In recumbent animal, convulsions can be controlled by administration of pentobarbitone sodium.

f. Rumenotomy may be performed to remove excessive amount of contaminated feed if the animal can tolerate surgery.

g. Fever can be controlled by cold water rinsing.

h. Some studies suggested that feeding of molasses reduces rumen pH and ammonia concentration and may be useful in reducing the risk of toxicity from urea.

Contraindications

Intravenous fluids containing glucoses should not be administered as they may produce hyperglycaemic signs.

Prevention:

a. Do not feed urea to hungry, dehydrated or malnourished animals or those with damaged livers.

b. Always start addition of urea to ruminant diets in small amounts and gradually increase it to a safe level.

c. Avoid feeds containing 3% urea or more in the DM as these are regarded as high-urea feeds. If required, give such feeds in restricted amounts, preferably spread over 12 hours or more of each day.

d. Do not feed urea if the main forage intake is dry, low in energy and protein, and high in fibre as during a drought or early summer. Mixing urea with molasses, fodder/sugar beet or good quality silage reduces the risk of poisoning.

e. Store, use and dispose of fertilizers and feeds containing urea carefully. Immediately clean up or disperse spillage, if any.

f. Do not cut the fodder or allow the animals to graze for a few days after application of urea or other nitrogen containing fertilizers.

Note : In ammonia gas toxicity, toxicokinetics and course of poisoning is different than urea toxicosis. Toxic concentration of ammonia can be released from a slurry pit or chicken house and may produce toxicosis in animals or birds confined to that place. Ammonia gas is a strong irritant to mucous membranes and enters the blood stream via lungs. Clinical signs include sniffing, coughing and keratoconjuctivitis. Severe pulmonary oedema and lung congestion occurs due to increased permeability of lung capillaries. It also causes alkalosis and compensatory acidosis. Death may result partly from asphyxia and partly from electrolyte and cellular metabolic action of ammonia. Terminal signs may resemble urea toxicosis. It requires symptomatic therapy and fresh air inhalation.

2. 4-Methylimidazole

4-Methylimidazole (4-MI) is a toxic by-product formed as a result of interaction of reducing sugars with ammonia during ammoniation of feed. Ammoniation of feed is mostly carried out to increase the feed value of forages. Ammoniated wheat straw, corn stalks and corn silage are less toxic because they contain low levels of reducing sugar; but molasses and in some cases high quality forages such as sorghum, alfalafa and cereal grains may produce a clinical syndrome known as "Bovine Bonkers Syndrome" when fed to cattle. The toxicosis of 4-methylimidazole is not common, but it may occur in adult cattle, calves and nursing calves (most commonly affected due to passage of toxic metabolites in milk).

4-Methylimidazole produces rapid or slow (few weeks) onset of toxicosis after start of giving treated feed. There is involvement of CNS and clinical signs include stampeding, ear twitching, champing, salivation, trembling, hyperexcitability, wild running, circling, convulsions and death. 4-Methylimidazole toxicosis does not produce specific necropsy lesions. Diagnosis of poisoning may be made from history of intake of ammoniated feed, clinical signs and identification of 4-MI in ration. Blood urea and ammonia levels remain normal. Pentobarbitone and acepromazine are helpful for controlling clinical signs. Thiamine (1-2 g, I.V. or I.M.) has been used as a non-specific neurological supportive therapy.

III. MISCELLANEOUS FEED ADDITIVES

1. Sodium Chloride (Salt, Common Salt)

Sodium chloride (common salt) is an essential nutrient for normal functioning of the body and is added to feed and ration of animals. It is an essential part of most animal fluids and plays important role in nerve conduction, muscle contraction, correct osmotic balance of extracellular fluid and absorption of other nutrients. Sodium chloride may become toxic when excessive quantities are ingested and intake of water is limited. If water is freely available, then salt poisoning is less severe. So term sodium chloride toxicity alone may not be accurate rather it is a condition that is considered to be water-deprivation-induced sodium chloride toxicosis. All species of animals including human beings are susceptible to the problem of salt poisoning and water deprivation, but poultry and pigs are most susceptible.

Properties: Sodium chloride (NaCl) or common salt is the chemical compound composed of elements chlorine (60.7%) and sodium (39.3%). Salt is widely and abundantly distributed in nature and occurs naturally as the mineral, halite (rock salt) and as mixed evaporites in salt lakes. It makes up nearly 80% of the dissolved material in seawater. Sodium chloride is readily soluble in water and insoluble or only slightly soluble in most other liquids. It forms small, transparent and colourless to white cubic crystals. It varies in colour from colourless, when pure, to white, grey or brownish, typical of rock salt (halite). Sodium chloride is sold in several different particle sizes (gradation) and forms, depending on the intended end use.

Sources of toxicity :

a. Salt is an essential component of food/feed. It is added to ration to increase or decrease the palatability. Inadvertent excessive use of salt in ration may lead to toxicosis in animals. Poisoning from over-ingestion may also arise when the salt is made freely available after a period of salt deprivation.

b. Ingestion of salt used for de-icing roads in winter may cause poisoning in ruminants. Such salts are usually deposited loosely in piles or containers alongside roads and are easily accessible to animals.

c. Water supplied from natural springs, deep wells and water contaminated with run-off from oil well drilling may contain high levels of sodium chloride.

d. Rock salt can be toxic to pet birds, particularly when it has contaminated water and food supplies. Dogs sometimes eat rock salt and get poisoned.

e. Excessive consumption of salty meat or meat flavoured with brines may occasionally cause poisoning in carnivores. Feeding of swill if it contains residues from bakeries, brine from butcher's shop, salt whey from cheese factories, and salted fish wastes may cause salt poisoning in animals, particularly pigs.

f. Exposure to hypersaline playa lakes can cause toxicity in waterfowl.

g. Overdose of saturated sodium chloride solution as emetic may cause toxicosis in small animals.

Factors affecting toxicity :

a. Sodium chloride poisoning can occur in all animals; however, pigs and chickens are affected most frequently, horses are next, followed by cattle. Sheep are less susceptible than horses and cattle and dogs are occasionally affected.

b. Heavy milking cows are highly susceptible to salt poisoning because of their unstable fluid and electrolyte status. Beef cattle and dry dairy cattle appear to be less susceptible than dairy cows in milk.

c. In poultry, young chicks are more susceptible due to their indiscriminate feeding behaviour, poor sense of taste and low plasma proteins than the adult birds.

d. In presence of water, large concentrations of sodium chloride (up to 13% of the ration of swine) can be tolerated without apparent ill effect. Deprivation of water due to any reason (mechanical failure of waterer, neglect, overcrowding, frozen water, etc.) enhances salt poisoning significantly.

e. Salt poisoning is more common in summer than winter and in semi-arid or arid areas than rain-fed areas. This is mainly due to less water availability, high temperature and low humidity in summer and in arid zones, all of which tend to increase water losses from the animal.

f. Salt hungry animal (animal that has been deprived of salt in diet) may take large amounts of salt in a single feeding and get overdosed.

g. Clinical signs may develop if enough salt is consumed in a short period as compared to intake of same amount of salt over a long period.

h. A sudden change from fresh water to salt water enhances salt toxicity, especially when the animal is hungry or unaccustomed to salt.

Toxicity: Toxicity of sodium chloride is often associated with water deprivation and is commonly called "water-deprivation-sodium ion toxicosis". If water intake is restricted, even a normal concentration of sodium chloride may produce toxicosis. On the other hand, if water is freely available even high salt may not create a problem because consumption of sufficient water facilitates excretion of sodium ions from body. In general, acute oral lethal dose of sodium chloride is about 2.2 g/kg in horses, cattle and swine, 6 g/kg in sheep, and 4 g/kg in dogs in conditions when water is not freely available. Toxic dose of salt as per cent of diet is 1.5-2 for cattle and sheep, 0.25 for pigs and 0.25-2 for poultry when drinking water is restricted and 10 for pigs and 5-10 for poultry when drinking water is freely available.

Toxicokinetics: Sodium chloride is rapidly absorbed from the GI tract and distributed throughout the body. The excess Na^+ in blood diffuses passively into the CSF, but requires active transport to be removed from the CSF. The surplus sodium ions in blood are excreted primarily by kidneys and little by skin and alimentary tract provided sufficient water is present in body. If the animal is unable to increase water consumption in response to the thirst generated by excess sodium (hypotonicity of blood), the excess of sodium in the blood produces toxicosis.

Mechanism of action: The exact molecular mechanisms of salt poisoning are not still clear.

Toxicity mainly occurs due to disturbance in both sodium and water balance.

a. Presence of large concentration of salt in the gut acts as a saline purgative and withdraws water from surrounding tissues to produce diarrhoea. Withdrawal of water from tissues results in dehydration. Sodium chloride in GI tract also causes mild irritation of mucosa, which contribute to diarrhoea.

b. Excess salt absorbed from the intestine results in hypertonicity of blood and hypernatraemia. Excess salt in the blood stream then tends to shrink capillary vascular endothelium and withdraws water from cells. Shrinkage of capillary endothelium in brain, meninges, kidneys and other organs results in increased capillary permeability, which causes escape of water from blood into interstitial space. The withdrawal of water from tissues into blood in an attempt to decrease the hypertonicity of blood results in intracellular dehydration. So the overall condition in salt poisoning is extracellular hyperosmolality and intracellular dehydration.

i. Shrinkage of capillary endothelial cells and altered capillary permeability in the brain and meninges enhance escape of water from blood to interstitial spaces and hence development of cerebral oedema. The high Na^+ in plasma and CSF also diffuses into brain cells, thus making them hypertonic to plasma and CSF. Water then enters the brain cells and overhydrates them. Excess of sodium ions in the brain cells also interferes with aerobic glycolysis and reduces the activity of sodium pump. Decreased activity of sodium pump to remove excess sodium from cells attracts more water due to osmotic gradient. The cerebral oedema and overhydration of brain cells (irreversible) are responsible for nervous derangement seen in salt poisoning. The oedema predominates in brain because of the rich vascular supply, but it may also be seen in other organs and tissues.

ii. Occurrence of hypertonicity of blood and hypernatraemia in salt poisoning result in shrinkage of kidney tubules and deposition of sodium crystals in the tubules. This results in anuria, uraemia, etc. Other signs like transient polyuria, hypersalivation, nasal secretions, hydropericardium, hydrothorax, ascites, etc. seen in salt poisoning occur due to excessive salt accumulation and subsequent water withdrawal in these organs. So in salt poisoning, major offender is sodium chloride but actual clinical signs and most of the lesions are due to water.

Clinical signs: Clinical signs are almost same in most mammals, although every animal may not manifest all of them. Signs of salt poisoning are mostly similar to other encephalopathic poisons. In pigs and other species, early signs are increased thirst, pruritus, salivation, serous nasal discharge, urinary inconsistence or polyuria (later anuria), diarrhoea (later constipation), vomiting, etc. Nervous signs may include hyperesthesia, partial or complete blindness or deafness, moving in circles, head pushing, muscle tremors, shivering or twitching and elicitable or intermittent generalised tonic or clonic-tonic seizures. Motor signs include incoordination, ataxia, swaying and walking backward. Morbidity varies due to salt intake, water availability and environmental conditions.

In cattle, additional clinical signs are belligerent behaviour, aggressiveness in getting to water supplies, bellowing as if in severe pain, and sucking in air as well as water with secondary bloat. A characteristic sign in cattle is dragging of the hind feet while walking, and in more severe cases knuckling of the fetlock joints. Dairy cows may develop acetonaemia. Poultry tend to manifest weakness and paralysis rather than motor excitement phenomenon.

Dependent signs in various species include fever, muffled heart and lung sounds from fluid in the pericardial sac and lungs, and dehydration. Death in salt poisoning may occur in several hours to few days. Death probably occurs due to combined metabolic lesions in vital organs and physical damage from oedema fluids in the brain. Rapid rehydration generally causes more acute neurological signs.

Post-mortem-findings: In pigs, blood filled pin-point ulcers are found on a markedly congested and inflamed gastric mucosa. Cattle have gastric inflammation or ulceration or both, oedema of skeletal muscles, hydropericardium, cerebral oedema and oedema of other tissues and organs. Oedema on ruminal surfaces is associated with haemorrhages in the area adjacent to gall bladder. In chicks, congestion of liver and oedema of various organs may be seen. Testes are oedematous and enlarged.

Microscopic lesions include congestion of GI tract, cerebral vascular endothelial proliferation and distended perivascular space. Cerebral oedema, early necrosis and malacia may be observed. Eosinophilic cuffs around vessels in cerebral cortex and adjacent meninges (eosinophilic meningoencephalitis) are almost a pathognomonic lesion of salt poisoning in pigs, particularly in first 48 hours. In cattle, dilation of mucosal and submucosal lymphatics in the duodenum and small foci of necrosis in the liver and renal medulla may be observed. Sometimes no gross necropsy lesions are evident.

Diagnosis: The history of salt or sodium compounds (i.e. sodium -propionate, -acetate, -carbonate) ingestion and relative water scarcity or deprivation with encephalic signs and post-mortem findings indicate salt poisoning particularly in pigs. Plasma and CSF concentrations of sodium >1 mEq/L, especially when CSF has a greater concentration than plasma, are indicative of salt poisoning. In the cerebrum >1800 ppm sodium (wet weight) is suggestive of toxicosis. If sodium chloride level exceeds 0.5%, 0.25% or 0.65% in stomach, small intestine and large intestine, respectively, salt poisoning is suspected. Laboratory analysis of feed and water is also necessary for confirmation.

Differential diagnosis should include infectious diseases, lead and other heavy metals (GI tract lesions are more severe), OC insecticides (fever but no thirst), OP insecticides (more parasympathetic signs) and trauma to brain. Animals that simply die of thirst may manifest weakness, stupor, collapse and death without convulsions.

Treatment and management: The ideal treatment for salt poisoning would be to pull sodium out of brain cells, CSF and tissues, so that sodium and water could enter the blood and then excreted in the urine. But there is no such treatment.

a. Limited intake of salt free water at frequent intervals may help in mild to moderate salt poisoning. If the animal is ambulatory, it may recover by itself with provision of small amounts of water. If the poisoning is severe, supply of drinking water in large quantity may aggravate the poisoning because excess water produces more cerebral oedema as the brain and CSF are already hypertonic with respect to blood.

b. In cattle and small animals, the temporary use of non-sodium hypertonic fluids (e.g. dextrose or other substance) may provide some help.

c. Symptomatic treatment like GI sedatives in case of gastroenteritis and sedatives in CNS stimulation should be instituted.

d. Offending feed or liquid should be immediately removed.

Prognosis: In ambulatory patients, chances of recovery are 50% or less. In severe, recumbent and convulsing animals, affected animals usually die regardless of the treatment.

BIBLIOGRAPHY

Bartik M and Piskac A (1981) Veterinary Toxicology. Elsevier Scientific Publishing Company, Amsterdam.

Beasley V (1999) Veterinary Toxicology. International Veterinary Information Service, Ithaca NY (www.ivis.org).

Bergland F (1978) Toxicological aspects of food-safety: Food additives. *Arch. Toxicol.* 1 : 33.

Burnstein JL (1998) Ionizing radiation. In: Emergency Toxicology. 2nd edn. Viccellio P (ed.) p 991. Lippincott-Raven Publishers, Philadelhia.

Cliver DO (1990) Food Borne Diseases. Academic Press, Inc., San Diego.

Concon JM (1988) Food Toxicology. Part B. Marcel Dekker, Inc. New York.

Conning DM (1995) Toxicology of food and food additives. In: General and Applied Toxicology.

Ballantyne B, Marrs T and Turner P (Eds.) p 1213. Macmillan Press Ltd., London.

Conning DM and Lansdown ABG (1983) Toxic Hazards in Food. Raven Press, New York.

Coombe NB and Hood AEM (1980) Fertilizer nitrogen effects on dairy cow health and performance. *Fert. Res.* 1 : 157.

Criver DO (!990) Food Borne Diseases. Academic Press, New York.

Finley JW and Schwass DE (1983) Xenobiotics in Foods and Feeds. American Chemical Society, Washington.

Jadhav SJ, Sharma RP and Salunkhe DK (1981) Naturally occurring toxic alkaloids in foods. *CRC Crit. Rev. Toxicol.* 9 : 21.

Kaur C and Brar RS (1996) Clinipathological studies on acute salt poisoning in broilers. *Ind. J. Vet. Path.* 20 : 150.

Kaur C, Sandhu BS, Sood N and Brar RS (1998) Effect of excess sodium chloride levels on testes in chickens. *Ind. J. Vet. Path.* 22 : 50.

Kotsonis FN, Burdock GA and Flamm WG (1996) Food toxicology. In: Casarett & Doull's Toxicology: The Basic Science of Poisons. 5th edn. Klaassen CD (Ed.) p 909. Mcgraw Hill Companies Inc., New York.

Lewis RJ Sr. (1989) Food Additives Handbook. Van Nostrand Reinhold, New York.

Loosli JK and McDonald IW (1968) Non-protein nitrogen in the nutrition of ruminants. FAO Agricultural Studies No. 73. FAO Corporate Document Repository, Rome. (http://www.fao.org/docrep/004/AC149E/AC149E00.HTM).

Lu FC and Kacew S (2002) Lu's Basic Toxicology: Fundamentals, Target Organs and Risk Assessment. Taylor & Francis, New York.

Miller K (1987) Toxicological Aspects of Food. Elsevier Applied Science, London.

Monier-Williams GW (1949). Trace Elements in Food. John Wiley and Sons, New York.

National Academy of Sciences (1960) The fluorosis problem in livestock production: A report of committee on Animal Nutrition. Publication 824. National Academy of Sciences - National Research Council, Washington D.C.

Osweiler GD (1996) Toxicology. Williams and Wilkins, Philadelphia.

Poulsen E (1978) Toxicological aspects of food safety: Introduction to the symposium. *Arch. Toxicol.* 1 : 15.

Radeleff RD (1970) Veterinary Toxicology. 2nd edn. Lea and Febiger, Philadelphia.

Rodostits O M, Gay C C, Blood D C and Hinchcliff K W (2000) Veterinary Medicine: A Textbook of the Diseases of Cattle, Sheep, Pigs, Goats and Horses. 9th edn. W. B. Saunders, London.

Rogers P (1999) Poisoning in cattle and sheep by urea, nitrates and nitrites: Sources, toxic doses, treatment and prevention. (http://homepage.eircom.net/~progers/ureanitr.htm).

Rosival I, Zwick K and Bartik M (1971) Utilization and toxicity of ammonia in ruminants. II. Attempt to influence the toxicity of ammonia by ion exchanger in the sodium cycle. *Acta Vet. Brno.* 40 : 301.

Salunkhe DK and Sharma RP (1984) Food Additives: A Benefit/Risk Dilemma. In: Modern Toxicology. Vol. II. The Adverse Effects of Xenobiotics. Gupta PK and Salunkhe DK (Eds.) p 131. Metropolitan Book Company, New Delhi.

Shibamoto T and Bjeldanes LF (1993) Introduction to Food Toxicology. Academic Press Inc., London.

Siller WG (1971) Cystic dilatation of seminiferous tubules, a sequel to sodium intoxication. *J. Path.* 107 : 191.

Stanton TL and Whittier J (2006) Urea and NPN for Cattle and Sheep. Colorado State University Extension. (www.ext.colostate.edu/pubs/livestk/01608.pdf).

Taylor AW (2003) Fertilizers. In: Encyclopedia of Agrochemicals. Vol 1. Plimmer JR, Gammon DW and Ragsdale NN (Eds.). p 483. John Wiley & Sons, Inc., New Jersey.

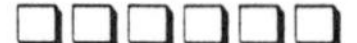

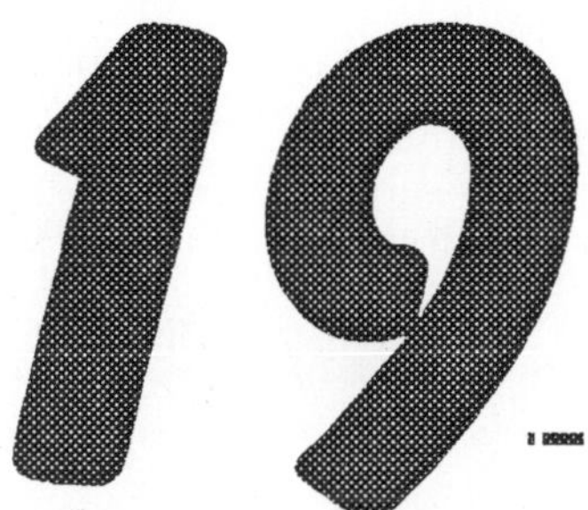

RADIATIONS

Types of radiation
 Ionizing radiations
 Non-ionizing radiations
Sources of radiation
Mechanism of action
Biological effects

Radiations are produced by disintegration of unstable naturally occurring or man-made elements. Radiations have been utilized for many beneficial effects, but direct or indirect exposure to ionizing radiations produce number of deleterious effects on health of animals. Ionizing radiations can cause different types of damages in mammalian systems including effects on both proliferative and non-proliferative tissues. Radiation exposure and injury require specific technical knowledge and handling because exposed animals generally act as reservoir of radioactivity that could be passed on to human beings through animal products and pose a serious threat to human health. Certain radioactive isotopes are among the most poisonous substances known with lethal dose being in microgrammes or less.

Types of radiation

Radiations are broadly of two types: Ionizing radiation and non-ionizing radiation.

1. Ionizing radiations

Ionizing radiations produce their effect by ionizing the biological molecules or atoms by knocking the electrons out of their orbit. This process of electron removal from atoms by ionizing radiation produces two electrically charged particles viz. negatively charged electrons and positively charged ions, both of which are toxic and may cause damage in living tissues. The ionizing radiations produce ionization either directly (called direct ionizing radiation) or indirectly (called indirect ionizing radiation). The direct ionizing radiations carry an electrical charge and cause ionization of molecules due to the mass and motion of the charged particle which imparts direct force to the electron in orbit e.g. alpha particles. Indirect ionizing radiations, in contrast, are not electrically charged, but they produce ionization by colliding with an atom which thereby liberates charged (ionized) particles e.g. all photon radiations and neutrons.

Ionizing radiations occur as either particles (e.g. alpha and beta particles) or electromagnetic rays (e.g. X-rays and gamma rays).

Particulate ionizing radiations: Particulate or particle radiations are the radiations of energy by means of fast-moving particles. Particle radiation can be emitted by an unstable atomic nucleus (radioactive decay) in the form of a charged particle (e.g. alpha and beta particle) or a non-charged particle (e.g. neutron). Charged particles interact strongly and ionize directly, whereas neutral particles interact less, ionize indirectly and penetrate farther.

a. *Alpha (α)-radiation (alpha-particle):* The alpha particle consists of two protons and two neutrons (double +ve charge) bound together into a particle identical to a helium nucleus. It arises from decay of unstable heavy atoms such as uranium, thorium, polonium and radium. The high mass and

2 positive charges result in large direct ionizing potential, but very little penetration. Therefore the alpha particles can not penetrate the skin easily, but pose a significant risk if inhaled or ingested as their great mass (and hence energy) produces significant tissue damage when in direct contact with tissues.

b. *Beta (β)-radiation (beta-particle):* The beta particle is a high energy, high speed electron that arises from conversion of a neutron to a proton in the nucleus. Common sources of beta-particles include ^{14}carbon, ^{32}phosphorus, ^{90}strontium and cathode ray tubes. The beta particles have a higher penetrating power up to 8 cm in tissues, but low ionizing power as compared to alpha particles. Beta particles are usually blocked by a thin light metal shield or several layers of cloth.

c. *Positron particle:* Positron is like a beta particle, but positively charged. It has the same mass as the beta particle, but it arises when a proton is converted to a neutron. Due to similarities between the two radiations, positrons are often included in beta-particles and the symbol β^- is used for beta particle and the symbol β^+ for positron (Beta particles, therefore, are also defined as high-energy electrons and positrons).

d. *Neutrons:* Neutron is an electron combined with proton which therefore has no charge. Neutrons are created in the fission chain reaction found in power reactors and atomic explosion. They readily penetrate, cause indirect ionization and can cause immense cellular damage due to their mass and speed. Neutron exposure can create radioisotopes in biological material, which can then decay and produce further damage.

e. *Proton:* Proton is a hydrogen ion. It is a potent ionizer, produced by neutron interactions.

Non-particulate ionizing radiations/ Electromagnetic radiations: Electromagnetic radiation is generally described as a self-propagating wave in space with electric and magnetic components. Electromagnetic radiation is classified into different types according to the frequency of the wave and includes gamma rays, X-rays and UV rays.

a. *Gamma (γ) radiation/ray:* Gamma rays are generally characterized as electromagnetic radiation (EMR) having the highest frequency and energy, and also the shortest wavelength, within the spectrum of EMR. Due to its high energy content, γ-radiation is able to cause serious damage when absorbed by living cells. It produces action via indirect ionization. Common sources of gamma rays emitter are ^{125}Iodine, ^{131}iodine, ^{60}cobalt and also X-ray and radiotherapy machines.

b. *X-ray:* X-rays are a form of electromagnetic radiation with a wavelength in the range of 10 nm to 0.01 nm. These are primarily used for diagnostic radiography and crystallography and are produced by X-ray machine. X-rays are a form of ionizing radiation and as such can be dangerous.

c. *Ultra Violet radiation:* Ultra Violet (UV) radiation is an electromagnetic radiation that lies within the wavelength range of 100-400nm. The UV wavelengths are divided into three types: UVA=400-315nm, UVB = 315-280nm, UVC = 280-100nm. In general, UVC is the most harmful and UVA is the least harmful. Naturally the Sun emits ultraviolet radiation in the UVA, UVB, and UVC bands, but because of absorption in the atmosphere's ozone layer, 99% of the ultraviolet radiation that reaches the Earth's surface is UVA. UV radiations have many industrial and other uses, which could be also a source of toxicity.

2. Non-ionizing radiations

Non-ionizing radiation refers to any type of electromagnetic radiation that does not carry enough energy to ionize atoms or molecules i.e. to completely remove an electron from atom or molecule. Non-ionizing radiation is thought to be essentially harmless below the levels that cause heating e.g. visible light, near UV-rays (ionizing to some molecules), infrared, microwaves and radio waves. The light from the Sun that reaches the earth is largely composed of non-ionizing radiation, with the notable exception of some ultraviolet rays.

Terms related to radiation

a. *Units of radiation:* Radiation dose to tissues is expressed in terms of quantity of absorbed energy (erg) per unit mass. The S.I. unit is the 'Gray (Gy)' which is defined as 1 joule of absorbed energy per kilogramme (1J/kg). The older unit of Rad (radiation absorbed dose), which is still in common use, is an absorbed dose of 0.01 joules of energy per kilogram of tissue. Thus one gray is equal to 100 rad. (1 Gy = 100 rad).

b. *Rem:* Rem (Radiation equivalent man) is the amount of any radiation that produces a biological effect equivalent to that resulting from 1 rad or 0.01 gray of gamma radiation. The unit rem takes into account the amount of damage caused to human tissue by the radiation. In general, one rem is equivalent to 1 rad, except for radiation sources such as neutrons or heavy nuclei, which cause greater damage to human tissue than other forms of radiation, and which therefore, will have a greater number of rem than rads for a given amount of radiation energy.

c. *Radioactive decay:* Radioactive decay is the decay of unstable isotopes by the subatomic particles and gamma or x-rays. Heavy elements generally decay by emission of alpha particles, while lighter elements generally decay by beta emission.

d. *Linear energy transfer:* Linear energy transfer (LET) is a measure of the rate at which energy is imparted to the absorbing medium per unit distance of track length. Radiations having higher LET (e.g. protons and alpha particle) are less penetrating but produce greater injury for a given absorbed dose than those having the low LET (e.g. x-rays and gamma rays).

e. *Irradiation:* It is a type of radiation exposure in which the patient's body is not contaminated with the radioactive material, so the radiation exposure does not produce continuing damage (except in case of a neutron emitter) to the patient itself or to other individuals once the patient is removed from the source.

f. *Surface contamination:* It is a type of radiation exposure in which the patient's body is actually physically contaminated with radioactive material, so the radiation exposure produces continuing damage to the patient as well as poses hazards to other individuals.

Sources of radiation

Animals may be exposed to radiations from various natural and man-made sources:

a. *Natural sources:* Several natural sources of radiation such as cosmic rays from space, disintegration of radioactive elements in Earth's crust and naturally occurring radio-active materials in the environment may give rise to the external or internal irradiation of animal body. Depletion of ozone layers in the atmosphere due to green house effect or other man made activities also enhances exposure to natural radiations through solar rays. The chances of exposure to the cosmic and solar radiations is generally more in the mountains than in the plains due to higher intensity of these rays at higher altitudes. Two decay products viz. ^{322}radon and ^{320}thoron of ^{238}uranium and ^{232}thorium, respectively account for about 54% of the earth's background radiation and dangerously pollute the atmosphere. In general the exposure from natural sources is low, except under specific circumstances like radon accumulating in a closed space.

b. *Nuclear weapons*: Nuclear weapons are very rich source of radiations. In the immediate vicinity of a nuclear explosion, the radiation effect is very less in comparison to damage caused by heat and blast. However, the widespread and long lasting effect of nuclear explosion is due to the fall out which is of three types:

   i. *Local fall out*: Particles caught up in the explosion become radioactive and fall in the near vicinity in few minutes to 24 hours.

   ii. *Tropospheric fall out*: Vapours are carried upward up to 10 km in troposphere, get condensed and carried to long distances and are deposited mainly by rains over a period of weeks and months.

iii. *Stratospheric fall out*: Some particles are carried upward into stratosphere, get deposited for years and then slowly come down.

Of the radioactive materials produced by an atomic explosion, a number of radionuclides like iodine–131, barium–140, strontium–89, strontium–90 and cesium–137 are likely to enter biological systems. Of these, strontium–90 and cesium–137 have greatest biological significance due to their long half-life.

c. *Nuclear power plants:* There are about 500 nuclear power plants worldwide with many operating with light-water coolant systems. This coolant water is radioactive and represents a hazard if released into the environment. Accidents in the nuclear reactors, as happened at Chernobyl, can release radioactive material into the environment and may affect large areas and population. This is equivalent to tropospheric fall out and a source of radiation.

d. *Industrial uses:* Radioisotopes and devices are widely used in industry for various purposes ranging from material analysis to food processing to chemical engineering. Improper transport or handling of radioisotopes may pose a hazard to workers and population nearby.

e. *Radioactive wastes:* Animals may be exposed to radiations due to ignorance and carelessness in the storage and dumping of radioactive materials.

f. *Diagnostic and therapeutic uses:* The use of x-rays and several radioactive isotopes in clinical research and therapy, if not monitored carefully, may expose animals to their harmful effects.

Factors affecting toxicity :

a. Mammalian cells are most sensitive to radiations during mitosis and in early G phase. Therefore, mammalian fertilized egg cell (zygote) is highly radiation sensitive. Resistance is usually greatest during the S phase; however, this depends upon the type of radiation.

b. Tissues with high rates of cell turnover are highly sensitive to the radiations, so rapidly proliferating stem cells of the intestinal epithelium and the haematopoietic system are highly sensitive and respond more rapidly to radiations than do less sensitive cells such as those in the lung and the basal layer of skin, which have low proliferative rates. Cells that divide only during embryogenesis are the least sensitive to the radiations.

c. When radiation is delivered at a low rate or in series of multiple fractions separated by several hours, the overall effect of cell-kill is usually less than that of an acute dose mainly due to the repair of sublethal injury.

d. Young and old persons and animals are more radiosensitive than young adults. Developing organisms (e.g. embryo and foetus) are more radiosensitive compared to adult ones.

Toxicity: The nature and severity of radiation induced toxicity can vary with type of radiation, magnitude of radiation dose and period over which it is delivered. In addition, age, sex and health status of the animal and, particularly, degree of post-irradiation care may affect the toxicity. A dose of 1 Gy of X-ray will cause about 2×10^5 separate ionizations within the mammalian cell. Of these, about 1 per cent occurs in the genomic material mainly due to breakage of DNA strands. Of many breaks that occur, almost all disappear within few hours, except a few (usually double strand breaks) which are mainly responsible for loss of cell viability and other sublethal injuries. The LD_{50} is expressed as $LD_{50/60}$ (i.e. dose that causes 50 per cent mortality within 60 days) in man and $LD_{50/30}$ (i.e. dose that causes 50 per cent mortality within 30 days) for most animal species. The LD_{50} for acute radiation exposure for humans is about 400 rem, while the LD_{90} is 1000 rem. A direct dose of >5000 rem will be lethal to humans within 1 hour mainly due to CNS effects.

Mechanism of action: The radiations owe their harmful effects in body due to the biochemical changes in tissues that in turn cause various physiological, histological and genetic changes. In the cell, most obvious changes are seen in nuclei than in other parts. The radiation induced toxicity represents a dynamic interaction with matter by direct or indirect processes. Accordingly, action of radiations can be studied under two subheadings: direct effects and indirect effects.

Direct effects: Direct effects of radiation involve transfer of radiation energy directly to the molecules of cells especially DNA, where there may be ionization, breakage of linkages, etc. Direct actions of different types of radiations are given below:

a. Beta-rays transfer their energy to the electrons of the atom in their path causing these electrons to fly away from their orbit, leaving the atom positively charged. Besides, β-rays may interact with the nuclei of atoms to produce electro-magnetic radiations similar to X-rays.

b. Fast and thermal neutrons being uncharged are highly penetrating in the biological tissues. They do not cause ionization directly but act by elastic scattering. In the elastic scattering, nuclei of atoms are kicked away by neutrons causing instability in them, which subsequently produce gamma-rays. This may kick-off another cycle and hence radioactivity is induced within the cells, especially in the nuclei of cells.

c. Alpha-rays produce both ionization (ejection of orbital electron from atom) and excitation (movement of electron from lower to higher orbit) in the molecules of material through which they pass.

d. X-rays and gamma-rays are non-particulate electro-magnetic radiations having tremendous amount of energy and high penetrating power. They produce their effect by following ways:

i. Photoelectric effect: When a low energy photon collides with an atom, all the energy is transferred to the electron which is ejected from the atom. The ejected photoelectron carries considerable kinetic energy and causes ionization of molecules.

ii. Pair-production: A high energy photon passing close to the nucleus of an atom may be completely absorbed accompanied with the ejection of a high energy e^- (electron) and a high energy e^+ (positron). This e^- and e^+ form a team called pair-production. The positron and electron lose energy in the medium, leading to chemical or physical changes.

Indirect effects:

a. Ion pairs: The ejection of electron in direct effect produces a positively charged ion. This ejected e^- is captured by another atom and hence a negatively charged ion is also formed. Thus a pair of ions i.e. positively charged (cation) and negatively charged (anion) is produced called ion pair. Significant events are produced by ion pairs. These ion pairs also rapidly interact with themselves and surrounding molecules to produce free radicals. Oxygen (O_2) present in large quantities in genetic material is one of the potent electron acceptor producing harmful effects.

$A \longrightarrow A^+ + e^-$ (e^- ejected from A)

$B \longrightarrow B^-$ (e^- captured by B)

Overall effect = $A^+ + B^-$ (ion pair)

b. Formation of free radical: Free radicals are electrically neutral molecules with an unpaired electron in their outer shell. The most fundamental effect of ionizing radiation on biological systems is the ionization of water with formation of free radicals H and OH. In this process, an ejected e^- from the oxygen atom of a molecule of water is captured by one H-atom of another water molecule producing ion-pair. In the presence of two other molecules of water, this ion-pair dissociates and produces two free radicals H and OH (Fig. 19.1). In the biological systems, the free radicals H or OH exist for only a fraction of second and react to form H_2O, H_2 or H_2O_2 or may react with macromolecules such as nucleic acids, amino acids, proteins, lipids, thiols or carbohydrates. The interaction of these free radicals or H_2O_2 with cellular macromolecules leads to a variety of genetic and non-genetic damages with loss of cell functions. Their interaction with genetic material may lead to DNA strands break, point mutation, and chromosomal aberration with subsequent loss of gene products coded for by that portion of DNA.

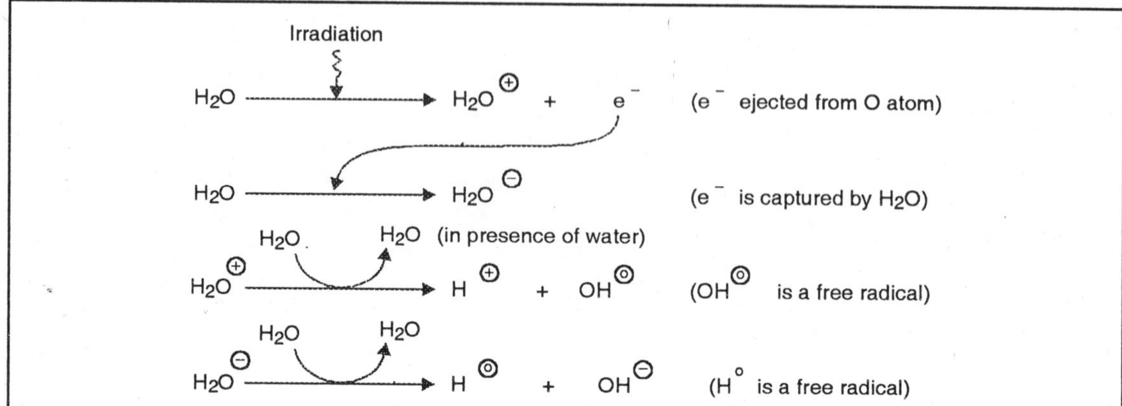

Fig.19.1. Postulated production of free radicals. The OH and H are free radicals and highly reactive. They produce H_2O_2 and organic peroxides which are highly reactive and produce biological effects.

If these genes are required by the cell to maintain itself, it will eventually result in cell death. Free radicals also result in peroxidation of biological membranes resulting in altered membrane permeability and subsequent loss of cellular functions.

Biological effects and clinical signs

Radiation causes damage to various macromolecules causing death of cells (non-genetic effect) or alterations in genetic material which are expressed in a later generation (genetic effect). Accordingly, biological effects of two types, non-genetic and genetic, have been described.

Non-genetic effects : Non-genetic radiation effects are due to the radiation-induced cell killings with the accompanying loss of functions for which the cells are responsible. Cell death is most likely to occur when the irradiated cells attempt to resume division. So tissues containing actively dividing cells tend to exhibit greater sensitivity to radiations than do those composed of fully differentiated cells with little or no mitotic activity. The severity and clinical expression of non-genetic effects differ widely, depending on whether an individual has received whole-body irradiation or partial-body irradiation.

a. Whole-body irradiation: Whole-body exposure at doses between a few and tens of grays of acute irradiation (delivered over a short-time interval) may result in early effects and delayed effects.

a. *Early effects:* Death may occur within few hours to few weeks following acute radiation exposure. The survival time and mode of death is dose-dependent. A dose of 100 Gy can cause death from neurological damage within few hours, 5-12 Gy can cause death from gastrointestinal injury within few days, and 2.5-5 Gy may cause death from irreversible damage to the haematopoietic system in several weeks. The prodromal syndrome develops shortly after irradiation and precedes the onset of neurological, gastrointestinal and haematopoietic syndromes.

i. *Prodromal syndrome:* It comprises the symptoms and signs that appear within 48 hours of irradiation (even within an hour), persists for few days and then gradually diminishes in intensity. It is mediated through the autonomic nervous system and includes clinical signs of anorexia, nausea, vomiting and fatigue at lower dose (4-5 Gy) and diarrhoea, fever, sweating, listlessness and apathy at higher dose.

ii. *Neurological syndrome:* It is seen following very high dose of radiation (>100 Gy) producing death from cerebrovascular damage in most mammalian species within 2 days. The syndrome is characterised by severe prodromal effects followed by transitory periods of depressed or enhanced motor activity. Severe nausea is followed by vomiting, disorientation, loss of coordination and muscular movement, respiratory distress, diarrhoea, convulsive seizures, coma and death. Though exact cause of death is not clear, an increase in the fluid content of brain due to leakage from small vessels creating a build-up of pressure inside the skull has been suggested as the cause of immediate death.

iii. *Gastro-intestinal syndrome:* This syndrome is characterised by prodromal phase followed by prolonged diarrhoea, loss of appetite, loss of fluid and electrolytes, dehydration, weight loss, gastric retention and decreased intestinal absorption. There is marked reduction in leucocytes; haemorrhages and bacteriaemia may occur, aggravating the injury and contributing to death. Sterilization of cells in the crypts prevents repopulation, villi begin to shrink and intestinal lining is eventually denuded of villi. Death occurs within 3-10 days due to the radiation-induced damage to the epithelium lining the GI tract.

iv. *Haematopoietic syndrome:* Proliferating haematopoietic stem cells are highly radiosensitive and are sterilized by radiation, thereby reducing the body's supply of red and white cells and platelets. Lymphocyte count is most sensitive index of radiation injury in the blood as neutrophils undergo interphase death with 50% decrease in number within 48 hours. Neutrophils initially show increase followed by dose-dependent fall. Platelet count usually decreases leading to bleeding. Approximately 3 weeks after irradiation, symptoms including chills, fatigues, ulceration of mouth, petechial haemorrhages of skin, fever, anaemia, etc. occur. Death usually occurs due to infection and depressed immunity.

b. *Delayed effects:* The clinical changes become apparent months or years after the whole-body irradiation. These include incidence of neoplasms, leukaemias, local tissue changes like lens opacity, shortening of life-span, etc. However, late effects are not much important in animals due to their short life-span.

i. *Carcinogenesis:* Radiation is effective in the treatment of cancer (sufficiently large doses) but is also acting as a carcinogen. For cancer induction, sublethal doses of radiation are important. Leukaemia is most frequently induced cancer. The latency period for leukaemia is 2-5 years, while for other tumours 10 or more years are required. Radiation carcinogenesis is thought to be a multistage process involving initiation, promotion and progression.

b. Partial-body irradiation: In partial-body irradiation, a part(s) of body or organ gets exposure from radiation.

i. *Skin:* Fall out on skin especially of β-radiation can lead to severe burns. It starts with oedema of skin leading to cell destruction, degenerative changes in basal layer and hair follicles, and fall of hair. The long-term effects of radiation on the skin, which develops months or years after exposure, include changes in pigmentation, atrophy of epidermis, sweat glands, sebaceous glands and hair follicles, fibrosis of dermis, increased susceptibility to trauma and chronic ulcerations.

ii. *Reproductive system:* The germ cells of the ovary and testis are very radiosensitive and their irradiation impairs fertility in both sexes in a dose-dependent manner. Cell division in the germinative epithelium of the testes stops at once. It causes death of spermatogonia (male germinative epithelium); so already developed cells undergo maturation without division. The sperm count drops after few days leading to azoospermia and sterility. Germ cell irradiation also increases mutation incidence in the offsprings (See genetic effects).

iii. *Digestive system:* The digestive system is usually involved after grazing on fall out pasture. There is inflammation and ulceration in the mouth and throat region and necrosis developing after high doses.

Salivary flow decreases due to damage to the salivary gland. The glandular mucosa of the stomach, small intestine and colon respond more rapidly and tolerate less radiation with development of ulceration and denudation of the affected mucosae. There is anorexia, diarrhoea and secondary infection. Damage to liver may produce hepatic failure, ascites and death.

iv. *Respiratory system:* Inhaled radioactive particles may lodge in the lungs and if insoluble, remain there for long time. In high doses, the earliest signs of radiation injury to the lungs are oedema and changes in blood circulation followed by pneumonitis within 1-3 months. In upper respiratory tract (nasopharynx, larynx, trachea, bronchi), there may be ulceration, atrophy and fibrosis.

v. *Nervous system:* Radiation-induced damage to the spinal cord, including demyelination and delayed necrosis of neurons, may occur between 6 months and 2 years of exposure leading to neurological signs like numbness, tingling, anaesthesia, paresthesia, weakness and paralysis. Necrosis of brain associated with demyelination and damage to cerebral vasculature may occur within 1-3 years and show neurological signs with death in some cases.

vi. *Endocrine system:* Endocrine glands including the thyroid, parathyroid, adrenal and pituitary glands have low cell turnover rates in adult animals and therefore are radiation resistant. In growing young animals, irradiation of thyroid gland by external gamma-radiation or internally deposited radio iodine can lead to hypothyroidism and growth retardation.

vii. *Urinary system:* Kidneys are highly radiosensitive followed by bladder and ureters. The kidneys shrink in size and the capsule thickens and adheres to cortex. In bladder, there may be inflammation, ulceration, fistula, fibrosis, contraction and urinary obstruction.

viii. *Musculoskeletal system:* Muscles, bones and cartilages are relatively resistant to the direct cytocidal actions of radiation. Damage to the bone-marrow may lead to anaemia, leucopenia, lymphopenia and tumour formation (delayed effect).

ix. *Eyes:* Exposure of eyes to the radiation may cause cataract, as lens of the eye is one of the most radio-sensitive tissues of the body.

Genetic effects : Damage to the germ cells may result in genetic mutation that is expressed in a later generation. Radiation induced hereditary effects may be dominant or recessive, appearing in the first or later generations involving changes in a single gene or in the gross structure of a chromosome (loss or addition of a chromosome, chromosome breakage and translocation). These genetic defects may lead to various abnormalities in the progenies like stillbirths, major congenital defects, sex chromosome abnormalities, mutations resulting in electrophoretic variations in blood proteins, tumours and leukaemias.

Post-mortem findings: Lesions may be present on the specific organ or system depending upon their exposure to the radiation. There may be gastroenteritis varying from haemorrhagic to ulcerative, ulceration of pharyngeal mucosa and pulmonary oedema, and all degrees of haemorrhages from petechiae and ecchymoses to haematomas and large extravasations. Degenerative lesions are present in all organs. All soft tissues, organs and bones of the body show the presence of radioactive material.

Special precautions must be taken in conducting a necropsy and disposal of radioactive organs.

Diagnosis: Diagnosis may be made from history of exposure to radiation or radioactive material, clinical signs and post-mortem lesions. Absolute lymphocyte count is considered the most useful screening measurement of total dose and prognosis. In humans, a lymphocyte count <1000 cells/ml^3 at 24 hours or <500 cells/ml^3 at 48 hours indicates severe exposure to radiation. An absolute lymphocyte count of over 1500 cells/ml^3 at 48 hours post-exposure generally rules out significant whole-body irradiation.

Treatment and management: There is no specific treatment of radiation intoxication. Symptomatic and supportive therapy is indicated under the supervision of a subject specialist.

a. Antibiotics should be used to treat secondary infections.

b. Fluid and electrolyte balance should be maintained by appropriate measures.

c. Corticosteroids and antihistaminic creams are indicated for skin ulcers and inflammation. Corticosteroids may decrease the severity of desquamation reaction but will have no effect on the erythema.

d. Fresh bone marrow cells transfusion may be undertaken in the haematopoietic syndrome to stimulate production of blood cells.

e. Parathyroid extracts and low calcium diets are recommended to increase the rate of excretion of radioactive material from the body.

Prognosis: Prognosis of radiation toxicity depends upon the dose of radiation and the extent of exposure. In high dose whole-body irradiation, the treatment may be hopeless.

BIBLIOGRAPHY

Adams GE and Wilson A (1995) Radiation toxicology. In: General and Applied Toxicology. Ballantyne B, Marrs T and Turner P (Eds.) p 1267. Macmillan Press Ltd., London.

Altman KI, Gerber GB and Okada S (1970) Radiation Biochemistry. Vol. II. Academic Press, New York.

Beasley V (1999) Forms of energy, chemicals and drugs that affect the digestive tract. In: Veterinary Toxicology. Beasley V (Ed.) p. 814. International Veterinary Information Service, Ithaca NY (www.ivis.org).

Casarett AP (1968) Radiation Biology. Prentice-Hall, Inc. New Jersey.

Clarke ECG and Clarke ML (1967) Garner's Veterinary Toxicology. 3rd edn. Williams and Wilkins, Baltimore.

Harley NH (1996) Toxic effects of radiation and radioactive materials. In: Casarett & Doull's Toxicology: The Basic Science of Poisons. 5th edn. Klaassen CD (Ed.) p 773. Mcgraw Hill Companies Inc., New York.

Kirk KM and Lyon MF (1984) Induction of congenital malformations in the offspring of male mice treated with X-rays at pre-meiotic and post-meiotic stages. *Mutat. Res.* 125 : 75.

Letavet AA and Kurlyandskaya EB (1970) The Toxicology of Radioactive Substances. Vol. 5. Zinc-65. Pergamon Press, Oxford.

Nomura T (1983) X-ray induced germ-line mutation leading to tumours. *Mutat. Res.* 121 : 59.

Pizzarello DJ and Witcofski RL (1967) Basic Radiation Biology. Lea and Febiger, Philadelphia.

Radeleff RD (1970) Veterinary Toxicology. 2nd edn. Lea and Febiger, Philadelphia.

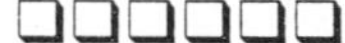

20 THERAPEUTIC AGENTS

Antibacterial drugs
- Sulphonamides
- Penicillins
- Aminoglycosides
- Tetracyclines
- Chloramphenicol
- Nitrofurans

Antiparasitic drugs
- Carbon tetrachloride
- Phenothiazine
- Ivermectin
- Levamisole
- Thiacetarsamide

Non-steroidal anti-inflammatory drugs
- Salicylates
- Phenylbutazone
- Paracetamol

Sedatives
- Chlorpromazine
- Benzodiazepines

Anti-histamines
- H_1-Histamine receptor antagonists
- H_2-Histamine receptor antagonists

A large number of veterinary and human drugs are available for dispensing, some of which may pose great potential for poisoning to pet and farm animals. In veterinary medicine, toxic effects occur mainly due to administration of an inappropriate drug in an inappropriate dosage to an inappropriate species. Use of human-label drugs in animal practice for which drug safety and efficacy data have not been established, use of multiple drugs simultaneously, or fixed dose drug combinations in animals also lead to toxic effects. In clinical practice, the toxic effect may occur even when a recommended drug is used at therapeutic doses mainly due to idiosyncrasy and individual variations. Aspirin is one of the drugs causing the largest number of deaths in cats. Sedative-hypnotics include a wide range of pharmacological agents used in the treatment of several CNS disorders. The number of poisoning cases from such therapeutic agents is large and it is not possible to discuss the toxicity of every drug available to animals. Accordingly, the present chapter describes toxicology of selected therapeutic agents commonly available and indiscriminately used in veterinary medicine.

I. ANTIBACTERIAL DRUGS

1. Sulphonamides

The sulphonamides are a group of complex synthetic organic chemical compounds having chemotherapeutic activity. The antibacterial activity of sulphonamides was first discovered by Domagk in 1935, who demonstrated that prontosil, an azo dye, is effective against streptococcal infection in mice. Sulphonamide toxicity can occur through individual dosing or therapeutic application in feed or water. Most cases result from overdosing the animals or feeding sulphonamides to animals that have limited water supply or high fluid losses as a result of diarrhoea.

Properties: The term sulphonamide (sulpha drug) is commonly used as a generic name for all derivatives of sulphanilamide. Sulphonamides are weak organic compounds which are sparingly soluble in water, but their sodium salts are water-soluble. They are highly soluble in alkaline solutions but are less soluble in acidic urine and some may even precipitate in the renal tubules of species having acidic urine (e.g. carnivores) leading to crystalluria and renal failure. Parenteral administration of sulphonamides can be painful, as the solutions of sulphonamides are strong alkaline solutions.

$$H_2N-C_6H_4-SO_2-NH-R$$

Fig.20.1. Basic structure of sulphonamides.

Toxicokinetics: Systemically acting sulphonamides are usually well absorbed (70-100%) following oral administration mainly from small intestine. The absorption rate is affected by the solubility of sulphonamides and presence of ingesta in the GI tract. After absorption, sulphonamides diffuse well into body tissues and fluids. The sulphonamides are primarily metabolised by acetylation by non-microsomal enzymes in liver and some other tissues. The acetylated metabolites can conjugate with glucuronic acid or sulphate. Sulphonamides also undergo hydroxylation, conjugation with glucuronic acid or sulphate, and cleavage of heterocyclic rings. Acetylation of sulphonamides reduces their solubility thus promoting crystallisation. In cattle, sulphonamides are more toxic due to extensive acetylation. Dogs lack the ability to acetylate sulphonamides, therefore, toxicity of sulphonamides is comparatively less in dogs. Sulphonamides or their metabolites are excreted mainly by kidneys through glomerular filtration, although renal tubular secretion and reabsorption also occur. Sulphonamides are excreted also in the tears, faeces, bile and sweat.

Gut-acting sulphonamides are poorly absorbed from the GI tract and are primarily eliminated in the faeces.

Mechanism of action: The antibacterial action of sulphonamides is mainly due to inhibition of folic acid synthesis in susceptible bacteria due to their structural resemblance to para-aminobenzoic acid (PABA). Sulphonamides generally produce selective toxicity on target microorganisms and do not affect animal cells because mammalian cells utilise the preformed folic acid and do not synthesise it in the body as in the bacteria. The mechanisms of toxicity are different and may include:

a. *Renal toxicity:* The renal toxicity of sulphonamides is attributable to their precipitation in the glomerular filtrate leading to crystallisation, haematuria and obstruction of renal tubules and ureter. Chances of crystalluria are more in dehydrated animals as the urine may contain drug concentrations above solubility limits resulting in crystal formation.

b. *Hypoprothrombinaemia:* Prolonged administration of certain sulphonamides may lead to vitamin K deficiency due to inhibition of enzyme vitamin K epoxide reductase. This results in hypoprothrombinaemia and deficiency of other vitamin K dependent clotting factors causing prolongation of bleeding and clotting time. It is mostly seen in poultry with sulphaquinoxaline.

c. *Keratoconjunctivitis sicca (KCS):* Prolonged treatment with certain sulphonamides (e.g. sulphasalazine, sulphadiazine and sulphamethoxazole) may cause keratoconjunctivitis sicca (dry eyes) in dogs. This occurs probably due to hypersensitivity reaction or due to direct lachrymotoxic effect of nitrogen-containing pyridine ring on the lachrymal acinar cells.

d. *Inhibition of carbonic anhydrous enzyme:* Prolonged administration of sulphonamides inhibit carbonic anhydrous enzyme resulting in accumulation of carbon dioxide leading to acidosis. Carbonic anhydrous is also involved in eggshell production in poultry, so its inhibition by sulphonamides may result in thin eggshells or even absence of eggshells.

e. *Hepatic necrosis*: Potentiated sulphonamide (sulphonamide + trimethoprim) therapy has been associated with development of hepatic necrosis in dogs. The exact mechanism responsible for this adverse effect is not known but is thought to occur from altered metabolism resulting in accumulation of hepatotoxic metabolites. The slow acetylation often results in increased sulphadehydroxylamine metabolite, which is hepatotoxic. Since dogs are slow acetylators, they are more susceptible to hepatic injury.

f. *Aplastic anaemia and thrombocytopenia:* Complete suppression of bone-marrow activity with anaemia, granulocytopenia, and thrombocytopenia may occur from a direct myelotoxic effect or due to an immune-mediated component. Reduction in serum folate concentration, presumably by inhibition of folate production by intestinal bacteria may also induce anaemia.

g. *Other effects:* Several other toxic effects of sulphonamides reported in domestic animals has been related to formation of methaemoglobin, peripheral neurotoxicity (in chickens and cattle), interference with thyroid hormone production resulting in iatrogenic hypothyroidism and goitre, anaphylactoid reactions, and interference with ruminal flora B-vitamin. Some sulphonamides (e.g. sulphamethazine) have been associated with development of tumours in laboratory animals. Development of kernicterus has been reported in human neonates and foetuses due to sulphonamide induced displacement of bilirubin from plasma proteins.

Clinical signs :

Acute toxicity: Acute toxicity may occur after large parenteral or oral doses of sulphonamides. Clinical signs of acute sulphonamide toxicosis include salivation, vomiting, diarrhoea and polypnoea. Other signs such as weakness, ataxia and spastic rigidity are less commonly seen. Rapid IV administration may lead to mydriasis, ataxia, blindness and convulsions. Rapid intravenous injection has also been associated with anaphylactoid reaction and acute drug shock with collapse and death.

Chronic toxicity: Prolonged administration of sulphonamides may induce toxic signs such as anorexia, depression, collapse, haematuria, albuminuria and oliguria. There may be defective blood coagulation, peripheral neuritis and reduced egg production. Additional signs in cattle may include mild transient agranulocytosis, haemolytic anaemia, leukopenia and reduced milk production. A hypersensitivity reaction similar to anaphylactic reaction with respiratory difficulty and urticaria may also occur after repeated exposure. Inhibition of iodine metabolism may result in goitre and thyroid hyperplasia.

Post-mortem findings: Sulphonamides do not produce specific necropsy lesions except for sulphonamide crystals in the renal pelvis and renal tubules in some animals. Kidneys may be gritty in texture when cut. Microscopic examination after necropsy may reveal sulphonamide crystals in the renal tubules and renal pelvis.

Diagnosis: Diagnosis of sulphonamide toxicosis may be made from history of administering the drug, clinical signs and post-mortem findings. Specimens of kidney tissue should be fixed in a slightly acidified formalin solution or in absolute ethanol to prevent dissolution of crystals. Concentration of sulphonamide in body tissues such as muscles, kidneys and liver above 20 ppm substantiates a diagnosis.

Treatment: Treatment of sulphonamide poisoning involves non-specific measures and supportive care.

a. In case of acute overdose, efforts should be made to evacuate the intestinal tract using emetic, lavage, saline cathartic and/ or adsorbent.

b. Efforts should be made to restore the renal functions with rehydration therapy. Normal saline and bicarbonate solution may be administered intravenously along with oral electrolytes and water.

c. Vitamin K_1 is indicated in cases of hypoprothrombinaemia and coagulation disorder.

d. Adrenaline and antihistamines are used to treat hypersensitivity and acute anaphylactoid reactions.

e. Further exposure to sulphonamide containing feed and water should be stopped immediately.

2. Penicillins

The penicillins are a large group of naturally occurring and semi-synthetic antibiotics. Many members of this group are drugs of choice for a large number of infectious diseases in animals. Penicillins are among the safest antimicrobial drugs, but hypersensitivity is an infrequent but serious adverse effect. Penicillins are considered to be one of the most common causes of drug allergy. Important members of the group include penicillin G, cloxacillin, amoxycillin, ampicillin, ticarcillin, carbenicillin and piperacillin

Toxicity: The LD_{50} of pure penicillin G in mice and anaesthetised cats by I.V. route is 3,500,000 and 500,000 units/kg body weight, respectively. In chickens, LD_{50} by I.M. route is more than 2,500,000 units/kg body weight.

a. *Hypersensitivity:* Hypersensitivity is the most important and serious adverse effect of penicillins. The major antigenic determinant of penicillin hypersensitivity reaction is its metabolite penicilloic acid, which reacts with proteins and serves as a haptan to cause an immune reaction. The hypersensitivity reactions vary from mild and transitory skin reactions to fatal anaphylactic shock. Acute allergic responses to penicillins have been seen in dogs and are characterised by salivation, shivering, vomiting, urticaria, etc. which appear within 15 minutes after the injection. Many allergic responses subside in a few hours. Pharyngitis or sore throat has also been observed in dogs after 4 days of penicillin therapy. In dairy cows, acute allergic reactions are characterised by laboured breathing, salivation and cutaneous oedema of head and perineal region. Dermatitis in animals also results from penicillins. Cross-allergic reactions between penicillins are well recognised.

b. *GI disturbances:* The use of broad-spectrum penicillins may cause GI disturbances, particularly diarrhoea and superinfection due to disruption of normal balance of GI microflora. It occurs mostly with those agents that are incompletely absorbed and have an extended antibacterial spectrum. Penicillins are also associated with occasional nausea, vomiting and anorexia.

c. *Platelet dysfunction:* Some penicillins (e.g., antipseudomonal penicillins) may cause thrombocytopenia and decreased agglutination. It is generally a concern when treating patients predisposed to haemorrhage or those receiving anticoagulant therapy.

d. *Organ toxicity:* Penicillins are irritating to the neuronal tissues and can provoke seizures, particularly when administered in high doses or when injected intrathecally. Epileptic patients are especially at risk. High doses or very prolonged use has been associated with neurotoxicity, particularly ataxia in dogs. As penicillins are accumulated in renal tissues at high concentrations, they have potential to cause acute interstitial nephritis.

e. *Cation toxicity:* Penicillins are generally administered as the sodium or potassium salt, therefore, cation toxicity is possible if larger quantities of drug are used. Sodium excess may aggravate the congestive heart failure. Rapid potassium-penicillin administration by IV route may precipitate hyperkalaemia.

Treatment: Treatment of anaphylactic reaction includes parenteral administration of adrenaline with other supportive measures. Minor allergic reactions subside after discontinuation of penicillin therapy. If a patient is allergic to penicillins, it is advised to use an alternative antibiotic.

3. Aminoglycosides

Aminoglycosides are a group of natural and semi-synthetic antibiotics having aminosugars linked to an aminocyclitol ring by glycosidic bond. They are mostly bactericidal drugs that share many chemical and pharmacological properties and have similar antibacterial spectrum and toxic effects. Important members of the group include streptomycin, neomycin, kanamycin, gentamicin, amikacin and tobramycin.

Toxicity: All aminoglycosides have potential to produce toxic effects, but the relative propensity differs. Nephrotoxicity, ototoxicity and neuromuscular blockade are important adverse effects observed with aminoglycosides.

a. *Nephrotoxicity:* Nephrotoxicity with aminoglycosides occurs as a result of excessive accumulation (40 to 50 times the levels in blood) of antibiotics by the proximal tubular cells in kidneys. As aminoglycosides are positively charged agents, they get attracted to negatively charged phospholipids of the renal membrane followed by their transport inside the tubular cells via pinocytosis. In renal tubules, the aminoglycosides get sequestered into lysosomes and also interact with cell organelles resulting in cellular death. The aminoglycosides can inhibit various essential enzymes like phospholipases, sphingomyelinases and ATPases. Inhibition of phospholipase, in particular, results in reduced synthesis of prostaglandins, diacyl glycerol and inositol triphosphate. As prostaglandins play important role in regulation of renal blood flow, their reduced synthesis has direct effect on the glomerular filtration. The nephrotoxicity produced by aminoglycosides is reversible in the initial stages because of the regenerative capacity of tubular epithelium, but on prolonged exposure the renal damage is permanent. Manifestations of nephrotoxicity include presence of enzymes of brush border in urine, proteinuria, presence of casts and low GFR. In later stages, collecting ducts loose ability to concentrate urine in response to antidiuretic hormone (ADH) resulting in polyuria. Among aminoglycosides, neomycin is most nephrotoxic followed by tobramycin and gentamicin; dihydrostreptomycin is least nephrotoxic.

b. *Ototoxicity:* Administration of aminoglycosides can produce both vesicular and auditory dysfunctions. Aminoglycosides get accumulated into perilymph and endolymph of the inner ear in a dose- and time- dependent manner. Once accumulated, their elimination from these fluids in very slow. Ototoxicity is greater when the plasma concentration of drug is persistently high. Ototoxicity once occurs is usually irreversible and results from progressive destruction of vestibular or cochlear sensory cells. Vestibular injury leads to nystagmus, incoordination, vertigo, head tilt, ataxia and loss of righting reflex in animals. Hearing impairment or deafness may be produced by permanent damage and loss of hair cells in the organ of Corti. Streptomycin is most vestibulotoxic followed by gentamicin, whereas neomycin is most ototoxic followed by kanamycin and amikacin. Cats are more susceptible to ototoxic effect of aminoglycosides than dogs. Impaired renal function increases chances of ototoxicity.

c. *Neuromuscular blockade:* All aminoglycosides have potential to produce neuromuscular blockade with curare-like action. The effect is produced mainly by interference with acetylcholine release from motor nerve endings, probably by antagonism of Ca^{++} that is normally required for exocytosis. Decrease in the sensitivity of post-synaptic sites to the neurotransmitter (ACh) has also been suggested. Neuromuscular blockade usually occurs after IV or IP administration of aminoglycosides, but can also be seen with other routes of drug administration. Neuromuscular blockade is not manifested ordinarily in normal clinical use of drugs. However, concomitant administration of neuromuscular blocking agents and general anaesthetics with aminoglycosides may substantially increase the risk of neuromuscular blockade. Muscular weakness, apnoea, respiratory arrest, etc., have been associated with aminoglycosides, particularly when used in very high doses. Neomycin and streptomycin have high propensity to cause neuromuscular blockade followed by kanamycin, amikacin and gentamicin; tobramycin is least likely to produce this effect.

d. *Other effects:* Aminoglycosides have low propensity to cause allergic reactions - both anaphylaxis and rash are rare. Administration of some aminoglycosides (e.g. streptomycin) may produce peripheral neuritis and dysfunction of optic nerve.

Treatment: Neuromuscular blockade may be treated by IV administration of calcium salts or neostigmine. Support of ventilation is essential. In experimental conditions, 4-aminopyridine has been found effective in reversing the adverse effects of aminoglycosides but its clinical usefulness is not certain. Nephrotoxicity of aminoglycosides can be prevented or minimised by avoiding use of potentially nephrotoxic aminoglycosides, ensuring adequate hydration status of patient and avoiding concurrent use of other nephrotoxic drugs.

4. Tetracyclines

Tetracyclines are a group of broad-spectrum antibiotics having a nucleus of four cyclic rings. They are obtained either naturally from soil actinomycetes or prepared semi-synthetically. Tetracyclines form insoluble chelate with divalent and trivalent cations like Ca^{++}, Mg^{++}, Fe^{+++}, and Al^{+++}. Important members include oxytetracycline, tetracycline, rolitetracycline, minocycline and doxycycline.

Toxicity: The tetracyclines have a relatively low toxicity at normal dosage levels. However, a number of adverse effects have been associated with tetracyclines.

a. *Gastrointestinal upsets:* All tetracyclines produce GI irritation to varying degree in some patients, particularly after oral administration. Anorexia, abdominal pain, diarrhoea, nausea and vomiting in small animals may occur. Superinfection by non-susceptible pathogens such as fungi, yeast and resistant bacteria is a possibility, which if occurs may lead to disturbances in the intestinal function with candidiasis, enterocolitis, or pseudomembranous colitis. The oral administration of tetracyclines may lead to fatal diarrhoea in horses and indigestion due to deleterious effect on rumen microbes in ruminants.

b. *Effect on bones/teeth:* Tetracyclines are deposited in growing teeth and bones due to their chelating properties with calcium. They form tetracycline-calcium orthophosphate complex, which inhibits calcification (e.g. hypoplastic dental enamel) and results in permanent discolouration (first yellowish then brownish) of the teeth. The stained and hypoplastic teeth are more prone to various degenerations. High concentrations of tetracyclines can interfere with the calcium deposition in bones and delay fracture healing. Given during pregnancy or in neonates, tetracyclines may cause temporary suppression of bone growth.

c. *Hepatotoxicity:* Tetracyclines in excessive doses can produce fatty infiltration of liver. Hepatotoxicity with jaundice due to large doses of tetracyclines has been reported in pregnant women and in some animals.

d. *Nephrotoxicity:* Tetracyclines are potentially nephrotoxic, particularly in the renal insufficiency. They may impair urinary concentrating ability in patients even with normal renal function. The administration of expired tetracycline products may lead to acute tubular nephrosis in animals. The inhibition of mammalian protein synthesis by tetracylines has catabolic effect resulting in increase in the blood urea nitrogen (BUN) levels.

e. *Hypersensitivity reactions:* Hypersensitivity reactions are not common with tetracyclines. Rarely, they may produce skin rashes, urticaria, pruritus and exfoliative dermatitis. Angioedema and anaphylaxis are extremely rare. Complete cross-sensitisation in exhibited by tetracyclines. Minocycline may be more likely to cause allergic drug reactions.

f. *Other effects:* Tetracyclines cause irritation on parenteral administration. Swelling, necrosis and yellow discolouration usually occur at injection site. The tetracyclines inhibit WBC chemotaxis and phagocytosis at injection sites, particularly when present in high concentrations. Tetracyclines may prolong blood coagulation either directly by chelating calcium or indirectly by depressing prothrombin synthesis due to depression of vitamin K by bacterial flora. Rapid intravenous administration of tetracyclines may result in hypotension, collapse and sudden death in animals. Other adverse effects caused by tetracyclines include drug fever in cats, photoallergic dermatitis in humans and antianabolic effect in many species.

Treatment: Treatment of tetracycline is symptomatic and supportive. Pre-treatment with calcium borogluconate and slow rate of IV infusion prevent unwanted effects on the cardiovascular system and sudden collapse. Effects on bones and teeth are generally permanent.

5. Chloramphenicol

Chloramphenicol is a broad-spectrum bacteriostatic antibiotic. It was initially obtained from *Streptomyces venezuelae* in 1947, but now is manufactured synthetically. Chloramphenicol is used in a variety of infections in veterinary medicine, particularly those caused by anaerobic bacteria.

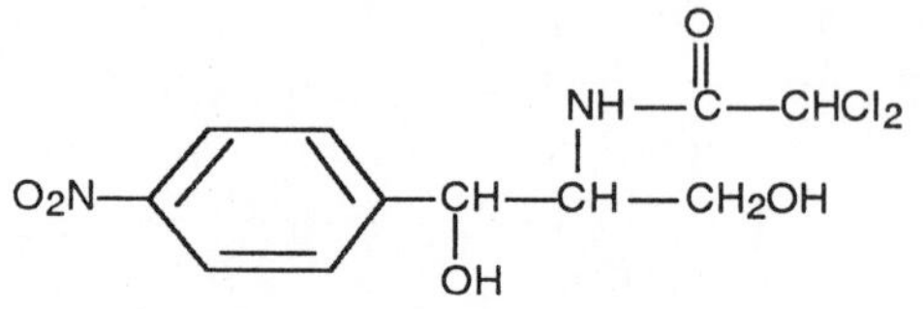

$$O_2N-C_6H_4-CH(OH)-CH(NH-C(=O)-CHCl_2)-CH_2OH$$

Fig. 20.2. Chemical structure of chloramphenicol.

Toxicity: Chloramphenicol has a low order of toxicity in domestic animals when used in recommended doses. However, it has been associated with serious adverse effects like bone marrow depression and aplastic anaemia.

a. *Bone marrow depression:* Chloramphenicol may produce dose-dependent (reversible) and dose-independent (irreversible) bone marrow depression. The reversible bone marrow depression may be observed in all species of animals, especially with prolonged use of the antibiotic. It occurs due to inhibition of mammalian mitochondrial protein synthesis in the bone marrow. The irreversible bone marrow-depression is a serious problem in humans, but does not appear to occur in domestic animals. It mainly results from formation of toxic intermediates associated with p-nitro group, which irreversibly damage the stem cells. The signs of bone marrow toxicity includes vacuolation of many of the early cells of myeloid and erythroid series, lymphopenia and neutropenia. In second irreversible form of bone marrow depression, aplastic anaemia develops and peripheral blood shows pancytopenia. The bone marrow is often hypoplastic or aplastic.
b. *Gastrointestinal effects:* Chloramphenicol may produce vomiting, diarrhoea and anorexia in animals. Use of chloramphenicol in neonatal calves leads to malabsorption syndrome associated with disruption of small intestine enterocytes.
c. *Hypersensitivity reactions:* Some dogs and cats may show hypersensitivity reactions to chloramphenicol with development of aplastic anaemia, similar to that observed after irreversible bone marrow depression. It may produce rashes and fever.
d. *Other effects:* Rapid IV infusion of chloramphenicol, especially that containing propylene glycol in formulation, may result in collapse, haemolysis and death in large animals. Chloramphenicol possesses some antianabolic effects in host animals to limited extent. In human neonates and premature infants, chloramphenicol produces Gray-baby syndrome characterised by vomiting, hypothermia, ashen grey cyanosis, cardiovascular collapse and death. It occurs due to accumulation of unconjugated chloramphenicol in body that blocks electron transport in liver, myocardium, and skeletal muscle. The human and animal neonates are deficient in microsomal enzymes and inadequately metabolise and excrete chloramphenicol.

Treatment: Treatment of chloramphenicol toxicosis is symptomatic and supportive. Chloramphenicol should be avoided in neonates because of less developed metabolising enzymes, especially in kittens. Chloramphenicol should not be given to nursing bitches and queens, particularly during the first week after parturition.

6. Nitrofurans

Nitrofurans are synthetic compounds that contain 5-nitrofuran ring. They are used primarily for their activity against gram-negative bacteria, but also have activity against gram-positive organisms. They have also been employed as antifungal and antiprotozoal drugs. Nitrofurazone and furazolidone are used as feed additives to treat bacterial enteritis in swine and as coccidiostat in chickens, turkeys and rabbits. The group comprises several agents, but only few are used efficaciously and safely in veterinary practices.

Nitrofurazone: The oral LD_{50} of nitrofurazone in rats in approximately 500 mg/kg body weight. Clinical signs are mainly neurological including irritability, tremors, weakness, convulsions and apnoea. In dogs, oral dosage of 50 mg/kg body weight causes neurological signs. In poultry, single oral dose of 150-200 mg/kg causes either depression or seizures in young chicks. Dairy calves given nitrofurazone in water > 30 mg/kg body weight in one study, developed acute clinical signs within 24-48 hours of the initial treatment characterised by opisthotonos, tremors, circling and intermittent seizures.

Furazolidone: Furazolidone toxicosis may be mediated by action on the Krebs cycle. Pyruvate and lactate are increased, possibly indicating a decreasing conversion of pyruvate to acetyl coenzyme A. In poultry, its continued use at 200 ppm in feed may reduce the hatchability of eggs; at 400 ppm it inhibits normal growth of young laying chickens with heamatocytological functions and depressed egg weights. Cardiomyopathy occurs at concentrations of 500-700 ppm. Cardiac hypertrophy in poultry is known as "round heart disease" and is characterised by increased moisture content and cardiac glycogen deposition. Mortality is correlated with increased heart : body weight ratio in chickens. In swine, furazolidone in high concentrations (> 600 ppm) cause mild ataxia with paresis of the hind limbs.

Treatment of nitrofuran toxicosis includes supportive therapy to correct renal insufficiency, dehydration or malnutrition. Good nursing care may be important for recovery.

II. ANTIPARASITIC DRUGS

1. Carbon Tetrachloride

Carbon tetrachloride was the first truly effective remedy to be introduced for treatment of fascioliasis. It is an industrial solvent and widely used in synthetic chemistry. In the early 20th century, carbon tetrachloride was widely used as a dry cleaning solvent and a refrigerant, and in fire extinguishers. Presently it is rarely used as anticestodal drug mainly due to its toxic effects and availability of better flukicidal agents.

Properties: Carbon tetrachloride (Tetrachloromethane; CCl_4) is a volatile, clear, non-inflammable liquid. It is soluble is organic solvents with burning taste and chloroform like odour. It is insoluble in water, but is readily miscible with alcohol, benzene, chloroform, ether and carbon disulphide. Although it does not occur naturally, carbon tetrachloride is ubiquitous in the environment. Its chemical stability results in an atmospheric half-life of 30 to 100 years.

Factors affecting toxicity:

a. *Weather:* Carbon tetrachloride is more toxic in cold weather as less evaporation of volatile CCl_4 occurs from lungs.

b. *Diets:* Diets high in protein increase the toxicity of carbon tetrachloride and diets low in protein decrease the toxicity. High fat diets increase toxicity of CCl_4 by enhancing its GI absorption.

c. *Plants:* Consumption of plants which are hepatotoxic or which contain oxalate tends to increase the effect of carbon tetrachloride on the liver.

d. *Species:* Carbon tetrachloride is highly toxic to swine, moderately toxic to sheep and cattle and less toxic to poultry.

e. *Body weight:* Fatty ewes and underweight animals are less tolerant to the toxic effects of carbon tetrachloride.

f. *Drug interactions:* Concurrent administration of carbon tetrachloride and microsomal enzyme inducers (e.g. phenobarbitone) markedly increases susceptibility to CCl_4 toxicity as more of the toxic metabolites are formed.

Toxicity: Toxicity of carbon tetrachloride depends on the species, dose and route of exposure. It is toxic to all mammals, especially to swine. Inhalation of CCl_4 for a few minutes to 3,000 ppm of carbon tetrachloride is tolerated while levels of 12,000 ppm for 15 minutes cause toxicity. The acute oral LD_{50} of CCl_4 in rats is 2,800 mg/kg. In mice, the LC_{50} of carbon tetrachloride in feed is about 10,000 ppm.

Toxicokinetics: Poisoning can occur from all routes including oral, inhalation and topical. Following oral exposure, CCl_4 is absorbed slowly from the intestine in unchanged form. After absorption, it is metabolised to active metabolites which are excreted through bile and urine. The biliary system returns the active metabolites to the intestine. Being volatile, elimination of carbon tetrachloride also occurs through expired air via lungs.

Mechanism of action: The exact mechanisms of carbon tetrachloride toxicity are not clearly known.

a. Carbon tetrachloride is a highly hepatotoxic agent and acts indirectly via formation of toxic metabolites. Carbon tetrachloride generates highly reactive trichloromethyl (CCl_3^-) and trichloromethyl peroxy (CCl_3COO^-) free radicals in liver with help of cytochrome P450 dependent monoxygenases. These free radicals (CCl_3^- and CCl_3COO^-) cause peroxidation of lipids and generation of secondary free radicals from these lipids. The lipid peroxidation causes breakdown of membrane structure and function causing cell death in more severe cases. The fatty infiltration of the liver, commonly seen in CCl_4 poisoning, is thought to develop as a result of the action of free alkyl radicals on biomembranes that in turn block exit of the lipoprotein micelles from the Golgi apparatus.

b. Carbon tetrachloride is an organic solvent and possesses defatting action. Its fat solvent property alters the permeability of cell wall as a result of which some essential substances (e.g. pyridine nucleotide coenzymes) come out of the cell.

c. In acute cases, death primarily occurs due to circulatory collapse and death. The exact mechanism of it is not known.

Clinical signs: Carbon tetrachloride produces both acute and delayed toxic effects. Manifestations of acute CCl_4 toxicity include CNS depression, dullness, diarrhoea, blood stained faeces, possible hypocalcaemia, incoordination, renal damage leading to anuria and azotemia, circulatory collapse, and death within 12-24 hours. Large dose of carbon tetrachloride is followed by narcosis similar to that associated with chloroform. Skin contact can lead to dermatitis through defatting action.

Delayed toxicity primarily occurs due to liver damage; kidney injury and visual disturbances may also occur. Clinical signs mentioned above along with icterus are generally delayed by 2-3 days and animal may die within 1-2 weeks. Although hepatic insufficiency is a prominent feature of delayed toxicity, death generally occurs due to renal damage.

Post-mortem findings: Post-mortem lesions include gastroenteritis confined especially to the abomasum and upper small intestine. Small amounts of CCl_4 produces fatty degeneration of the liver and large amount may produce hepatic cell necrosis. The effects of CCl_4 on hepatocytes, depending on dose and exposure time, are manifested histologically as hepatic steatosis (e.g. fatty infiltration), centrilobular necrosis and ultimately cirrhosis. Renal damage may be seen in form of congestion and necrosis in renal tubular epithelium. The hepatic and renal lesions are observed only in delayed toxicity and not in acute cases.

Diagnosis: Diagnosis of carbon tetrachloride poisoning may be made from history of administering CCl_4 as drug, clinical signs and lesions.

Treatment and management: Treatment of CCl_4 overdosage is symptomatic and supportive. Treatment in recent oral exposure involves administration of gastric or rumen lavage, activated charcoal and a saline cathartic. The delayed hepatotoxic effect of CCl_4 can be suppressed to some degree by IV dextrose solution or IV calcium borogluconate therapy. Osmotic diuretics and fluids are used to increase urine out put.

2. Phenothiazine

Phenothiazine (PTZ) is one of the early drugs with a fairly wide range of activity against GI nematodes. It is used in continuous low-level feeding programmes for ruminants and horses. The toxicity of phenothiazine has limited or prevented its use in swine, dogs, cats and some other species. It is stable when dry but easily oxidises when wet. Phenothiazine is almost insoluble in water (1: 800,000), so it is used as suspension (single drench) or powder for addition to feed or incorporation in salt or mineral (*i.e.* continuous daily low-level medication).

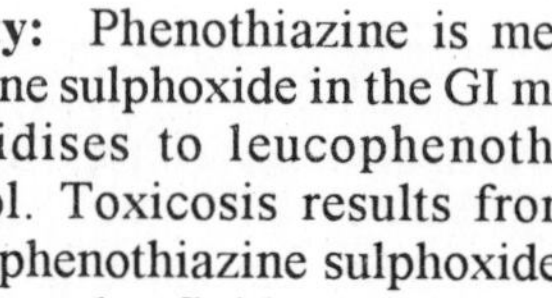

Fig.20.3. Chemical structure of phenothiazine (PTZ).

Toxicity: Phenothiazine is metabolised to phenothiazine sulphoxide in the GI mucosa which further oxidises to leucophenothiazine and leucothionol. Toxicosis results from excessive amounts of phenothiazine sulphoxide which may permeate to ocular fluids and dermis, producing photophobia and photosensitisation. Healthy animals tolerate phenothiazine therapy while debilitated and anaemic animals are more susceptible. Of the animals, sheep, goats and birds are resistant to toxic effects. Cattle and swine are susceptible and horses are most susceptible among domestic animals. In horses, generally a lethal dose is < 50 g for an adult horse and 30 g for a young horse when they are weak and anaemic, while 500 g has been without effect in healthy animals.

Toxic signs of phenothiazine poisoning in horses include dullness, weakness, anorexia followed by oliguria, colic, constipation, fever and rapid pulse. Signs related to haemolysis of erythrocytes include icterus, anaemia and haemoglobinuria. Haemolysis probably occurs due to activation of lysolecithin enzyme in the blood. Phenothiazine may also produce photosensitization in some species, especially in calves and lambs, at high dosages. Photosensitization mainly occurs due to saturation of liver with phenothiazine sulphoxide that goes into circulation and acts as photodynamic compound in presence of sunlight. Photosensitisation signs in ruminants (not in horses) include reddening and thickening of ears, muzzle, and other non-pigmented areas of the skin, with later development of scabs.

Treatment and management: Treatment of phenothiazine toxicity in the horses is aimed primarily at replenishing lost RBCs by transfusing blood. The photosensitised animals should be kept away from direct sunlight. Other supportive and symptomatic therapy may also be used.

3. Ivermectin

Ivermectin is a semi-synthetic agent derived from the natural avermectins. It is a commonly used endectocide in veterinary medicine. It is useful against GI roundworms and lungworms in horses, ruminants and pigs and heartworms (mainly preventive) in dogs and cats. It is also used as an ectoparasiticide against mange mites, lice, grubs and horn flies. It occurs as an off-white to yellowish powder and is highly lipophilic.

Toxicity: Ivermectin has high margin of safety in cattle, horses and some other species, but some breeds of dogs are highly susceptible to it. In dogs, toxicity is predominantly seen in rough-haired Collie breed but may occur in other breeds as well. Beagle dogs can tolerate an oral dose of 2 mg/kg ivermectin without clinical signs, but Collies show toxic signs of tremors, mydriasis and death even at oral dose of 0.1-0.2 mg/kg. The toxic signs in dogs include mydriasis, salivation, ataxia, tremors, paresis, stupor, recumbency and coma. Dogs may also exhibit a shock-like reaction when ivermectin is used as a microfilaricide, presumably due to hypersensitivity reaction associated with dying microfilaria. Neonatal pigs are also susceptible to ivermectin toxicity presumably due to more permeability of blood-brain barrier to ivermectin. In horses, swelling and pruritus at the ventral mid-line may be seen about 24 hours after ivermectin dosing due to a hypersensitivity reaction to dead parasites. Ivermectin in birds has been associated with lethargy and anorexia. There are no characteristic lesions in ivermectin poisoned animals.

Treatment and management: Overdosage of ivermectin may be treated by supportive and symptomatic therapy. Intravenous administration of physostigmine may provide some relief for dogs suffering from severe ivermectin toxicity. Adrenaline is indicated for acute anaphylactic reactions.

4. Levamisole

Levamisole is an imidazothiazole anthelmintic having broad range of antinematodal activity in numerous host species. Commercially available levamisole is actually the l-isomer of dl-tetramisole. Levamisole HCl occurs as a white to pale cream coloured, odourless, crystalline powder. It is highly soluble in water so can be used as injection. Levamisole acts as autonomic ganglionic stimulant (cholinomimetic) and causes activation of parasympathetic and sympathetic nervous systems.

Toxicity: Levamisole has a relatively narrow safety margin (T.I. ≈ 5-6), but is still tolerated at recommended dosages. The clinical signs of toxicity are extension of its antiparasitic action and include both muscarinic and nicotinic cholinergic signs like salivation, constriction of pupil, muscle tremors, excitation, ataxia, colic, diarrhoea, urination, dyspnoea, transient coughing and collapse. Death usually occurs as a result of asphyxia due to respiratory paralysis. Signs of levamisole overdosage often mimic those of organophosphorus insecticide poisoning. Levamisole may cause pain and inflammation at the injection site, but usually it is transient. The

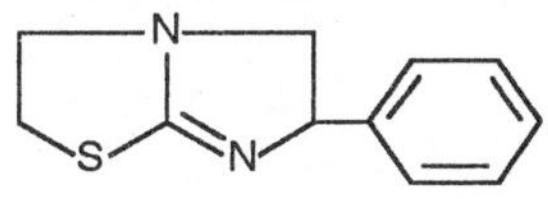

N S N

Fig.20.4. Chemical structure of levamisole.

horses and dogs are more susceptible to the adverse effects of levamisole. Levamisole is considered to be more toxic when administered parenterally than when given orally or topically. Intravenous administration is particularly hazardous and is never practised.

Treatment and management: Acute toxicity of levamisole is treated mainly with supportive and symptomatic therapy. Decontamination with emetics, gastric lavage, activated charcoal or saline cathartic is recommended if possible within 1-2 hour of ingestion. Atropine sulphate can alleviate acute signs. Hexamethonium, an autonomic ganglionic blocker, can also inhibit the action of levamisole. Intravenous fluids, oxygen and artificial respiration may be administered, if required.

5. Thiacetarsamide

Thiacetarsamide (Thiacetarcemide; arsenamide) sodium is an organic arsenical compound. It is used to kill adult heartworms (*Dirofilaria immitis*) in dogs and has no efficacy against immature heartworms or any other nematode. It is available commercially as one percent buffered injectable solution.

Toxicity: Thiacetarsamide has a narrow margin of safety. Adverse effects related to arsenic toxicity may develop during therapy that may be severe and life threatening. Adverse effects in dogs may include persistent vomiting, anorexia, icterus, hepatotoxicity, nephrotoxicity and thrombocytopenia. Severe local reactions with tissue sloughing and phlebitis may occur, if thiacetarsamide is injected extravascularly. Thromboembolic pneumonia with signs of coughing, dyspnoea, haemoptysis, fever and lethargy may result as the dead heartworms accumulate, usually in the caudal lung lobes. Thiacetarsamide induced renal failure is more likely in dogs with previously compromised renal function.

Treatment and management: Dimercaprol (British anti-lewisite) can be used as an antidote to thiacetarsamide overdosage. Glucocorticoids have been recommended to treat signs of pulmonary thromboembolism, although the use of glucocorticoids in thiacetarsamide therapy in controversial.

III. NON-STEROIDAL ANTI-INFLAMMATORY DRUGS

1. Salicylates

Salicylate group of compounds include aspirin (acetylsalicylic acid), sodium salicylate and salicylic acid. Aspirin is the most commonly used analgesic, antipyretic and anti-inflammatory agent. Sodium salicylate in addition to analgesic and antipyretic actions has antirheumatic action which is important in animals and human beings. Salicylic acid is restricted almost entirely to external application because of its extremely irritant action on the gastric mucosa.

Properties: Aspirin (Acetylsalicylic acid; ASA) is the salicylate ester of salicylic acid. Bayer first developed aspirin in 1899, and since then it remains the standard reference for non-opioid analgesics. It occurs as a white crystalline substance. It is stable in dry air but hydrolyses to salicylic acid and acetic acid in moist air. It is slightly soluble in water and freely soluble in alcohol.

Toxicity: Salicylates are derivatives of phenol, which is known to be toxic to cats. In cats, even low doses of aspirin (<50 mg/kg) produces toxic hepatitis in 50% of the animals. Aspirin administered orally (60 mg/kg) every 4 hours in the cat is lethal within 32 hours. Haematemesis and gastric ulcer perforation have been reported in dogs receiving 100-300 mg/kg/day of aspirin orally for 1-4 weeks. At a lower dose of 50 mg/kg/12 hours, vomiting was observed in dogs approximately 2 hours after each dose.

Toxicokinetics: Aspirin is easily absorbed from the stomach and proximal small intestine in monogastric animals, although rate of absorption is dependent on factors like stomach contents, gastric emptying and gastric pH. During and after the absorption, most of aspirin is hydrolysed to

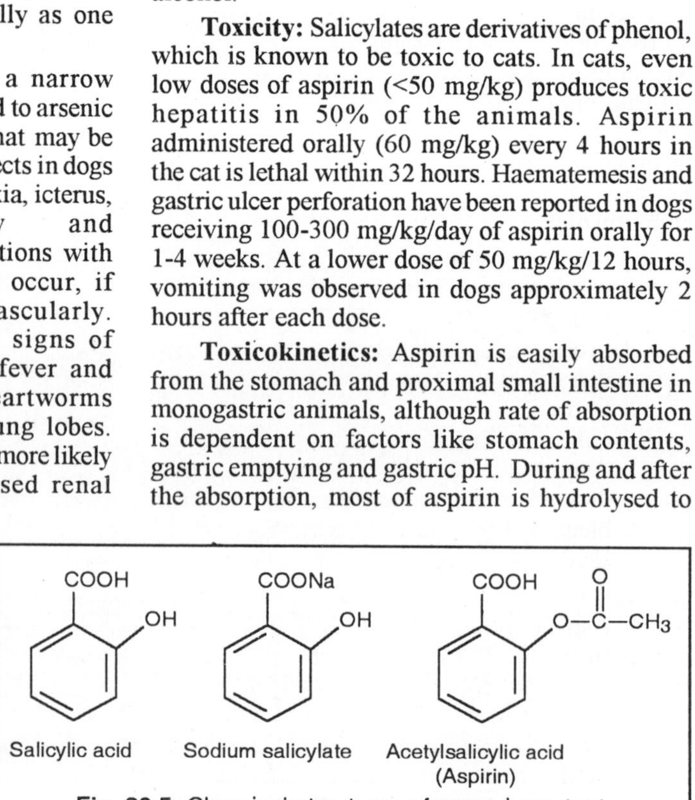

COOH, OH — Salicylic acid

COONa, OH — Sodium salicylate

COOH, O–C(=O)–CH_3 — Acetylsalicylic acid (Aspirin)

Fig. 20.5. Chemical structures of some important salicylate analgesics and antipyretics.

salicylic acid (salicylate) and acetic acid by esterases present in tissues and blood. Salicylate becomes extensively bound (~ 70%) to plasma albumin. It is widely distributed in body and penetrates into synovial fluid, peritoneal fluid, saliva and milk, and readily crosses the placental barrier, although diffusion across the blood-brain barrier is limited. Aspirin and other salicylates are metabolised in the liver primarily by conjugation with glucuronic acid and glycine, and also by some other metabolic pathways. Some salicylic acid is also excreted unchanged. Neonatal animals (less than 30 days) and cats are less able to metabolise and excrete salicylates. Excretion of salicylate and its metabolites occur mainly via kidneys by glomerular filtration and renal tubular secretion. In general, plasma half-life in herbivores is about 1 hour and in cats it is about 30 hours. The elimination of aspirin is dose-dependent; therefore accumulation of toxic levels in plasma and tissue may occur readily with high doses. Alkalisation of urine promotes excretion.

Mechanism of action: Aspirin generally acts by virtue of its content of salicylic acid, although some of its unique effects are due to its capacity to acetylate proteins. As with most other NSAIDs, both the therapeutic and unwanted effects of aspirin and other salicylates are primarily due to inhibition of cyclooxygenase enzyme activity and consequent inhibition of prostaglandins synthesis.

a. Inhibition of prostaglandin synthesis in GI tract results in increased gastric acid secretion and diminished mucus protection. This may cause epigastric distress, nausea and vomiting. The ion trapping of drug in gastric mucosal cell enhances gastric irritation and toxicity. Aspirin produces a dose-related gastric ulceration and haemorrhage. The gastric bleeding may be painless and frequently leads to blood loss in the stool and occasionally to ion-deficiency anaemia.

b. Aspirin, even in small doses, irreversibly inhibits the platelet cyclooxygenase enzyme and the subsequent synthesis of thromboxane A_2. As a result of decreased TXA_2, platelet aggregation time is reduced producing an anticoagulant effect with a prolonged bleeding time. Long-term use of large dose decreases synthesis of clotting factors in liver and predisposes patient to bleeding.

c. At high doses, aspirin and other salicylates may uncouple oxidative phosphorylation and may cause hyperglycaemia and glycosuria. Occasionally hypoglycaemia is seen.

d. Aspirin is a derivative of phenol, so it is not readily metabolized in cats. Therefore, it is more toxic to cats than other species.

Clinical signs :

Acute toxicity: Toxic doses of aspirin cause gastric or intestinal irritation, epigastric distress, nausea, vomiting and/or anorexia. High doses may produce hyperventilation, gastric lesions, hepatitis and suppression of erythropoiesis in bone marrow in some cases. Toxic doses cause a centrally mediated hyperpnoea and alkalosis followed by respiratory depression, acidosis, circulatory collapse, hyperpyrexia (due to uncoupling of oxidative phosphorylation), convulsions, coma and death. Death occurs mainly due to the respiratory failure. Anaemia with Heinz bodies and reduced RBC production is observed in cats. Aspirin and other salicylates cross the placenta quickly and may produce incidence of stillbirths in high doses (500-1200 mg/kg). Aspirin has shown to be teratogenic in animal studies.

Chronic toxicity: Chronic toxicity of salicylates includes lethargy, episodic hyperpnoea, respiratory alkalosis, decreased blood prothrombin concentration and tinnitus. The most important adverse effect of aspirin is gastric mucosal damage and peptic ulceration with varying degree of occult GI blood loss. In human beings, repeated high doses of aspirin produce a syndrome called salicylism characterised by dizziness, tinnitus, vertigo, reversible impairment of hearing and vision, excitement, hyperventilation and electrolyte imbalance. Hypersensitivity reactions including rashes, skin eruptions, urticaria, etc. can also be observed in some cases. In humans, aspirin administration has been implicated in the aetiology of 'Reye's syndrome' in infants and children suffering from viral infection characterised by liver damage and encephalopathy. Therefore, aspirin is not given in pyrexia of unknown origin in children below 12 years.

Post-mortem findings: Necropsy findings in acute and subacute salicylate poisonings include degeneration or necrosis of surface epithelium and mucosal haemorrhages. Intracellular mucin is reduced in damaged and regenerating epithelium.

Diagnosis: Diagnosis of aspirin and other salicylate poisoning is based on history of excessive exposure to salicylates, clinical signs and lesions. Blood or serum salicylate concentrations may help in establishing the diagnosis and extent of poisoning. In cats, blood concentration of 60 mg/dl has been associated with death.

Treatment and management: Treatment of aspirin and other salicylates poisoning involves detoxification and supportive therapy.

a. Very recent exposure may be treated with emetic or gastric lavage. Activated charcoal and saline cathartic may also be used.

b. Sodium bicarbonate orally or sodium lactate solution intravenously is advised to combat acidosis.

c. Intravenous glucose may be needed if the animal is hypoglycaemic.

d. Whole blood transfusions may be used if significant haemorrhage has occurred.

e. Misoprostol, a prostaglandin-E_1 derivative, may help prevent aspirin-induced gastric ulcers.

f. Sucralfate should be given if gastric erosions have occurred due to salicylate therapy.

2. Phenylbutazone

Phenylbutazone is a synthetic pyrazolone derivative that was introduced into human medicine in 1949 for treatment of rheumatoid arthritis and other musculoskeletal disorders. It is weakly acidic and lipophilic NSAID, which is mainly approved for use in horses and dogs. It has analgesic, antipyretic and anti-inflammatory properties, but is more toxic than aspirin that limits its clinical use.

Toxicity: Similar to other NSAIDs, phenylbutazone acts by inhibiting cyclooxygenase activity and hence the synthesis of prostaglandins. It also scavenges toxic oxygen radicals. In horses, phenylbutazone produces oedema, ulceration of large intestine, diarrhoea, anorexia and necrosis of hepatic vein, especially after prolonged use or high doses. Foals with a heavy parasite burden or that are undernourished and ponies are more susceptible to the development of adverse effects. Gastrointestinal ulceration, haemorrhage, biliary stasis and proximal tubule damage have been reported in dogs. Although thought to be less toxic to dogs (due to relatively short elimination half-life), phenylbutazone has been associated with blood dyscrasias in dogs and cats. Manifestations of acute overdosage with phenylbutazone include a prompt acidosis with compensatory hyperventilation, seizures, coma, severe fall in blood pressure and symptoms of renal failure (oliguria, proteinuria and haematuria) and liver injury (hepatomegaly and jaundice). In horses, a dose of phenylbutazone only three times higher than the therapeutic dosage may cause dilation and degeneration of the walls of small veins.

Treatment and management: Phenylbutazone toxicity should be treated with detoxification and supportive therapy. Intravenous diazepam may be used to help control seizures. The use of H_2-blocker, misoprostol (PGE analogue) or sucralfate has been suggested in treating the GI effects.

3. Paracetamol

Paracetamol (Acetaminophen) is a para-aminophenol derivative that possesses analgesic and antipyretic effects similar to aspirin, but is not an anti-inflammatory agent. Paracetamol is very popular for use in human patients because it is well tolerated and lacks many of the side effects of aspirin, but has limited application in veterinary practice mainly due to toxicity associated with paracetamol administration, especially in cats. Cats lack the specific glucuronyl transferase required to conjugate paracetamol, so there is formation of reactive metabolites.

Toxicity: Paracetamol is safe in recommended therapeutic doses and is well tolerated in humans, but its use in dogs may cause renal, hepatic, GI and haematological effects. Paracetamol in high doses may cause severe liver and kidney damage through electrophilic metabolite. Paracetamol poisoning is common in cats, because it is frequently administered by owner themselves due to easy availability of the drug at homes. Toxic manifestation of paracetamol includes cyanosis, Heinz body anaemia, methaemoglobinaemia, jaundice, liver failure and facial oedema. Paracetamol acting via active metabolites oxidises haemoglobin to methaemoglobin and sulphaemoglobin, shortens life of erythrocytes, and can cause frank haemolysis. The cyanotic conditions occur due to hypoxia associated with conversion of haemoglobin to methaemoglobin. Haemolysis of red blood cells is responsible for anaemia (Heinz bodies) and haemoglobinuria. Jaundice is attributed to both lysis of erythrocytes and hepatic necrosis. Paracetamol is often fatal in cats.

Treatment and management: Treatment of toxicity or overdosage of paracetamol in cats and dogs involve standard detoxification and supportive measures. Acetylcysteine (150 mg/kg, IV or PO initially followed by 70 mg/kg, PO every 4 hours for 5 to 7 treatments) can reduce extent of liver injury or methaemoglobin in dogs and cats by providing an alternate substrate for conjugation with the reactive metabolite of paracetamol. Glucocorticoids and antihistamines are contraindicated.

IV. SEDATIVES

1. Chlorpromazine

Chlorpromazine HCl is a phenothiazine derivative used mainly as sedative, pre-anaesthetic and neuroleptic. Although chlorpromazine has been superseded as a sedative by acepromazine and some other drugs, it is still considered the prototype phenothiazine agent.

Properties: Chlorpromazine is a 2-chloro-10-(3-dimethyl amino propyl)- phenothiazine. It occurs as a white to slightly creamy white odourless, bitter tasting crystalline powder. Its hydrochloride salt is very soluble in water and is usually used. Chlorpromazine has a wide range of activity arising from its depressant effects on the CNS and on various central neurotransmitters receptors.

Toxicity: In dogs, I.V. administration of 1.5 mg/kg chlorpromazine produces moderate depression and ataxia which last for 6-12 hours. When a dose of 3 mg/kg is given intravenously, it produces marked CNS depression and ataxia for 24-48 hours. Prolonged treatment may produce ocular lesions. Chlorpromazine produces undesirable effects in horses and is not advocated in equine practice.

Toxicokinetics: Chlorpromazine is absorbed rapidly after oral administration, but undergoes extensive first pass metabolism in the liver. The drug is also well absorbed after IM injection. It is distributed throughout body and brain concentrations are higher than those in plasma. The drug is metabolised mainly in the liver and kidneys

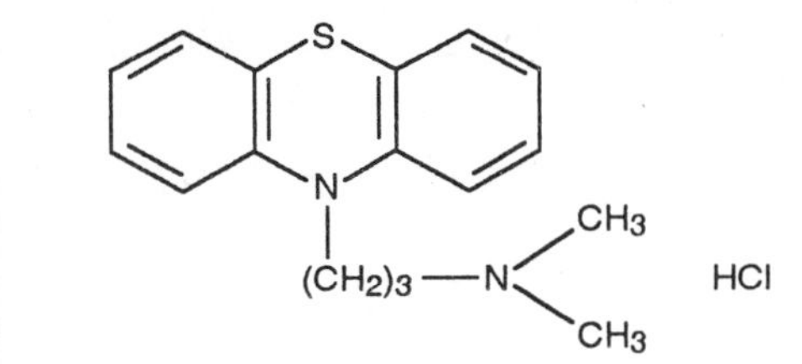

S
N
$(CH_2)_3$ — N
CH_3
CH_3
HCl

Fig. 20.6. Chemical structure of chlorpromazine hydrochloride.

by hydroxylation and glucuronide conjugation. The biological half-life of chlorpromazine is estimated to be 6 hours in dogs. Chlorpromazine is reported to stimulate hepatic microsomal enzyme activity in animals.

Mechanism of action: Chlorpromazine and other phenothiazine sedatives act by blocking variety of receptors including cholinergic-muscarinic, H_1-histaminic, alpha-adrenergic and 5-hydroxytryptaminergic receptors. Chlorpromazine has potent action on dopamine receptor, especially D_2- dopamine receptor blocking action. It is thought to depress portions of the reticular activating system that assists in control of body temperature, basal metabolic rate, emesis, vasomotor tone, hormonal balance, and alertness. Dopaminergic receptors in the basal ganglia appear to cause the extrapyramidal symptoms. Effect on alpha-adrenoceptor, muscarinic receptor, 5-HT receptor and histamine-receptor may supplement to adverse-effect profile.

Clinical signs :

Acute toxicity: Clinical signs of acute chlorpromazine toxicity include lethargy, dullness, sedation, incoordination, unsteady gait and ataxia. This is followed by animal sinking backwards on its hocks and then lunging forward in an uncoordinated manner. The horse may stumble and fall, then stand and continue lunging and rearing. This violent reaction (incoordination and excitement) alternates with periods of sedation. Because of this reaction, chlorpromazine is rarely used in equine medicine today. Additional signs of chlorpromazine toxicity in animals include fall in blood pressure, hypothermia, protrusion of nictating membrane, thrombocytopenia and platelet dysfunction. Chlorpromazine produces extrapyramidal symptoms in cats in high doses, which are characterised by tremors, shivering, diarrhoea and loss of righting reflex. Lethargy, diarrhoea and loss of anal sphincter tone may also be seen. Cardiovascular collapse, secondary to bradycardia and hypotension, has been reported in all major species. Dogs, particularly Boxer breed, are more sensitive to these effects than other species.

Chronic toxicity: Signs of chronic toxicity include all of the above mentioned signs plus leukopenia, granulocytopenia, agranulocytosis, jaundice, drowsiness, dizziness, fatigue, dryness of mouth, urinary retention, constipation, etc.

Treatment and management: Acute poisoning of chlorpromazine should be treated symptomatically. Seizures may be controlled with barbiturates or diazepam. Parkinsonian symptoms, if present, should be treated and further use of phenothiazine sedative discontinued immediately. The administration of adrenaline hydrochloride is contraindicated whenever phenothiazine drugs are used.

2. Benzodiazepines

The benzodiazepines are amongst the most widely used CNS drugs. These are used extensively as hypnotic-sedative, anxiolytic, anticonvulsant, muscle relaxant, appetite stimulant and anaesthetic/pre-anaesthetic agents in humans and animals. Important benzodiazepines include diazepam, oxazepam, clorazepate and midazolam. Diazepam is the most commonly used benzodiazepine in veterinary practice and is the representative of this class of drugs. Benzodiazepines act by augmenting the effects of $GABA_A$ receptors and increasing the chloride conductance in the central nervous system.

Toxicity: Benzodiazepines in normal sedating doses may produce variable responses in different species. In horses, diazepam may cause muscle fasciculation, weakness, ataxia and even recumbency due to skeletal muscle relaxation. Cats may exhibit behaviour changes (irritability, depression or aberrant demeanour), while dogs may show extremely variable responses like excitement. Effects of diazepam overdoses are generally limited to significant CNS depression (confusion, decreased reflexes and prolonged sleep) without serious depression of respiratory or cardiovascular function. However in the presence of other CNS depressants, it may cause severe respiratory depression. Diazepam should not be used in the Greyhound (and possibly other related breeds) due to hyperaesthesia, CNS excitation, ataxia, struggling, etc. produced by the drug.

Long-term use of diazepam may interfere with the learning and memory in small animals and may produce disinhibition in dogs. In cats, chronic use of diazepam is believed to be associated with liver damage and may have diabetogenic effect. In human beings and animals, diazepam seems to have much the same tendency to produce physical dependence as do other hypnotic-sedatives (e.g. barbiturates) though it is less liable to produce tolerance. The withdrawal syndrome (e.g. anxiety, tremors and loss of appetite) after prolonged use in both man and animals is generally slower in onset and less intense than barbiturates, probably because of the long-plasma half-lives of diazepam and its metabolites.

Treatment and management: Treatment of acute toxicity of diazepam consists of supportive and symptomatic measures only. Flumazenil, a selective benzodiazepine antagonist, may be used for reversal of central sedative effects of the benzodiazepines overdosage.

V. ANTI-HISTAMINES

Histamine receptor antagonists or antihistamines are drugs, which competitively block action of histamine at the histamine receptor sites. Depending on their affinity for histamine receptor subtypes, these drugs are broadly classified into two groups: H_1-receptor antagonists and H_2-receptor antagonists.

1. H_1-Histamine Receptor Antagonists

The H_1-receptor antagonists comprise a large group of agents that selectively inhibit H_1 receptors. These agents are sometimes referred to as classic or conventional antihistamines (antihistaminics) because they were the first to be discovered. These agents are widely used in the treatment of allergic disorders, prevention of motion sickness and as an adjunct in systemic anaphylaxis. Some of the more frequently used H_1-antihistamine drugs are diphenhydramine, pyrilamine, dimenhydrinate and promethazine.

Properties: Most H_1-receptor antagonists are substituted ethylamines. The first generation H_1-antagonists are mostly lipid soluble so they easily enter CNS and produce sedation and other central effects. In contrast, the newer H_1-receptor, often called the second-generation H_1-receptor antagonists or non-sedating antihistamines, do not cross the blood-brain barrier and hence have no CNS depressing effect.

Toxicokinetics: Most H_1 receptor antagonists are lipid soluble amines hence they are readily absorbed on oral or parenteral administration. The first generation H_1 antagonists are widely distributed in body and enter brain; the newer non-sedating second generation compounds penetrate brain poorly. Most H_1-receptor antagonists are metabolised by hydroxylation in liver and are capable of inducing the hepatic microsomal enzyme system. On repeated administration, many H_1 antagonists induce their own metabolism. The potency, duration of action and extent of biotransformation are related to the type of H_1 antagonist.

Mechanism of action: The H_1-receptor antagonists act by competitively antagonising the actions of histamine at H_1-receptor sites. These drugs block all actions of histamine except for those mediated solely by H_2-receptors. In addition to H_1-receptor blocking action, many of these drugs tend to block muscarinic receptors and a few drugs also adrenergic or serotonin receptors, which are mainly responsible for their adverse effects.

Toxicity: The incidence and severity of adverse effects vary with the preparation and the individual agent. The H_1-histamine receptor antagonists produce sedation, diminished alertness, lethargy, somnolence and ataxia due to CNS depression. Various intestinal disorders include anorexia, nausea, vomiting, constipation or diarrhoea when antihistamines are given orally for a prolonged period. The anticholinergic effects are expressed by dry mouth, dysuria, pupillary dilation, blurred vision and tachycardia. Depression of bone marrow, leucopenia and agranulocytosis occur rarely. In higher doses, hyperexcitability, muscular twitching, convulsions, opisthotonos, coma, nervous signs and circulatory collapse are seen. Death may occur due to respiratory failure. Some agents (e.g. piperazines) are found to be teratogenic in animals.

Treatment and management: Treatment of acute antihistamine toxicity is symptomatic. Use of sedative or ultrashort-acting barbiturates may be of value in case of hyperexcitation and convulsions. A care should be observed during therapy because when the excitement phase ends, a sedative phase begins which may complicate the toxicity due to excessive sedation.

2. H_2-Histamine Receptor Antagonists

The H_2-Histamine receptor antagonists competitively inhibit the interaction of histamine with H_2-histamine receptors and block gastric acid secretion elicited by histamine. These drugs include cimetidine, ranitidine and famotidine.

Toxicity: There have been number of reported side effects in man, but incidence of serious toxicity from H_2- histamine receptor antagonists is limited in animals. The adverse effects in human beings with cimetidine are dizziness, headache, nausea, myalgia, skin rashes and itching. Large IV doses can produce arrhythmias, bradycardia and cardiac arrest. Cimetidine (not other H_2-antagonists) possesses anti-androgenic action, decreases metabolism of oestradiol and increases plasma prolactin concentration. Its prolonged use may produce gynaecomastia, loss of libido, impotence and temporary decrease in sperm count. Rarely, reversible bone marrow depression, hepatitis or anaphylaxis may also be observed. Cimetidine also inhibits the activity of cytochrome P-450, thereby slowing metabolism of many drugs. A clinically important disadvantage of cimetidine described in human patients is relapse of gastroduodenal ulceration due to rebound hypersecretion of gastric acid after the therapy is discontinued.

Adverse effects of ranitidine and other H_2-histamine blockers appear to be very rare in animals at the dosages generally used. Although some side effects (e.g. confusion, headache, diarrhoea/ constipation) have been reported in human beings, the limited clinical experience in animals have not indicated any serious toxic manifestation from ranitidine.

Treatment and management: Treatment of acute H_2-histamine receptor blocker toxicity is only symptomatic and supportive.

BIBLIOGRAPHY

Adams H R (2001) Veterinary Pharmacology and Therapeutics. 8th edn. Iowa State Univ. Press, Iowa.

Barragry T B (1994) Veterinary Drug Therapy. Lea & Febiger, Philadelphia.

Beasley V (1999) Veterinary Toxicology. International Veterinary Information Service, Ithaca NY (www.ivis.org).

Bircharad S J and Sherding R G (2000) Saunder's Manual of Small Animal Practice. W. B. Saunders, Philadelphia.

Bishop Y (1998) The Veterinary Formulary. 4th edn. Pharmaceutical Press, London.

Bonagura J (1995) Current Veterinary Therapy. XII : Small Animal Practice. W. B. Saunders, Philadelphia.

Booth D M (2001) Small Animal Clinical Pharmacology and Therapeutics. W. B. Saunders Comp., Philadelphia.

Campbell W C (1989) Ivermectin and Abamectin. Springer-verlag, New York.

Hjelle JJ and Graner GF (1986) Acetaminophen-induced toxicosis in dogs and cats. *J. Am. Vet. Med. Assoc.* 188 : 742.

Kore AM (1990) Toxicology of non-steroidal anti-inflammatory drugs. *Vet. Clin. North Am: Small Anim Pract.* 20 : 419.

Lewis D T, Merchant S R and Neer T M (1995) Ivermectin toxicosis in a kitten. J. Am. Vet. Med. Assoc. 205 : 584-586.

Lovell RA (1990) Ivermectin and piperazine toxicoses in dogs and cats. *Vet. Clin. North Am: Small Anim Pract.* 20 : 453.

Lu FC and Kacew S (2002) Lu's Basic Toxicology: Fundamentals, Target Organs and Risk Assessment. Taylor & Francis, New York.

Osweiler GD (1996) Toxicology. Williams and Wilkins, Philadelphia.

Papich MG (1990) Toxicoses from over-the-counter human drugs. *Vet. Clin. North Am: Small Anim Pract.* 20 : 431.

Plumb DC (1999) Veterinary Drug Handbook. 3rd edn. Iowa State Univ. Press, Ames.

Pratt W B and Fekety R (1986) The Antimicrobial Drugs. Oxford Univ. Press, New York.

Prescott JF and Baggot JD (1993) Antimicrobial Therapy in Veterinary Medicine. Iowa State Univ. Press, Ames.

Sandhu HS and Rampal S (2006) Essentials of Veterinary Pharmacology and Therapeutics. Kalyani Publishers, Ludhiana-New Delhi.

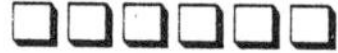

INDEX

A

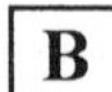

C

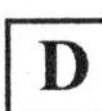

E

F

G

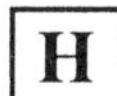

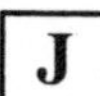

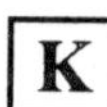

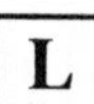

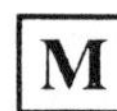

N

O

Q

R

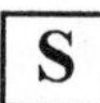

T

U

V

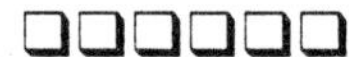